For many women, the midlife transition, with its accompanying shifts, changes in relationships (such as aging parents anc increased awareness of the health challenges that may prese... also provides a powerful opportunity to reassess and reengage with lifestyle factors that can improve health and well-being. Building on the previous *PAVING the Path to Wellness Workbook* by Drs. Frates, Tollefson, and Comander, this new program provides thoughtful questions that invite self-reflection and evidence-based information on the latest science regarding movement, nutrition, social connection, meaning, and purpose, as well as tools and strategies to support women in the implementation of practices that contribute to thriving in midlife and beyond. The depth and breadth of experience from the authors in their personal and professional lives and working with thousands of women is evident in this practical, thoughtful, and compassionate guide. This program is a great resource for both patients and clinicians.

Cindy Geyer, MD, FACLM, DipABLM, American College of Lifestyle Medicine Women's Health Member Interest Group co-chair, Lifestyle, Integrative, and Functional Medicine Physician, UltraWellness Center

Every woman who wants to feel good about herself, while being empowered to live her healthiest life, should read this book. Solid information and self-reflective activities, presented in a gentle and welcoming way, will inspire and guide the reader to choose her own path towards better health—through midlife and beyond.

Robyn Stuhr, MA, ACSM-CEP, Vice President, Exercise is Medicine®, American College of Sports Medicine

PAVING a Woman's Path Through Menopause and Beyond is an extraordinary book and course as it breaks down so many of the sociocultural barriers that impede women to thrive and reach their performance potential in the face of changing health conditions. Moving, eating well, and being mindful of yourself and the environment around you are key steps to finding peace, wellness, and health. The steps they have laid out are based on scientific evidence and boots-on-the-ground patient experiences. The theory and practice merge to create a fabulous resource for all women!

Stacy T. Sims, PhD, Female Athlete Performance Physiologist, author of *ROAR* and *Next Level*

Women in midlife and beyond are bombarded with multiple stressors: aging parents, children or childlessness, health issues, work, and home issues. To live a healthy and vibrant life, women must regroup and address their own wellness. The Paving the Path to Wellness Program is an amazing guide for women on this journey. The importance of nutritious food, sleep, mindfulness/stress reduction, and movement/exercise cannot be overemphasized, and will reap benefits in every aspect of health and disease prevention. These elements—just a few of the 12 components in the PAVING STEPSS program—will enrich your physical, emotional, and spiritual health. For a new beginning to the rest of your life, I highly endorse this program!

Deborah Kwolek, MD, FACP, NCMP, Lead, Women's Health and Sex- and Gender- Based Medicine Program, Massachusetts General Hospital

PAVING

A **WOMAN**'S PATH THROUGH **MENOPAUSE** AND **BEYOND**

Michelle Tollefson, MD
Beth Frates, MD
Amy Comander, MD

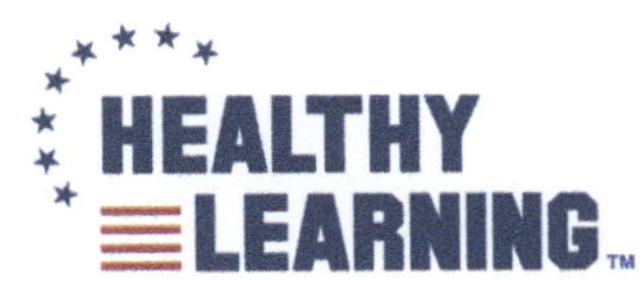

ISBN: 978-1-60679-580-4
Book layout: Cheery Sugabo
Cover design: Cheery Sugabo
Front cover photo: Sabrina Bracher/Shutterstock.com

Healthy Learning
P.O. Box 1828
Monterey, CA 93942
www.healthylearning.com

DEDICATION

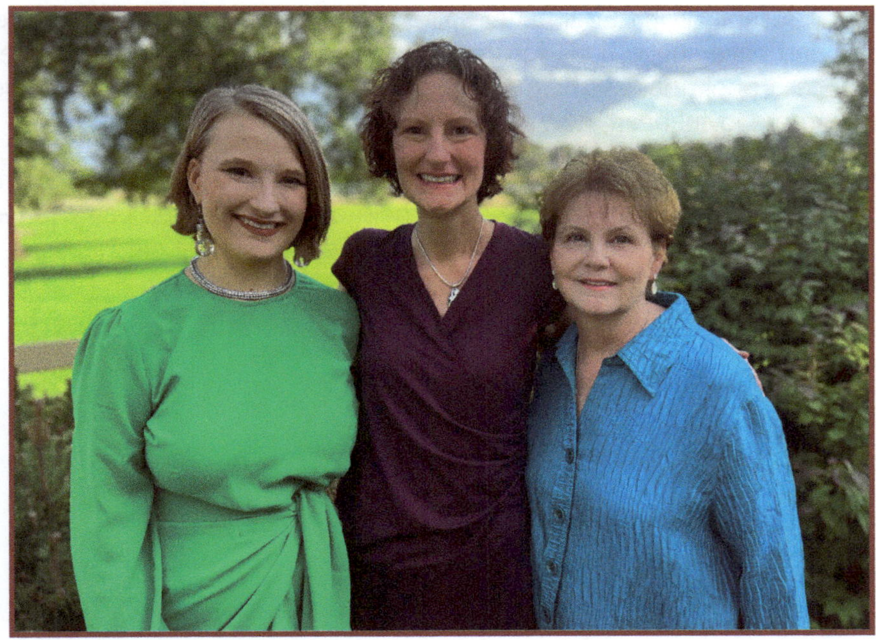

This book is dedicated to my mom, whose joyful heart, spirit, and strength made me the woman I am today, and to my daughter, whose joyful heart, spirit, and strength will continue to impact the world for decades to come.

—Michelle Tollefson

ACKNOWLEDGMENTS

We would like to thank the women who helped us create this book for you. Becky Gerken, Judy Joseph, Darla Eisenhauer-Spires, and Carol Jensen reviewed the initial manuscript and gave suggestions for improvement. Their recommendations enabled us to produce a book that will help women have a healthier body, a more peaceful mind, and a more joyful heart, now and for decades to come.

We would also like to thank our family and friends who supported us as we wrote this workbook. Their love and support allow us to help others pave their paths to wellness, through our books and the PAVING the Path to Wellness non-profit organization.

CONTENTS

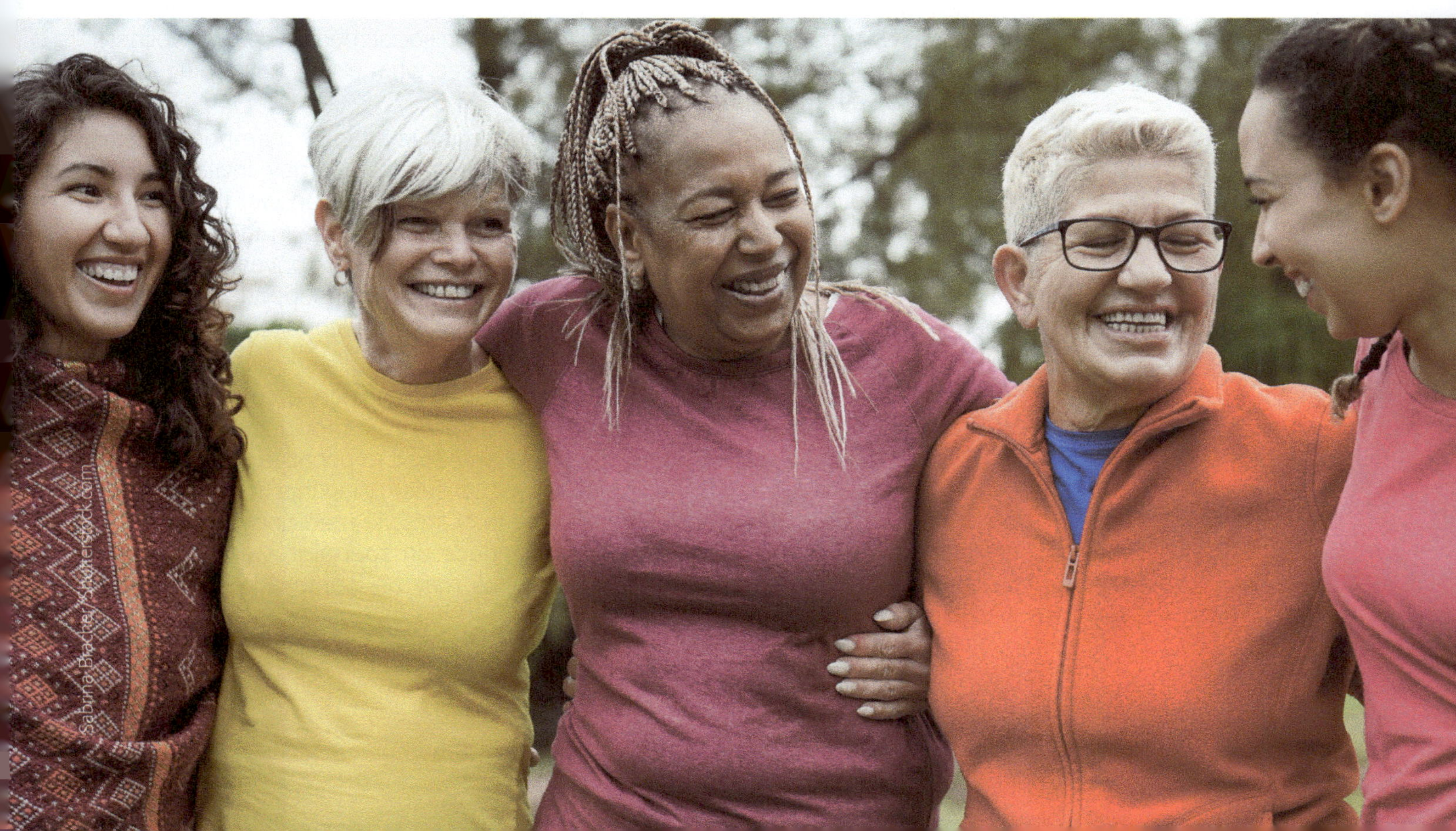

PREFACE

Lifestyle medicine pioneer, physiatrist, and Harvard Medical School faculty Dr. Beth Frates developed the PAVING the Path to Wellness Program at Spaulding Rehabilitation Hospital in 2012 for stroke survivors. It consisted of 12 weekly, in-person sessions attended by patients who had experienced a stroke and their partner or support person. Since that time, it has been offered both in-person and online, in small groups and larger groups, for healthcare clinicians and patients, business executives and employees, to people in the United States and worldwide.

Subsequently, Dr. Amy Comander, a breast oncologist and the Director of Lifestyle Medicine at the Massachusetts General Hospital Cancer Center, collaborated with Dr. Frates to develop and offer PAVING the Path to Wellness to breast cancer survivors. After finishing chemotherapy for breast cancer, Dr. Michelle Tollefson joined one of Dr. Comander's online groups and was so inspired by her personal experience with the program that she offered it to other breast cancer survivors in her home state of Colorado.

Drs. Frates, Comander, and Tollefson joined together to co-author the *PAVING the Path to Wellness Workbook.* In collaboration with Valeria Tivnan and Christina Dougherty, they also founded a non-profit organization called PAVING the Path to Wellness, which receives all proceeds from this book and the original workbook. The non-profit organization's mission is to help all people thrive with a healthy body, peaceful mind, and joyful heart.

You can use this book in several ways:

- Book only—This book can be used by yourself as you go along a personal wellness journey. In addition, you may want to check out the PAVING the Path to Wellness website at www.pavingwellness.org and follow us on social media, @pavingwellness on Twitter, or @paving.wellness on Instagram to see what else is happening in the PAVING the Path to Wellness organization.
- Book with others—If you belong to a book club or have a family member or friend working on their well-being who wants to join you on this journey, invite them to get a book and come along. You can go through the chapters, answer the prompts individually, or use them as the basis for engaging discussions. In fact, you could use the reflection questions and prompts to engage in deeper conversations about purpose, energy, and social connections with others. Social support is beneficial when you're trying to live your best life and embrace healthy lifestyle habits so having someone with you on the journey is wonderful.
- Educator options—If you are a teacher or professor of a college course, master's program, PhD program, medical school, or other healthcare provider school, where students are learning vast amounts of material and need to prioritize their own self-care to optimally learn and also care for others, consider using this book. This book could even be used as part of a healthy lifestyle or lifestyle medicine course. If you are a group facilitator, a community health education specialist, wellness coach, personal trainer, or nutrition specialist, this book may be helpful when you meet with clients one-on-one or as part of a group.

- Book with a concurrent PAVING the Path to Wellness group—If you're enrolled in a PAVING the Path to Wellness group that is using this book, either in-person or online, your leader will let you know how to use the book. You will likely read each chapter and reflect upon its questions prior to the live group discussion covering the same topic. Your leader can give you further insight into the subject, knowing that you've already read the information in this text, and engage the group in discussions regarding the material. If you are not part of a PAVING the Path to Wellness group in-person or online, and you want to learn more, visit www.pavingwellness.org or email us at info@pavingwellness.org for more information.

This book contains content beyond what you may have already learned in the *PAVING the Path to Wellness Workbook*. If you haven't already read that book, you may want to purchase it, as it contains information that directly aligns with this content, but is not specific to menopause, midlife, and more mature women.

In this book, like the original *PAVING the Path to Wellness Workbook*, you'll read about the 12 PAVING STEPSS and answer questions that help you learn more about yourself and enhance your wellness journey. You are encouraged to write your answers in the book, but if you're someone who prefers to reflect on the questions and not write, that's fine too. You are not being graded. This is your journey, and you know what is best for you. You can read the book cover to cover, or visit the chapters whose topics are calling you.

The COACH Approach acronym, created by Dr. Beth Frates, which stands for curiosity, openness, appreciation, compassion, and honesty, will be used to help you to better understand each of the 12 aspects of PAVING.

In each chapter, Dr. Michelle Tollefson will share insights that she's gained through working with countless women as an obstetrician-gynecologist. Her patients have allowed her to understand common concerns and struggles faced by menopausal, midlife, and more mature women. She also understands what it's like to go through menopause, after having abruptly entered menopause during her treatment for breast cancer. Her personal experience gives her additional insight that she brings to this book.

Even if you've already taken the PAVING Questionnaire in the past, we invite you to visit www.pavingwellness.org and take the PAVING the Path to Wellness Questionnaire online. You will receive your scores at the end of the questionnaire. You can record them and compare them with your results when you take it again after completing this book or at any time in the future.

If you prefer to take the PAVING Questionnaire in a paper format, you are welcome to do so. There is no right or wrong answer to these questions. This tool allows you to determine what areas you want to focus on and will help you better understand yourself at this "snapshot" in time. When you retake the questionnaire, it will likely be different. Also, there should be no shame, blame, or guilt associated with taking this survey. Its purpose is to help you along your wellness journey. Don't compare yourself to others or what you think you "should" be doing. You are here now, learning about well-being, which is all that matters.

If any information covered in the book brings up past trauma and mental health concerns, such as depression, addiction, anxiety, extreme stress, eating disorders, or other issues that could benefit from support, reach out for help. You can call your primary care provider or a local doctor, reach out to a mental health professional, such as a counselor or therapist, or call a mental health hotline at 1-800-662-HELP (4357). Please get the help that you need.

In addition, various medical conditions will be discussed in this book. It is important to note that this book does not take the place of medical advice. We want you to stay connected with your doctor(s) and other healthcare team member(s) and follow their advice. We believe that everyone should have a primary care provider (physician, nurse practitioner, or physician's assistant) who can oversee their medical care and connect them with other health-related resources. If you don't have a primary care provider, you are encouraged to reach out to one in your community and schedule an appointment.

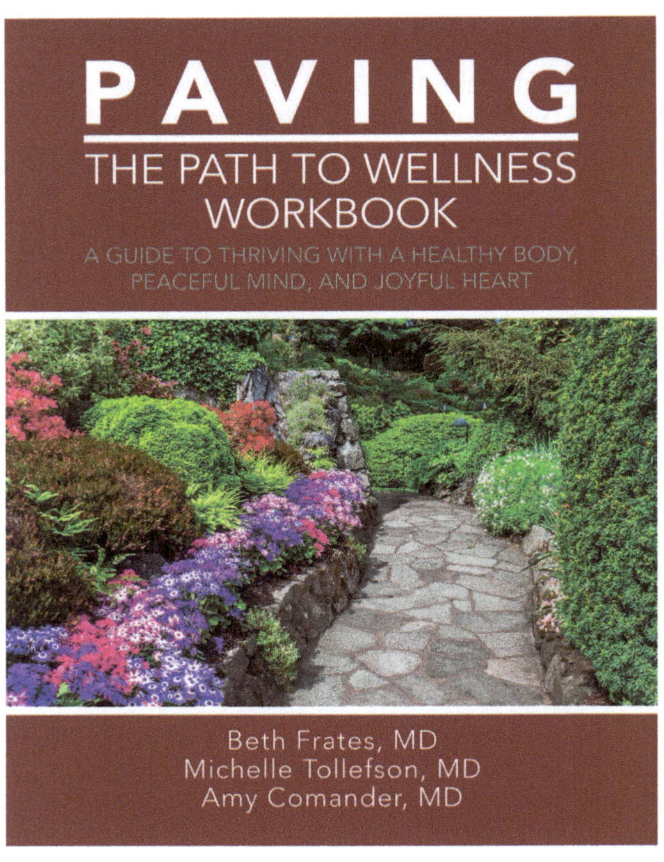

CHAPTER 1
THRIVE, NOT MERELY SURVIVE

Thriving. That's what we want for you. Don't sit back and settle for a good enough life where you are merely surviving. You are meant to thrive.

The World Health Organization defines healthy aging as "the process of developing and maintaining the functional ability that enables well-being in older age" (1). This book will help you wherever you are in your well-being journey. Whether you are just starting the menopausal transition or finished it decades ago, this book is for you. It is for women everywhere, those currently going through the menopausal transition or who have gone through it, and want to live their best lives.

You likely want to live a long vibrant life, engaging with your community, having strong relationships with loved ones, moving easily around your environment, and possessing the energy to live a meaningful life. Thriving looks different for each woman. You may have chronic health conditions, physical limitations, environmental challenges, or chronic stress that make your life challenging. While the PAVING the Path to Wellness program can't remove these challenges, it can help you live a life where your body is as healthy as possible for you, where your mind is more peaceful, and where your heart is more joyful.

It's incredible how many women still feel like their genes completely determine their fate, when, as midlife or more mature women, they have a tremendous amount of control over how they age. The daily choices they make regarding what food they fuel their body with, what movement they engage in, whether they prioritize sleep, and how they manage stress, significantly impact how they age. Age is just a number. More important than your age is how you act, feel, and live your daily life. This book will be your roadmap as you PAVE your Path to Wellness, one healthy lifestyle choice at a time.

The PAVING the Path to Wellness program is comprised of 12 components. You can remember these 12 steps through the following acronym PAVING STEPSS:

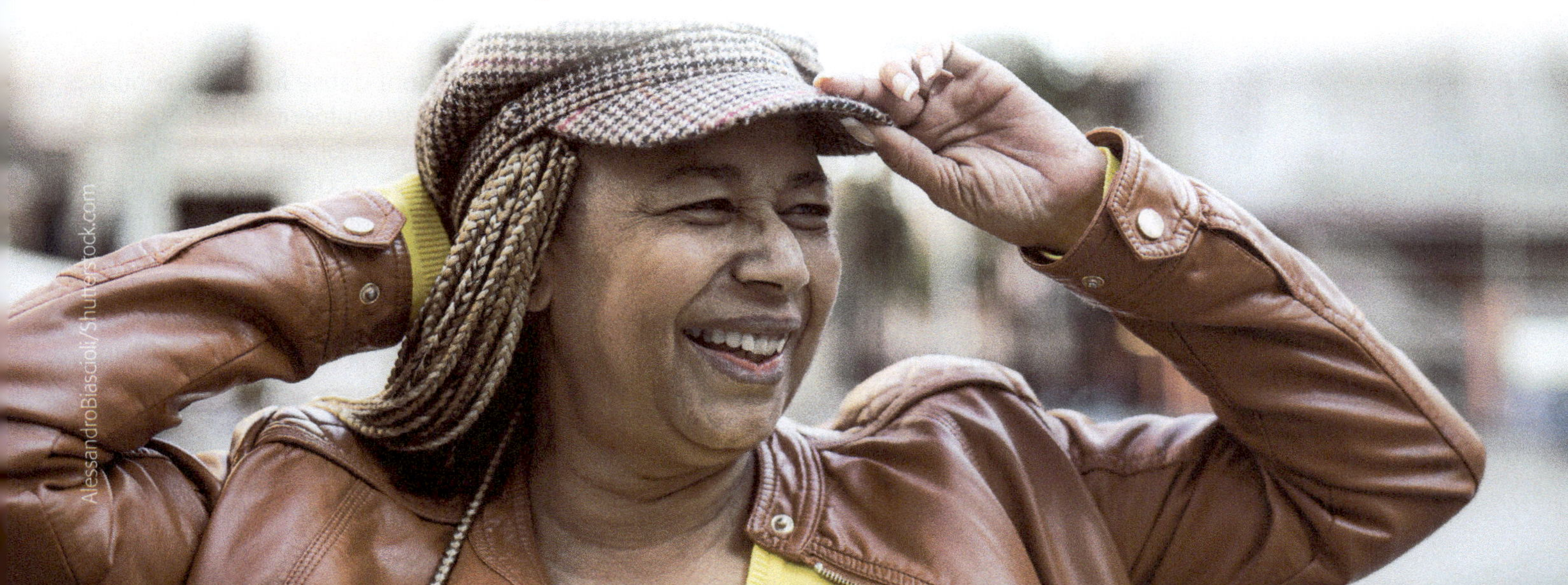
AlessandroBiascioli/Shutterstock.com

P Physical Activity
A Attitude
V Variety
I Investigations
N Nutrition
G Goals
S Stress Resiliency
T Time Outs
E Energy
P Purpose
S Sleep
S Social Connection

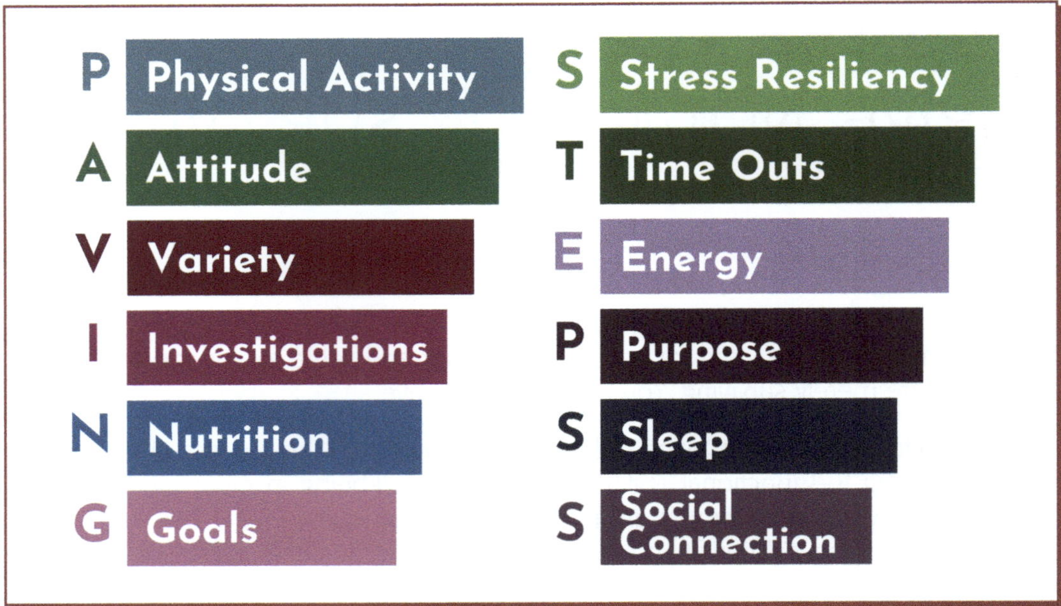

Figure 1-1

❑ P.A.V.I.N.G.

- *PHYSICAL ACTIVITY:* As you age, you tend to lose muscle, so resistance exercise becomes extra important to support your brain health, maintain muscle strength, stay independent, and keep your bones strong. Most women could benefit from adding more movement to their lives, so you'll also receive tips to help you move more throughout the day.
- *ATTITUDE:* Having a more peaceful mind and joyful heart is a beautiful goal for every woman. Attitude plays a significant role in this. In the attitude chapter, you'll explore your attitudes toward aging and your body, and better understand how they impact your health. You'll also learn ways to have a perspective that enables you to thrive.
- *VARIETY:* Variety supports brain health, so you'll learn how to use this principle to keep your brain sharp. You'll also explore how variation in your leisure activities can enhance your well-being. In addition, you'll learn to use variety to grow more fully into your authentic self.
- *INVESTIGATION:* This chapter will investigate menopause and midlife symptoms that you may be experiencing. You'll read about healthy lifestyle habits that can sometimes help with those symptoms too.
- *NUTRITION:* Nourishing your body with high-quality, nutrient-dense food is essential to age well. Fueling your body with foods containing phytonutrients, antioxidants, vitamins, and minerals will help you be healthy and strong. Incorporating abundant fruits, vegetables, whole grains, beans, lentils, nuts, seeds, soy foods, and fermented foods will be discussed, as well as the recommended daily intake of calcium, fiber, protein, and fluids.
- *GOALS:* The chapter on goals covers breaking free from boredom and increasing fun in your life through the use of goal-setting. The chapter that covers goals that are SMART in more ways than one. It also explores using goals to support well-being during midlife transitions and creating goals to increase your chances of attaining and sustaining the type of future you want.

❑ S.T.E.P.S.S.:

- *SLEEP:* It's typical that attaining restorative sleep becomes more challenging as you age. Therefore, it's vitally important that you have information on what to do during the day to increase your chances of getting sound sleep at night. You'll learn about handling middle-of-the-night trips to the bathroom as well as other sleep guidelines.
- *TIME-OUTS:* You need time-outs to refresh and recharge. This chapter explores the multitasking trap and how you can manage your time to best support having a peaceful mind and a joyful heart. Taking time to nurture your spiritual well-being is another focus of this chapter.
- *ENERGY:* Fatigue is prevalent in midlife and more mature women. This chapter looks at avoiding energy drainers as well as incorporating more energy boosters into your daily schedule. Discussing energy management and the "Spoon Theory" will help you more mindfully use your energy throughout the day.
- *PURPOSE:* Purpose often shifts for midlife and more mature women. Understanding your unique goals, values, experiences, passions, and expertise can help you discover a new purpose or refine a purpose that you may already have. This chapter covers how learning to tell your personal story and using your struggles to guide your purpose, can be fulfilling and inspiring.
- *STRESS:* This chapter explores chronic stress during menopause, midlife, and beyond, and how this negatively impacts physical and mental health. You'll also learn how thoughts impact your behaviors and how you can use your environment to support having a peaceful mind.
- *SOCIAL CONNECTION:* This chapter covers emotional intimacy and sexual health. In addition, you'll receive suggestions for creating new social connections, improving your current relationships, and strategies to decrease loneliness.

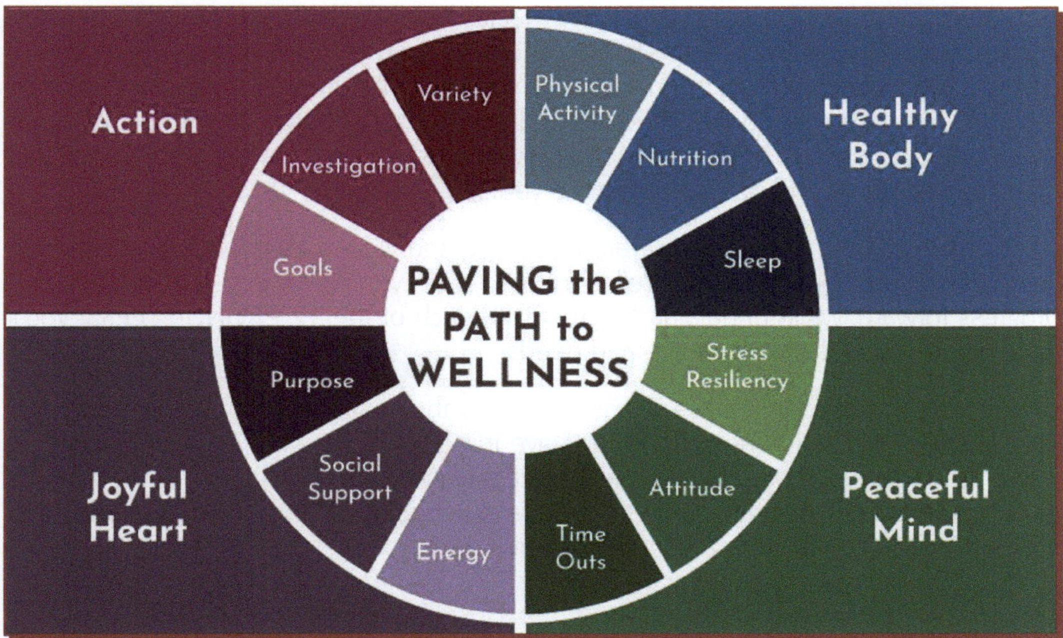

Figure 1-2

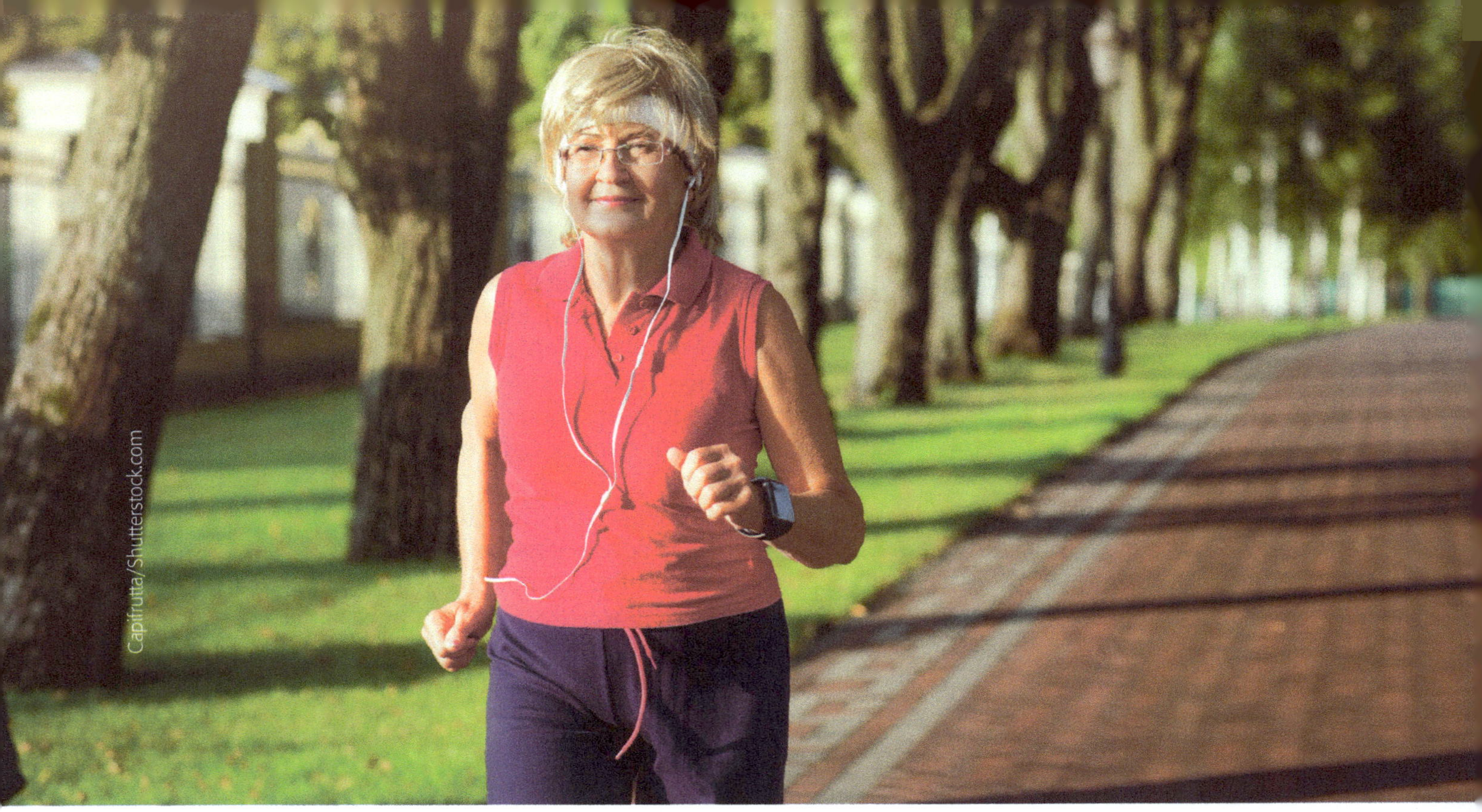

We have worked with countless midlife women throughout our years as clinicians and understand the challenges and concerns of midlife and more mature women. We also appreciate the immense wisdom that midlife and more mature women have accumulated through a lifetime of experiences. Through tapping into your strengths, values, passion, and lived experiences, we believe you have the potential to thrive, even if you feel like you're currently just surviving.

As three female physicians, we know what it's like to be a woman in today's society, juggling expectations and responsibilities, and wearing many "hats" each day. Some of us have also gone through menopause. It's hard to prioritize self-care with packed schedules and long to-do lists, frequently draining energy before bedtime. We know that it's hard, and we're here to support you with practical tips throughout the book that have worked for us and other women like yourself.

Being academic physicians, we are fascinated and guided by the evidence, and will share that throughout the book. We'll also try to meet you where you are and help you progress forward, while understanding that with each of the 12 PAVING STEPSS, you'll have different levels of knowledge and needs.

Like the female patients we've cared for over the years, we know you want to live your best life. We feel honored that you have this book in your hands and are ready to begin this journey. Prepare to take these next steps with us on your well-being journey, as you embrace this beautiful time in your life as a midlife or more mature woman and commit to focusing on your personal self-care.

Reference

1. World Health Organization, Decade of Healthy Ageing: 2020-2030. Updated March, 1, 2019. Accessed online www.who.int June 4, 2022.

CHAPTER 2
PHYSICAL ACTIVITY

Physical Activity Throughout Menopause, Midlife, and Beyond

Acronym—PHYSICAL ACTIVITY

Prioritize
Health
You
Strength
Include
Challenge
Aerobic
Laugh
Adapt
Connect
Time
Incorporate
Variations
Intensity
Try
Youthful

PAVING
THE PATH
to wellness

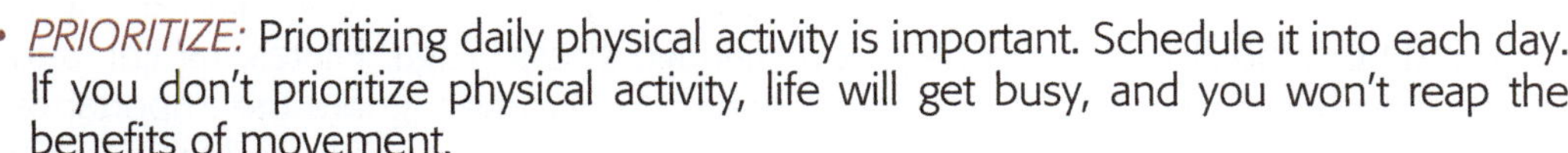

- *PRIORITIZE:* Prioritizing daily physical activity is important. Schedule it into each day. If you don't prioritize physical activity, life will get busy, and you won't reap the benefits of movement.
- *HEALTH:* Regular physical activity supports physical and mental health. Conversely, too little aerobic exercise and excessive sedentary time will harm your physical and emotional well-being. Talk to your healthcare provider about how movement supports your health and get clearance if needed.
- *YOU:* You are the only person who matters when it comes to your exercise routine. Don't worry about what other people are doing or compare yourself to others. It doesn't matter what you wear or what you look like when you exercise. Move like you want to move. Be mindful of how different types of exercise make you feel. For example, you can keep a journal where you track what kind of movement you engage in and how you feel when it is done. Don't be surprised if you notice that your energy increases and your mood improves as you move more.
- *STRENGTH:* Strength training at least twice a week on non-consecutive days builds muscle, keeps your bones strong, may decrease hot flashes, and supports remaining independent for decades to come.
- *INCLUDE:* Include others in your physical activity plans. For example, invite a friend to go on a walk with you, try a group class, or join a team at your local recreation center. You get two pillars (social connection and physical activity) in one.

- *CHALLENGE:* Don't get stuck in an exercise rut. Challenge yourself by participating in new activities that require more skill or endurance. For example, you can compete against yourself to try to run faster, use more resistance on a stationary bicycle, or take a more advanced Zumba class.
- *AEROBIC:* Get your heart pumping with aerobic activity on most days of the week. All movement is beneficial, but your body reaps the most rewards when you regularly engage in exercise that gets your heart pumping.
- *LAUGH:* Incorporate physical activity that makes you laugh, is fun, and is enjoyable. If you find fun activities, you're more likely to continue to engage in them. For example, pick up that hula hoop or try a belly dancing class with a friend.

- *ADAPT:* Adapt physical activities to meet your needs. If you're feeling exhausted, exercise at a reduced capacity. If you can't run due to physical limitations, try walking. If you can't walk, stretch in your chair. If you can't go to the gym for resistance training, lift cans of food.
- *CONNECT:* Connect with organizations and groups that support physical activity in your community and online. Many communities and recreation centers have groups that do physical activities together. Explore social media and online to connect with others who like your activities.
- *TIME:* Track your time to ensure that you get adequate movement each week. Every minute counts. Aim for 150+ minutes of at least moderate-intensity aerobic activity each week. Get up, stretch, and move, if you've been sitting for an hour.
- *INCORPORATE:* Incorporate some physical activity that helps your balance, supports mind-body health, and can help you manage stress. Yoga, Pilates, tai chi, and qi gong are examples of such activities. Oftentimes, women ignore the importance of balance. However, it is critical as you age, because if you stumble and fall, you could fracture a bone which may lead to loss of mobility and possibly independence.
- *VARIATIONS:* Once you've found an activity you enjoy, consider what variations you can make to that activity to add variety. If you enjoy riding your bicycle, try a different path, ride further than you usually do, or register for a bicycle race. Mix it up to keep your exercise routine interesting. Remember, variety is the spice of life.
- *INTENSITY:* Move at an intensity that enhances your health. Though you can benefit from any movement, being active at an intensity that will allow you to talk but not sing can help you even more than exercising at a low intensity.
- *TRY:* Try new things. You'll never know if you enjoy out-of-the-box activities, such as tae kwon do or tap dancing classes, if you don't try. Explore classes at your local recreation center and push yourself outside your comfort zone. You're never too old to learn something new. Your body and brain love novelty. Try including family members or friends. You can also try exercising at different times of the day to see what best resonates with you and your body. Try exercising in nature and see how you feel.
- *YOUTHFUL:* Be aware that you can be youthful at any age. When you are engaged with purpose, you exude youthful vitality. Exercise helps you have the energy you need to participate in the activities you enjoy. The key is to find activities you enjoy and stick with them. When you feel fit, you are also more likely to feel youthful.

Imagine your ideal self at 80, 90, or 100. Are you sitting on your couch immobile all day, or does your desired vision for yourself involve you being physically active and able to move easily? If you're like most middle-aged or more mature women we know, you want to be physically active as you age, which is possible for most women. However, this involves challenging the stereotype of a frail, unhealthy, sedentary older woman sitting in her rocking chair, knitting all day. Hopefully, you will help shatter this stereotype by showing the world what it means to be a physically active midlife or more mature woman, embracing movement and reaping the benefits of exercise to the age of 100 and beyond. You may not have exercised in decades, have never lifted a weight, or the thought of breaking a sweat while exercising may be enough to make you skip this chapter. On the other hand, regardless of where you are on the exercise spectrum, you are invited to explore this chapter to discover ways to have a stronger body, a more peaceful mind, and a more joyful heart through physical activity.

Exercise is vital throughout life; however, it's even more critical for women who are menopausal, during midlife, and beyond. As women age and their estrogen levels decrease, weight gain often occurs, and the risk of chronic medical conditions, such as heart disease, stroke, type 2 diabetes, osteoporosis, dementia, and cancer increase. What if there was a medication that could increase your quality of life and decrease your risk of every medical condition just listed? Of course, you would want to take it. Luckily, research shows that exercise can do all of this and more. It also decreases your fall risk, increases the chances that you'll live independently throughout your life, and helps manage midlife stress. In addition, many menopausal women suffer from mood changes, brain fog, fatigue, and muscle aches. Physical activity can help ease these symptoms too.

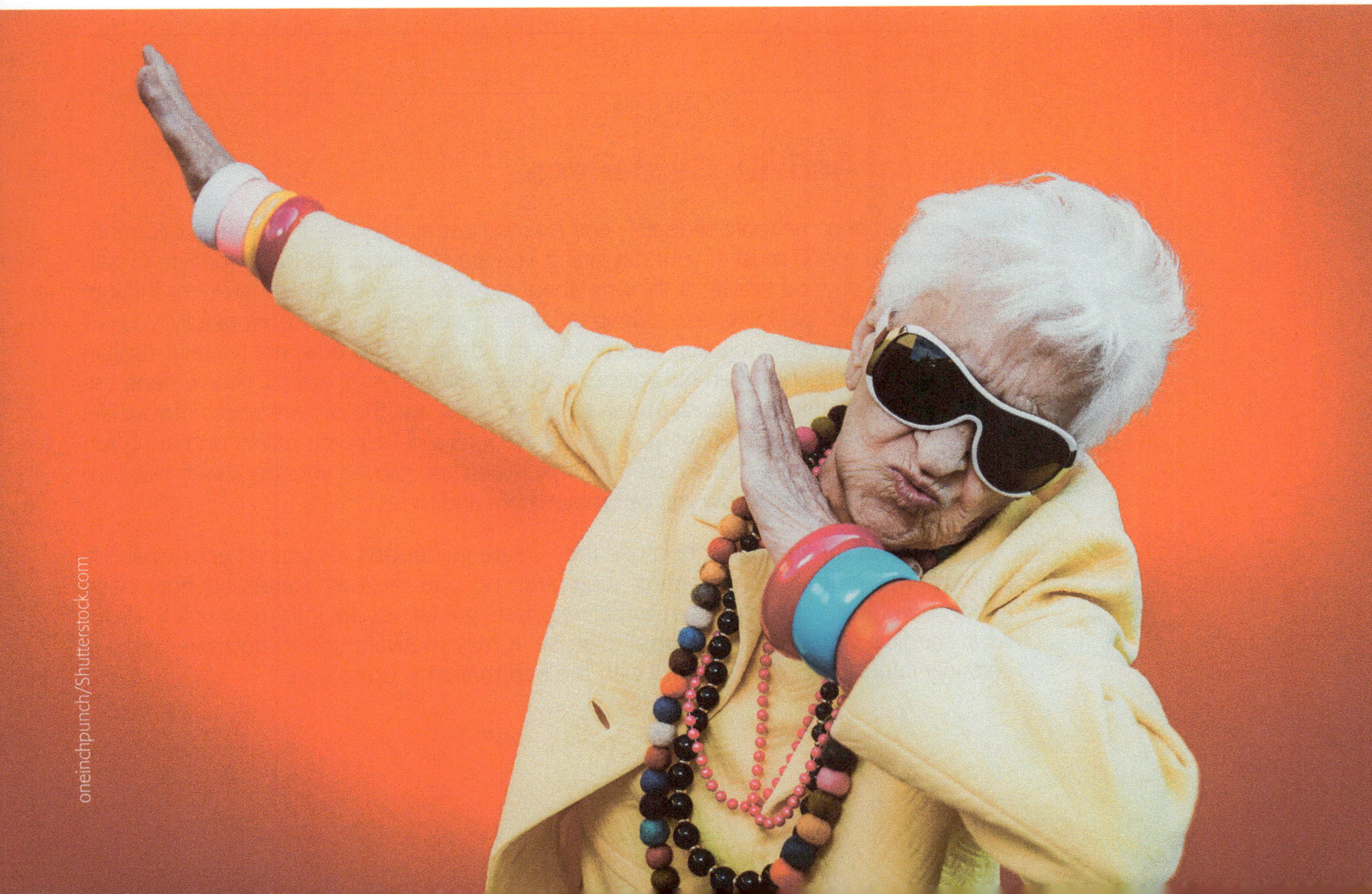

oneinchpunch/Shutterstock.com

Physical activity also supports achieving or maintaining a healthy weight. However, movement is vital for much more than weight. In addition, weight changes can be deceptive, especially when starting a new exercise program. For a variety of reasons, women may not lose a significant amount of weight initially, even though their clothes may loosen. Rather than the number on the scale, be mindful of how you feel physically, your mood, and your energy level. These are significant indicators that moving more is paying off regardless of weight.

Hopefully, with all this information, you're inspired to move more and sit less. Imagine your ideal self in your 80s, 90s, or at 100.

❑ What role is physical activity playing in your life at this age? Are you living independently? Are you walking with ease? Explain.

____

____

____

❑ What role do you believe physical activity will need to play in your life moving forward to help you reach your goals?

____

____

____

Physical Activity Guidelines

Most women become more sedentary and exercise less as they age. If you are not currently exercising and spend most of your day sitting, you are not alone. It is never too late to gain benefits from physical activity. If thinking about exercise makes you feel guilty or think of what you "should" be doing, take a deep breath and give yourself grace. Hopefully, you will be motivated to exercise regularly after reading this chapter. Guilt does not typically result in lifelong behavior change. Remind yourself that regarding physical activity, you've done the best you could to this point, based upon what you knew and the circumstances of your life. Then, move in a way that brings you joy. This chapter will help you reflect on having fun while moving and return to the days and times when you moved your body with freedom and glee. Read on to see how you can move more and sit less.

Guidelines are important because they create guideposts for you on your wellness journey. This journey is not one of judgment; no one receives grades on how close or far away they are from the guidelines. Use guidelines to inform yourself about what medical studies tell you about exercise. It may motivate you to do more and will certainly inform you. What you do with the information is up to you.

The Physical Activity Guidelines for Americans recommend that most women engage in at least 150 minutes (two and a half hours) of moderate-intensity aerobic physical activity, spread throughout the week. When exercising at a moderate intensity, you should be able to talk but not sing. You can benefit further by going beyond this recommendation by increasing the intensity or duration of the movement. Every minute of moderate-intensity physical activity counts toward this 150-minute goal. For example, walking quickly from your car into the store or working in your yard counts toward the goal. You can also consider these minutes leading toward your goal if you do a minute of jumping jacks or marching during a commercial break. The point is to look for ways to sneak in a little extra movement throughout your day.

If you aren't already exercising or if you have any medical conditions, check with your doctor before starting a new exercise program, so that they can help you find a physical activity that is safe for you. Your health status and medical conditions may limit what you can safely do. However, rarely will a woman not benefit from some form of physical activity. So, if you're reading this and need clearance from your doctor or primary care provider, put the book down, call their office, and let them know that you want to ensure that you exercise safely. They'll be thrilled that you reached out.

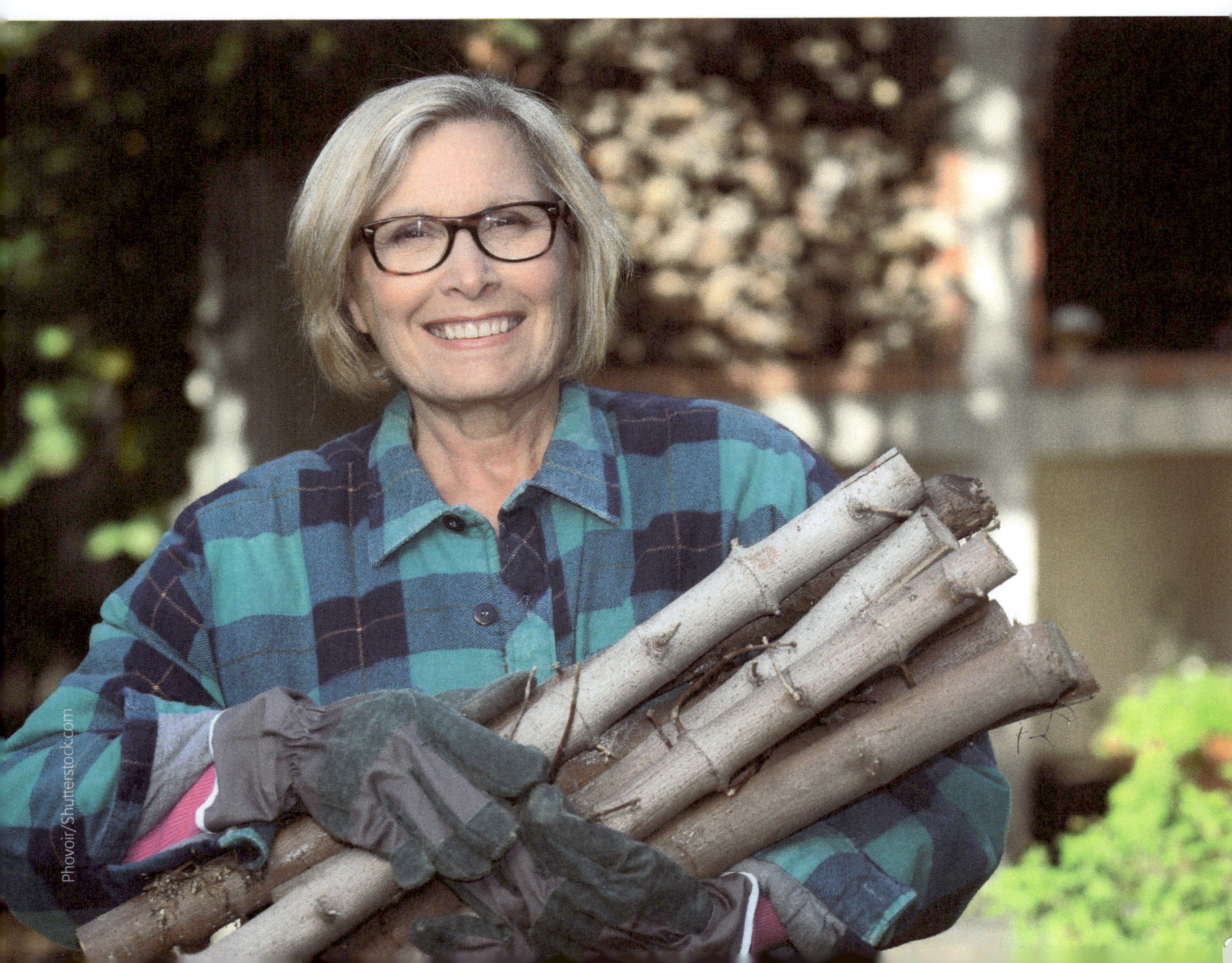
Phovoir/Shutterstock.com

Exercise Log

For the next week, keep track of your movement. Include the date, the type of physical activity, the intensity, and the duration of the activity (refer to Table 2-1).

Date	Type of Movement	Intensity (light, moderate, or vigorous)	Duration

Table 2-1. A sample exercise log

- ❑ Based on your movement log, are you meeting the recommendation of being physically active at a moderate intensity for at least 150 minutes each week?

- ❑ If not, does this encourage you to increase your physical activity gradually?

- ❑ If you are already meeting this recommendation, do you want to make any changes regarding your aerobic activity (such as changing the type, intensity, frequency, or duration)?

It is good to start low and go slow when initiating a new physical activity routine. For example, if you haven't exercised in years, do not attempt to run a road race, such as a 10K or a marathon, when you start out. Running a road race may be an appropriate goal, but you must gradually build up your endurance to train safely. Also, like most women, you want to gain every benefit possible for every minute you spend sweating or lifting weights. For this reason and safety, working with a physical therapist or certified personal trainer who can create or modify a physical activity regimen just for you is a great way to start. To create an individualized plan, they can review your medical conditions, personal limitations, aerobic and resistance training history, goals, and types of movement you enjoy.

Wherever you are on the physical activity spectrum, think about how you can move more and sit less today and throughout this week. Small changes over time can lead to significant change. For example, physical activity for some women may involve standing from a sitting position ten times daily and lifting food cans as weights, while they watch television. For others, it may include playing competitive tennis, hula hooping while watching TV, taking a weekly yoga class, or lifting weights at a gym twice a week. Also, most women do not need to meet with a physical therapist or personal trainer. If your doctor clears you to exercise, and you feel comfortable starting an exercise routine, that's alright.

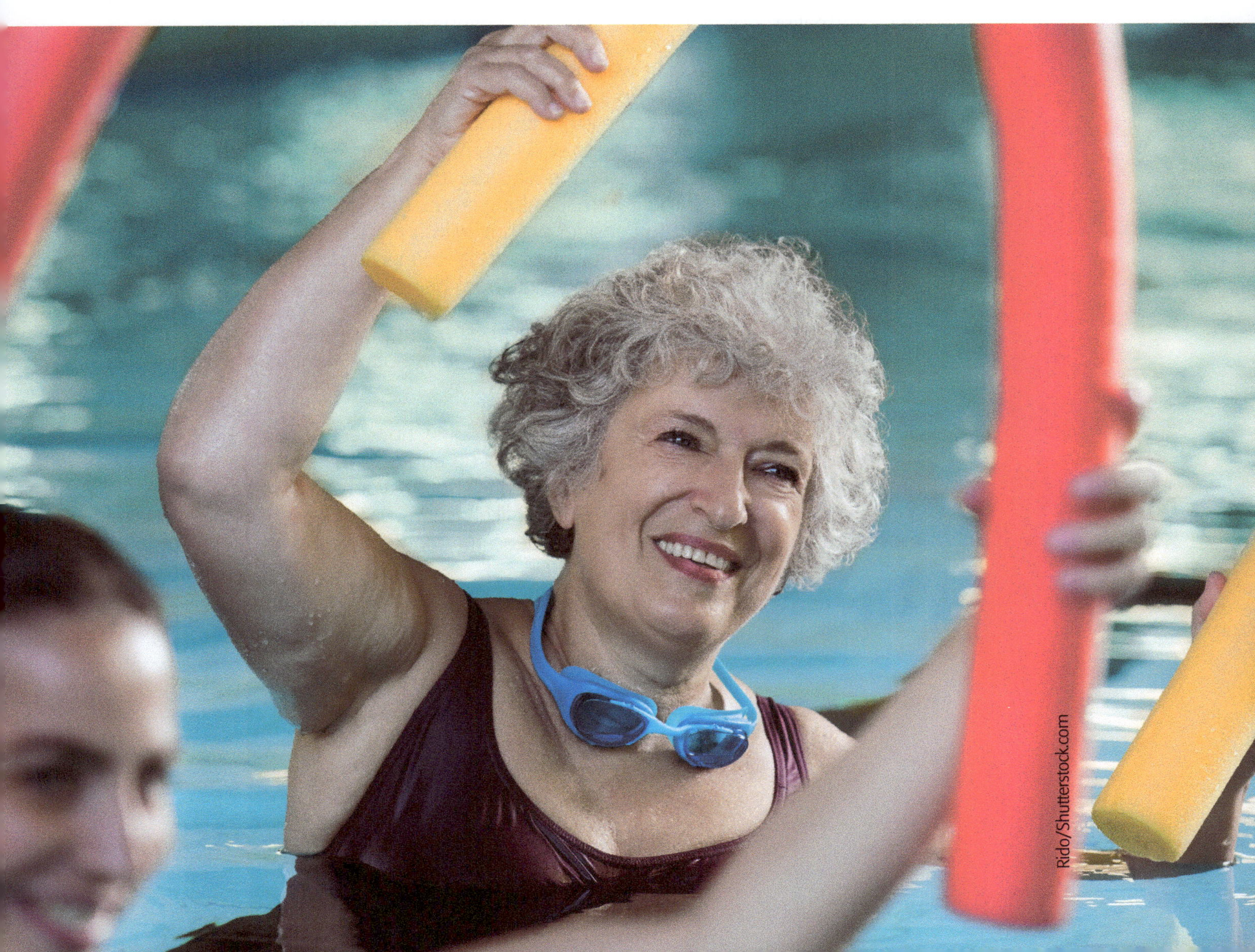

Rido/Shutterstock.com

Walking

You may want to run and hide when you hear the word exercise. Many women do not enjoy nor gravitate toward gyms or typical formal exercise classes and activities. Whether or not you are one of these women, you can likely benefit from walking more and sitting less.

Walking is an activity that almost any woman of any age and stage can do. You don't need special equipment (though a good pair of athletic shoes is worth investing in if you don't already have some). You can walk almost anywhere, whether exploring your neighborhood paths and hiking trails in the summer or walking on an indoor track or in a shopping mall in the winter.

You can start at a comfortable pace, and when you are ready for more of a challenge, walk a little faster or longer. Some women enjoy tracking their number of steps on their walk or throughout the day. You can use an old-fashioned, inexpensive pedometer. However, many smartphones and watches will also record your steps. If you want to record how many steps you took or how long it took you to walk a certain distance, you can follow your number of steps or the time you spent walking to see how you progress. There are many wearable devices that can track heart rate, steps, duration of time, and other measures that you may want to monitor. For some women, this information can help inspire them to continue to move more.

If you're hesitant to start walking more or the thought of moving more intimidates you, convince yourself to get up and walk a few steps. Once you are up and moving, you may find that walking a little more is not too hard. Often getting started is the hardest part. If you struggle with the motivation to walk, you may want to keep your athletic shoes out so that they are easily accessible and remind you to take walks. Finding a friend or partner to walk with, or joining a more formal walking group, may be just what you need to stay motivated. You may want to consider walking with a friend who has a dog. If you walk with someone, you will benefit from both social connection and the physical activity. If you can walk outdoors, you will also benefit from being in nature.

Although the research doesn't definitively show that walking decreases hot flashes, it has been shown to improve quality of life and support mental health. It also is associated with a reduced risk of chronic disease.

Don't worry about what other people are doing, how fast or far they are walking, or what you feel like you "should" be doing; get up and take that first step. This is a place of no shame, blame, or guilt. You shouldn't "should" yourself. This is a "should" free zone. After that, the rest of the steps will likely seem easier. Just remind yourself that moving more supports a healthy body, peaceful mind, and joyful heart.

- [ ] How do you feel about walking more to improve your physical fitness?

____

____

____

- [ ] What would help you walk more (e.g., asking a friend to join you, buying new walking shoes, finding a nearby walking trail, etc.)?

____

____

____

Jogging (Running)

Jogging is another viable method of exercising for some women during menopause, midlife, and beyond. Jogging can be a particularly positive way to be physically active, because like walking, running is a normal, natural human function. Furthermore, except for a pair of appropriately cushioned shoes, the requirements for running are minimal, e.g., a place (virtually anywhere) and a time to jog (most any time—mornings, afternoons, or evenings—when the climate and the external lighting permits).

Jogging (running at a relatively leisure pace) is a type of movement in which both feet are regularly off the ground at the same time, as opposed to walking, which entails having one foot on the ground at a given time. It should also be noted that you don't need to run fast or every day to reap the benefits of jogging. In addition, age is not a barrier to running. In reality, the number of older women among the more than eight million individuals who jog or run regularly in the United States is substantial.

The list of evidence-based benefits of jogging, which also apply to several other forms of moderate-intensity exercise, includes the following:

- Enhances bone density.
- Improves an individual's ability to engage in activities of daily living.
- Lowers blood pressure.
- Raises stamina.
- Helps control body weight.
- Decreases risk for diabetes.
- Boosts mental health (e.g., reduces stress, as well as feelings of depression and anxiety).
- Improves cognitive functioning (memory and ability to learn).
- Offers social benefits (e.g., a social connection), when undertaken with others.
- Extends a person's life span.

The point to remember is that jogging, as a form of exercise, can be an effective way to help develop and/or maintain your physical and mental health. Unfortunately, it can also be a source of injury. The likelihood and degree of those injuries depend on a variety of factors, including whether you ask your body to do too much, too soon. In this regard, all runners (particularly those individuals just starting their jogging regimen) are encouraged to "listen to their bodies." Similar to walking, the consensus recommendation is to start low, go slow. Accordingly, if it is (for whatever reason) uncomfortable for you to jog for 10 uninterrupted minutes, consider jogging for however long you can and then walk for a few minutes, before completing your 10-minute target run.

- ❑ What time of the day could you jog that best accommodates your interests and needs?

____

____

____

- ❑ What factors would affect your decision of where to run (e.g., convenience, accessibility, safety, etc.)? Keep in mind that there is no best location for where to run. It's an individual decision.

____

____

____

Options

In addition to walking and jogging, there are other forms of exercising that can help you combat the challenges of aging, including the following non-inclusive list:

- Bicycling
- Calisthenics
- Dancing
- Hiking
- Jumping rope
- Lifetime sports
- Pilates
- Skiing
- Swimming/water exercise
- Yoga

The point is that wishful thinking won't improve your health. In fact, the basic strategy for enhancing your level of well-being is very straightforward—sit less and move more. Do what you like and like what you do. Commit to being fit.

Not Enough Time to Move More

A common barrier to physical activity for midlife and more mature women is difficulty finding adequate time for physical activity. If you struggle with finding time to move more, consider scheduling time on your calendar devoted specifically to movement. Whether it's a formal water aerobics or a Zumba class or a block of time for you to take a neighborhood walk, it deserves protected time on your schedule.

Also, remember that every minute of movement counts. So even if you don't have time for an hour-long workout, move for whatever time you have. Ten minutes, five minutes, or even one minute is good for your body and mind.

If even thinking about physical activity is enough to make you sweat, think about how you can add a few more minutes of gentle movement to your day. Whether stretching, walking, jogging, swimming, or some form of exercise you find enjoyable, your body will thank you and benefit from the time you've dedicated to moving more.

- [ ] Do you find that a lack of time gets in the way of moving more?

____

____

____

- [ ] If so, what could you do to address this?

____

____

____

Resistance Training

A number of women do not embrace lifting weights at a gym, so you're not alone, if you're part of this group. But the literature is clear. During menopause and beyond, women gain significant health benefits from performing resistance exercise.

Loss of estrogen contributes to decreased muscle mass and increased fat mass, typically seen in women who have gone through menopause and don't engage in resistance training. When women lose lean muscle mass, resting metabolic rate (the calories burned while doing nothing but just breathing) decreases, leading to weight gain (typically about 10 pounds), if the individual continues to eat and move at a level as they did before this change. Although aerobic activity is essential for health, it is not sufficient to prevent muscle loss after menopause. Doing resistance training with resistance bands, hand weights at home, weight machines at a gym, or using the weight of your body (e.g., lunges and planks) strengthens muscles. Resistance training not only increases your level of muscular fitness, but also your metabolic rate, life satisfaction, and positive well-being. Furthermore, if you suffer from hot flashes and night sweats, research shows that resistance training helps. It's surprising how much medical research demonstrates the power of resistance training to diminish hot flashes and night sweats symptoms.

Ideally, you should engage in resistance training about two to three times a week with at least a day in between. Whether using exercise bands, handheld weights, or equipment at a gym, aim to complete about 8-12 repetitions of the activity, expecting your muscles to feel very tired by the end of the set. Doing two to three sets of each exercise will allow you to strengthen each muscle group you are using.

If you are new to resistance training or have medical conditions or limitations, you should work with a certified personal trainer or a physical therapist to create an individualized muscle strengthening routine. You can also watch videos online to learn how to perform simple resistance training exercises at home. In that regard, you should visit the American College of Sports Medicine or the American Council on Exercise websites to explore their resources. The Mayo Clinic also has a collection of strength training videos online that you can watch. In addition, many community recreation centers, YMCAs, and health systems offer training on their equipment or have classes that you can take that will lead to enhancing your level of muscular fitness.

Eating an adequate amount of protein each day is also extra important, as protein is needed for repairing, strengthening, and building lean muscle. Fueling yourself with high-quality, nutrient-dense foods will help you optimize your workout time to reap the full benefits from your work. Consider eating pre- and post-workout snacks that include some protein and carbohydrates. For example, apples with nut butter, a handful of almonds and some carrots, or edamame and a banana would make an excellent pre- or post-workout snack. Also, remember to stay well hydrated while working out. As you age, thirst typically decreases. Get in the habit of bringing a water bottle to the gym, as well as to wherever you go. Staying adequately hydrated will give you the energy to move throughout your day.

If you're interested in learning more about a healthy lifestyle through menopause and beyond, Dr. Stacy Sims's book *Next Level* (1) is an excellent resource. The resistance training and cardio workout sections can help you understand their role in improving your physical fitness.

❑ Do you currently engage in resistance training at least twice a week?

____

____

____

____

❑ If not, do you want to start or increase the resistance training you are doing? What will be your next steps?

____

____

____

____

❑ If you are already engaging in resistance training, do you want to make any changes (consider the type of resistance training, frequency, and intensity)?

____

____

____

____

Balance Training

With aging, your risk of falling increases. While a fall as a child may have led to a scraped knee, a fall as an older adult can lead to a fracture. Furthermore it is one of the leading causes of loss of independence in older women. However, certain types of physical activity can improve your balance and decrease your chances of falling. Studies show that any activity that elicits muscle strengthening can have a positive effect on balance. You can also practice standing from a sitting position, walking heel to toe, or balancing on one leg while holding onto a stable chair. In addition, there are wobble boards and balance balls that some women enjoy using to improve their stability.

Ideally, women should practice balance training or engage in balance-promoting physical activities a few times a week. It is crucial to engage in balance training that does not lead to a fall while you are training. Working with a certified personal trainer (such as one certified through ACE or ACSM) or a physical therapist can be beneficial, if you have any medical conditions or physical limitations. You may also want to explore at-home balance training exercise videos found online.

❑ Do you engage in balance-promoting exercises every week?

____

____

____

❑ If not, do you want to start doing physical activity that supports balance? What would you like to try?

____

____

____

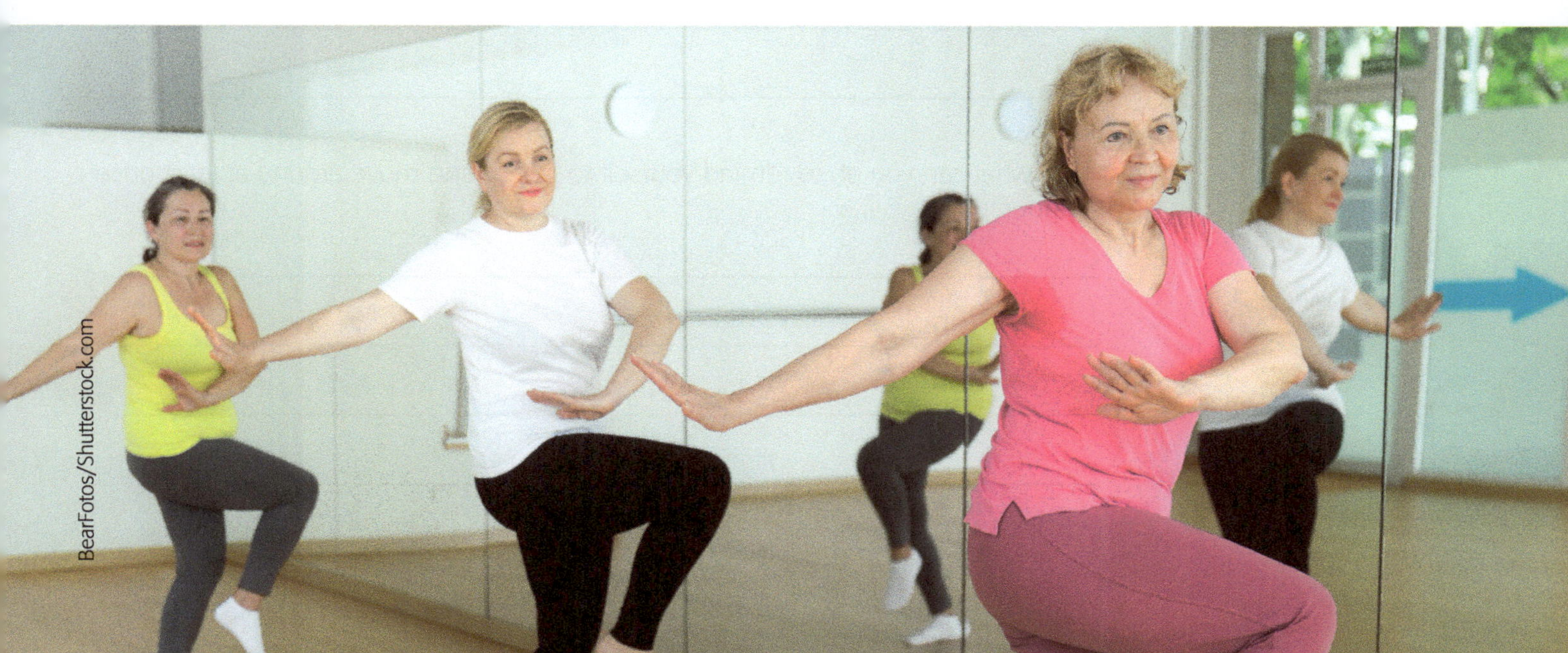

❑ If you already engage in balance-promoting exercises, is there anything you want to change with your routine?

___

___

___

Exercise Bursts and Sedentary Time

Women typically become more sedentary as they age. Even if you do 30 minutes of aerobic exercise in the morning, it is detrimental to your health to spend most of your day sitting. Spending most of your day being sedentary is associated with an increased risk of cardiovascular disease, diabetes, metabolic syndrome, obesity, and early death. Increased sedentary time also predicts more nighttime hot flashes and night sweats, independent of whatever time you might spend doing aerobic activity.

You can increase your active time and decrease your sedentary time in whatever way works best for you. Engaging in moderate or vigorous physical activity that interrupts prolonged sitting improves cardiovascular and metabolic health. Even doing 15-30 seconds of moderate-to-vigorous movement is beneficial, if you can safely move at this intensity.

Consider setting a timer to remind you to get up and move a little at least every hour (or at least every 30 minutes, if you have diabetes). Whether you move for under a minute at a vigorous level, walk around your living room, or stand to stretch, an exercise burst can improve your health. If you aren't already exercising at a vigorous level or have chronic conditions, check with your physician before engaging in vigorous activity.

❑ Do you sit for prolonged periods without standing to stretch and move?

___

___

___

___

❑ If so, what can you do to remind yourself to get up and move around at least once an hour?

___

___

___

___

Kegels/Pelvic Floor Muscle Exercises

The pelvic floor muscles form a sling, supporting the uterus, vagina, bladder, and rectum. Unfortunately, as women age and their estrogen levels decrease with menopause, these muscles typically weaken, often leading to stress urinary incontinence (leaking urine when coughing, sneezing, or even exercising). The situation may negatively impact their sexual health. Luckily, these muscles can be strengthened through pelvic floor muscle exercises, sometimes called Kegels. Strengthening the pelvic floor muscles increases circulation, sometimes reduces stress urinary incontinence, and supports sexual health through increased blood flow. In addition, adequate circulation to the pelvic floor can increase genital arousal, vaginal lubrication, and orgasm.

To strengthen these muscles, contract the muscles you would use if you were trying to stop urinating midstream. Though stopping urination midstream routinely is not recommended, it may be beneficial to try it once, if you have problems identifying what muscles to contract. You should feel the muscles draw inward and upward when contracting them. If you are unsure if you are tightening the correct muscles, you can insert a clean finger about an inch into the vagina and try to contract the pelvic floor muscles. You should feel the muscles tighten around your finger. Once you've identified the muscles, tighten and hold the contraction for about three seconds and then release for three seconds and repeat ten times. Try to do these three times a day.

Eventually, you can work up to holding the contraction for more extended periods of time (for example, ten seconds at a time). In addition to prolonged contractions, you can do quick, strong contractions as fast as you can. Try doing ten quick contractions and then taking a break before repeating. If you are uncertain whether you are contracting the right muscles, or are having any pelvic discomfort or incontinence, see your physician or a physical therapist with expertise in pelvic floor work.

❏ After reading the aforementioned information, is there anything you want to do to improve the strength of your pelvic floor muscles?

____

____

____

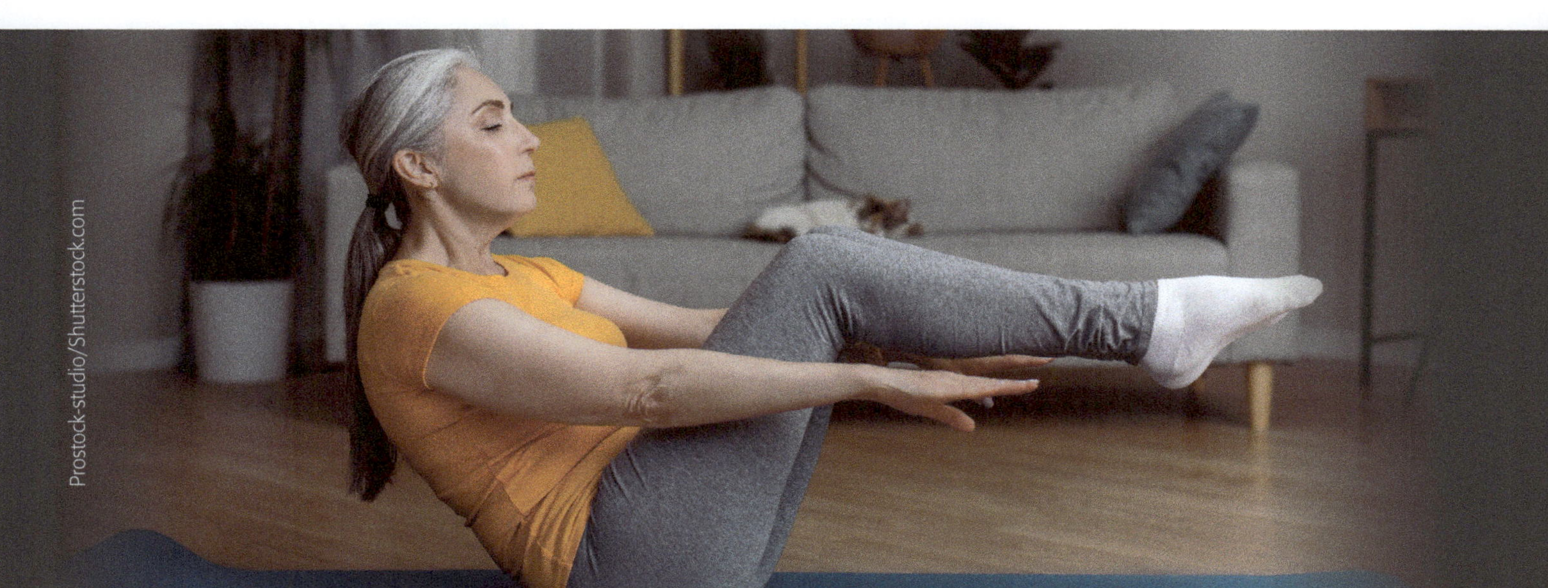

Prostock-studio/Shutterstock.com

Core Strength

Although Kegels are important for pelvic floor muscle health, keeping your core muscles strong is also important. If your core muscles are weak, your pelvic floor muscles may weaken even more and will have to compensate for your weak core muscles and, as a result, work overtime. Your core muscles are your abdominal and back muscles that attach to your pelvis and spine. The Mayo Clinic's website explains how to properly do "core strength exercises," such as abdominal crunches and planks. In addition to helping protect your pelvic floor, a strong core improves balance, decreases the risk of falls and breaking bones, and increases your chances of maintaining independence long-term.

A strong core also helps your posture. Back pain becomes more common with age. Having strong core muscles supports improved posture. When you have good posture, your shoulders are not rounded over, and your muscles are working to support your body in a way that does not promote back pain. Good posture may even increase confidence and self-esteem in some women. WebMD's website on Posture Exercises details exercises that you can do at home whether you want to improve your posture or just maintain the good posture you already have.

- ❑ After reading this information, is there anything you want to do to improve your level of core muscle fitness? If so, what is it?

  ____

  ____

  ____

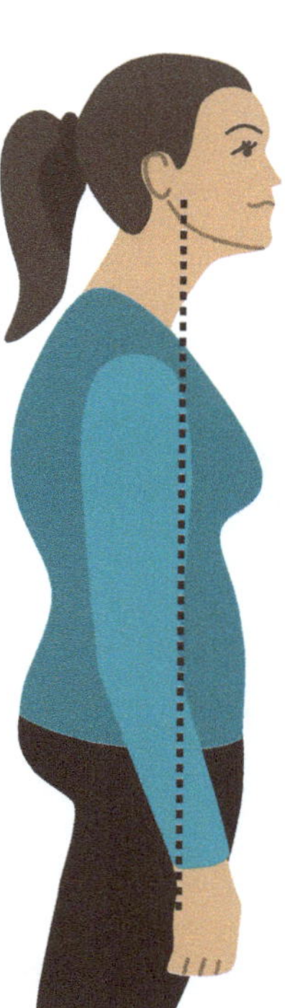

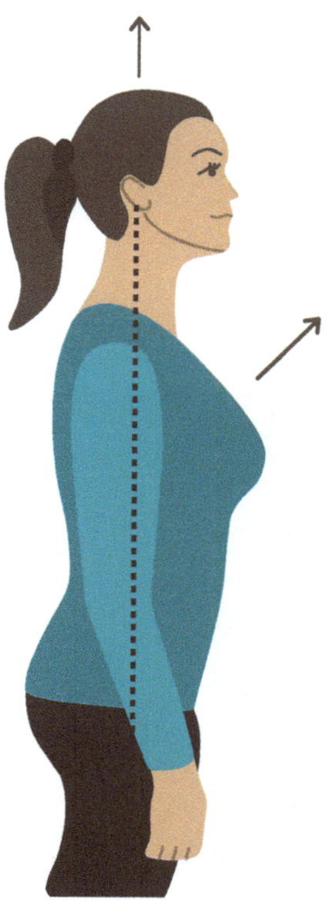

Olli Turho/Shutterstock.com

Movement and Bone Health

Just as your bones need vitamin D and calcium to be strong, they also need regular physical activity. As women go through menopause, the rate at which bone loss occurs accelerates. If a woman loses enough of her bone mass, she can get osteopenia or osteoporosis (weak bones associated with an increased fracture risk).

If you have osteopenia or osteoporosis, you should talk to a physical therapist or your healthcare provider before starting an exercise routine, as you do not want to injure your bones by engaging in exercise that is not appropriate for you.

If you want to prevent getting osteopenia and osteoporosis and are already cleared to exercise, consider doing movement that stimulates your bones to stay strong. Engaging in weight-bearing exercises where you must work against gravity to move, such as walking, jogging, going up stairs, hiking, and doing Zumba, encourages your bones to remain strong. Although swimming and water aerobics are great forms of physical activity, they don't stimulate your bones as much as other activities. Your bones also benefit by performing resistance exercises, such as using resistance bands, working out on weight machines, or lifting weights. The resistance afforded by these exercises challenges your bones and helps them become stronger. Hopefully, at least, it also decreases the amount of bone loss.

In addition to weight-bearing exercises and resistance training, your bones also respond well to jumping, hopping, or skipping, where the bones receive stimuli from jumps. As with most intense forms of physical activity, talk with your healthcare provider or a certified personal trainer before engaging in this type of movement.

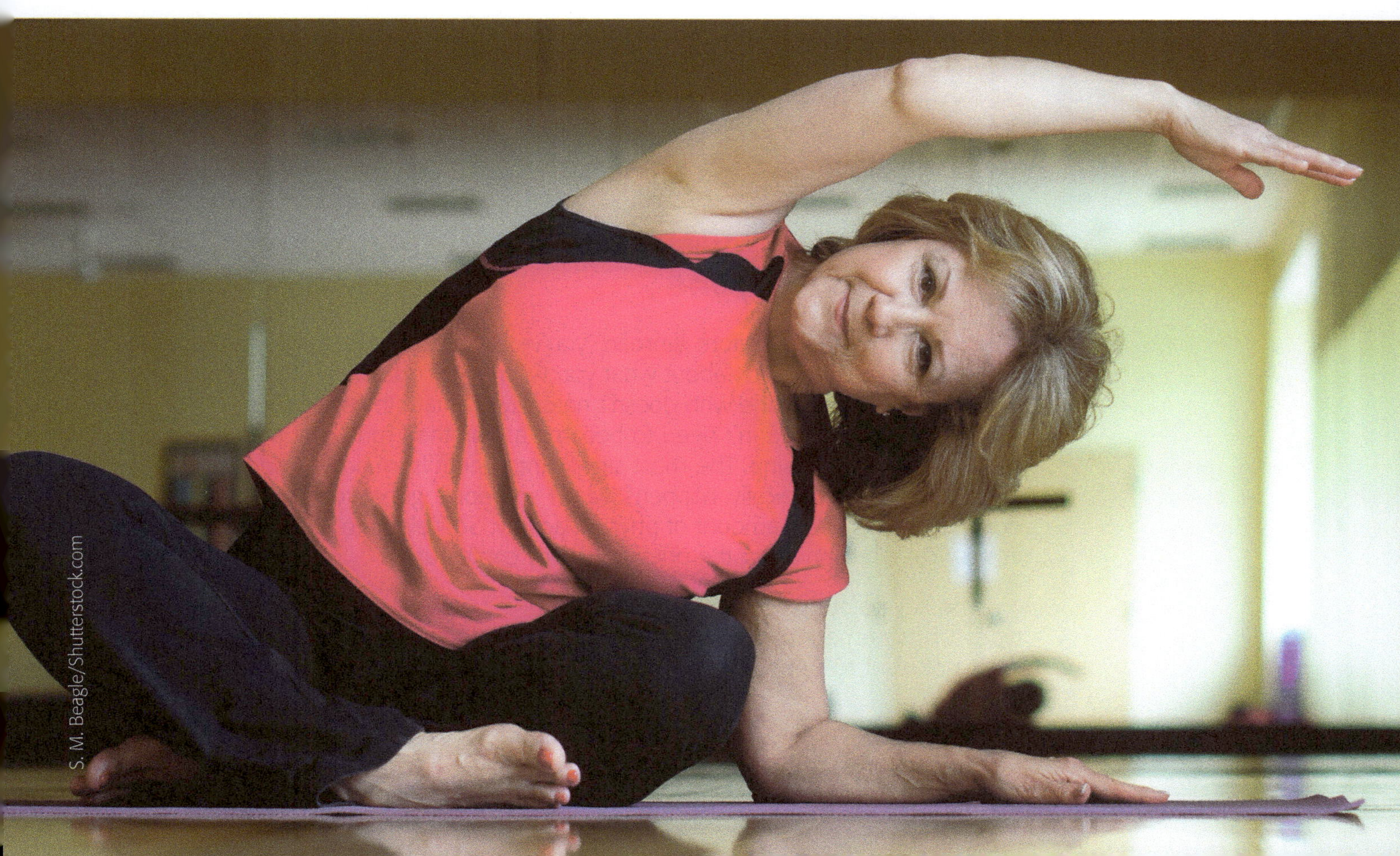

S. M. Beagle/Shutterstock.com

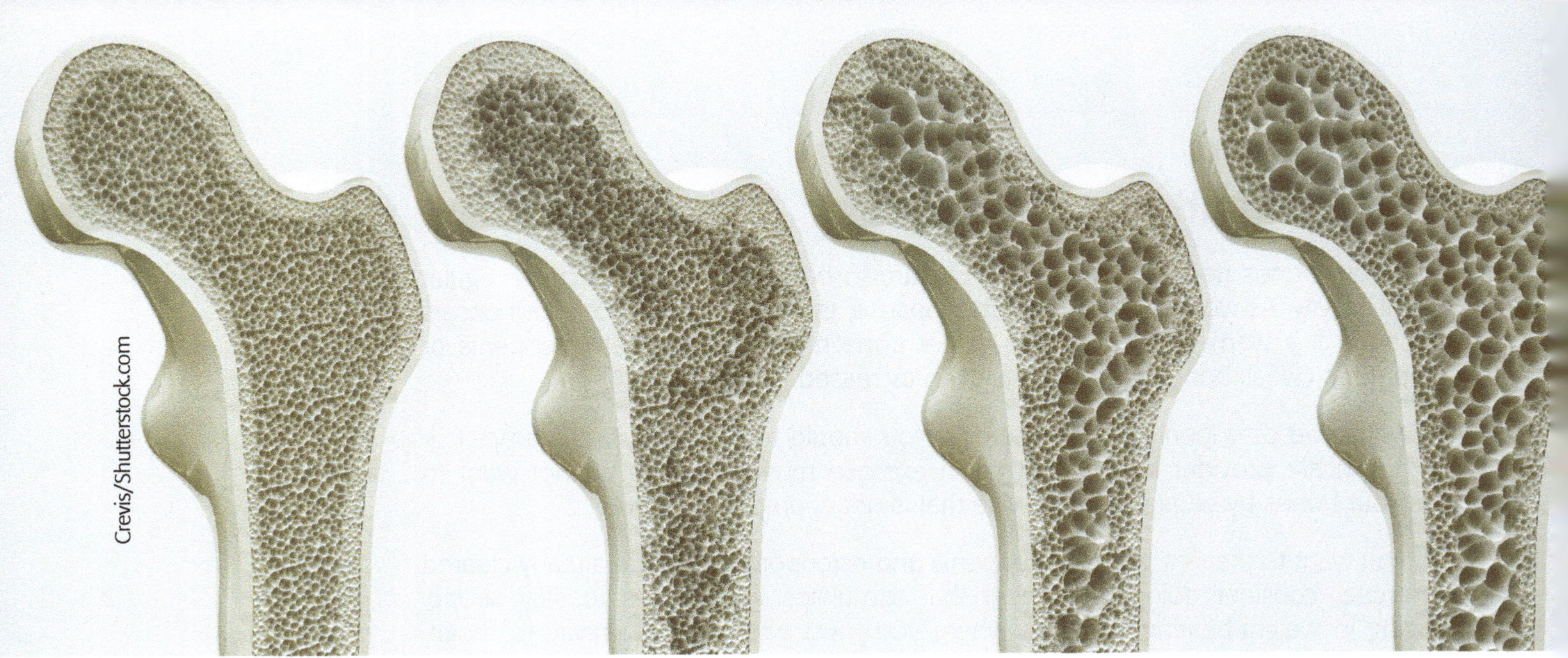

Crevis/Shutterstock.com

❏ Are you engaging in movement that supports your bone health?

❏ Is there anything you want to change concernig your physical activity to take care of your bones?

Moving More and Sitting Less During Menopause, Midlife, and Beyond

As a midlife or more mature woman, you've had experiences with movement and likely have strong opinions about what you will or won't do when it comes to physical activity. If you're someone who doesn't naturally gravitate toward exercise, don't worry, you're not alone. You don't need to become a marathon runner or a triathlete to gain the benefits of exercising. The most significant benefit from adding additional minutes of aerobic activity typically happens when someone goes from being sedentary to doing even a minimal amount of physical activity. So, celebrate every time you "move" in the right direction along the physical activity continuum.

The key point that you need to remember is to review your life and consider what types of movement you enjoy the most. For example, maybe you're someone who does not want to sweat while doing aerobic activity. For you, water aerobics may suit you best. Or, you may be someone who can't stay motivated by doing exercise alone. Signing up for a regular class, where you join others to do Zumba, for example, may inspire you to move more.

❑ What type of physical activity have you enjoyed in the past? Consider your childhood, adolescence, young adulthood, and recently.

____

____

____

❑ What can you learn from your past that would help you design a plan to be more physically active to work well for you with your individual preferences and circumstances?

____

____

____

The following list offers ideas of things that you could learn, add to your current plan, or that might assist you with your physical activity. As you review the list, put a star next to those that resonate with you.

- Infuse joy in your move-to-improve efforts.
- Be kind to yourself.
- Congratulate yourself for any physical activity you might do.
- Look for ways to sit less and move more throughout the day.
- Ask a partner or a friend to join you.
- Explore a local park or the trails around your home.
- Try a new form of physical activity.
- Visit your recreation center to see what opportunities they offer.
- Wear comfortable and supportive athletic shoes.
- Start low and go slow.
- Don't compare yourself to others.
- Find some new fun workout clothes to wear.
- Don't underestimate the power of walking.
- Track your movement or resistance training so that you can see your progress.
- Use an activity tracking monitor such as your phone, watch, or another device.
- Join a group competition.
- Enjoy being outdoors and moving.
- Set a timer to remind yourself to stand and move after sitting for an hour.
- Drink plenty of water to stay well hydrated.
- Try activities that you used to enjoy as a child.
- Take a class that involves physical activity.

- [ ] After reviewing the aforementioned ideas, is there anything you want to do to incorporate more fun or variety into your physical activity regimen? Also, consider ideas you have that were not in the aforementioned list.

____

____

____

Lessons on Moving More From the Blue Zones

The blue zones are the five locations in the world with the highest concentrations of centenarians (people who live until at least 100 years old), with relatively low levels of chronic diseases, such as cardiovascular disease, type 2 diabetes, and some cancers. They are the places where people are living healthier and longer.

In the blue zones, people aren't healthy due to a complicated exercise regimen or going to the gym daily. Instead, their environments encourage frequent movement throughout the day. Many older people in the blue zones grow and care for their gardens. In addition, they stay busy caring for younger generations, doing household chores, riding their bicycles, and/or walking throughout their community.

In Okinawa, Japan, one of the blue zones, people traditionally sat on floor mats rather than chairs or couches. Frequently sitting on the floor and returning to standing requires muscle strength, balance, and flexibility, which typically decrease with age. Sitting on the floor without back support also encourages good posture. Although younger generations are not following this tradition as much as the older generations, it is still beneficial to learn the value of sitting on the floor from this traditional practice.

Although you likely do not live in a blue zone, you can set up your home to encourage more movement. Maybe you create an area in your home with pillows on the floor that encourage you to sit on the ground, rather than on your sofa. If you don't already have a garden, consider planting one. Not only will it require regular movement to plant, care for, and harvest, but you'll also reap the benefits of having fresh produce available. Try to do household projects or chores that require manual labor, such as raking leaves, shoveling snow, or mowing the yard, rather than using a snow blower or riding a lawnmower.

The individuals who live in the blue zones regularly walk in their neighborhoods. Think about the places that you go to throughout your day. Maybe, you drive to a coffee shop nearby that you could try walking to next time. Perhaps, you drive down the street to a friend's house or your mailbox when you could easily walk or bike there instead. Consider exploring your bicycle and walking trails, neighborhood parks, and other areas of your neighborhood in which you don't typically spend your time. Think of it as an adventure that also supports your health.

The longest-living people in the blue zones don't typically sit for hours upon hours. Instead, they are up and moving at least every half hour. Consider setting a reminder on your phone, an alarm, or a timer to remind you to get up and move, if you've been sitting for over an hour or even 30 minutes. Try to do whatever you can to move more and sit less throughout your day, and you'll be able to gain some of the benefits of the centenarians who live in the blue zones. For more information about the blue zones and the health practices associated with longevity in these regions, read Dan Buettner's book, *Blue Zones: 9 Lessons for Living Longer From the People Who've Lived the Longest* (2) or any of his other books on the blue zones. Buettner and the Blue Zones™ company continue to help people around the globe lead healthier lives by learning from blue zone research. You can also visit the website www.bluezones.com to learn more.

❑ How does your home encourage physical activity?

___

___

___

❑ In what ways does your home discourage physical activity?

___

___

___

___

❑ What did you learn from the information on the blue zones that you could use to increase your physical activity in your own home or community?

___

___

___

___

❑ Is there a goal you want to set to help you put this information into practice soon?

___

___

___

___

Be Smart With Your Movement

Although you may have been able to run a mile without warming up as a teen, you are now older and wiser. To get the full benefits of physical activity and avoid injury, it is crucial to be smart with your movement by adhering to the following tips:

- If you are starting a new exercise routine or have medical problems, get clearance from your primary care provider first.
- If you have chest pain, shortness of breath, or experience bothersome symptoms while exercising, stop and seek medical attention.
- Be mindful of the temperature when you exercise, wear proper clothing for the weather, and stop if you get too hot or too cold.
- Stay adequately hydrated while working out. Consider keeping a water bottle close by while exercising.
- Wear comfortable clothes that will help prevent you from overheating.
- Invest in athletic shoes that will protect your feet and give you proper support.
- Consider at least initially working with a certified personal trainer or physical therapist to help you exercise in a way that is best suited to your individual needs, limitations, and preferences.
- Start slowly and gradually increase your level of intensity or the length of time that you exercise.
- Always warm up and cool down after exercising.
- Get up slowly and carefully when standing, as dizziness when standing is more common with age.
- Listen to your body. If a movement hurts, you don't feel good, or something doesn't seem right, stop exercising.
- Allow adequate rest and recovery between exercise sessions. If you are doing strength/resistance training, allow at least one day of recovery between sessions.
- Use proper form when exercising to decrease your chances of injury, as well as to avoid compromising the benefits from doing a particular exercise. If you don't know how to do a particular movement or use a piece of equipment, ask someone with expertise, such as a certified professional trainer.
- Don't hold your breath for prolonged periods when exercising. Remember to breathe as you normally would.
- Eat healthy food that will keep you adequately fueled throughout your activity.
- Prioritize sleep, as your muscles need rest to rebuild and recover fully.

❑ Is there anything you want to change with your physical activity routine to ensure you are moving safely?

____

____

____

____

Coaching Yourself on Physical Activity With the COACH Approach

You can support yourself on the PAVING the Path to Wellness journey by coaching yourself to be healthier, one step at a time. The following is a list of questions to consider while coaching yourself to enjoy movement throughout the day. The acronym COACH (C – curiosity. O – openness. A – appreciation. C – compassion. H – honesty) is used to help you better understand the COACH approach to physical activity.

CURIOSITY

You need to get curious and learn more about your relationship with exercise. Why do you think you feel the way you do about exercise and physical activity in general? For example, maybe you've resisted movement because it is uncomfortable, painful, or you don't like sweating. Perhaps you've had a negative attitude toward exercise because you see it as something that society tells you that you "should" do. Maybe you've had a bad experience with movement in the past.

- ❑ Why do you embrace or resist aerobic activity or resistance training?

____

____

____

____

- ❑ What needs to be in place for you to move at least 10 minutes more daily than you currently do, five days a week?

____

____

____

____

- ❑ What reminders can you use to remind you to sit less and move at least once an hour?

____

____

____

____

- ❑ Whom can you connect with and share your goals about exercise?

____

____

____

OPENNESS

Changing behaviors can be challenging, even if they are healthy lifestyle behaviors that you want to adopt. The following questions are designed to help you explore your openness to changing your attitudes and behaviors around exercise.

- ❑ How can you be more open to learning about and trying different types of physical activity?

____

____

____

- ❑ What would you need to know or do to change your attitudes toward exercise or embrace new types of physical activity?

____

____

____

- ❑ What would it take for you to look at movement with a new lens, one without shame, blame, or guilt?

____

____

____

- ❑ What steps could you take to leave the past behind and start a new journey with movement and joy?

____

____

____

APPRECIATION

Your body is unique. It helps you move throughout your day, getting you from where you are to where you want to go. Unfortunately, women often take physical movement for granted until an injury, illness, or health condition limits their activity.

- ❑ How can you appreciate what your body has done for you by physically moving you through each day of your life?

  ____

  ____

  ____

- ❑ When thinking about movement, what benefits to your mind, body, and soul do you look forward to experiencing after engaging in physical activity?

  ____

  ____

  ____

  ____

- ❑ When was the last time you were routinely physically active? How can you replicate those circumstances?

  ____

  ____

  ____

  ____

- ❑ What step can you take to add a few minutes of physical activity to your day and celebrate that?

  ____

  ____

  ____

  ____

- ❑ What is your favorite way to savor success, and how can you use that in your exercise journey?

____

____

____

COMPASSION

For midlife and more mature women, thinking about exercise often involves feeling like they "should" be doing something that they're not doing or doing something better than they are currently. Women often share compassion for everyone except themselves.

- ❑ How can you show compassion toward yourself in your thoughts and actions, for where you are with exercise and potential physical limitations?

____

____

____

- ❑ When you talk to yourself about exercise, speak to yourself the same way you would speak to a good friend. Knowing that no program, person, or journey is perfect, how can you look at your relationship with physical activity with love and understanding?

____

____

____

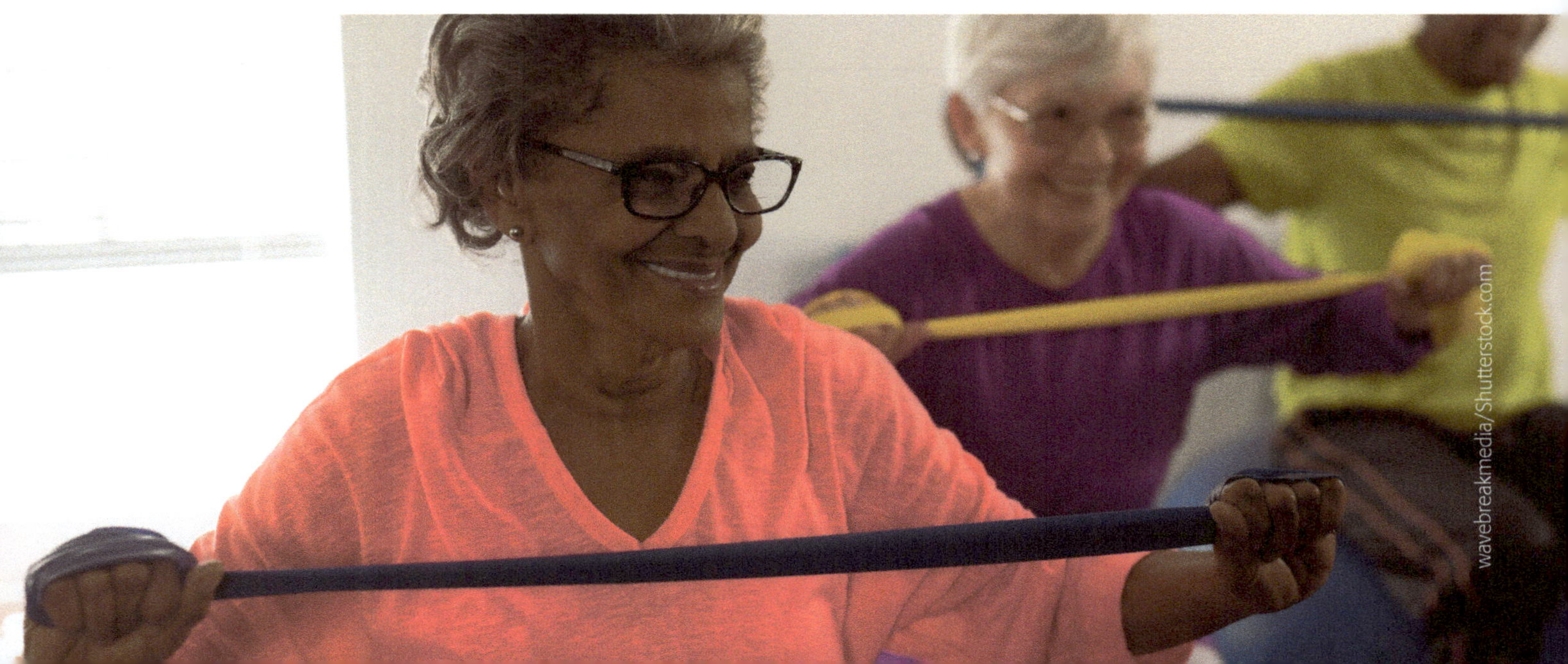
wavebreakmedia/Shutterstock.com

❑ Imperfections create each person's beauty and wisdom that can inspire and inform steps forward. So what is it about the journey that inspires and informs you?

____

____

____

____

HONESTY

It can be hard to consider whether your lack of physical activity or being too sedentary harms your physical and mental health. However, honesty in this area is essential if you want to PAVE your Path to Wellness.

❑ Based on an honest assessment of your current physical activity habits, what do you need to do to improve your health through physical activity?

____

____

____

____

❑ What obstacles are holding you back from enjoying routine movement (e.g., aerobic, resistance, balance)?

____

____

____

____

❑ What are you afraid of concerning physical activity?

____

____

____

____

- ❑ Suppose you had the opportunity to participate in any possible exercise, and there were no barriers in your way (financial, logistical, or physical). What would you choose to do (maybe hiking a colossal mountain, paddleboard yoga, mountain biking, belly dancing, golfing, roller skating)?

  ___

  ___

  ___

- ❑ Even if you cannot do the desired activity, what can you do that would give you a similar sense of satisfaction? Be honest with yourself.

  ___

  ___

  ___

Physical Activity Wrap-Up

As you conclude this chapter, consider society's stereotype of a frail, inactive, older woman sitting quietly in the corner watching TV. After reading this chapter, hopefully, you're ready to join in helping shatter this stereotype. Menopause, midlife, and beyond are ideal for reevaluating all physical activity areas in your life, including aerobic activity, resistance/muscle-strengthening activities, balance training, decreasing sedentary activity, and pelvic floor muscle exercises. Always remember that physical activity on a regular basis is an essential component of PAVING the Path to a healthy body, peaceful mind, and joyful heart, now and for years to come.

References

1. Sims ST, Yeager S. *Next Level: Your Guide to Kicking Ass, Feeling Great, and Crushing Goals Through Menopause and Beyond.* Rodale Books, NY; 2022.
2. Buettner D. *The Blue Zones: 9 Lessons for Living Longer From the People Who've Lived the Longest.* National Geographic Books: Washington, D.C.; 2012.

CHAPTER 3
ATTITUDE

Attitude Throughout Menopause, Midlife, and Beyond

Acronym—ATTITUDE

Action	**Teach**
Truth	**Understanding**
Tells	**Daily**
Improvement	**Energizes**

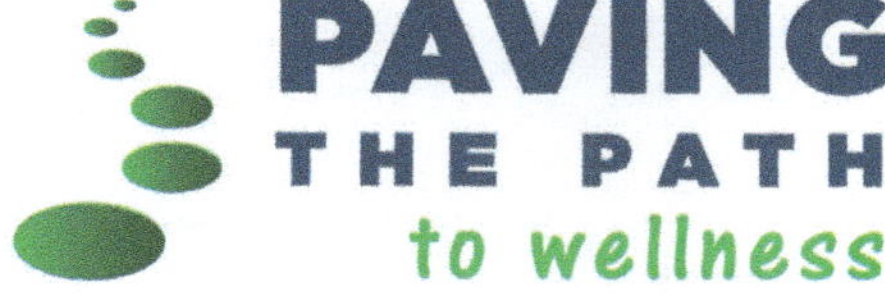

- *ACTION:* Your attitude impacts your actions. Be mindful of your attitude and its influence on your actions and interactions with others.
- *TRUTH:* If you are struggling with an attitude, ask yourself if you're basing your attitude on true beliefs or false assumptions. Your negative and self-critical attitudes often come from premises not based upon the truth. Check-in with your truth.
- *TELLS:* Your attitude tells others about who you are, what you think of them, and how you view the world. Make sure that the attitude you are broadcasting to others about yourself aligns with what you want to say to people.
- *IMPROVEMENT:* You should embrace an attitude of improvement. A growth-mindset attitude focuses on what you can learn from challenging times or setbacks and ultimately leads to reaching higher ground.
- *TEACH:* Your attitude is an influential teacher, if you reflect upon what it is trying to teach you. Pause and check in regularly with your attitude to uncover whether you can learn from it. For example, your attitude may tell you that you need connection, more "downtime," or that you need to spend more time doing self-care.
- *UNDERSTANDING:* When you struggle with a problematic attitude, you need to give yourself grace and compassion. Nobody has a positive mood at all times. Do what you can to support yourself during this challenging time, and remember that moods come and go.
- *DAILY:* It's easy to go through the day without reflecting upon your attitude. Start by checking in with your attitude daily and set an intention that aligns with the mindset that you hope to embrace as you go through your daily activities.
- *ENERGIZES:* A positive attitude energizes yourself, as well as those around you. Of course, you can't always have an optimistic outlook, but when possible, work to have an attitude that will be a source of positivity for you and those you love.

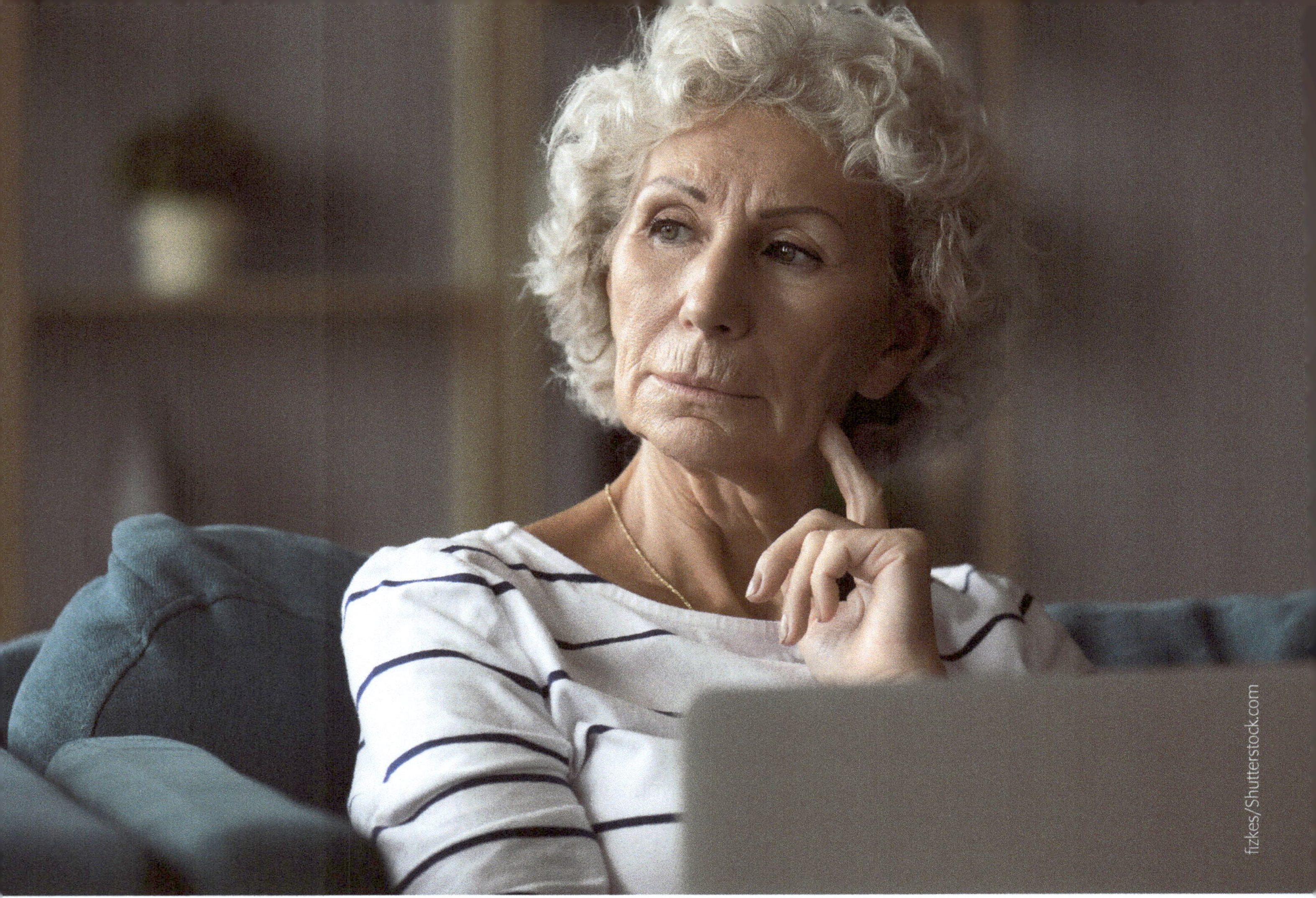

Attitude—Understanding the Basics

The *Oxford Dictionary of English* defines attitude as "a settled way of thinking or feeling about someone or something, typically reflected in a person's behavior" (1). Your attitude impacts how you view the world. Your thoughts, beliefs, and perception of yourself and others directly impact your attitudes, for better or for worse.

Although some women express positivity toward approaching and going through menopause, many others experience frustration, confusion, and sadness. It is challenging to have a positive attitude toward menopause and aging, when this transition is not honored by society. Unfortunately, ageism, fueled by the beauty industry, is typical in today's society. Ageism also suggests that menopausal and more mature women should be quiet and not disrupt the status quo. The PAVING the Path to Wellness Program not only embraces midlife and more mature women's wisdom, beauty, and power, it also supports a joyous journey through a health-promoting attitude, knowledge, and community.

Though female ageism is common in 21st century America, honoring the wisdom and beauty of aging women is the norm in many cultures and before our current times. A number of powerful women are working to change negative menopause stereotypes, including Michelle Obama, Maria Shriver, Whoopi Goldberg, and Oprah Winfrey. You are invited to challenge the status quo and age in the way you want to age, regardless of society's narrative. To embrace and thrive as a midlife or more mature female requires an attitude that embraces this journey. As you challenge the status quo, you'll tend to become more vocal and advocate for your needs. In the process, as you redefine the beautiful diversity in which women age, you'll pave the way for women who come after you to age in a way that supports their authentic selves too.

Throughout this chapter, you'll explore your attitudes toward menopause, aging bodies, health, and other aspects of life. When considering your past, current, and future attitudes, avoid thinking of them as "good" or "bad." For example, if you're going through a very sad or difficult time in your life, it is unlikely that you'll consistently have a joyful attitude. Likewise, when exploring your moods, it's not with the intention that you should try to pretend that you're always happy, as you want your attitude to be authentic. Also, try to avoid telling yourself that you "should" have a particular attitude. Guilt does not support well-being.

This chapter intends to teach you how to coach yourself to adopt and sustain a healthy, more optimistic, grateful, and growth mindset attitude. Keep in mind that always having a positive attitude is not realistic nor authentic. Having a healthy mindset and attitude will aid you in coaching yourself to adopt and sustain healthy lifestyle habits. In addition, having a positive, yet realistic, attitude that looks toward possibilities while acknowledging potential limitations can propel you to reach your goals. By the end of this chapter, you'll hopefully be ready to break even more stereotypes about aging women with an attitude that allows you to grow into your authentic self and experience all that life offers.

Coaching Yourself on Attitude With the COACH Approach

You don't have control over everything, but you do have control over your attitude. In other words, while you may not be able to control your circumstances, you can change what you focus on, which directly impacts your attitude. Coach yourself to have a mindset that supports your well-being.

Sometimes, women realize that they're feeling negative about everything. When they are in a bad mood, even their favorite people, places, or favorite activities can't change their negativity. However, the wisdom of their years can help them move through this negativity, if they take the time to coach themselves through it. Like your feelings, moods come and go. So, if you can pause and be mindful of a mood that you don't wish to continue, you can coach yourself beyond this temporary attitude toward a better mental place at your own pace.

- ❏ Dig deep and think about all the factors that have influenced your attitudes in life. What have you learned from your family, your friends, your education, and your life experiences?

____

____

____

CURIOSITY

Before you can change your mood for the better, you need to get curious about your attitude.

- ❑ How would you describe your attitude over the last week, month, and year?

- ❑ What formed your attitudes toward menopause and aging?

- ❑ What beliefs are you embracing that are holding you back?

- ❑ Do you desire to challenge your beliefs about menopause and aging to increase the vitality you feel at your age?

- ❑ How would having a different attitude change how you feel about yourself, engaging in healthy lifestyle behaviors, relationships with others, or joy in life?

- ❑ Do you have a model or example of someone in your life or whom you know who aged in a way that you want to model? If so, describe them.

____

____

____

- ❑ What beliefs, activities, and interactions typically improve your attitude?

____

____

____

- ❑ List ways to deal with the people who surround you, places you spend time, or self-talk you engage in to improve your attitude.

____

____

____

OPENNESS

Changing your attitude requires openness to an attitude adjustment.

- ❑ Select an attitude(s) that you want to change.

____

____

____

- ❑ What is motivating you to change this attitude?

____

____

____

❑ What do you want to learn, discuss, or change in your life to explore this attitude adjustment?

____

____

____

Perhaps, you are embracing an attitude that is keeping you from being healthy, content, and joyful. For example, maybe you have a negative attitude toward exercise that is not serving you well, or you feel that weight gain is inevitable for midlife women.

❑ What would empower you to let go of this attitude?

____

____

____

❑ What obstacle might be in your way of an attitude adjustment? Maybe, you have a spouse, friend, or family member who reinforces the negative belief that women are always moody and beyond their prime after menopause.

____

____

____

❑ How can you address this obstacle?

____

____

____

❑ If there are no obstacles in your way, what can you do today to work on your attitude?

____

____

____

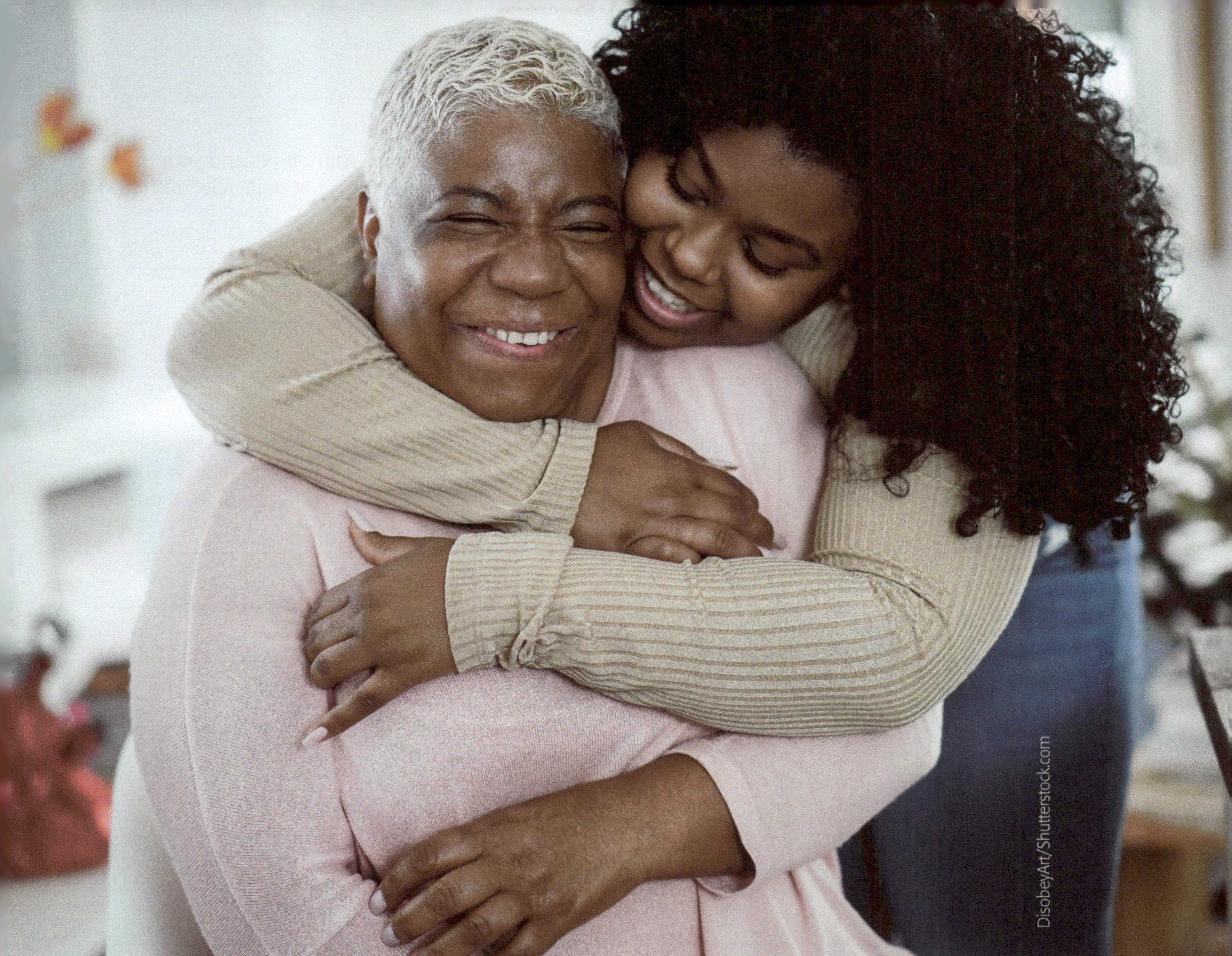

DisobeyArt/Shutterstock.com

APPRECIATION

Your attitude does not only impact yourself. It can affect others. Understanding what is at the root of negative or health-defeating attitudes and how they negatively impact others can motivate you to change them.

- ❑ How do your attitudes negatively impact others? Be gentle with yourself while considering this and give yourself grace. This can be difficult to think about, if you are completely honest with yourself. Nobody has health-promoting and uplifting attitudes all the time.

  ____

  ____

  ____

- ❑ Take a moment to appreciate how your relationships with others and your life may change if you change your attitude. What would improve in your relationship(s) if you made an attitude adjustment?

  ____

  ____

  ____

- ❑ A charismatic adult is someone who energizes you and gives you strength whenever you are around them. Take the time here to appreciate these people in your life. Who are the charismatic adults in your life, and why are you grateful for them?

  ____

  ____

  ____

- ❑ Take some time to appreciate those who come to you in their time of need and allow you to lead and share your inner wisdom with them. For whom are you a charismatic adult?

  ____

  ____

  ____

- ❑ Next, reflect upon how you've changed your attitudes in the past. What strengths and resources have you used?

  ____

  ____

  ____

- ❑ How can you use these strengths and resources to help you when you need an attitude change?

  ____

  ____

  ____

- ❑ What you appreciate tends to appreciate. What are attributes of your attitude for which you are grateful?

____

____

____

- ❑ How can you foster or increase these attributes?

____

____

____

COMPASSION

You've answered many difficult questions when going through the COACH approach, while focusing on your attitude. You may have uncovered some attitudes that aren't serving you well, and may negatively impact your health and your relationships. Take a few deep breaths and feel compassion for yourself. Most people have times in their lives when they adopt a self-defeating behavior. Everyone has those moments. For some, these moments meld into months, and for others, maybe even years. It's best to address these disempowering feelings and attitudes before they gain momentum and become a mountain rather than a molehill.

Feel compassion for the negative or health-defeating attitudes that you may have. They do not define you. They are only attitudes, and attitudes can change. You have done the best that you could do with your knowledge, your situations, and what you have experienced. If you find this challenging, think about how you would feel toward a good friend struggling with their attitudes and trying to improve them. You would not want them to feel guilty or discouraged. Instead, you would like them to feel inspired to continue reaching for higher ground and healthier attitudes.

- ❑ Please take a moment to write about how difficult it is to live in a society that is often ageist and undervalues menopausal, midlife, and more mature women. Feel compassion for yourself and other women who have aged in this environment. Express yourself fully here with writing, drawing, a picture, or a photograph. Include whatever speaks to you.

____

____

____

Sometimes, talking to a loved one or advocate can help put things into perspective, if you struggle. If you don't have a mental health professional but feel you could benefit from connecting with one, talk to your primary care provider or a healthcare practitioner and ask them for a referral. If you are in crisis, call 911 or reach out to a crisis hotline at 1-800-273-8255.

❑ How can you show compassion toward yourself and others for your attitudes in the past, present, and future?

____

____

____

____

Changing an attitude may take time. Be gentle with yourself. It's a process.

HONESTY

On occasion, it can be challenging to identify what attitudes are not positive or are not serving you or others well. You are more likely to have a positive attitude adjustment, if you can be completely honest with yourself while thinking about your attitude.

❑ After honest reflection, would you benefit from talking with a trusted loved one, friend, or mental health professional about your feelings, attitudes, and past or current situations? If so, what steps can you take to reach out?

____

____

____

____

If comfortable, you could ask your family and friends how they view your attitude toward life, aging, or menopause. Not that their view is the only thing you should consider, but it may help you better understand yourself by learning what sorts of attitudes you are expressing to others. You will only know this by asking others.

Take this time to be truthful with yourself when you are going down the wrong path and need to adjust your attitude. Then, take responsibility for your attitudes and your ability to change.

When you notice that your attitude is harming how you feel, your health, or your relationships with others, you now know how to use the COACH approach to change your attitude. With practice, you'll hopefully notice when you're headed in the wrong direction and quickly get back on the path to wellness.

Tapping Into Wisdom

When you notice that your attitude is not supporting your well-being, you can tap into your wisdom to shift your attitude.

Think of all you have learned this past year, decade, and since the beginning of your life. You are constantly learning and maturing. As a child and teen, you likely thought in terms of "black and white," while now you understand there is a lot more "gray," and that rarely is something as simple as it seems on the surface. As you age, you also tend to understand better what you can control and what is beyond your control. You have the wisdom of knowing what helped you in the past when you've struggled with an attitude problem.

If you can identify something that triggered a negative attitude, consider using a growth mindset-thought pattern to move beyond this attitude. Consider how you can use what you are going through to teach yourself or others. Realizing the lesson you can learn from the experience can hopefully propel you into a health-promoting attitude. You can also think of how you've used positivity, gratitude, optimism, enthusiasm, and expecting the best in the past to modify your attitude. See if you can use these experiences to guide your well-being this time too.

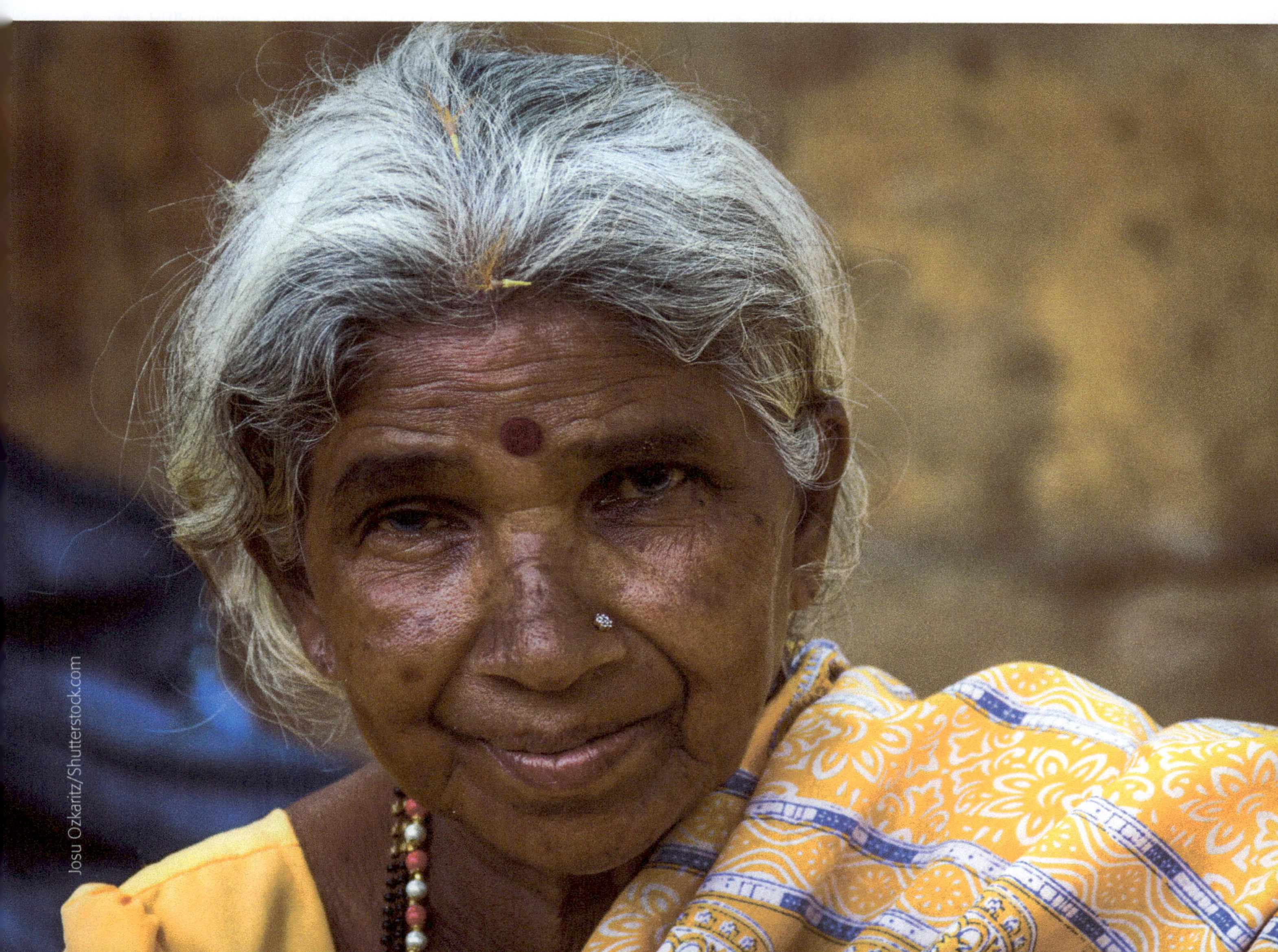
Josu Ozkaritz/Shutterstock.com

Healthy Attitude Support Through Lifestyle Behaviors

It's hard to have a positive, health-promoting attitude about anything when you are overly tired or stressed. Likewise, when you are physically unfit, aren't surrounded by positive people, have been sedentary, or when you're eating unhealthy foods, it is also more challenging to have a good attitude. Sometimes, you experience extreme stress or sadness. It can be almost impossible to have a good attitude during these times. That's okay.

Having a fake outward positive attitude is not desirable either. During those difficult times, give yourself grace and do what you can to support yourself and move forward. These topics will be addressed later in this book.

Moving beyond those challenges may involve lifestyle modifications, such as eating high-quality foods, engaging in physical activity on a regular basis, using stress management techniques, prioritizing sleep, avoiding risky substances, and connecting with supportive people in your life. On occasion, either you just need time or you may need professional support.

Words of Wisdom From Dr. Michelle Tollefson

Having a positive attitude toward menopause in our society is challenging. As a gynecologist, I have worked with countless women who have successfully navigated menopause with wisdom, health, and beauty. I educated them about menopausal symptoms, counseled them about hormone replacement therapy, and tried to empower them to optimize their health during this transition time and beyond. However, I have also heard from many women who were surprised by the symptoms caused by hormonal changes, felt dismissed by their employers and coworkers when discussing hot flashes, and thought they were being pushed toward the side by a culture that did not honor middle age and more mature women.

According to research, a positive attitude toward aging is associated with improved physical and mental health and decreased anxiety and depression (2). The authors of this study suggest challenging negative stereotypes around aging to support overall health.

Whether you are approaching the menopause transition or went through that part of your journey years ago, I want to encourage everyone to change the societal attitude toward this normal transition time in the female lifespan.

Having accurate information about the menopausal transition also supports a more positive attitude during this time. The following is a list of symptoms that many women experience during the menopausal transition. Of course, every woman's experience is different. Rarely will a woman not experience any of these symptoms. In reality, most women experience several or more. For some women, the symptoms are mild, and for others, they can significantly impact their quality of life.

As you read the list, note the symptoms you are experiencing and any others that you've noticed. Then, I encourage you to talk with your gynecologist or another healthcare practitioner about your symptoms to get individualized education and support. Common symptoms will be addressed in more detail in the investigation chapter—literally investigating how you feel and what can support you in this time.

- Hot flashes
- Night sweats
- Vaginal dryness
- Decreased interest in sex
- Mood swings
- Feeling anxious or sad
- Weight gain
- Decreased energy
- Dry skin
- Hair changes
- Musculoskeletal pain
- Irregular menstrual bleeding
- Urinary incontinence
- And other symptoms

Your attitude toward the menopausal transition can impact your experience. Reminding yourself that other women have experienced these symptoms can help you realize that you are not alone. Have compassion for yourself and your body as you go through this natural life process. Remember that the menopausal transition does not last forever and that hot flashes signify that your body is functioning. Remember that you are going through a communal experience that women traverse during their lifespans. Also, when you experience these symptoms, use them as a reminder to engage in self-care and consider what you can do to support yourself during this time.

You are encouraged to openly discuss menopausal symptoms with others, rather than feeling like you should hide them. Many women feel the need to hide and minimize their menopausal symptoms. However, consider that any female you are with will either go through menopause eventually, is going through it now, or has already gone through it. Openly acknowledging your menopausal symptoms, including hot flashes, may help change the stigma around menopausal symptoms for women who will come after you. If you are experiencing a hot flash, move through it in whatever way is best for you at that moment. For many women, wearing layers of clothing or carrying a fan is beneficial. Other women prefer to stand and walk, take a few slow relaxing breaths, and let it pass. Consider acknowledging it if you are in a group or you may prefer not to mention it. Regardless of how you choose to handle it, do not be embarrassed. Hot flashes are a normal part of the menopausal transition that most women experience.

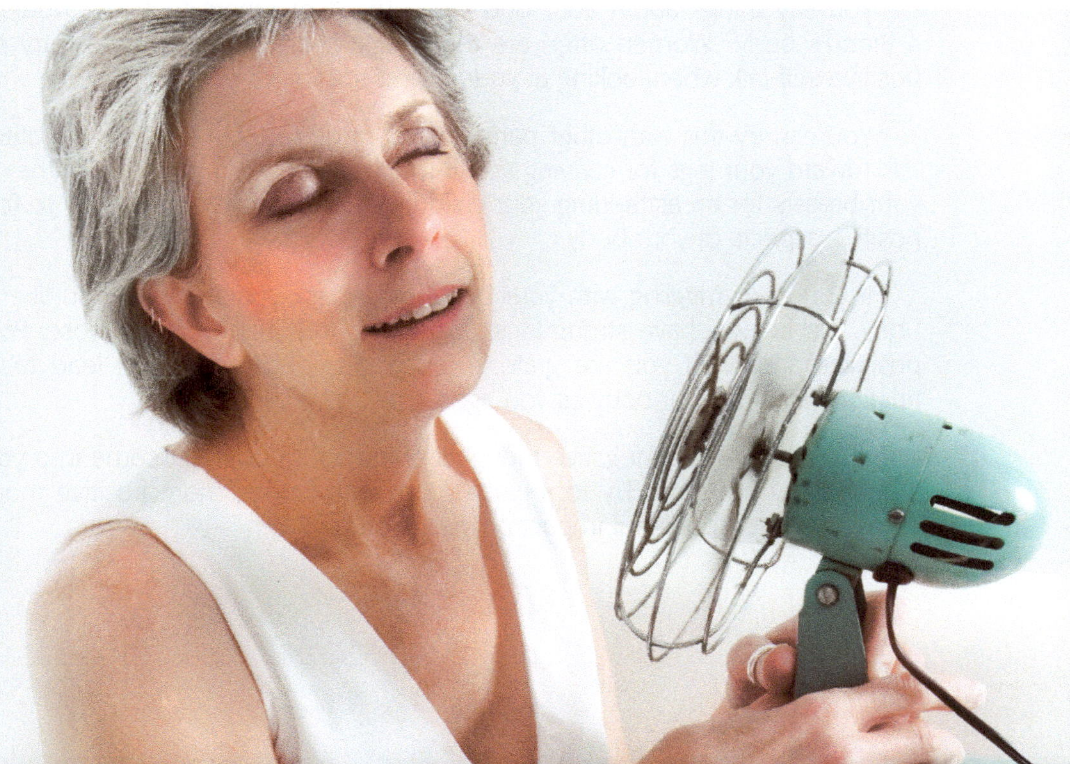

Attitude Toward Your Body

Consider all that your physical body has done for you by moving you throughout your life. The human body is a masterpiece that moves you throughout your days and allows you to interact with others. Many women experience physical changes during the menopausal transition and after. Sometimes these changes can cause women to have a negative attitude toward their bodies, especially women who have struggled before with negative body-image issues.

As body dissatisfaction increases, self-esteem and quality of life decrease. Body dissatisfaction is also associated with increased depression and anxiety in menopausal and post-menopausal women. Try not to compare yourself to others or listen to the marketing that tells you that you "should" look a certain way or feel a specific way about your body. Just as your personality is unique, so is your body. It would be boring if women all looked the same or didn't have any wrinkles. Try to practice self-compassion toward your body.

As you age and your appearance changes, there are practices that you can engage in that support a body-positive attitude, including the following:

- Engaging in aerobic activity daily
- Strength training two to three times a week
- Trying yoga or another mind-body movement
- Stretching
- Engaging in body-positive self-talk
- Eating nourishing foods
- Getting out in nature and appreciating the beauty of nature in various forms
- Expressing gratitude for a body that functions and is old enough to go through menopause
- Connecting with a friend or family member over the phone or in person who is already supporting body positivity

Consider your self-talk about your body or how you talk about your body to others. Do you say things about your body to yourself or others that you would say about a friend's body? Women often are their worst critics. This next week, try engaging in positive self-talk when looking at your face in the mirror each day.

You can try this with other parts of your body too. Try expressing gratitude in self-talk toward your legs for carrying you throughout life, your arms for all they have held, your breasts for breastfeeding your children (if you breastfed), etc. Try to focus on the positive aspects of your body.

If you are struggling with your body image, ask yourself what you like about your body. Maybe you have strong legs, or you like the shape of your nose. Focus on the positives and what you are grateful for, and hopefully, this will lead to a healthier relationship with your body as you age.

Also, be aware of negative thoughts about your body that come into your mind or that you say out loud. Try to replace these with kinder, more positive thoughts. Your thoughts have a powerful impact on your attitude.

Having a body-positive attitude does not mean that you don't care about how you look. Instead, having a positive attitude about your body supports your desire to do what you can to care for your body through healthy lifestyle behaviors. Give yourself grace and remember, you want to work with your body and not against it, and a body-positive attitude supports this.

If you are struggling with your body image or weight after this, talk to your healthcare practitioner for additional support. Don't suffer alone. Help is available, and health professionals are there to support you.

❑ Does your self-talk help you to appreciate the beauty of your body?

____

____

____

❑ How could you change your self-talk to support body positivity for yourself?

____

____

____

Whether you're approaching menopause or went through it decades ago, hopefully, you'll challenge negative stereotypes of women. If you want to wear a bikini, do it! If you want to wear high heels and glitter eyeshadow, do it! Don't mold yourself into a particular image or try to act how you think society or someone wants you to act. You are intended to live into your whole self, and if that challenges society's script, that's great. Nobody's body is perfect. As a woman, consider committing to not judging other women based on appearances. Women should lift each other up and support one another, as everyone lives into their authentic selves.

Among the ways to support a positive attitude in midlife and beyond are the following:

- Listen to uplifting music.
- Look through old photos.
- Do something spontaneous.
- Do something fun.
- Reach out to someone that you haven't connected with this past year.
- Do something that you used to enjoy as a child but haven't done recently.
- Forgive, forget, and move on quickly, so you can enjoy the present.
- Try to expect the best in people, circumstances, etc.
- Check-in with yourself, and then plan something to support your attitude.
- Plan an activity with someone whose presence enlivens you.
- Get outside and spend time in nature.

- Volunteer.
- Do something to help the world.
- Read an uplifting book.
- Listen to an inspiring podcast.
- Engage in a creative activity, like painting or photography, where you can control the beauty of what you see.
- If you are able and interested, go sledding, snowshoeing, kayaking, paddleboarding, hula hooping, jumping rope, riding a bicycle with a helmet, jumping in puddles, or blowing bubbles.
- Get out of your home and spend time around people.
- Visit your local community center or YMCA.
- Do something that supports your spiritual well-being.

❑ Which of the aforementioned ideas would you like to use this week to stimulate your attitude?

____

____

____

Attitude Wrap-Up

As you move along your life journey, having an attitude of self-compassion and empowerment will hopefully help you thrive as you age.

- Try to take the high road at every turn.
- Try to find the silver lining in challenging situations.
- Try to work with people to make progress, even when things are dim and dismal for you and others.
- Try to embrace a new, health-promoting attitude as you pave your path to wellness.

Instead of growing old, think about growing wise, growing well, and growing into your authentic self.

References

1. Stevenson A, editor. *Oxford Dictionary of English*, New York: Oxford University Press; 2010.
2. Bryant C, et al. The relationship between attitudes to aging and physical and mental health in older adults. *International Psychogeriatrics*. October 2012; 24(10):1674-83.

CHAPTER 4
VARIETY

Variety Throughout Menopause, Midlife, and Beyond

Acronym—VARIETY

Volunteer
Action
Research
Imagine
Education
Tasks
Yesterday

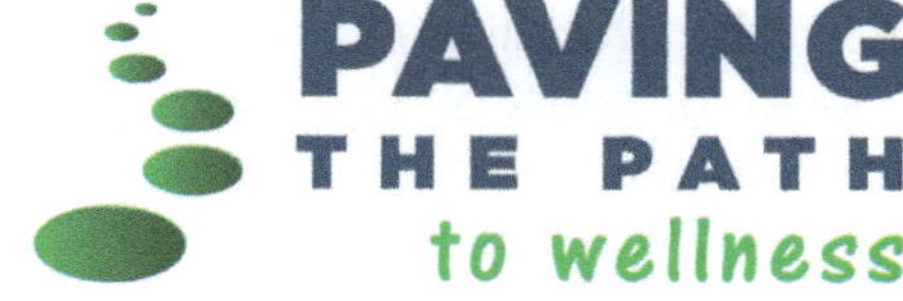

- *VOLUNTEER:* Volunteering in your community is a great way to add variety to your life. Don't stay quiet if you see someone in need or realize that you could assist someone. Volunteer to help. Others will be glad that you did.
- *ACTION:* It's easy to continue doing what you've always done. Take action and sign up for a new class, say hello to a stranger, or order a different dish at your favorite restaurant. Don't sit on the sidelines of life. Take action and mix it up. Don't wait until tomorrow. Take action today.
- *RESEARCH:* Research different opportunities in your community. Become an investigator and explore how you want to add variety to your life. You may never know what options exist if you don't research what is there.
- *IMAGINE:* Imagine how to make an activity or interaction better. Close your eyes and envision how it could be improved. Then take action. For example, if your day involves running errands, maybe you could invite a friend to go along or visit a favorite store while you are out. Imagine the possibilities.
- *EDUCATION:* Regularly learning new things and expanding your knowledge through education is beneficial for lifelong brain health. Learning can entail a variety of formats, for example, learn a new skill online by watching videos, signing up for an art class, or taking a local college course. The world is waiting to teach you new things.
- *TASKS:* All women have tasks that they do that aren't necessarily exciting, like washing dishes and doing laundry. Try adding variety to these tasks. You can make some of the mundane parts of life take on a new life. For example, try singing while you wash the dishes. Listen to a new podcast while doing laundry. It doesn't matter what you do; just add variety to change things up.
- *YESTERDAY:* Look at what you did yesterday, last month, and years ago to add variety to your life. Maybe you haven't played your guitar in years, or you haven't connected with a friend from college in over a decade. Your past contains a treasure trove of ideas for adding variety to your future.

Variety—Understanding the Basics

While this chapter is going to be exciting, monotony is part of life. Brushing your teeth, taking out the trash, and doing laundry are routine parts of the day that women don't usually view as exhilarating. Even though you'll always have monotonous things on your "to-do" list, you can look for ways to decrease boredom and increase joy in your life.

Engaging in a diverse range of activities has been shown to improve cognitive function, memory, and executive function (e.g., flexible thinking, planning, problem-solving, organization, and self-control). Exposure to various experiences, activities, people, and locations encourages your brain to build new connections between brain cells, improving your brain's structure and function over time.

When you think of stereotypes of women beyond the menopausal transition, you may think of a "little old lady" watching game shows or a woman in her rocking chair, knitting for hours on end. While knitting is a beautiful way to stimulate your brain, it is just one creative activity among many that you could experience each day. You may not know menopausal or more mature women who fit the "little old lady" stereotype. Yet you probably know many women in this age group who could benefit from increased variety. Take the challenge to actively look for ways to diversify the experiences in your life, as you break yet another stereotype of midlife and more mature women.

Think of the range of women you know who have experienced the menopause transition. Consider the wisdom they have accumulated and how they creatively thrive. The world needs their knowledge and generativity. So, now is your time to shine, share what you have learned with others, learn from other midlife and more mature women, and look for opportunities to increase variety and joy.

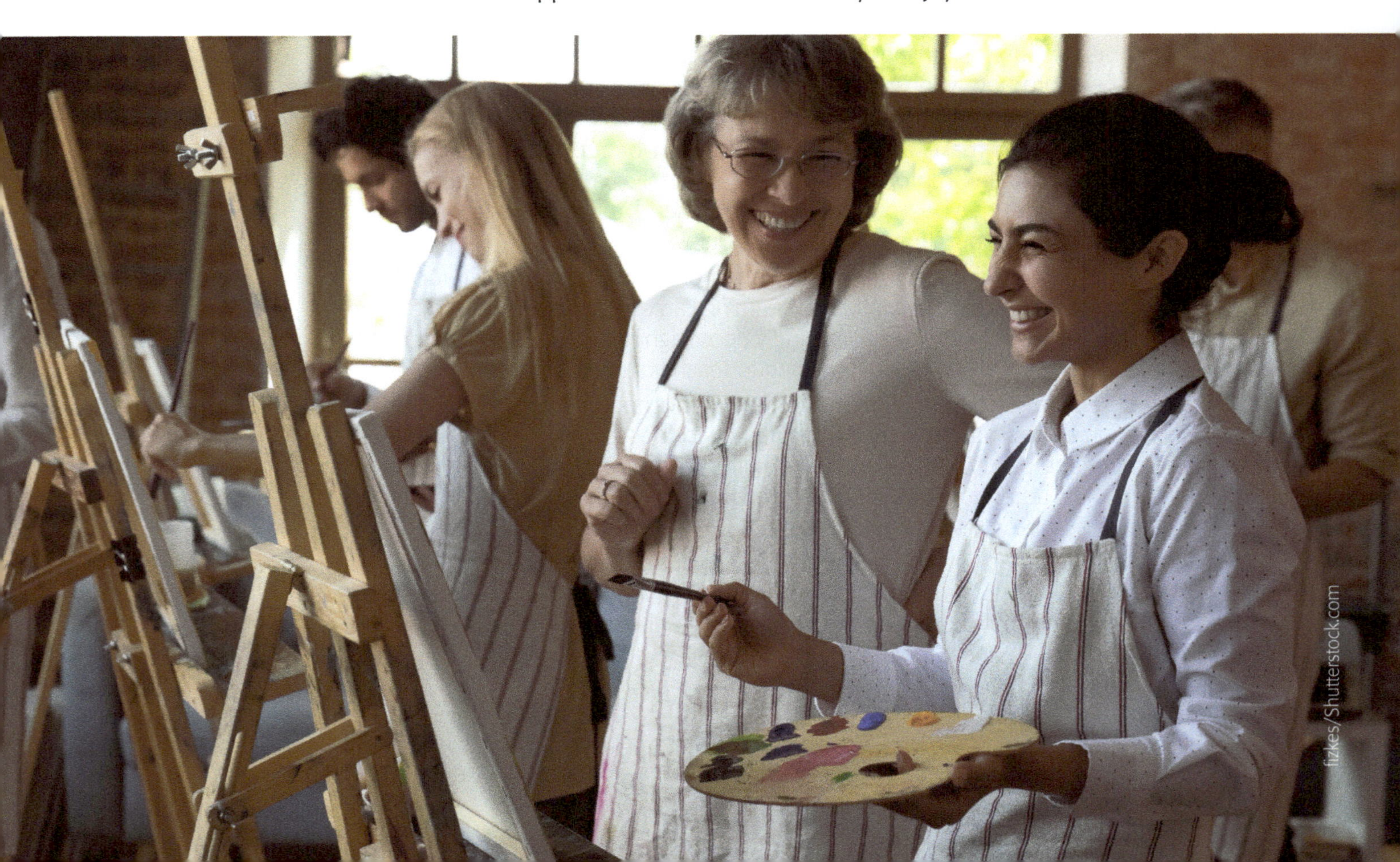

fizkes/Shutterstock.com

You may be thinking that you are too old. You are not. Maybe you feel it's selfish to focus on diversifying your experiences to add joy, awe, and wonder to your life. It's not selfish. If you're like most women who are going through or who have gone through menopause, you've spent years serving others: your partner, children, parents, siblings, friends, employer, colleagues, and more. Now is the time to think about what type of experiences you want. You are not done. If you're reading this book, you are still breathing, you are still living, and this world has new things for you to learn and experience. Embrace all that life offers, as you increase variety in your daily life.

Variety for Brain Health

Engaging in a diverse range of activities appears to improve cognitive health. Adults who engage in different activities adjust to situations, events, and people, which leads to modification of behavior and the use of a wide variety of skills. Research on over 7,000 midlife people in the United States over ten years showed that participants who engaged in greater activity diversity or increased their activity diversity had higher overall cognitive and executive functioning (1). They also had improved memory. This study examined diversity in paid and volunteer work, interaction with children, doing chores, engaging in leisure and physical activities, and informally helping others. This research highlights how variety results in mental stimulation and adaptation.

THE REASONS WHY VARIETY IS IMPORTANT TO MENTAL AND BRAIN HEALTH:

- Helps develop an attitude and mindset of curiosity.
- Improves brain function.
- Increases stress resilience.
- Enhances performance in mentally challenging activities.
- Improves memory.
- Increases cognitive reserve (may help compensate for early Alzheimer's disease).
- Reduces risk of cognitive decline.
- Increases social networks.
- Supports greater psychological well-being.
- Decreases boredom which has been linked with depression and anxiety.
- Decreases restlessness.
- Can increase energy.
- Makes life more satisfying.
- May decrease the risk of substance use and binge eating.

WAYS TO SUPPORT BRAIN HEALTH THROUGH VARIETY:

(Note: Please read this list of options and mark the ones that are appealing to you.)

- Look at your community recreation center's schedule of activities and try an activity that appeals to you or join a group.
- Call a friend whom you haven't talked to in over five years.
- Watch a movie in a genre that you don't typically view, for example, try a comedy or documentary film.
- Run or walk in the exact opposite loop that you usually do.
- Take a new route when driving somewhere you often go.

- Explore a grocery store that you don't typically frequent and discover what healthy options and brands they may carry that you haven't tried before.
- Try a different dress style. For example, if you consistently wear dresses, try pants, or if you continually wear monochrome colors, try a pattern.
- Try a new restaurant that serves an ethnic cuisine you don't typically eat.
- Enrich your environment by changing a room in your home to be more stimulating.
- Attend a concert or theater production.
- Buy a new plant and nurture it.
- Learn something new, for example, read a book on a topic you don't typically read.
- Listen to a new podcast.
- Try a new type of leisure activity every month.
- Take photographs while on a nature walk.
- Visit an animal shelter.
- Go to a museum.
- Turn off the television and study something new.
- While engaging in a monotonous activity, like sorting laundry or washing dishes, make it more exciting by listening to music.
- Interact with different people, for example, by joining a new organization or taking a group class.
- Consider getting paid for your work, if you aren't already doing so.
- Find ways to interact with children, your relatives, or by volunteering at a school or a community-based organization.
- Think of ways to switch up your chores.
- Try volunteering through diverse activities or a non-profit organization.
- Try a new type of physical activity every month.
- When outside your home, look for ways to informally help people.
- Visit new places in your community, state, or beyond.
- Look for ways to decrease physically passive activities.
- Visit the library to find new things to learn.
- Explore the internet and increase your knowledge about a new topic.
- Go to your local park and take a hike.

What would you add?

- ______________________________________
- ______________________________________
- ______________________________________

❑ What have you always wanted to do but haven't tried?

____

____

____

❑ Why are you waiting?

____

____

____

____

Hobbies, Leisure Activities, Flow, and Variety

Consider the last time you did a new activity because you thought it would be fun. If you're like many midlife and more mature women, you'll find it challenging to think of something that fits this description. Your brain craves variety and flow. Mihaly Csikszentmihalyi highlighted the concept of "flow" in his research and writings. Flow occurs when the challenge you face aligns beautifully with your skills pertaining to the challenge. When you are in flow, time may seem to stop. You are focused on the experience and not necessarily the result. You are not doing something because you "should" do it or to meet someone else's expectations. Engaging in behavior where you rise to a challenge, using your unique skill set, can lead you to experience flow.

For you, a flow experience is likely different from a flow experience for someone else. Just as you have different talents, skill sets, and things that you enjoy, you also have various activities that bring you into a flow state. You may already engage in activities where you experience flow but, perhaps, could incorporate variety to experience even greater flow.

The hobbies that you enjoyed as a child, as a young adult, or enjoy now can give you clues as to what activities will bring you into flow. If you haven't recently tried an activity you enjoyed years ago, try it again, if it is safe. For example, if you loved coloring with crayons as a child, maybe you could find a video that shares some adult coloring tips, purchase a set of crayons and an adult coloring book, and see if coloring brings you joy.

It's also beneficial to incorporate some challenges where you can bring your skills to the activity. For example, could you view some adult crayon art, take a coloring course, and use your new skills to create your art? Remember, it's not about the result but enjoying the process and experiencing flow. If coloring doesn't interest you, maybe another creative outlet, such as a pottery, glass blowing, or painting class, would. For example, learning to play the clarinet, or taking a ballet class would create an opportunity for flow, as your skills match the level of challenge.

Your brain wants variety, and trying various new (or old) hobbies and leisure activities can add joy to your life and challenge your mind. Consider participating in activities because you want to be in the moment, fully absorbed in that activity, not because you've always done it or enjoy the result. You are deserving of joyful, flow-filled experiences. Look for ways to learn new hobbies and leisure activities through online or in-person classes at your local YMCA, library, community center, or college. Talk to your friends about what brings them flow and consider joining them.

Don't just stop after doing this once. Consider trying to engage in a new flow-producing experience every month. It may take some investigation, and you may realize that an activity you thought you would enjoy isn't as fun as you had imagined. That's alright. You have incorporated brain health-enhancing variety in your life and learned more about yourself. Now you have this knowledge as you look for another way to increase variety and flow experiences through hobbies, work, and leisure activities in the future.

Connection and Variety

Dr. Ned Hallowell, a world-renowned psychiatrist, connection expert, and author, explained in his book *Connect: 12 Vital Ties That Open Your Heart, Lengthen Your Life, and Deepen Your Soul* that the importance of connections extends beyond your family and friend groups (2). His inventory of a connected life involves relationships with the following:

- Family
- Neighborhood
- Friends
- Work
- The past
- Nature/outdoors
- Pets/animals
- Art and beauty
- Activities, hobbies, past times
- Information and ideas
- Institutions, clubs, organizations, other groups
- Spiritual connection
- Connection to self
- Connection to life
- Other connections

Although connections will be covered later in this book, at this time, you need to focus on increasing variety in your relationships.

❑ When you read through this list, are there specific areas where you feel well connected and others where you feel disconnected?

____

____

____

Next, return to the list and check those items where you feel like you have a strong connection. Put an X by the areas where you want to improve your connection. Keep in mind that it's normal to feel connected to some of these areas and disconnected from others. Increasing your connections' depth and breadth (variety) can boost your well-being.

There are an infinite number of ways to add variety through connection. For example, if you aren't feeling very connected with your neighborhood, you could reach out to a family you've never met with a plate of cookies and a warm greeting. You could also read an informative book in your neighborhood park, which would support connection with your neighborhood, nature, and information. In addition, incorporating variety through contact with art and beauty could occur through visiting an art museum or attending a concert.

As you read through the aforementioned list, think of ways to add variety to your life through these areas of connection. Doing so will likely bring you joy and support your brain health and overall emotional well-being.

Growing Into Your Authentic Self With Variety

Your self-image naturally evolves as you age. As you traverse menopause and the years beyond, your self-image will continue to develop. Hopefully, as you age, your self-image aligns with your true self.

Keep in mind that it's normal to have areas that may need work, as you grow into your authentic self during menopause, midlife, and beyond. At these stages in life, many women feel less fear of failure and feel like they no longer need to fill the roles that others have put on them. Embrace this time, without morphing yourself into the person you think you "should" be or that others want you to be. You are meant to thrive during this time in your life and beyond. As you grow more fully into your authentic self, variety can support this transition and your well-being.

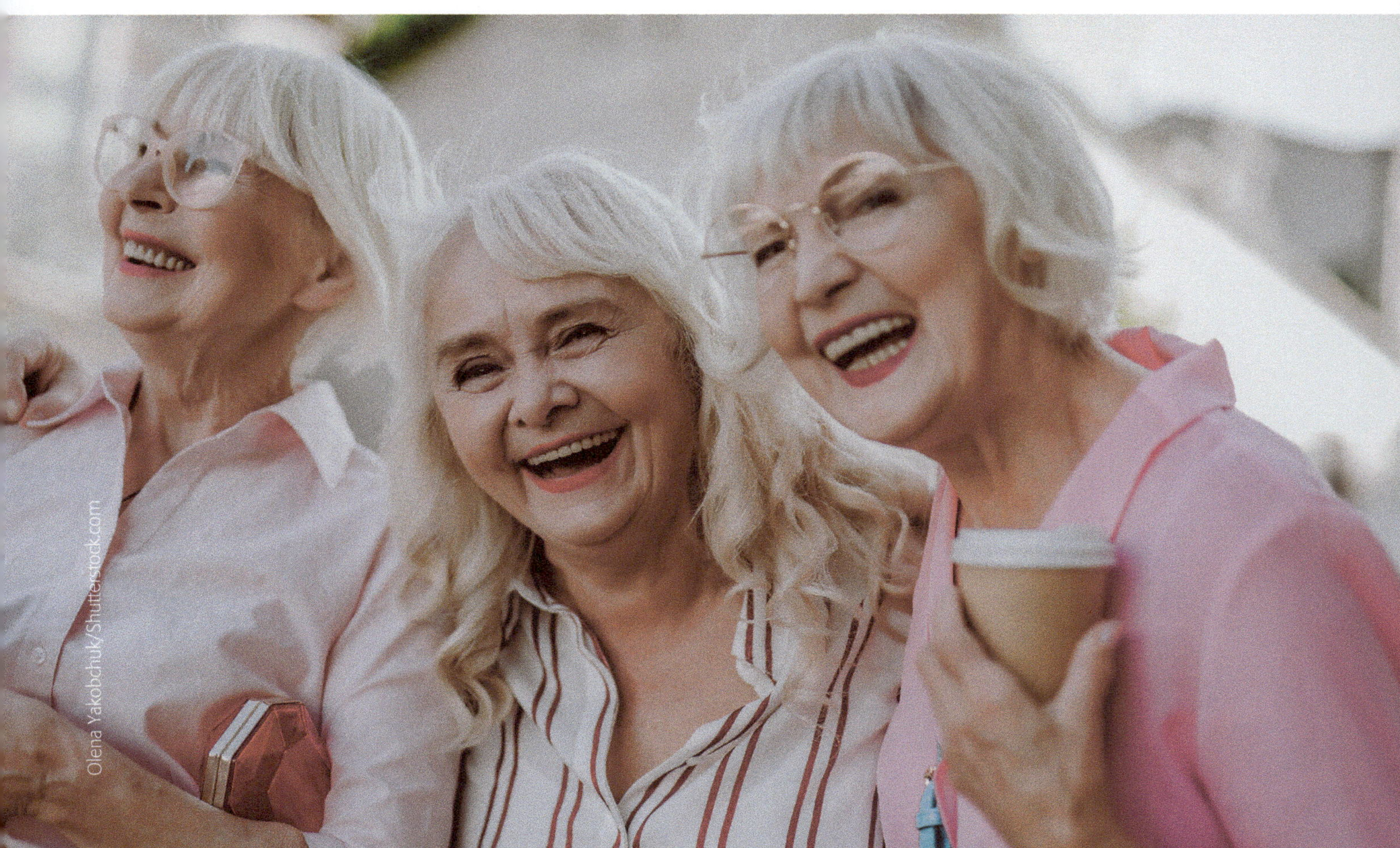

Olena Yakobchuk/Shutterstock.com

- [ ] Envision yourself as someone who has fully grown into their authentic self. What would you be thinking, doing, or experiencing that would be different from what you are doing now?

____

____

____

Incorporating a variety of experiences, thoughts, or connections with people who support you will increase awe and wonder during your life journey.

As you grow into your authentic self as you age, try to push yourself out of your comfort zone. Trust your intuition. Trust that it's alright to try something new. For example, maybe your authentic self spends time in nature, serves others, or spends more time focused on spiritual health. When you feel your authentic self differs from your current state, it's a signal that it's time to add variety.

As you use variety to get closer to your authentic self, you can experience confidence and pride as a middle-age or more mature woman. You can feel proud of the work that you are doing to infuse awe and wonder into your world.

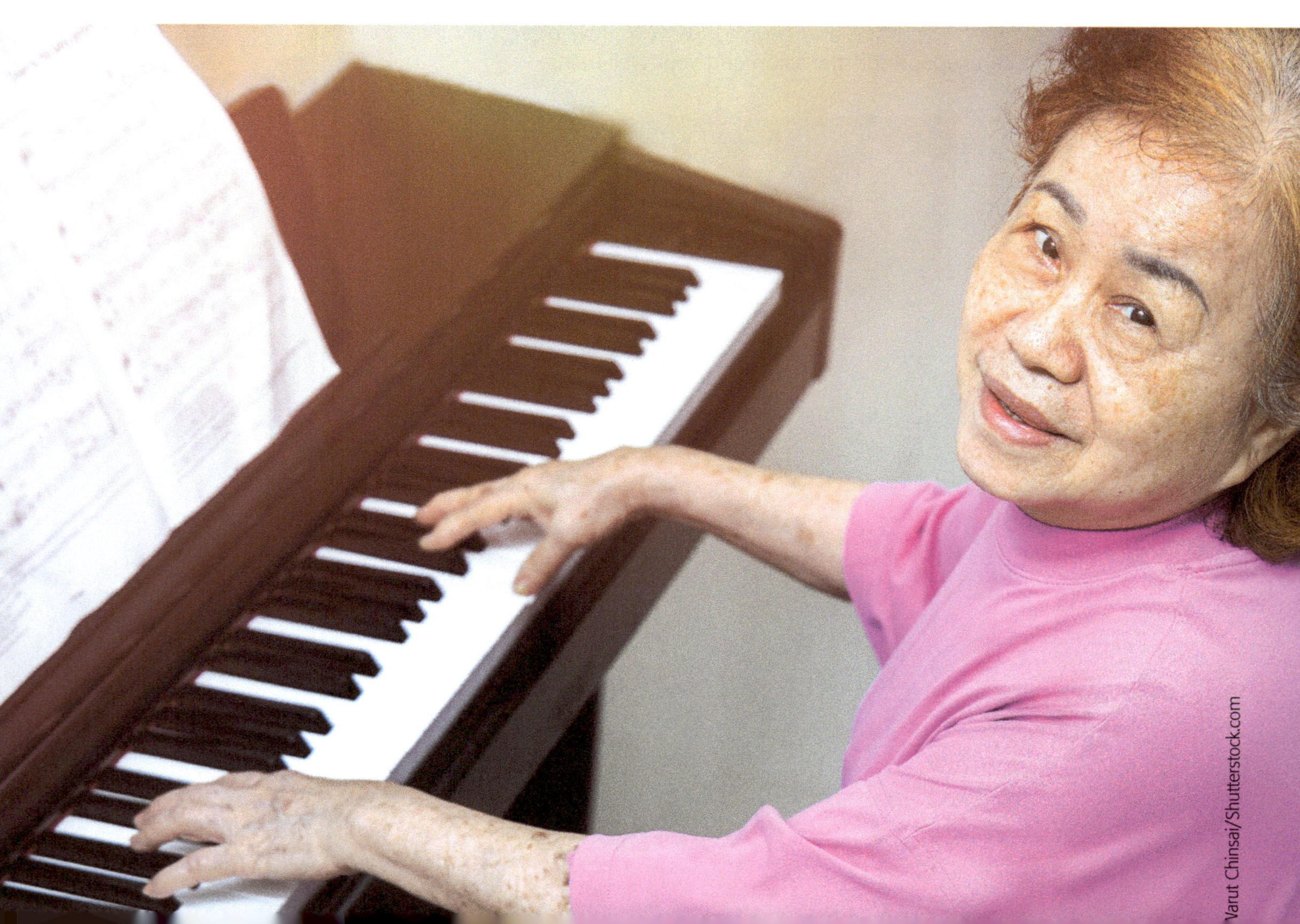

Varut Chinsai/Shutterstock.com

Coaching Yourself on Variety With the COACH Approach

When you realize that you need more variety in your life, you can coach yourself through the COACH approach. Usually, variety doesn't happen by chance but through planned experiences, activities, and interactions. So, rather than waiting for life to increase variety for you, you can coach yourself to a happier, healthier, more joyful life filled with variety. Using the acronym COACH can be helpful in that regard.

CURIOSITY

In this fast-paced society, it's easy for your life to become so filled with routine tasks and obligations that you don't have a chance to consider where you need increased variety in your life. The COACH approach can help you with this.

❑ What areas in your life are dull, boring, or could benefit from more variety?

____

____

____

❑ What do you want to do about these dull areas to increase variety?

____

____

____

❑ What varied activities have brought you flow or glimpses of joy in the past?

____

____

____

❑ How could you use variety to experience activities that are similar to but different from these past activities?

____

____

____

- ❑ Take a moment to create a flow timeline. List or draw what activities brought you into a flow state on the timeline. Then, identify your favorite activities at that time. Have fun while you complete this flow timeline.

Childhood	Adolescence	Young Adulthood	Now

Table 4-1. Flow timeline

- ❑ What did you learn from reflecting on your flow timeline?

____

____

____

OPENNESS

Being open to growing into your authentic self is powerful. If you are not open to this transformation, positive growth will not occur. There is no shame, blame, or guilt in this process. For example, if you have always wanted to belly dance, look for a local class or online lesson and give it a try.

- ❑ What do you feel embarrassed about wanting to try?

____

____

____

____

- ❑ Explore what it is that creates this sense of embarrassment.

- ❑ What would you say if your friend wanted to try this activity?

- ❑ How does your openness to adding variety to your activities and experiences impact your happiness, joy, and well-being?

- ❑ How does your fear, embarrassment, or judgmental nature prevent you from trying new things?

- ❑ What mindset would you need to change to add variety to your experiences, activities, and connections?

- [ ] If no one was watching, what would you try?

APPRECIATION

Appreciation for the diversity in life and the variety of opportunities hopefully increases as you age. This sense of gratitude can be fostered and enhance your well-being.

- [ ] Identify someone you know who is an excellent example of fearlessly trying new experiences. What can you learn from them?

- [ ] Would connecting with them help you move forward with your experimentation? Explain.

- [ ] Consider times when you stepped out of your comfort zone and discovered something new that you enjoyed. Describe the experiences.

- [ ] What strengths do you have that can empower you to try something new? This could be the support of family and friends. On the other hand, it could be that you are creative, have a growth mindset, or have a sense of humor and can laugh at yourself.

- [ ] Think of ways that your life already benefits from variety. Are you expressing gratitude for these areas of your life? If not, can you start this now?

____

____

____

- [ ] Now, think about and describe the things you are grateful for that have steered your course in an unexpected direction that has provided great joy and variety to your life.

____

____

____

COMPASSION

Women are often the most critical of themselves. Self-criticism does not nurture an attitude that fosters variety. Compassion for yourself, as you try new things, can increase your openness to variety.

- [ ] Are you compassionate with yourself when you try a new activity and fail?

____

____

____

- [ ] What would you tell a friend if they tried something new and failed?

____

____

____

- [ ] How could you change your mindset to be one of growth or one that is more compassionate as you try various new things?

____

____

____

- ❑ Write a compassionate statement that supports that it's okay if you have a mishap when trying something new.

___

___

___

- ❑ How can you reduce your anxiety around trying something new, e.g., have a friend join you, take a class, or gather more information? Realize that this is not the end of the world if it doesn't work out.

___

___

___

- ❑ The next time you feel like shaming, blaming, or guilting yourself, treat yourself like a dear friend. What do you need to put in place to make this a reality?

___

___

___

HONESTY

- ❑ What is holding you back from trying new things and adding more variety to your life? Be honest with yourself.

___

___

___

- ❑ Do you feel judged by people or continued judgment from people in your past? If so, what can you do to diminish these feelings?

___

___

___

- ❑ Everyone has insecurities. What are yours?

- ❑ How have these insecurities kept you from increasing variety in your life, experiencing flow, and growing into your authentic self?

- ❑ After honest reflection, consider if and why you care what your friends and colleagues think of you and what you do. How does this impact whether you embrace variety or continue with only what you have done before?

- ❑ In what areas do you excel? List as many as you can. Try to get to at least 10.

- ❑ What type of compliments do you receive? Why do you think this happens? Be honest.

- [ ] When you see something good, beautiful, or wise in others, do you compliment them?

____

____

____

Honest, encouraging feedback can help people achieve more than they thought possible. By appreciating your unique talents and those of the people around you, you'll create an environment of continual growth.

Variety Wrap-Up

Hopefully, this chapter helped you reflect upon utilizing variety to support your health. As you incorporate more variety into your life, you may initially feel insecurity or self-doubt. Remember that you are not alone. It's normal to feel apprehension or uncertainty as you try new things.

Remind yourself of the importance of experiencing diverse activities and interactions with others and your world. It's worth pushing yourself out of your comfort zone to reap the benefits of increased variety. Remember to adopt a growth mindset where mishaps are opportunities to learn and grow. You will experience bumps, but these can help you understand and fortify yourself for future endeavors. As you incorporate more variety into your life, you'll likely inspire others around you to try new things and spread the benefits of variety far and wide.

References

1. Lee S, Charles ST, Almeida DM. Change is good for the brain: activity diversity and cognitive functioning across adulthood. *The Journal of Gerontology*: Series B. 2021 Jul;76(6):1036-48.
2. Hallowell EM. *Connect: 12 vital ties that open your heart, lengthen your life, and deepen your soul.* New York: Simon and Schuster; 2001.

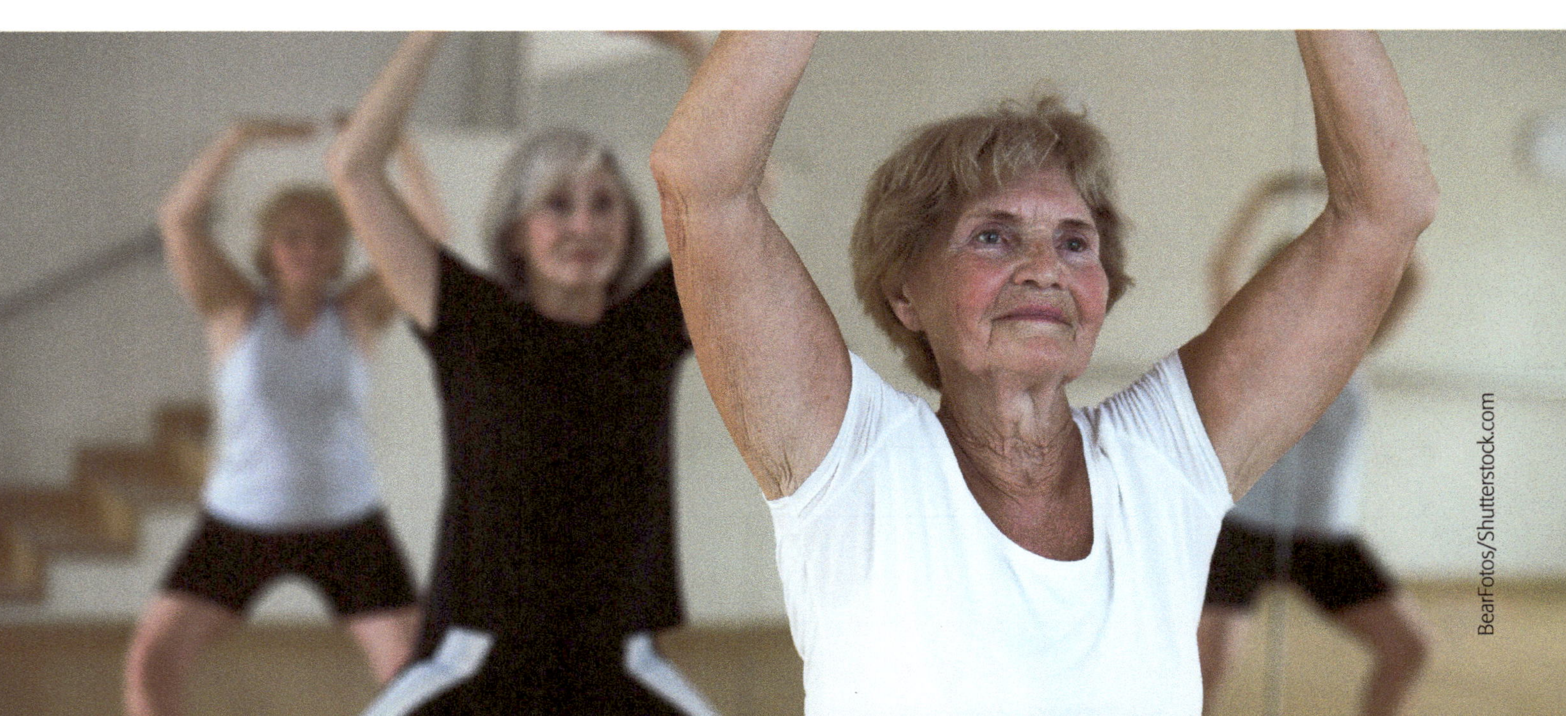

BearFotos/Shutterstock.com

CHAPTER 5

INVESTIGATION

Investigation Throughout Menopause, Midlife, and Beyond

Acronym—INVESTIGATION

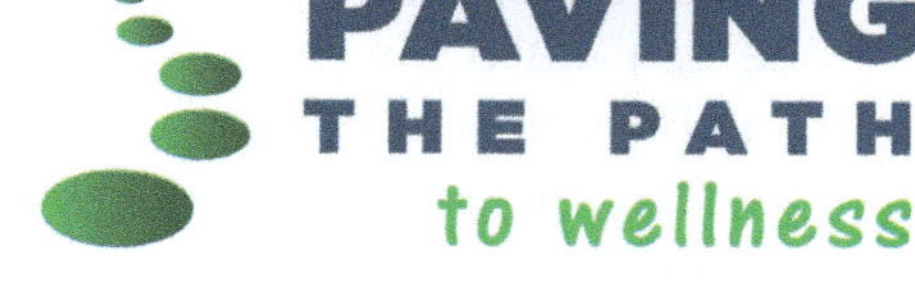

Interests	**Growth**
Now	**Appreciation**
Values	**Time**
Environment	**Inclusion**
Spirituality	**Options**
Talents	**Notes**
Innovation	

- *INTERESTS:* Start with your interests and try to learn more about them. If you're interested in crocheting, investigate new patterns, local classes, or online tutorials. Let your interests guide you as you take your investigation to the next level.
- *NOW:* The time is now to investigate. Learn more about yourself, what interests you, what opportunities there are in your community, and what you like. Don't wait and let more time pass by. There's no time like the present. Investigate now.
- *VALUES:* Research topics that align with your values. Maybe there are specific causes or organizations that you want to explore. Investigate ways to get involved in activities or learn more about these causes. Let your values guide your investigations.
- *ENVIRONMENT:* Investigate your environment. Explore your neighborhood, your community, and your state. Many women travel to remote locations but have never visited local tourist attractions or the beautiful natural attractions nearby. Become a detective and see what your environment has to offer.
- *SPIRITUALITY:* Investigate ways to support your spiritual well-being. There may be ways to help your spiritual well-being that you aren't aware of in your community or online. Social media, podcasts, books, and online videos are just some formats you can investigate to support your spirituality.
- *TALENTS:* Use your talents to help others. You have skills that the world will appreciate. Your abilities can make the world a better place. Sometimes, you must investigate how to use your talents and gifts in order to utilize them fully.
- *INNOVATION:* Most people see problems every day but often don't pause to reflect on how they can use innovation to address these issues. Investigate. Research and see if you can fix that problem that's bothered you for years.

- *GROWTH:* When you investigate something, you grow into a more well-rounded person, and your brain grows too. You form new connections between the cells in your brain when you learn. You are never too old to learn something new. Your brain wants you to continue growing throughout your life.
- *APPRECIATION:* Appreciate the investigation process. Enjoy the journey. There does not always have to be an end goal. For example, if you're interested in birds, appreciate the process of learning more about birds. Appreciate the PAVING the Path to Wellness journey as you investigate what healthy habits work best for you.
- *TIME:* Dedicate time to investigate and learn new things. Make space in your day for gaining new knowledge. For example, it takes time to learn a new language, play a new instrument, or feel comfortable with a new type of exercise. Stick with it and give it time. Don't rush it.
- *INCLUSION:* Include others in your investigations. Consider asking someone to join you as you take a new class or learn a new skill. Investigating with a friend or loved one can make the process even more rewarding. The next time you're learning something new, see if you can include anyone else.
- *OPTIONS:* As you start your day, ask yourself what options you have for the tasks that you need to do. You may have a certain way you planned on accomplishing those tasks, but can you investigate a new way to go about the job? You often don't know all your options until you do some research.
- *NOTES:* Take notes during your investigation. It's easy to forget what you've learned. You may want to take a small notebook with you wherever you go, so that if you think of a topic you want to investigate, or if you learn something new, you'll have a place to record it. You can also keep ideas in the "notes" application on your phone.

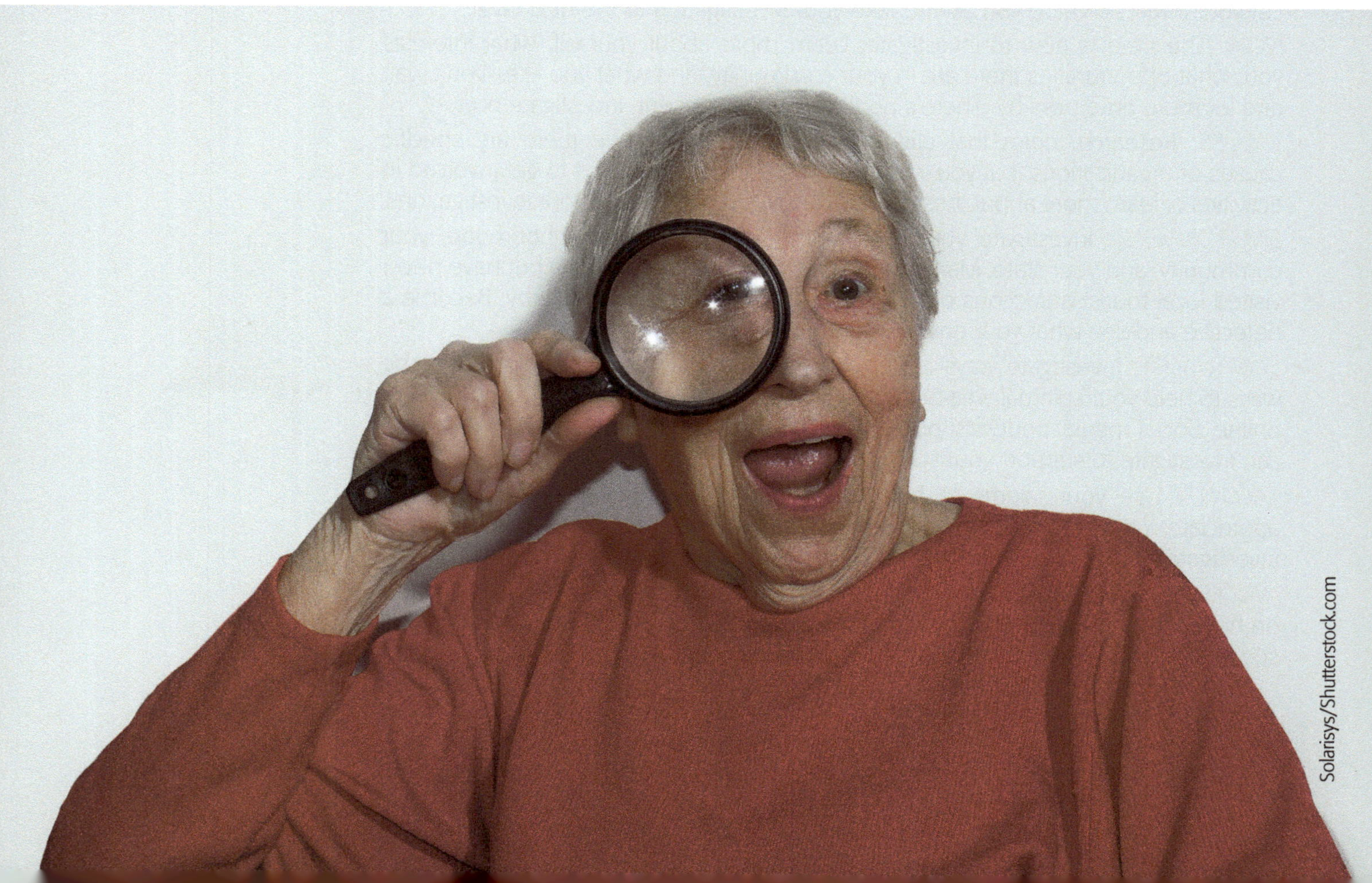

Solarisys/Shutterstock.com

Investigation—Understanding the Basics

Passage through menopause is part of your natural journey as a woman. Cessation of menstruation for 12 consecutive months, typically around age 51 in the United States, signals the official start of menopause (1). However, many women experience symptoms associated with the menopausal transition in their 40s, several years before menstruation stops. In addition, it's common for women to have symptoms attributed to menopause for many years after menopause. A few symptoms, such as hot flashes, typically last for several years. Some women experience none, while others have hot flashes for more than a decade. Other symptoms become more common with age, such as urinary incontinence and vaginal dryness. Throughout this chapter, you will investigate strategies for addressing common symptoms that peri-menopausal and post-menopausal women experience.

Just as your personality and body are unique, so are your menopausal experiences. Although covering all menopause-related symptoms is beyond the scope of this chapter, this chapter investigates many of the most common symptoms, along with evidence-based information on potential therapies. This book should not replace medical advice from your physician or other healthcare providers. If you are experiencing symptoms that are covered in this chapter or have other concerns, please get in touch with your healthcare provider for support. You may think that your situation doesn't warrant a clinical visit. In this case, reach out to the healthcare practitioner's office and share your problem, because it may be something they can address on the phone or over Zoom. On the other hand, it may require a clinic visit, and it's good to handle these situations earlier rather than later.

Words of Wisdom From Dr. Michelle Tollefson

After working with women for years, I've realized that as a society, we do a poor job of educating women about typical menopause-related symptoms. Even if they are very healthy, most women will experience some symptoms related to menopause that they wish they could avoid. Remember, going through menopause is healthy!

Menopause is a natural part of the female lifecycle. Sometimes it may not feel beautiful, and you long to be symptom-free. However, you must remember that women naturally reach a phase where the ovaries cease to ovulate each month. Healthy habits will help diminish the severity of some symptoms. Still, even women following all the guidelines for healthy living will experience some symptoms due to the decrease in estrogen associated with the cessation of ovulation and menstruation. Women should not feel ashamed of menopausal symptoms.

Sometimes just knowing that the symptoms are part of the normal menopausal transition and not the result of a feared disease can relieve unnecessary anxiety. For example, frequently, I see women who worry that the brain fog they are experiencing with the onset of menopause is due to early-stage dementia. However, it typically is due to menopause and will self-resolve with time. Other women benefit from knowing that they are not alone with what they are experiencing. This factor is true for the many women I see who struggle with mood fluctuations or decreased interest in sexual activity during this time. I reassure them that many other women experience (but don't discuss) these symptoms. Privateness can lead women to feel alone in their experience, increasing their suffering.

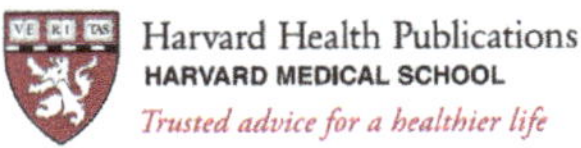

PAVING the Path to Wellness

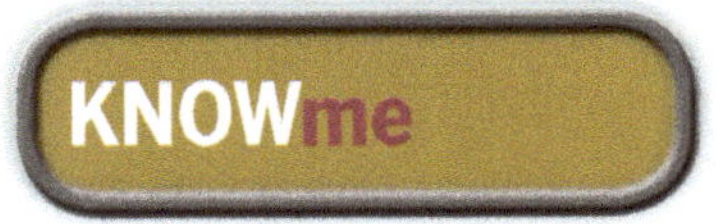

Measuring your Overall Wellness Using the PAVING Wheel

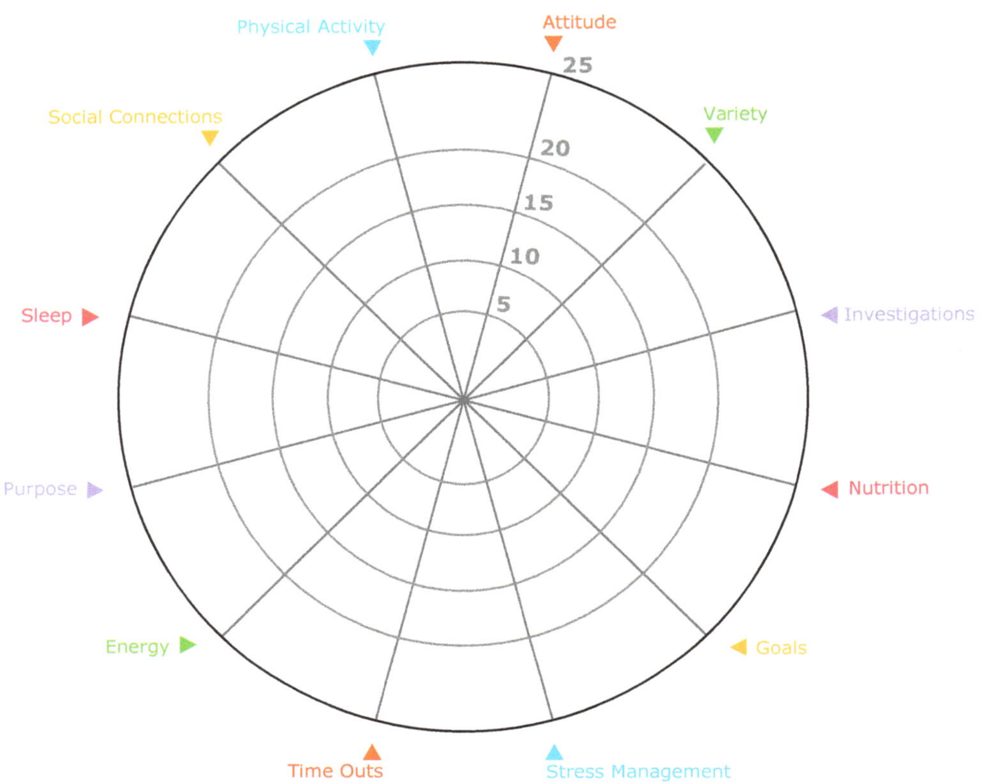

HOW TO USE THIS PAVING WHEEL

SCORE Plot your total scores for each component of the PAVING Wheel.

CONNECT Connect your scores.

EVALUATE Use the resulting PAVING Wheel (see example to the right) to evaluate areas where you may want to improve and consult the corresponding Module for more guidance.

RE-EVALUATE regularly by re-using this PAVING Wheel whenever you want to gauge your overall wellness and areas where you may want to improve.

EXAMPLE

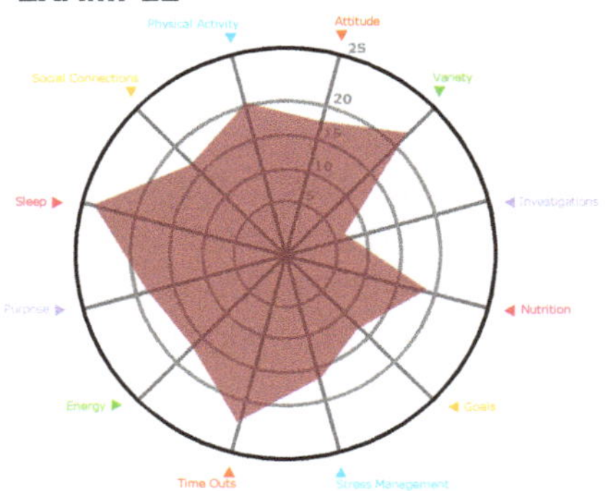

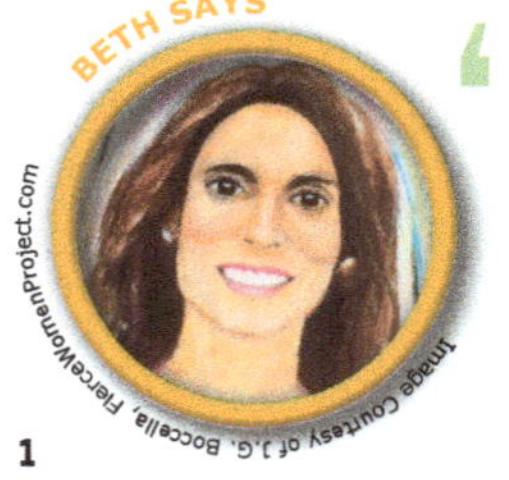

"There are no right or wrong answers. No scores are good or bad. Using the PAVING Wheel is for you alone to assess your Wellness and identify areas to improve your own personal Wellness."

1

Figure 5-1. PAVING the Path to Wellness questionnaire

INSTRUCTIONS Rank each item on a scale of 1-5. The Key is below. Calculate the subtotal of each of the 12 sections and plot them on the PAVING Wheel on page 1.

1	**Never** do this	2	Only **rarely** do this	3	**Sometimes** do this	4	**Often** do this	5	Do this regularly as **part of my routine**

MODULE 1 Physical Activity	
	I exercise 5 days in the week for about a half an hour.
	I enjoy myself when I exercise.
	I perform strength training exercises twice a week.
	I perform flexibility exercises routinely.
	I perform balance exercises routinely.
Physical Activity Total:	

MODULE 1 Stress	
	I have learned about stress and its effect on the mind and body.
	I am familiar with stress reduction techniques, and I use at least one when I feel that I am anxious, annoyed, or worried.
	I know about stress resiliency, and I practice enhancing my resiliency on a regular basis.
	I don't get angry easily.
	I meditate, take deep breaths, practice yoga, or do mindfulness based stress reduction (MBSR) regularly.
Stress Total:	

MODULE 2 Attitude	
	I use mistakes as opportunities to learn and grow.
	I write thank you notes or express my gratitude verbally.
	I celebrate success when it happens.
	I concentrate on the task at hand fully without distraction.
	I am optimistic about the day.
Attitude Total:	

MODULE 2 Time outs	
	If I sit for over an hour, I stand up and take a break for five minutes each hour.
	If I feel frustrated and annoyed, I take a few deep breaths to calm down.
	I take my vacation every year.
	When I am at home, I make sure to turn off my computer and put my work projects away at least for an hour at dinner time.
	After working on the same project for a few hours, I step away from it to get perspective on it.
Time Outs Total:	

MODULE 3 Variety	
	I do a variety of different exercises.
	I try to have a rainbow of colors on my plate.
	I enjoy a variety of fruits and vegetables.
	I like to try new activities.
	I spend time and connect with a wide range of friends.
Variety Total:	

MODULE 3 Energy	
	I have a friend who I know energizes me.
	I have identified at least one activity that brings me joy and energy.
	I am able to avoid situations and people that drain my energy.
	I only drink two cups of coffee a day.
	I don't rely on sugar/sweets or cookies for a quick energy fix.
Energy Total:	

MODULE 4 Investigations	
	I perform mini experiments on myself regularly.
	I am curious as to what foods are good for my body.
	I am curious as to what effect physical activity has on my body.
	I read about the latest research findings in medicine, nutrition, sleep, stress management, and/or exercise.
	I talk about health with family and friends.
Investigations Total:	

MODULE 4 Purpose	
	I feel that I have a clear purpose in life.
	I am able to prioritize my activities and projects easily.
	I make sure that my activities and projects are in alignment with my values.
	I have identified the people and activities that are most important to me.
	I am using my strengths to fulfill my purpose.
Purpose Total:	

MODULE 5 Nutrition	
	I eat 4 fruits a day.
	I eat 5 or more vegetables a day.
	I know proper portions for protein, carbohydrates, and fats, and I eat those portions.
	I think about the food that I eat and ask myself if it is good for my body.
	I view food as fuel, as medicine, and enjoyment too.
Nutrition Total:	

MODULE 5 Sleep	
	I sleep 7-8 hours a night.
	I don't drink coffee after noon time.
	I have a bedtime routine in which I relax before bed.
	I don't sleep with my phone on in the bedroom.
	I take 20 minute naps when I am over tired.
Sleep Total:	

MODULE 6 Goals	
	I set long-term goals for myself, share them with someone, and review them.
	I set three-month goals for myself, share them with someone, and work toward them.
	I set monthly goals and share them with someone.
	I set weekly goals and share them with someone.
	I set daily goals for myself and keep myself accountable for them.
Goals Total:	

MODULE 6 Social	
	I can name at least one person who brings me strength.
	I am involved with a group (activity, exercise class, art class, religious affiliation or the like)
	I visit with friends on the phone or in person at least 5 times a week.
	I have a healthy relationship with my spouse, partner, or best friend.
	I have a pet or plant that I can nurture and spend time with every day.
Social Total:	

2

Figure 5-1. PAVING the Path to Wellness questionnaire (cont.)

One of the most rewarding aspects of my profession is helping patients investigate, manage, and decrease discomfort from menopausal symptoms, especially when they didn't even know that treatment was available. From urinary incontinence to vaginal dryness, brain fog to dry skin, and decreased interest in sexual activity to night sweats, the severity of the symptoms can often be reduced and, in some cases, eliminated.

Investigation is the key. If you don't reach out to your healthcare provider and ask for their assistance, they will not be able to help you. I encourage you to make a list of what is bothering you and make a plan of action to address these with the appropriate health professionals. No problem is too big, too small, or too private to be discussed with a caring member of the healthcare team.

Gynecologists have expertise with menopausal symptoms, sexual health, and other female-specific conditions. Your primary care doctor, however, should be able to hear your concerns and guide you in the right direction, even if they don't manage your specific problem. Don't be embarrassed and don't delay. Your health professionals care about you and want to help you, but they'll never be able to assist you, if you don't take the first step and ask for help. Join your healthcare provider in investigating the symptoms you are experiencing. You deserve it! Make your appointment today!

Prioritize Your Health

Women commonly prioritize the health of their children, their partner, and aging parents above their personal health. However, regardless of your past priorities, NOW is the time to investigate areas of your life needing attention and prioritize YOUR physical and mental well-being.

Investigating Your Health

As you use investigation to improve your health, it is beneficial to better understand where you are currently with your overall health. Although you may have previously completed the PAVING Wheel assessment in the *PAVING the Path to Wellness Workbook*, consider taking it again. While investigating your health, completing this PAVING Wheel assessment is an ideal place to start.

Pause and complete the PAVING Wheel now. You can obtain more copies of the PAVING Wheel at www.pavingwellness.org.

You are encouraged to schedule an annual wellness exam if you haven't had one in the past year, by reaching out to your primary care physician or provider. If you don't have a primary care provider, now is a great time to establish care. You may want to ask your family and friends for recommendations concerning a primary care provider or reach out to a clinic, after determining which doctors your insurance covers. You can call your insurance company and ask for a list of physicians covered by your insurance plan. If you don't have health insurance, reach out to a local community health clinic to discuss your options for care.

Next, consider whether you have any health concerns that you haven't discussed with a healthcare provider. Maybe you have a lingering pain in your shoulder that started a few months ago, or you've noticed your eyesight isn't as good as it used to be at night.

Don't suffer by yourself. To investigate this issue, reach out to your primary care provider or specialist. Investing in your health is worth the effort! If you've seen a healthcare provider for this concern and didn't feel your needs were adequately addressed or didn't resolve the problem, reach out to that provider again or see another healthcare provider. Getting a second opinion may be just what you need, or your previous healthcare practitioner may have another idea for addressing your issue. Don't give up! Investigations take time. Ask about other potential treatment options. Maybe a referral to a physical therapist or dietitian could help, or perhaps you may need a new medication.

The human body is complex, and the investigations required to get to the root cause of a problem can also be complicated. If you don't talk with your healthcare provider, you won't fully understand your treatment options. Even if you decide to do nothing and wait, at least you will be better educated moving forward.

Initially, you need to make a list of your medical concerns, questions, and symptoms:

____

____

____

____

____

____

Using your list, complete the chart (Table 5-1). You may need to investigate to determine which healthcare practitioner to contact and choose a plan of action—for example, check with your primary care doctor to see if you should see them or

Medical Concern, Question, or Symptom	Healthcare Practitioner to Contact	Plan of Action

Table 5-1. An example of a healthcare plan of action chart

someone else about your shoulder discomfort. Also, maybe you were previously given a recommendation by a healthcare provider that you didn't follow through with but are ready to do so now. If there are appointments that you need to make or recommendations you haven't followed, consider listing them in the chart to address them. If you are unsure of whom to contact or don't have a plan of action, start by reaching out to your primary care provider's office.

Seeing your primary care physician or provider is extremely important; however, it's essential to ensure that you also address other areas of your health.

- ❏ *DENTAL CARE:* When was your last dental cleaning and check-up? If it has been more than six months since your last check-up, you may want to schedule a visit now.

  ____

  ____

  ____

  ____

- ❏ *EYE CARE:* When was your last eye check-up? Do you need to call your optometrist or ophthalmologist to schedule an exam?

  ____

  ____

  ____

  ____

- ❏ Many women focus on their physical health but forget to address their mental health, unless they have a significant problem. How is your mental health right now? Consider your mood, anxiety, depression, stress, or history of mental health concerns.

  ____

  ____

  ____

  ____

❑ Would you benefit from talking to a mental health professional about these concerns? If you have a mental health professional (counselor, therapist, psychotherapist, psychiatrist, marital counselor, etc.), consider reaching out to them. You can also contact your primary care provider first.

____

____

____

It can be challenging to be vulnerable when sharing your mental health concerns, especially when you are struggling, but help is available, and there are people who want to help you. A social worker or health navigator may be able to help too.

❑ Who will you reach out to for any mental health concerns if you have any currently? If you aren't struggling now, write down who you would reach out to if you have a mental health concern in the future?

____

____

____

If you are struggling with a mental health problem and don't have someone to help you if you are in crisis, call your local crisis line or go to the emergency department. If you or someone you know is considering suicide, call the suicide hotline immediately at 800-273-8255. Someone is there 24 hours a day, 7 days a week, 365 days a year.

Menopausal Symptoms

Although hot flashes are just one menopausal symptom, they often get the most attention. Many medications exist to treat menopausal symptoms, but the category most frequently used is hormone replacement therapy (HRT). Controversy and misinformation about HRT abounds, so even after reviewing Table 5-2, reach out to your doctor or primary care provider to discuss HRT if you want to learn more and consider its potential use.

Gynecologists have extensive training in this area though other primary care providers usually have some training in this area also. Therefore, they often feel comfortable discussing hormone replacement therapy risks and benefits, as well as treating patients with it. Just ask your healthcare provider.

A list of common menopausal symptoms and lifestyle modifications that may help you manage the symptoms are detailed in Table 5-3. The symptoms are often caused or exacerbated by fluctuating hormones or low estrogen levels. Although hormone changes are typically the cause of these symptoms, they may be due to conditions not related to menopause and may require investigation with your healthcare provider. Also, lifestyle changes may not necessarily improve the symptoms.

Reason for hormone replacement therapy use	• Often used for treating vasomotor symptoms (hot flashes and night sweats) in menopausal women. • May use it vaginally to treat genital and urinary symptoms.
Bioidentical hormone replacement therapy	• Chemical structure is the same or very close to the structure of hormones made by the body. • Can come from a compounding pharmacy or be made conventionally.
Non-hormonal medications	• Hormones (usually estrogen and a progestin) are typically used for treating menopausal symptoms, but non-hormonal medications, such as paroxetine, may also be used to treat hot flashes and night sweats.
Compounded or conventionally prepared hormones	• Compounded hormones are prepared in a compounding pharmacy. • Compounded bioidentical hormones have similar risks to non-compounded hormones (conventional) plus additional risks. • The American College of Obstetricians and Gynecologists recommends conventional hormone therapy over compounded hormone therapy, due to additional risks of compounded hormones. • The American College of Obstetricians and Gynecologists notes the lack of safety and efficacy research for compounded hormones, as well as potential variation in potency and purity.
Vaginal vs. non-vaginal	• Vaginal estrogen creams, tablets, and flexible vaginal rings, release a low dose of hormones to the vagina and surrounding tissues without the high systemic levels seen with non-vaginal delivery systems. • Often used when women have urogenital symptoms but don't need or want treatment for hot flashes and night sweats. • May sometimes be appropriate for use even if systemic hormone replacement therapy is contraindicated.
Delivery route	• Oral medications • Skin (transdermal): often recommended for women with chronic medical conditions such as high blood pressure or cholesterol • Vaginal: ring, tablet, or cream with a low level of estrogen delivered to surrounding tissues • Implants/pellets
Why do many women need to use a progestin/ progesterone	• If a woman has a uterus, a progestin is needed to decrease the risk of uterine cancer, which is significantly increased, if a woman with a uterus takes estrogen without a progestin.
Risks and benefits of hormone replacement therapy (HRT)	• All hormone replacement therapy has some level of risk. • Talk with your doctor or healthcare provider about your risks with hormone replacement therapy, if you are interested in potentially using it. • HRT is contraindicated in some conditions. • Many healthy women use HRT for several years after entering menopause, where the benefit exceeds the risk (determined through an individual risk assessment and discussion with their healthcare practitioner). • Risks seem to increase with a prolonged duration of therapy. • Long-term use of systemic (non-vaginal) HRT is not usually recommended. • Likely increased risk of breast cancer, cardiovascular disease, blood clots, and stroke with systemic long-term use • General recommendation is to use the lowest effective dose to treat hot flashes and night sweats for the shortest time needed. • HRT is not recommended for prevention of chronic disease. • Benefits are that it usually decreases vasomotor symptoms (hot flashes and night sweats), it treats genitourinary syndrome of menopause, and it may support bone health and reduce colorectal cancer risk.

Table 5-2. Hormone replacement therapy overview (2)

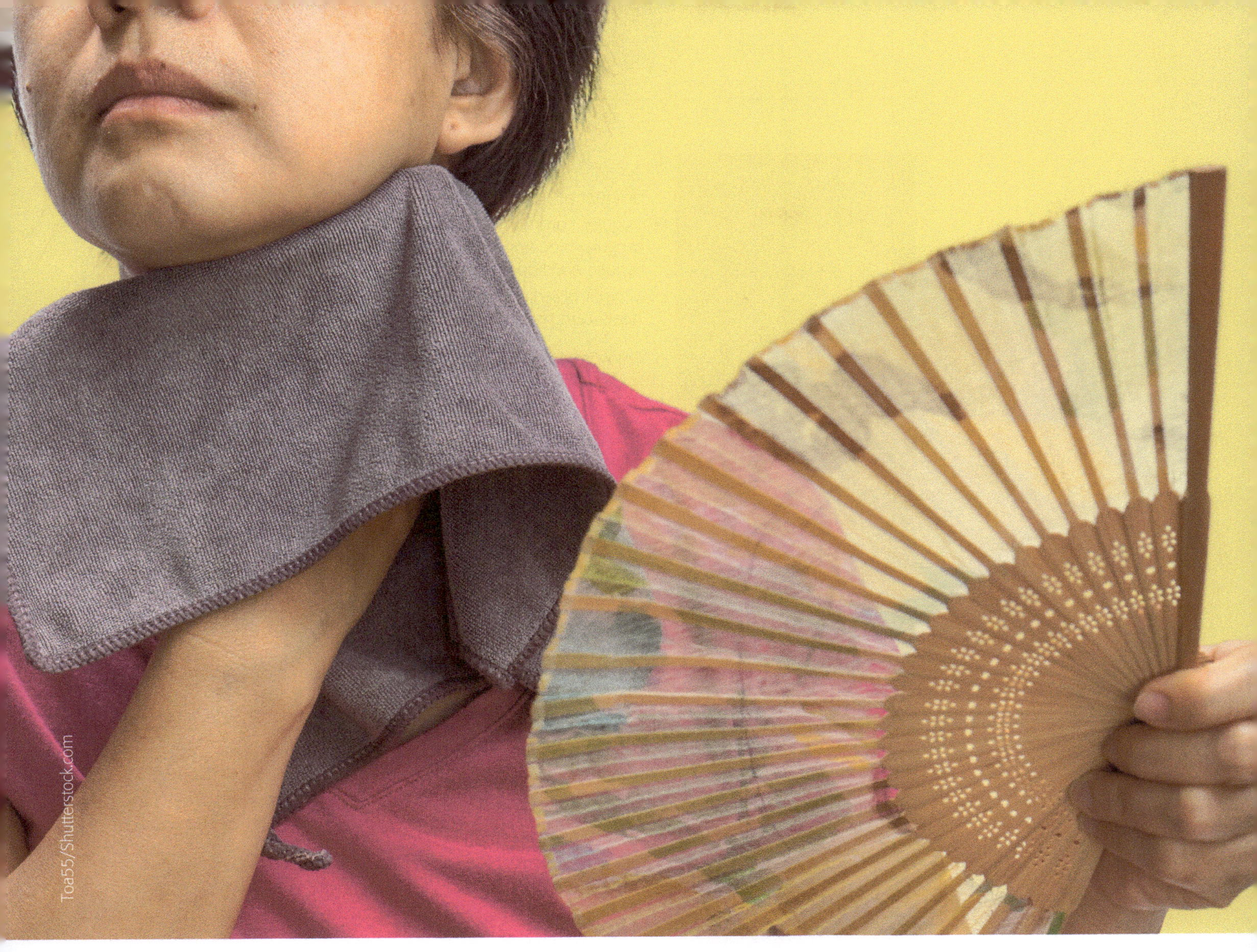

Toa55/Shutterstock.com

It is also important to be aware that the menopausal transition may be a time of increased stress for various reasons. Furthermore, menopausal symptoms may even increase this stress as well, as they become more severe due to stress. However, addressing them can help you feel like you have some control. Please work with your healthcare team to investigate the cause and best treatment for any symptoms that you experience.

❑ Are you experiencing any menopausal symptoms listed in Table 5-3 that you would like to address? If so, explain what next steps you will take.

Symptom	Lifestyle modifications
Irregular vaginal bleeding	• Before menopause, periods may become irregular in timing and amount of blood flow. • Regular communication with your doctor is vital during this time as irregular bleeding is not always due to being perimenopausal and may require additional workup to rule out other conditions. • Vaginal bleeding after menopause should be investigated. Call your healthcare provider.
Hot flashes and night sweats	• Enjoy drinking soy milk or eating soy foods such as tofu, tempeh, miso, and edamame. • Engage in physical activity—30 minutes at least three times a week. • Try yoga or tai chi. • Layer your clothes so you can remove layers, as needed. • Try dry wick sleepwear, clothes, sheets, and pillowcases. • If you smoke, try to stop. Ask for help, if needed. • Drink cool beverages. • Try cooling your environment. • Avoid warm environments, hot foods, and beverages, if they trigger symptoms for you. • Try stress management behaviors. • Consider doing cognitive-behavioral therapy. • Meditate. • Practice mindfulness-based stress reduction. • If desired, discuss hormone replacement therapy with your healthcare provider. • Note, there is no consistent evidence for using black cohosh, red clover, or vitamin E to help control hot flashes and night sweats.
Sleep problems	• Get regular aerobic exercise but don't exercise close to bedtime. • Keep your bedroom cool, dark, and quiet. • Avoid or limit alcohol and caffeine. • Don't use tobacco. • Wear moisture-wicking or thin sleepwear. • Try having multiple layers of sheets on your bed. • Relax with yoga, tai chi, or meditation. • Treat any underlying problems such as sleep apnea or restless leg syndrome.
Fatigue	• Prioritize sleep. • Get adequate exercise. • Decrease sedentary behavior. • Avoid ultra-processed foods that can lead to a sugar crash and decreased energy. • Manage stress in a healthy manner. • Avoid alcohol consumption.
Aches and pains	• Get adequate exercise and physical activity. • Eat foods that decrease inflammation, such as fruits, vegetables, and whole grains. • Avoid ultra-processed foods. • Consider heat therapy, such as a heating pad or a warm bath. • Practice relaxation techniques. • Prioritize sleep. • Investigate and treat the underlying problem with your healthcare provider.

Table 5-3. A list of common menopausal symptoms and lifestyle modifications that may be helpful in managing these symptoms

Urinary tract infections (UTI)	• Contact a healthcare provider if you have UTI symptoms. The following list of action items in this section may decrease the risk of a UTI, but they won't treat a UTI. • Maintain adequate hydration. • Don't delay urinating when you feel an urge to urinate. • Try to fully empty your bladder when urinating. • Try unsweetened cranberry juice (not cocktail) or cranberry supplements, as there is a possibility they may help. • Urinate before and immediately after having vaginal intercourse. • When using the bathroom, wipe from front to back. • Use antibiotics when they are prescribed.
Urinary incontinence	• Exercise most days of the week. • Regularly do kegel exercises—pelvic floor muscle training (discussed in the physical activity chapter). • Avoid drinking very large amounts of liquid in a short period of time. • Avoid constipation. • Consider vaginal incontinence tampons. • Disposable underwear and pads. • Urinate regularly. • Consider seeing a gynecologist or urogynecologist for more information on potential treatments, such as vaginal pessaries, medications, or surgery.
Genitourinary syndrome of menopause, which may include vaginal dryness, irritation, discomfort during intercourse, and urinary tract symptoms	• Hormone replacement therapy: usually vaginally but sometimes systemic if also having hot flashes • Ospemifene: medication that helps with urogenital symptoms • Prasterone: non-estrogen medication for urogenital symptoms • Use of vaginal lubricants during intercourse • Use of vaginal moisturizers • Potentially soy foods
Mood changes, such as anxiety, sadness, decreased motivation, irritability, and mood swings	• Get adequate exercise. • Yoga and tai-chi may help. • Meditate and use stress management techniques. • Prioritize sleep. • Eat a high-quality diet. • Medication management • Assistance from a mental health professional • Reach out to a crisis line immediately if you are having suicidal thoughts or are in crisis (800-273-8255).
Body image	• Exercise improves body image, regardless of weight (both aerobic exercise and strength training). • Connection with the body through yoga or tai-chi • Relaxation exercises • Cognitive-behavioral therapy • Practicing gratitude and self-compassion • Engaging in social activity

Table 5-3. A list of common menopausal symptoms and lifestyle modifications that may be helpful in managing these symptoms (cont.)

Fun Investigation Ideas During Menopause

You are never too old to have fun and enjoy your wellness journey. Read the following list of fun investigation ideas and put a star next to ones you may want to explore:

- Genealogy
- National parks in your area or potential vacation locations
- How to cook something you've never cooked before
- How to care for plants
- How to knit or do needlepoint
- Research your ethnic background.
- How to fix ____ (insert something that needs fixing in your house)
- Who can fix _____ (maybe you can't or don't want to fix it)
- Classes at your local community center, YMCA, or college (many colleges offer free or reduced-rate classes for seniors)
- Nearby towns—go to the visitor's center, try to explore the city as if it were your first time visiting.
- Holiday traditions in various cultures
- How to do a craft you've never done before
- Visit the library and look at non-fiction books to find something to investigate.
- How to do origami
- Journaling
- Writing your memoir to publish or to share with family and friends
- Mentoring young women in a school you graduated from or a local organization
- Starting or joining a book club
- Joke books
- How to do a magic trick
- How to play a new card game or board game
- How to play chess, backgammon, or scrabble
- Crossword puzzles or word searches
- How to play a new sport
- How to learn a new skill on the computer
- What podcasts exist on some of your favorite topics
- Your or others' religious/spiritual beliefs

Circle five of the aforementioned ideas that you put a star next to that you might consider trying. List some specific next steps you will take to begin your investigations.

Coaching Yourself on Investigations With the COACH Approach

Reflect upon your recently completed PAVING Wheel, and then answer the following questions.

CURIOSITY

PAVING WHEEL QUESTIONS:

- ❑ How does your current wheel compare to how it would have been had you completed it a few years ago?

  ____

  ____

  ____

- ❑ What areas of the wheel typically stay the same or stable for you, and in what other areas do you often fluctuate? Why do you think this happens?

  ____

  ____

  ____

- ❑ What areas of your wheel do you feel called to address now?

  ____

  ____

  ____

- ❑ If there are certain areas that you don't want to address now, even though your score was lower in this area, why do you think you don't want to focus on these areas now? Remember, there is no right or wrong way to do this.

  ____

  ____

  ____

MENOPAUSAL SYMPTOM QUESTIONS:

Instead of being angry and annoyed, remember to bring your curious self to the forefront when experiencing menopausal symptoms. For example, consider what you could do if you are speaking to your boss, at dinner with friends, or in a grocery store, and get a hot flash. For example, you could:

- Take a "bathroom" break. Get yourself comfortable, take deep breaths, and run your hands under cold water, possibly putting some on the back of your neck. Take the time that you need.

- Carry on and focus on the meeting at hand, let the symptoms take their course naturally, and take off a sweater or coat, if you are wearing layers to make yourself more comfortable.
- If you feel comfortable with the person, explain the situation and carry on with the project or conversation in a suitable way.
- Take five deep, slow breaths and realize that this is temporary and will pass. Try to focus on a pleasant memory, something you are grateful for, or be mindful of what else is around you, such as a flowering plant, music in the background, the smell of coffee, or a photograph of your child.
- Drink a cold beverage and see if this makes you feel better.
- Phone, text, or Zoom with an understanding friend to talk about your symptoms or anything else you may wish to share.
- Use a hand fan, make a paper fan, or go outside, if there is a breeze.

❑ List several things that you would feel comfortable doing during a hot flash.

____

____

____

You could consider trying one or more of the suggested seven items or some of your own ideas. Be curious about how they work for you. Keep in mind that you are the experiment and the experimenter. You can use the menopausal symptom as a trigger to take a healthy break, connect with a friend, hydrate, listen to music, or do something else that is soothing. In that case, the menopausal symptoms can help lead you to areas of wellness that you may not have explored that day. Curiosity is key to better understanding yourself and your symptoms, and appreciating the beauty of the aging body, as well as the wisdom learned through this process.

Next is a great time to consider a symptom diary to aid in your investigations (refer to Table 5-4). This could be for hot flashes, urinary incontinence, or mood changes. Write down the symptom, time, day, and what you were previously doing that may have contributed to the symptom. Then, record what you did to help relieve the symptom and whether it worked.

Symptom description	Time of day	Previous activity	Intervention	Results	Lessons learned

Table 5-4. An example of a symptom diary

❑ What did you learn from your symptom diary? Consider sharing this with your healthcare provider.

OPENNESS

PAVING WHEEL QUESTIONS:

Be open to considering areas you may not have thought about before, such as your purpose in your life, energy levels, and attitude. For example, if you scored low on physical activity, this is an opportunity to explore your feelings about exercise and the fears, desires, and dreams you may have in this area.

❑ Describe one of the areas that makes you uncomfortable and why.

Keep in mind the wheel does not always need to be perfect. One may question whether it can ever be perfect. It's about being open and aware of where you are now with these 12 steps.

❑ What are you surprised by after completing your wheel?

❑ Where are you doing well on your wheel right now?

- ❑ What areas of your wheel do you want to work on now? These may not be the lowest areas you scored, as it does not matter what you scored. Instead, these may intrigue and entice you to explore further. List your thoughts.

  ____

  ____

  ____

MENOPAUSAL SYMPTOM QUESTIONS:

- ❑ Experiencing menopausal symptoms is normal, and there should be no shame, blame, or guilt attached to any symptom, the duration of the symptom, or the success or failure of an intervention. This is all part of living and part of healthy aging. However, if you feel angry, guilty, or shameful, share your thoughts in an expressive writing paragraph.

  ____

  ____

  ____

Some people fear that these symptoms (such as mood changes, night sweats, or urinary incontinence) will never go away or that there is nothing that can be done. If this is you, talk to a friend or get help from a healthcare provider. Being anxious or worried about the duration of your symptom and menopause, in general, is expected. Still, excessive devotion of time to this concern is a sign that maybe you are becoming trapped by your fear. Let this be a signal to let you seek help.

- ❑ Are you open to seeking help from healthcare practitioners when you have a physical problem?

  ____

  ____

  ____

- ❑ Are you open to seeking help from mental health professionals when you have a mental health problem?

  ____

  ____

  ____

- ❑ If you don't feel open to either one, explain why you think this barrier exists.

- ❑ If not, what could help you be more open to discussing these with the appropriate professionals, such as a gynecologist or a therapist?

APPRECIATION

PAVING WHEEL QUESTIONS:

Look at the questions where you scored high on the PAVING Wheel and savor your self-care success in these areas.

- ❑ If you know that you would have scored high in these steps in the past, describe that.

- ❑ What strengths do you have now that can empower you to tackle the steps on this wheel that are troubling you?

- ❑ Describe a time in your life when you met a challenge and were successful.

- ❑ Look back at your previous answer, pull out the strengths you used during that example, and list them.

____

____

____

- ❑ Who is in your life who supports you, allowing you to score high in the social connection section of the PAVING Wheel? What is it about those people and what they do that helps you feel supported? Spend a moment to sit in that warmth and love, knowing how lucky you are to have these people in your life.

____

____

____

MENOPAUSAL SYMPTOM QUESTIONS:

If you weren't going through menopause by the time you were in your 60s, your Ob-Gyn would be concerned for your health, as your body would likely not be aging healthfully. In addition, they may wonder if you had uterine cancer and want to investigate any vaginal bleeding further.

- ❑ Do you appreciate that your body goes through a normal healthy process and progression? Explain.

____

____

____

____

- ❑ When considering your life currently, for what do you feel gratitude? You don't have to be completely healthy to appreciate the level of fitness that you do have.

____

____

____

____

- ❑ In what ways can you share your appreciation with your family, friends, and community who support you and your health? For example, do you want to send them a thank you note? Do you want to bring them fresh flowers? Do you want to share a homemade meal or dine out at a restaurant with your friend?

- ❑ Do you appreciate reading this book and reflecting on these questions (with a community of PAVING participants if you are in a group)? Explain.

COMPASSION

PAVING WHEEL QUESTIONS:

- ❑ Consider your answers to the PAVING Wheel questionnaire. What area is the most challenging or complex for you currently? How can you express compassion to yourself for this area where you are struggling?

- ❑ What would you say to a friend about their wheel if it looked the same as yours and they asked for feedback? What comments would you share?

- ❑ It's important to realize that you are not striving for scores of 5 for every question or a score of 25 with every section on the PAVING Wheel questionnaire. You are simply learning and exploring how you live and prioritizing your self-care during this time in your life. If you feel shame, blame, or guilt, what do you need to do to free yourself from these disruptive feelings that hold you back?

  ____

  ____

  ____

  ____

- ❑ Consider your past and where you are now by showing compassion and understanding to yourself. Allow yourself to envision the wheel of your future. What are you hoping your wheel will look like in six months?

  ____

  ____

  ____

  ____

- ❑ Are there specific areas of the PAVING Wheel questionnaire where you need to extend kindness to yourself? Remember to speak to yourself the way that you would a good friend.

  ____

  ____

  ____

Do you find it challenging to be compassionate to yourself in all areas of the PAVING Wheel? If so, it might be a good idea to reach out to a friend, loved one, or healthcare provider to further your understanding of your feelings. For example, you may have joined a gym multiple times in your life or committed to exercise classes that you were unable to follow through with for various reasons. This happens to most people, and you should not feel ashamed.

Setting yourself up for success is the key. Looking at what did not work in the past and using the information about the classes you signed up for or the gym that you joined, and finding out what did not work for you, will help you navigate your physical activity for the future. You may not need a gym or exercise class. You may just need an exercise buddy to work with you. It's a waste of time to shame, blame, or guilt yourself about the past. Leave it behind and work on strategies for the future.

❑ Were there specific things like caring for a sick child or family member or addressing your medical diagnosis that demanded your attention and took time away from many aspects of this PAVING Wheel?

____

____

____

MENOPAUSAL SYMPTOM QUESTIONS:

❑ Do you have compassion for the limitations that your body currently has? Explain.

____

____

____

❑ How can you show increased understanding for yourself regarding your limitations, aging body, etc.? Explain.

____

____

____

❑ How can you have compassion for your past experiences and how you have handled your self-care in your past?

____

____

____

____

Major stressors like moving, changing jobs, financial challenges, difficulty in relationships, divorce, separation, and COVID-19 crises, can all play a part in your ability to focus on yourself and your healthy habits. If you have been managing some of these stressful life events, it's important to acknowledge these are major life strains and that you have made it through them. Finding the time to focus on yourself now and work on your self-care will even help you manage any residual issues that you may be experiencing from these significant life stressors.

- [ ] What do you think you need to feel more compassion for yourself if you have been experiencing or are experiencing these or other life stressors?

____

____

____

HONESTY

PAVING WHEEL QUESTIONS:

- [ ] Did you answer the questions honestly on the PAVING Wheel, or were you answering them to satisfy others or gain a higher score? If so, consider redoing the wheel if you weren't simply sharing your gut reactions and real-life experiences. But, again, this is not about getting an A in a class. It's about truly understanding the being that is you.

____

____

____

- [ ] Even if you are being honest with your answers on the PAVING Wheel, are there areas of the Wheel where you try to impress, satisfy, or please others by saying you're doing things that you aren't doing, like exercising or not eating junk food late at night?

____

____

____

____

- [ ] Are you being honest with your healthcare provider about your behaviors? Now is the time for honesty. People can only help you if you tell them what is going on. You can only help yourself if you are honest with yourself.

____

____

____

____

MENOPAUSAL SYMPTOM QUESTIONS:

- ❏ Some women harbor fears about the aging process. If this is you, please share your concerns.

  ____

  ____

  ____

- ❏ What are you not investigating or learning more about that would benefit your health somehow? For example, how to make your home safer to decrease the risk of falls or how to reduce your risk of breast cancer.

  ____

  ____

  ____

  ____

- ❏ Why have you avoided taking care of certain areas of your health?

  ____

  ____

  ____

  ____

Investigation Wrap-Up

Life is a journey with treasures and lessons waiting to be discovered. Openness to learning more about yourself and investigating areas of your life where you are struggling can lead to tremendous growth. As you move forward, when you encounter new symptoms or struggles, consider what you can learn from these experiences. Investigation is a tool that can lead to increased self-awareness, improved health, and greater joy along your journey.

You have a unique treasure chest of celebrations, successes, struggles, and tribulations. Each is a gem, a different jewel that carries its own power and strength. They make you who you are. Celebrate the successes and treasure the unique gems that come from struggles, such as supporting a family member with dementia or having a breast cancer diagnosis. Each challenge you've experienced has marked you significantly and made you the strong woman you are today. Discover your treasures and jewels, and wear your beautiful jewel necklace, highlighting all you have been through.

Create your necklace and then consider the following:

- ❑ What are the shiny diamonds that are your celebrations that you've enjoyed up until this point?

____

____

____

____

- ❑ What are other gemstones that represent difficult times you've endured?

____

____

____

____

- ❑ How have these struggles made you stronger, wiser, more resilient, and the woman you are today?

____

____

____

References

1. American College of Obstetricians and Gynecologists (ACOG). Practice Bulletin No. 141: management of menopausal symptoms. *Obstet Gynecol.* 2014 Jan;123(1):202-16, reaffirmed 2016, correction can be found in *Obstet Gynecol* 2016 Jan;127(1):166
2. Levine, Elliot M., Menopause. *DynaMed.* Retrieved May 14, 2022, from https://www-dynamed-com.aurarialibrary.idm.oclc.org/condition/menopause#GUID-203D73A1-AE49-4815-BFFB-D431E2FB16EF

CHAPTER 6
NUTRITION

Nutrition Throughout Menopause, Midlife, and Beyond

Acronym—NUTRITION

Natural
Understand
Try
Recipes
Inspiration
Taste
Individualize
Open
Nourish

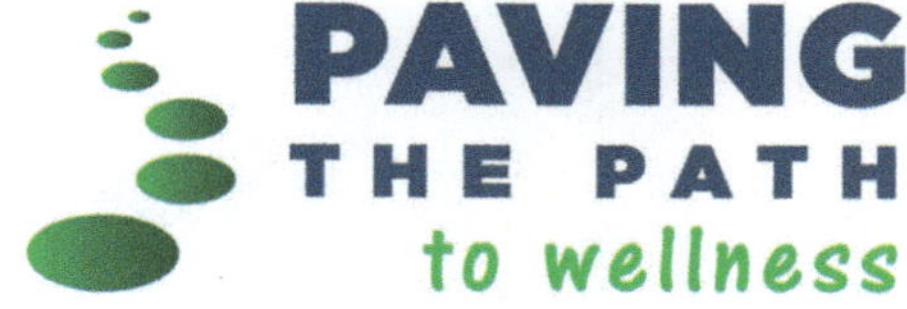

- *NATURAL:* Eat natural foods, foods that come from plants. Most of your food should be recognizable as something that came from a plant, from the ground. If it's fluorescent pink candy, blue ice cream, or black frosting, it's not natural and not nutritious.
- *UNDERSTAND:* Understand the dietary guidelines. You should know how much fiber, calcium, protein, and iron you need each day for optimal health. You can talk with your primary care provider or a registered dietitian to understand if you should modify your diet due to medical conditions.
- *TRY:* Try new types of cuisine and season your food with spices and fresh herbs. When you're at the grocery store, try purchasing fruits and vegetables that you've never tried before. Enjoy healthy plant-based protein sources, such as beans, lentils, and nuts. If you've never tried them, give them a try!
- *RECIPES:* Have fun exploring recipes in cookbooks at the library, bookstore, or online. You can search sites with words such as recipe and healthy, vegan, vegetarian, tofu, lentils, inexpensive, and easy, to find recipes that meet your needs. Even though lifestyle medicine experts don't usually use the terms vegetarian and vegan as they focus on what you aren't eating instead of what you ARE eating, they can be helpful in recipe searches.
- *INSPIRATION:* Get inspiration from your favorite dishes and look for ways to make a healthier version of them. Just because you are trying to eat healthier doesn't mean that you can't enjoy your favorite meals. Look for recipes that substitute plant protein for meat or modify the recipe to decrease the added sugar and saturated fat.
- *TASTE:* You want to eat delicious food that brings you joy! It takes a while for your tastes to change, so be patient as you try new healthy foods and ways of cooking. The more you expose yourself to new foods, the more accustomed you become to their tastes. Don't be surprised if fruit tastes sweeter, and you don't need the salt shaker anymore.

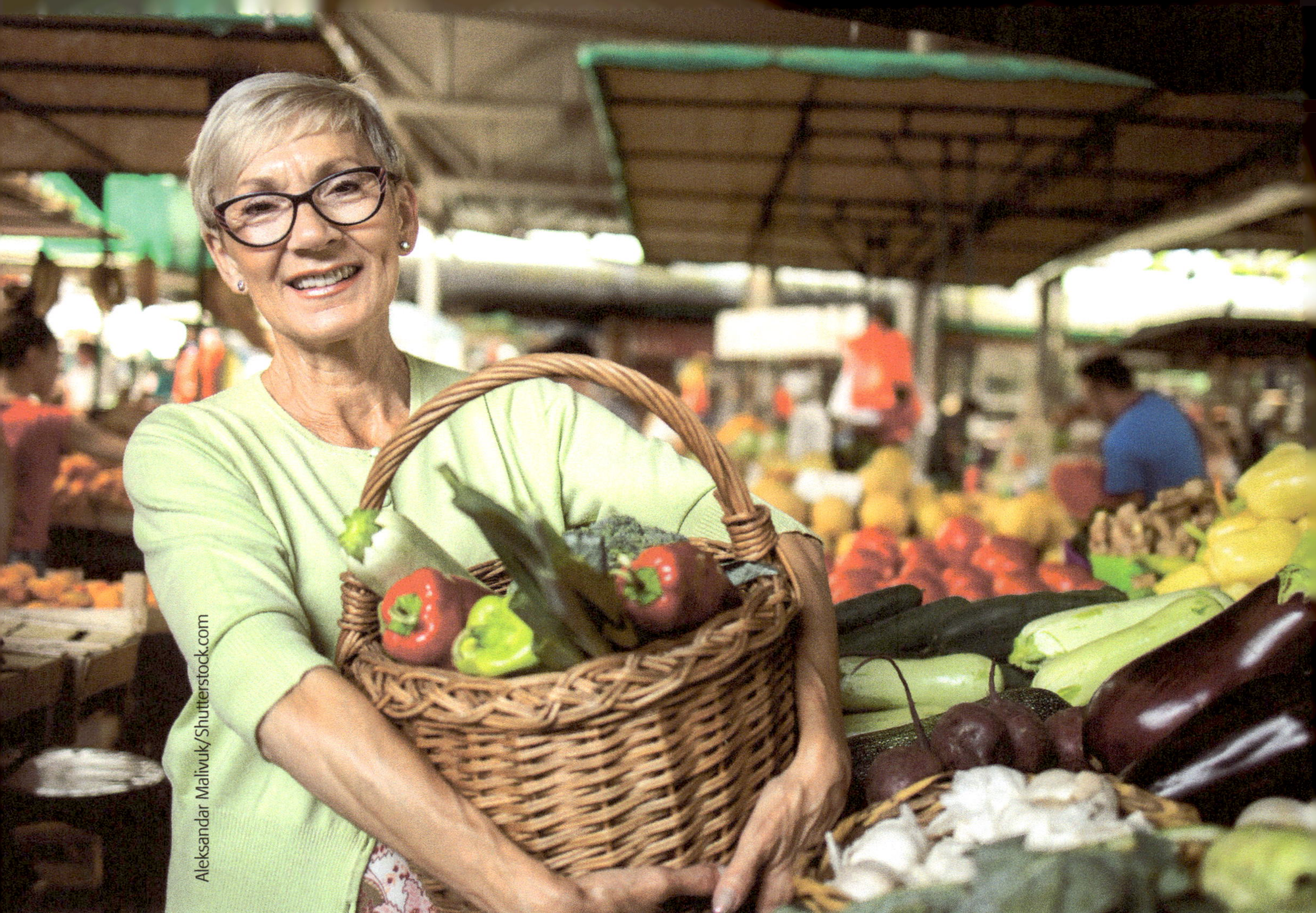
Aleksandar Malivuk/Shutterstock.com

- *INDIVIDUALIZE:* Only you know your schedule, your tastes, your needs, and what will work well for you and your family. If you have time to cook on the weekends but not on weekdays, batch cook on the weekends. If your family goes out to dinner, join them but look for healthier options that you will enjoy. If you want to eat broccoli for breakfast and oatmeal for dinner, do it. It's up to you.
- *OPEN:* Be open to changing what and how you eat. Your eating habits are deeply rooted in your family upbringing, culture, and society, and change can be challenging. However, openness to trying new foods, eating mindfully, and learning more about nutrition can help you along your wellness journey.
- *NOURISH:* Nourish yourself with high-quality, nutrient-dense foods. You can nourish yourself with every meal you eat and every bite you take. Your body and mind will have the energy needed for optimal functioning when you eat nourishing food.

Nutrition—Understanding the Basics

By the time you reach menopause, if you're eating three times daily, you've likely eaten over 55,000 meals. Over this time, you've developed a relationship with your food. The culture you come from, the environment you grew up in, your family's food traditions, and your taste preferences likely impact your food choices more than any nutrition knowledge.

Also, as a middle-aged or more mature woman, you've been exposed to a barrage of nutrition messages telling you what you "should" and "shouldn't" eat. You've likely seen advertisements for the latest super-food to cure all your problems. Nutrition research and health gurus often contradict one another. When you overlay this with society's emphasis on a female body stereotype that is not typical of most American women and a diet industry focused on selling weight loss plans, pills, and procedures with the promise of achieving this body shape, it's obvious why many women have a complicated relationship with food.

This chapter contains evidence-based information about nutrition for middle-aged and more mature women, empowering you to choose the right path. If you are one of those women who have struggled with healthy eating and viewing food as nourishment, or if you are interested in optimizing your nutrition to address menopause symptoms, by the end of this chapter, you'll be ready to savor a variety of delicious foods. It's never too late to revise your relationship with food or learn tasty new recipes, nurturing yourself one bite at a time.

Food is fuel for your body. It gives you the energy you need to be physically active each day. Without adequate nutrition, your body and mind will suffer. Eating a high-quality diet supports your immune system, decreases your chances of getting infections, and keeps your heart healthy and bones strong, while also helping your memory and mood.

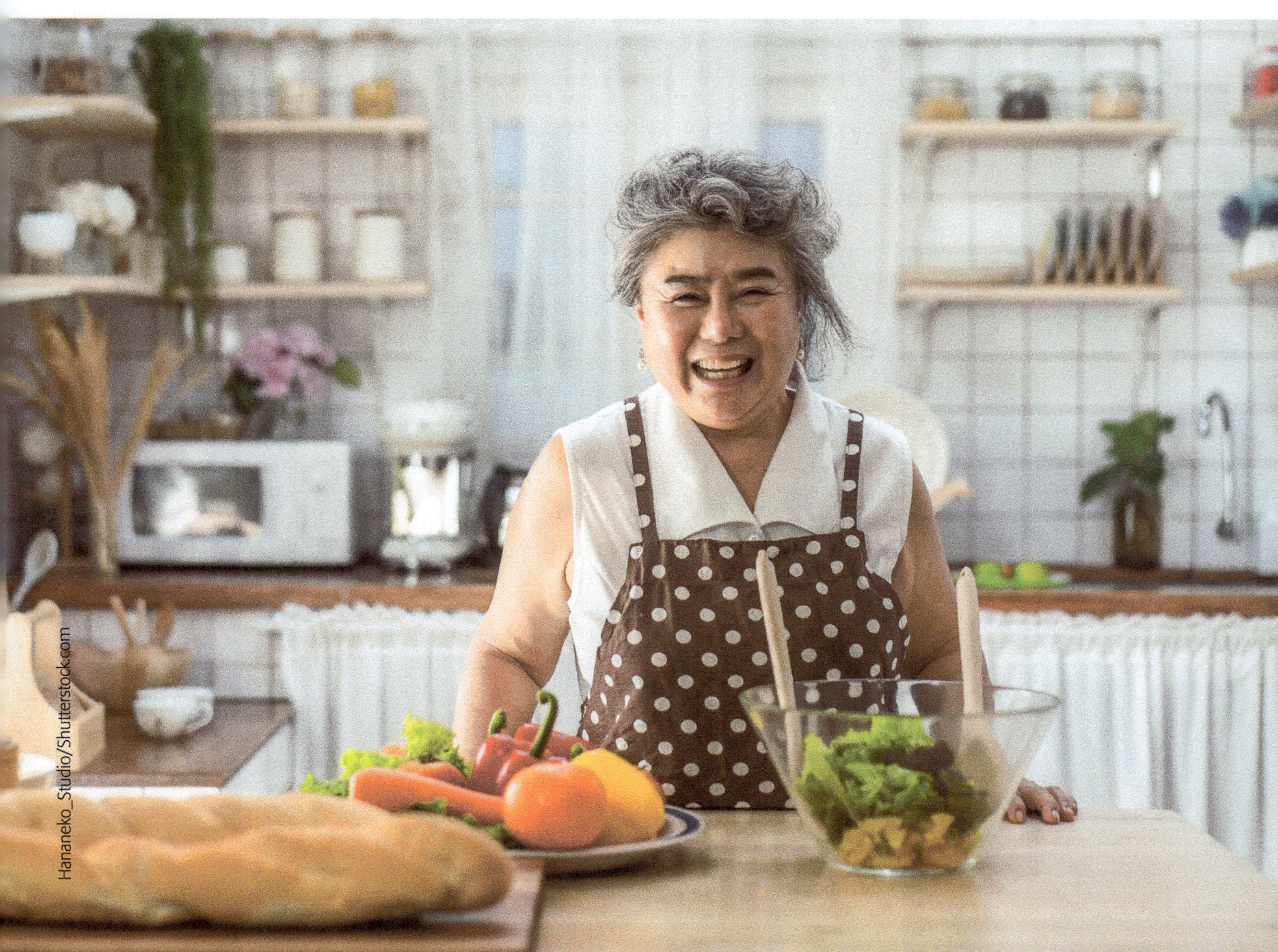

Hananeko_Studio/Shutterstock.com

Food also impacts your risk of getting type 2 diabetes, cardiovascular disease, hypertension, high cholesterol, mood disorders, dementia, and some cancers. Even if you're living with one of these conditions, the food you eat still impacts your risk for other chronic diseases and may even improve your health. Talk with your doctor(s) about the impact of diet on your health. Consider asking them for a referral to a registered dietitian. These health professionals have advanced training in food science and can co-create an individualized food plan to best support your health.

This is meant to be a joy-filled journey, as you learn how food can impact your health now and for decades. This may be when you can think about what foods YOU enjoy, that YOU want to try, or what foods are best for YOUR health. While raising children, it is easy to focus on finding foods that they will quickly eat between finishing their homework and heading to sport's practice.

Often, moms don't want to waste food, so they'll eat the leftover macaroni and cheese or bagel, thinking this may suffice for a healthy dinner, but it doesn't. While juggling a demanding work schedule, you may not have had the time that you hopefully have now to pause and consider what food truly nourishes you. Maybe you can take a cooking class, try a different ethnic cuisine that you've never tried, plant a garden, or find new recipes on Pinterest.

Midlife offers the potential to find joy in cooking, pleasure in eating, and experiment with preparing delicious foods that support your health and well-being. However, even though you may have the time to cook, you may not be interested. In this case, you can consider researching companies that provide the ingredients for healthy, whole-food, plant-based meals and, in some cases, provide the cooked meals ready for reheating.

Words of Wisdom From Dr. Michelle Tollefson

As I began to incorporate more lifestyle medicine into my gynecology practice, it was exciting to see the impact nutrition could have on the lives of my menopausal patients. While training to be a doctor specializing in women's health, I wasn't exposed to learning about the power of food as medicine for most conditions, especially not menopause. Although I knew how to prescribe hormone replacement therapy and could discuss the individualized risks and benefits with patients, I had no evidence-based dietary recommendations for my menopausal patients as a new doctor.

While exploring the women's health-focused nutrition literature, I read a number of studies that highlighted the importance of a high-quality, nutrient-rich diet for menopausal women. As I learned more, I eagerly shared this knowledge with my patients. At first, I wondered if women would want to make significant dietary changes to address symptoms, like hot flashes or mood changes. Still, I quickly learned that many of my patients were "hungry" for evidence-based nutrition information. As a result, some of my favorite patient visits have been when women return to follow-up, eager to share how healthier eating impacted their symptoms and improved other health issues such as constipation and acne.

While not a panacea for all menopausal problems, dietary changes are often beneficial for women addressing common menopause symptoms, as well as other medical conditions.

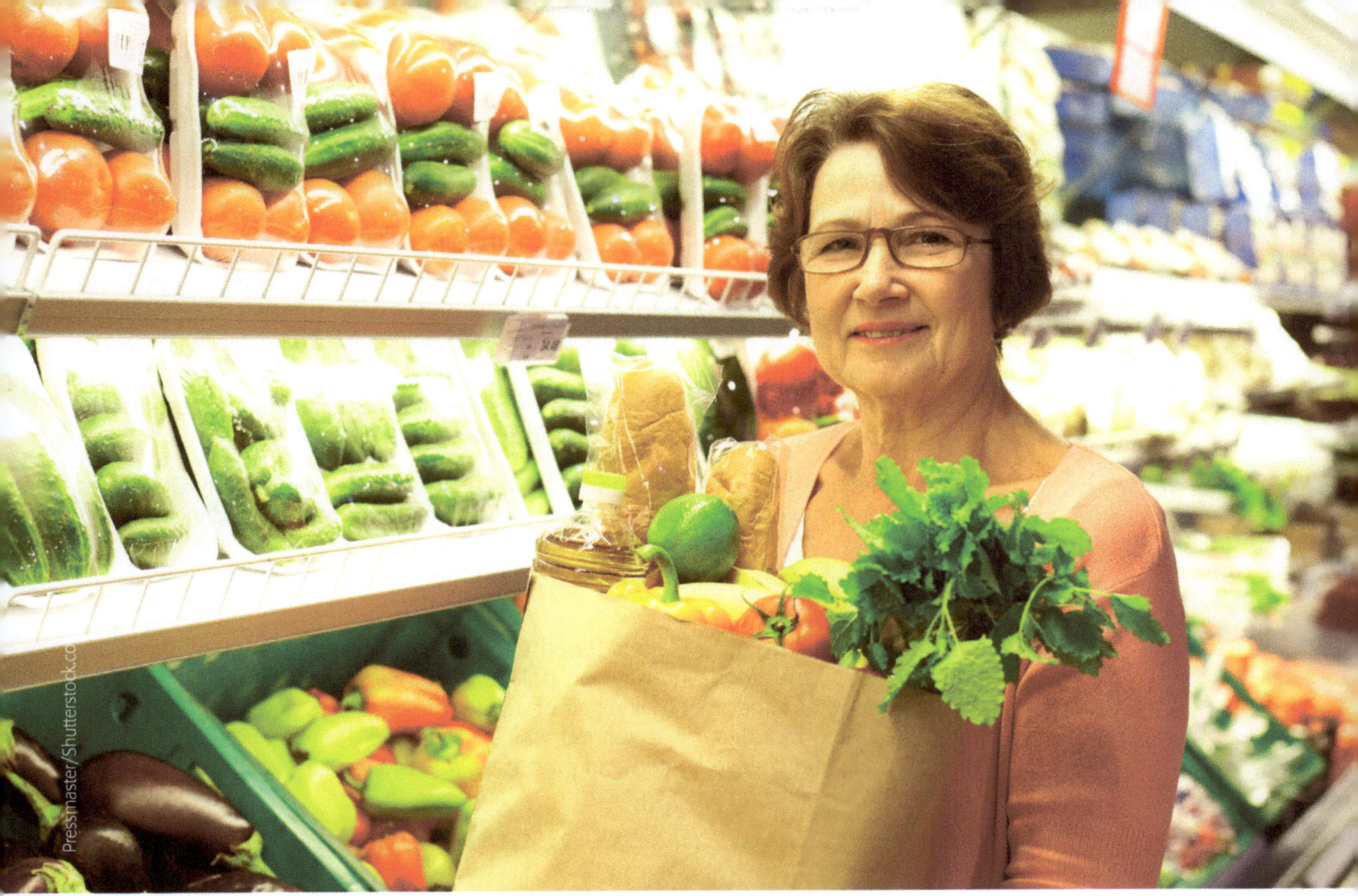

Nutrition Guidelines

The Dietary Guidelines for Americans (DGA) 2020-2025 highlight nutrition recommendations for midlife women. (1) The Dietary Guidelines for Americans encourage us to "make every bite count," with recommendations for all age groups as follows:

- Healthy eating is essential throughout the female lifespan.
- Eating nutrient-dense foods and beverages is important.
- Customize food choices according to personal preferences, budgets, and cultural traditions.
- Be mindful of calories while eating nutrient-dense foods.
- Limit alcoholic beverages, as well as foods high in added sugars, saturated fat, and salt.

The Dietary Guidelines for Americans also has the following guidance for older adult women:

1. Calorie needs typically decline with age, so it is extra important to ensure that nutrient-dense foods fill these calories.
2. Try to eat about two to three cups of vegetables daily and 1½-2 cups of fruit.
3. Eat a variety of vegetables, including dark leafy greens, red and orange vegetables, beans, peas, and lentils.
4. Make the majority of your grain intake whole grains.
5. Limit added sugars to no more than 10 percent of your total calories.

6. Limit saturated fat to no more than 10 percent of your total calories.
7. Limit sodium to no more than 2,300 mg daily.
8. Discuss all supplement use with your healthcare provider.
9. Talk with your healthcare provider about vitamin B12 as absorption decreases with age, and your doctor may recommend supplementation. This factor is especially important for people who eat plant-based, vegetarian, or vegan diets.
10. Calcium and vitamin D intake and possible supplementation are beneficial to discuss with your healthcare provider too.

*It should be noted that although industry and politics influence the Dietary Guidelines for Americans, you can still look to these guidelines for some general guidance.

Harvard Healthy Eating Plate

The Harvard Healthy Eating Plate is based upon the latest science, without significant influence from the food industry or politics. The Harvard Healthy Eating plate emphasizes water rather than dairy, half of a plate of vegetables and fruit. A variety of whole grains are included, while refined grains are limited. Protein should be healthy with red meat and cheese limited and processed meats avoided. Healthy oils, such as olive oil, have a place on this graphic too.

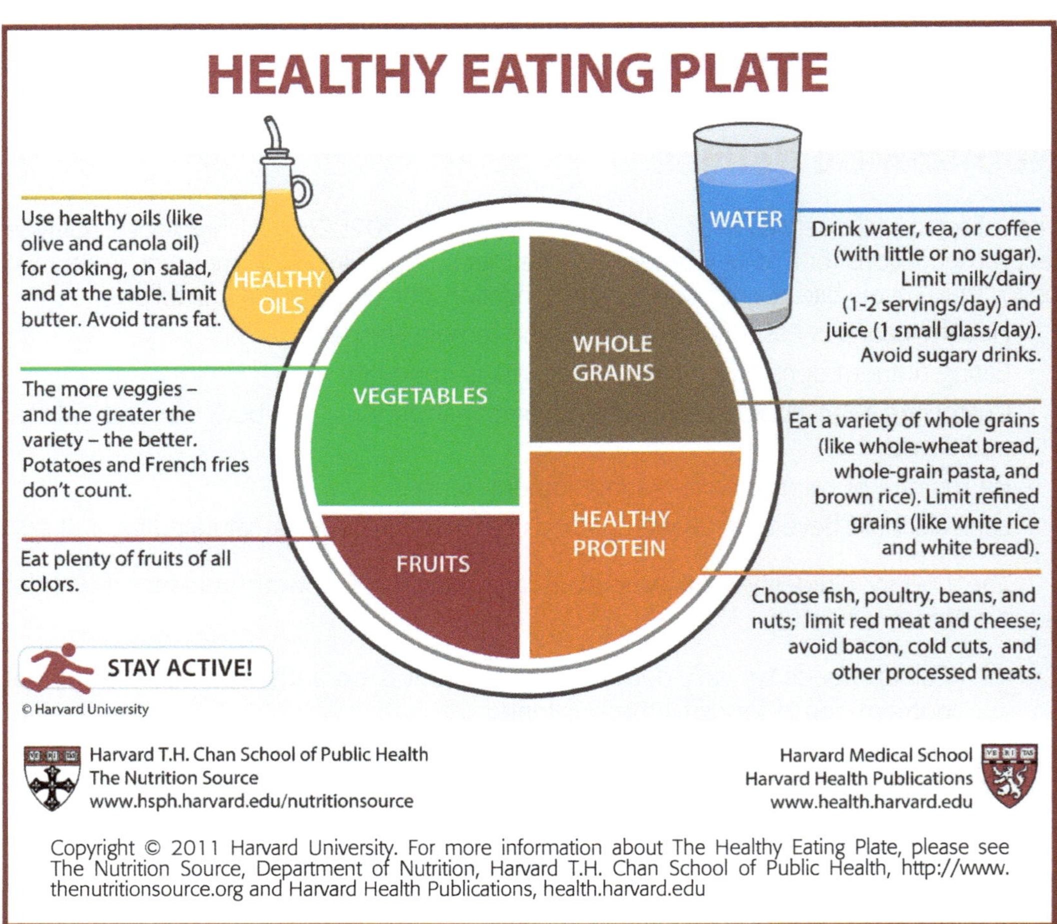

Figure 6-1. The Harvard Healthy Eating Plate

Healthy Dietary Pattern

A healthy eating style that benefits the heart, blood vessels, brain, and entire body positively helps menopausal women. Although there are many different dietary patterns, most of those recognized as being health-promoting by nutrition experts have many of the following attributes in common:

LIMIT OR AVOID:

- Ultra-processed foods
- Fried and fast-foods
- Foods with added sugars
- Foods high in saturated fat
- Foods with added salt
- Sugar-sweetened beverages
- Red and processed meat
- Refined grains
- Excessive alcohol intake

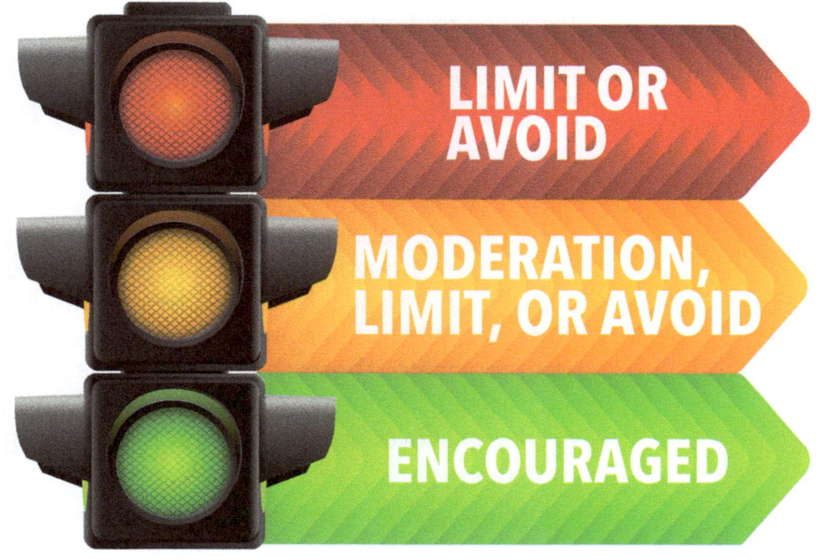

M.Stasy/Shutterstock.com

MODERATION, LIMIT, OR AVOID:

If you choose to eat these foods, do so only in moderation. They are not required for a healthy diet.

- Low-fat dairy products
- Seafood and fish
- Poultry

ENCOURAGED:

- Eat predominantly whole or minimally processed foods.
- Eat a variety (a rainbow) of plant-based foods.
- Enjoy vegetables and fruits.
- Make all or most of your grains whole grains.
- Use herbs and spices when cooking.
- Enjoy plant-based sources of protein such as beans, peas, lentils, seeds, and nuts.
- Consider enjoying soy-based foods such as tofu, soymilk, and tempeh.
- Get most of your nutrients from foods rather than from supplements, unless directed by your healthcare provider.
- Stay hydrated with water, while also enjoying tea and coffee, if desired.

Protein

Adequate protein intake is vital for midlife and more mature women, as lean muscle mass typically decreases in post-menopausal women, and protein is essential for maintaining or gaining lean muscle. Unfortunately, many women do not get enough protein in their diets. The recommended daily allowance (RDA) of protein for women is 46 grams daily. Getting 15-30 grams of protein at every meal is often recommended. You can consume dietary protein by eating nuts, seeds, tofu, soymilk, beans, peas, lentils, whole grains, seafood, and fortified soy products, as well as animal products. The DGA state that older adults can often benefit from incorporating a wider variety of protein sources. Americans typically overconsume meat, poultry, and eggs, while lentils, beans, peas, seafood, dairy, and fortified soy alternatives are often under-consumed according to the DGA.

Prebiotics, Probiotics, Salt, and Fiber

PREBIOTICS

Prebiotics are food for your gut bacteria. They have fiber that your gut bacteria can digest, even though you cannot digest this fiber without the bacteria. These important bacteria are essential for overall health, and it is important to keep them well fed. The bacteria feed on fiber and create short-chain fatty acids, including acetate, butyrate, and propionate. These short-chain fatty acids help regulate your energy, glucose, lipid metabolism, immunity, inflammation, cancer risk, and mood. Some prebiotic foods that gut bacteria love include those on the following list:

- Onions
- Whole grain bread
- Artichokes
- Leeks
- Soybeans
- Bananas
- Garlic

PROBIOTICS

Probiotics are live microorganisms that are intended to have health benefits when you consume them or apply them to your body. Among the reasons a high-quality probiotic can be a good thing are that they can boost energy levels, improve digestive health, help combat fatigue and stress, and reduce the symptoms of a variety of illnesses. Note: you should try to get your probiotics from food, rather than probiotic supplements, unless directed by your doctor.

- Kefir
- Yogurt (look for plant-based yogurts with added healthy bacteria)
- Sauerkraut
- Miso
- Pickles (look for pickles without vinegar in the refrigerated section of your grocery store)
- Kimchi
- Kombucha
- Tempeh
- Natto

SALT

Salt, also referred to as sodium chloride, is a mineral that is used to flavor food. While too much salt in your diet can be harmful, so can too little. Research has found that salt plays a vital role in helping ensure that you're well-hydrated and you maintain an appropriate level of electrolyte balance. Then again, consuming too much has been linked to high blood pressure, as well as an enhanced risk of heart disease, stroke, and kidney disease.

In reality, you want to keep your salt intake at 2,300 mg or less a day. Rather than adding salt into your recipes, just lightly put it on the finished dish before eating.

FIBER

Fiber is a type of carbohydrate that your body can't digest. As a result, when eaten, it passes through your body undigested. As such, fiber has a host of health-related benefits, including reducing your risk of both heart disease and type 2 diabetes.

While fiber has many health benefits, middle-aged women often don't experience all of its benefits due to fiber deficiency. After age 50, women should eat at least 21 grams of fiber daily. Fiber is abundant in plant-based foods, such as fruits, vegetables, beans, legumes, and whole grains. Fiber-rich cereals are another great source of fiber. Check the label.

Among the potential benefits of fiber are the following:

- Increases the feeling of fullness (may help with weight loss if overweight).
- Decreases blood sugar spikes.
- Supports the health of your gut microbiome (good bacteria in your intestines).
- Improves cholesterol.
- Decreases the risk of heart disease.
- Decreases the risk of type 2 diabetes.
- May reduce the risk of some types of cancer.

It should be noted that it's important to distinguish between fiber and carbohydrates. Remember that vegetables and fruits are, in fact, carbohydrates. In the case of diabetes, someone may need to limit their starchy vegetables and simple carbohydrates to control their blood sugars. Cookies, cakes, pastries, muffins, chips, white bagels and pasta, and other ultra-processed sweets are simple carbohydrates. They should not be in the same category as vegetables when considering carbohydrates.

The point to remember is that if you aren't used to eating a lot of fiber, start increasing the amount of fiber you eat slowly, and soon you'll be getting the benefits of a fiber-rich diet.

Full Plate Living is a nutrition program that promotes a high-fiber approach to healthy eating, highlighting the consumption of whole, unprocessed plant foods. Full Plate Living helps people add more whole plant-based foods to meals they're already eating. It's a small-step approach that can lead to big health outcomes and is a completely free service provided by the non-profit Ardmore Institute of Health. To learn more, visit www.fullplateliving.org/physicians.

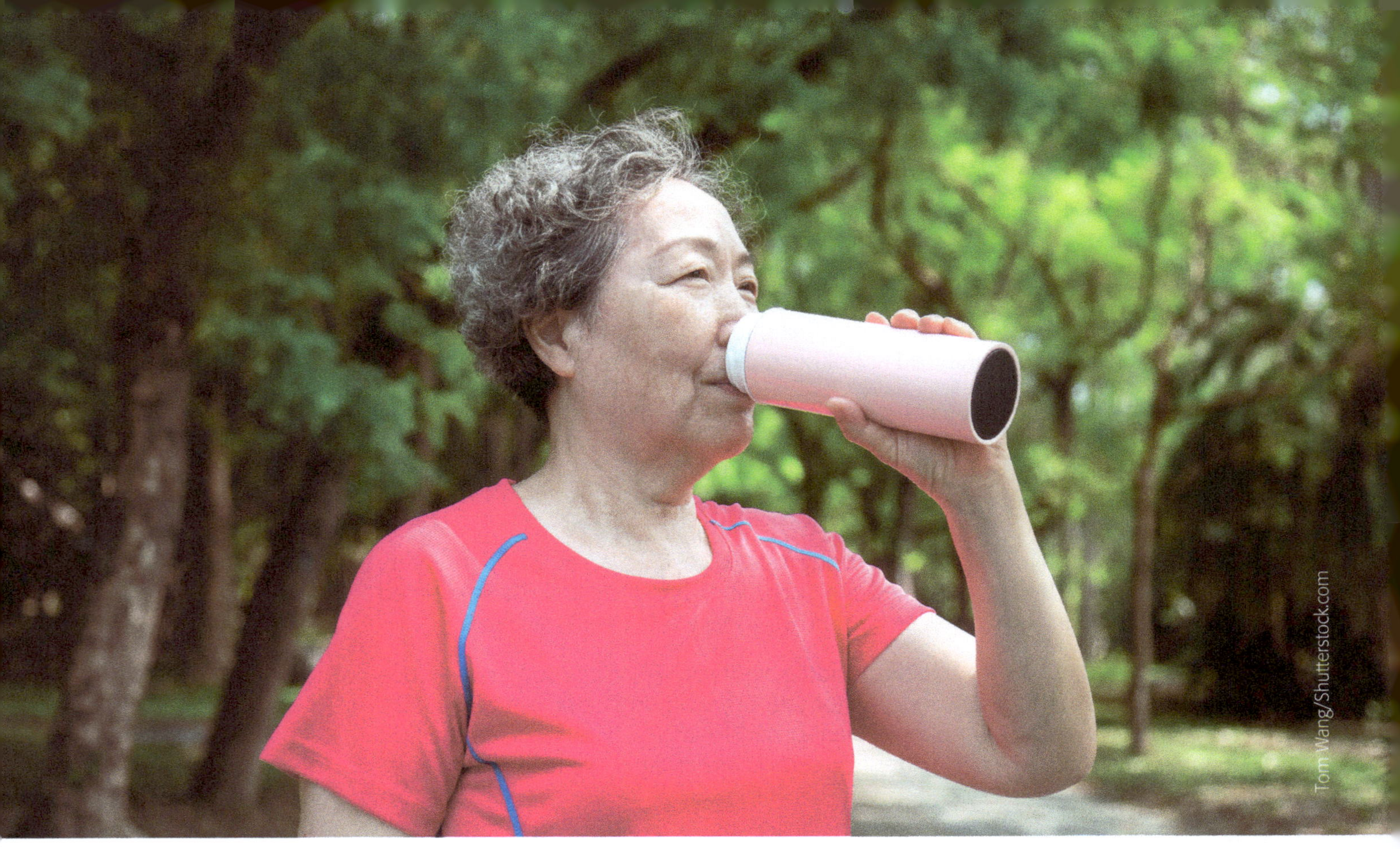

Tom Wang/Shutterstock.com

Fluid Intake

As women age, the sensation of thirst typically decreases. Be mindful of your daily fluid intake to ensure it is adequate. There are a variety of recommendations, including drinking eight, eight-oz glasses of water a day, about 2.7 liters each day, or a percentage of your body weight per day. The point is to drink enough water to be well-hydrated. If you urinate and your urine is pale, you are likely well-hydrated. If you are not urinating more than once or twice daily and your urine is yellow or darker yellow, you are likely dehydrated. Brain fog, dizziness, feeling dizzy when standing, fatigue, and constipation are common symptoms of dehydration. Again, rehydrating with water is the best remedy.

Most women do not usually require electrolyte drinks for daily hydration. On the other hand, contact your doctor if you've been sick, have diarrhea, are vomiting, or are sweating heavily. You may benefit from an electrolyte drink. You should avoid any drinks with dyes or other chemicals.

Remember that fruit juices, herbal teas, fruits, and vegetables contain water. Coffee, tea, soft drinks, such as Coke and Pepsi, and energy drinks are caffeinated drinks. Caffeine is a diuretic. In other words, they make you urinate more. Their impact on your hydration status is, therefore, more complicated.

Some women restrict the amount of fluid they drink near bedtime to avoid getting up in the middle of the night to use the bathroom. In this case, it is essential to get adequate fluid intake in the morning and afternoon, if you do not drink much fluid near bedtime.

Even though it's crucial to get adequate water intake, you should not exceed the recommended amount. It can lead to hyponatremia (a dangerously low salt level in your blood).

Protein Intake Journal

You should keep a record of how much protein you get for a day. Then, you should repeat this for several days to better understand your average daily protein intake. Remember, the recommended daily allowance (RDA) of protein for women is 46 grams daily. You can use the sample protein intake journal, shown in Table 6-1, to facilitate your effort to determine how much protein you're consuming daily. Keep in mind that you may need to do a quick Internet search to find how much protein or fiber is in a particular food.

Date	Food	Amount of Protein

Table 6-1. A sample daily protein intake journal

Fiber Intake Journal

Similar to your protein intake, you can employ a fiber intake journal to record how much fiber you are getting each day. If you repeat this for several days, you'll have a better idea of whether you're getting the recommended amount of fiber each day. Your aim should be to eat at least 21 grams of fiber each day, unless otherwise directed by a healthcare practitioner. It is important to note that if you aren't already getting this amount, you should slowly increase your fiber intake, rather than changing it rapidly.

Date	Food	Amount of Fiber

Table 6-2. A sample daily fiber intake journal

Fluid Intake Journal

You can also record the type of beverages you drink each day and the approximate amount of fluid you drink (refer to table 6-3). It is important to be aware that while 2.7 liters per day is the recommended fluid intake for women, much of this comes from fruits and vegetables.

Date	Beverage	Amount

Table 6-3. A sample fluid intake journal

- ❑ Do you want to change your diet based on your fiber, protein, and fluid journals? Explain.

____

____

____

Bone Health

Bone mass is the weight of all of the bones in your body, as measured in grams. Given the numerous roles that bones play in your body (providing structure, protecting organs, anchoring muscles, and storing calcium), it is important that you do whatever you can to prevent or slow your bone loss. If you don't, your risk of developing osteoporosis (a condition in which the bones become weak and brittle and as a result more prone to fracturing) increases.

Bone mass declines more rapidly after a woman goes through menopause. If bone mass gets too low, bones become fragile enough to be diagnosed with osteopenia or osteoporosis (very low bone mineral density), putting you at higher risk for bone fractures, falls, pain, and a loss of independent living. In addition to exercise, what you eat impacts bone health significantly. Women need calcium and vitamin D for bone health. Although most women typically think of dairy products like milk and yogurt when discussing calcium, non-dairy milk is often fortified with calcium. In addition, calcium fortifies some cereals and orange juice. You can also get calcium from green leafy vegetables, soybeans, almonds, figs, and tofu.

Women over age 50 should be getting at least 1200 mg/day of calcium each day. You may benefit from tracking how much calcium you get for a few days to better understand your typical daily calcium intake. If it is below 1200 mg daily, you should talk to your healthcare provider about calcium to determine if supplementation is right for you. Some research has shown that there may be risks to taking calcium supplements, so it's important to discuss your situation with your healthcare provider to determine what is best for you. If you take calcium supplements, taking them with a meal is best for absorption, as well as getting it throughout the day rather than taking it all at once.

Vitamin D is also essential for healthy bones. You can find vitamin D in fortified foods and drinks, such as fortified orange juice, dairy and non-dairy milk, salmon, swordfish, and tuna. Your body needs vitamin D to absorb calcium adequately. If you don't have sufficient vitamin D, you may eat or drink enough calcium-rich foods or take calcium supplements but not get the full benefits.

Women aged 51-70 should be getting 600 IU/day of vitamin D, and over age 70, the National Academy of Medicine recommends 800 IU/day. Many women need more than this amount to have adequate serum levels of vitamin D. Your body makes vitamin D when exposed to sunlight. Still, vitamin D levels are often low despite spending time in the sun due to many confounding factors. Discussing vitamin D with your healthcare provider is also crucial for bone and overall health. We encourage you to ask your doctor about getting your vitamin D level checked.

Excessive salt can also negatively impact bone health. Limiting excessive salt, caffeine, and alcohol consumption are three additional diet-related ways to support bone health and get adequate calcium and vitamin D.

Calcium Intake Journal

Tracking the amount of calcium in your foods for a few days can be helpful for you to better understand your typical daily calcium intake (refer to table 6-4). In addition, make sure you include supplements your healthcare provider has recommended, if you take a calcium supplement or multivitamin with calcium.

Date and Time	Food	Amount of Calcium

Table 6-4. A sample calcium intake journal

❏ Based on the results of your calcium journal, do you want to make any changes to your diet or talk to your healthcare practitioner? Explain.

____

____

____

Weight Management for Women

Discussing body weight can be a sensitive subject for many women, but it is essential to consider, given that a person's body weight impacts many facets of health for midlife and more mature women. If you struggle with your weight, you are not alone. Decreased calorie requirements and decreased muscle mass that often occur with menopause may lead to weight gain, if you don't modify your diet. As discussed in the chapter on physical activity, you can maintain your level of lean muscle mass (and in a few instances, even increase the amount of lean muscle you have) by engaging in regular physical activity, resistance exercises, and eating a healthy diet with adequate protein.

In addition to increasing the risk of many lifestyle-related chronic conditions, such as type 2 diabetes, cardiovascular disease, hypertension, high cholesterol, stroke, and breast cancer, having an overweight or obese body mass index (BMI) also makes it more challenging to control these conditions, if you develop them. Being overweight or obese also impacts menopause-related symptoms. For example, hot flashes and night sweats are more common for post-menopausal women with overweight or obese BMIs. In addition, urinary incontinence, sexual dysfunction, and menopausal muscle and joint pain are also more common in women who are overweight.

Body mass index (BMI) is a reference point that physicians use to better understand the impact of weight on someone's health. It creates categories meant to inform healthcare providers about risks and possible interventions. For example, to qualify for specific procedures or medications, a physician must document that a patient has a particular BMI.

It is important to note that a person's BMI does not define them. It is a medical reference point. Some people are very muscular and thus have a higher BMI. To fully and adequately counsel on any weight issues, a woman needs to be understood beyond her BMI. Researchers use BMI to better understand health at a population level. Neither weight nor BMI defines a woman. Therefore, there is no need to work in these classifications and categories to make strides in how you feel about yourself.

Strategies, such as being mindful of caloric intake, eating nutrient-dense foods, watching portion sizes, avoiding the sugar cycle, and eating mindfully, are beneficial for menopausal women trying to maintain or achieve a healthy weight. In addition to nutrition, getting adequate sleep and engaging in physical activity on a regular basis (aerobic and resistance exercise) support a healthy weight.

Unfortunately, it is challenging for many women with an overweight or obese BMI to achieve and sustain a weight that is in the healthy range and supports optimal health. If you are struggling with your weight (over- or underweight), please reach out to your healthcare team for help. There is no shame, blame, or guilt for asking for help with your weight.

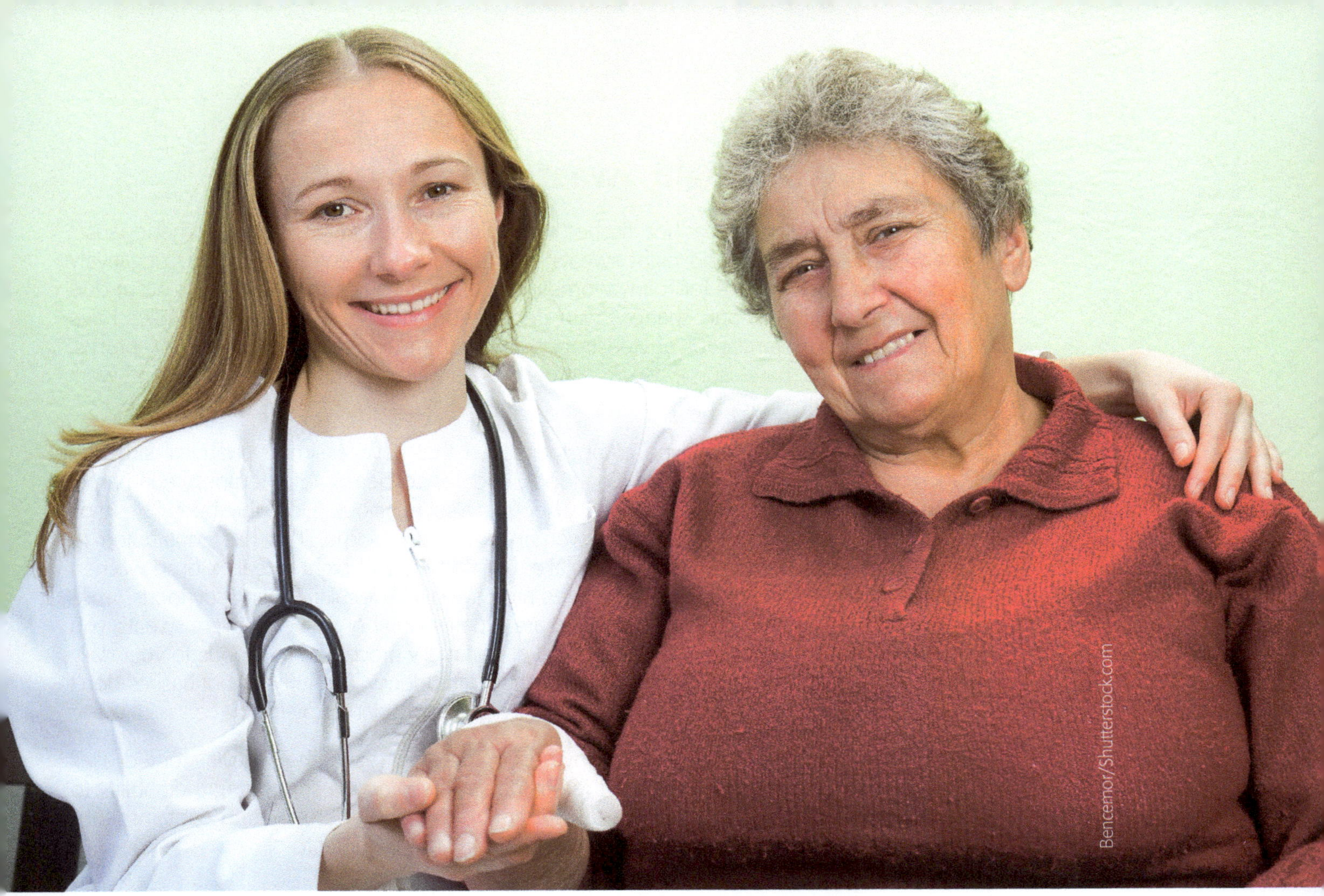
Bencemor/Shutterstock.com

Your physician or primary care provider can likely assist you and refer you to other helpful healthcare team members, such as registered dietitians, nutritionists, physical therapists, personal trainers, or mental health professionals to help you manage stress. If your healthcare provider and team members are talking to you about weight in a way that bothers you and makes you want to shut down, it's best to relay that to them for many reasons. One is that they likely genuinely want to help you. However, it's possible they haven't learned how to communicate compassionately and in an empowering way around body image and sensitivities about weight. If you speak up, you will help yourself and many other patients who likely feel the same way.

Wellness or health coaches can also support you with making the behavior changes needed to achieve a healthy weight. Your healthcare provider may refer you to a physician with expertise in obesity medicine or weight loss. Some physicians are board-certified in obesity medicine. In addition, some women benefit from prescription medication support through a doctor to help them achieve a healthier weight. You won't know what your options are unless you ask. Many insurances plans cover these referrals and medications.

Support for weight loss can also come through communities, such as Forks Over Knives, the Physicians Committee for Responsible Medicine, the McDougall Program, Full Plate Living, WW (Weight Watchers), Nutrisystem, and Jenny Craig. There are also online platforms available, such as Noom, that focus on the behavior component of eating and weight loss. Your local community center or YMCA may have resources too.

Hot Flashes, Night Sweats, and Soy

Most women experience hot flashes and night sweats during the perimenopausal transition. Hot flashes and night sweats are more than an annoyance. They negatively impact the quality of life for many women. Since hot flashes and night sweats occur due to menopausal hormone changes with decreased estrogen, a number of studies have examined the potential for phytoestrogen-containing foods to impact these symptoms. Phytoestrogens have some weak estrogenic activity in parts of the body but work differently in other areas.

Soy isoflavones are a type of phytoestrogen that have a similar chemical structure to estrogen made by your body. Soy foods, such as soybeans, tofu, tempeh, edamame, and soymilk, contain soy isoflavones. They are also nutritious. How the body uses soy isoflavones differs, depending on a woman's gut microbiome. This has contributed to inconclusive research on dietary soy intake, hot flashes, and night sweats. Some women experience relief from their hot flashes and night sweats by regularly eating soy foods, while others do not experience a change. If you are experiencing hot flashes or night sweats, you may consider adding one to three servings of minimally processed soy foods to your daily diet and see if it impacts your hot flash severity or frequency. Even if your hot flashes don't decrease, you will still benefit from eating this high-quality plant protein source.

Lignans are another group of phytoestrogens that researchers have studied. Flax seeds are rich in lignans. Although there is no strong evidence supporting their ability to impact hot flashes, ground flax seeds are antioxidant and fiber-rich, and contain heart-healthy omega-3 fatty acids. In addition, they may lower cholesterol.

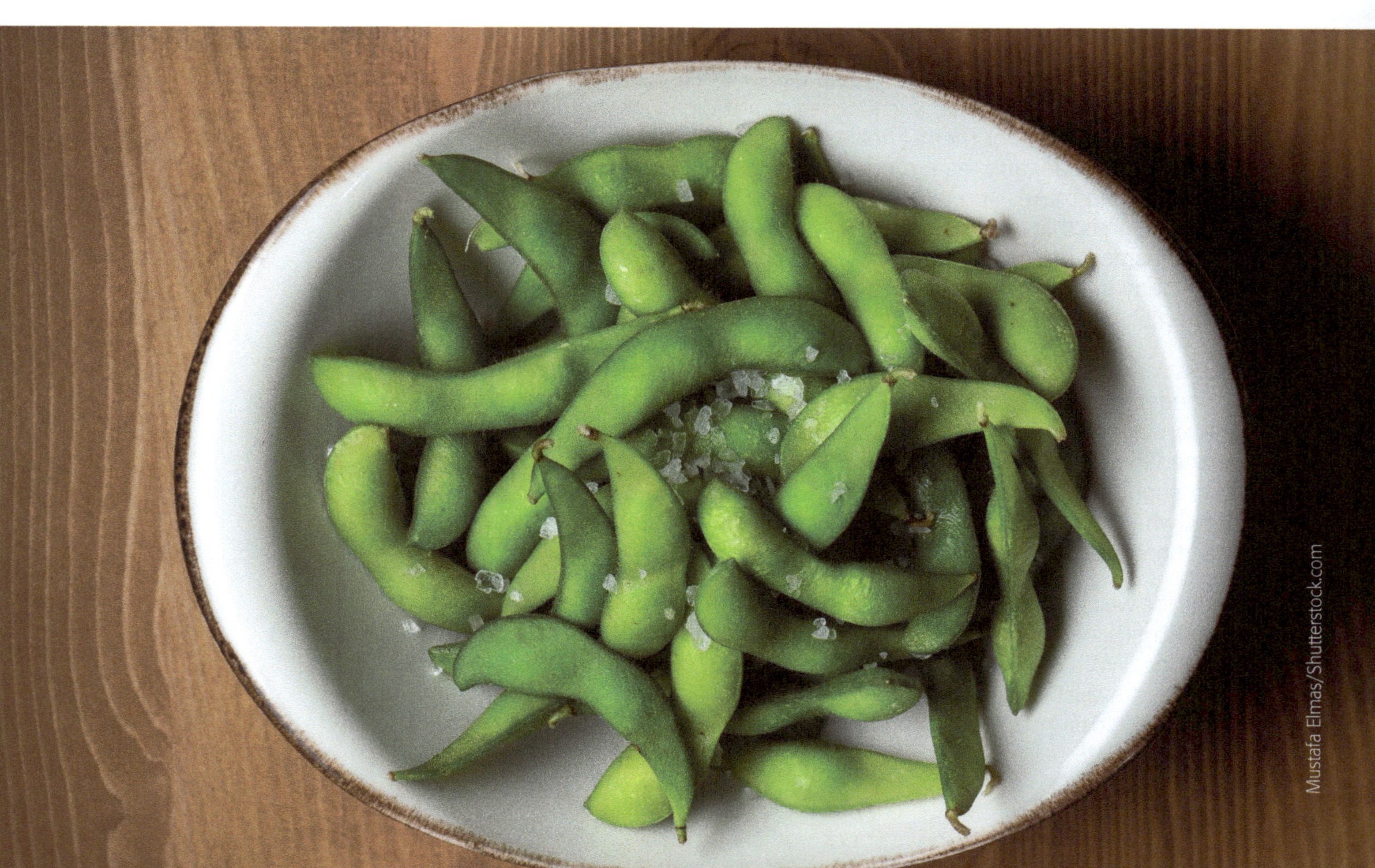

Mustafa Elmas/Shutterstock.com

Many women use soy supplements, isolates, extracts, and powder to decrease hot flashes and night sweats. Unfortunately, the supplement industry is not regulated. Therefore, soy supplements do not have the same standardization and oversight as prescription medications. The research on their safety and efficacy is also mixed. Non-dietary soy supplementation may decrease hot flashes and night sweats for some women, but you should talk with your doctor about their use concerning their potential risks and contraindications, as they are not safe for everyone.

Among the dietary changes to consider if you experience hot flashes and night sweats are the following:

- Avoid hot drinks (potential trigger).
- Be mindful of alcohol intake (potential trigger).
- Limit caffeine intake (possible trigger).
- Be mindful of spicy foods (potential trigger).
- Drink cool beverages and stay adequately hydrated.
- Explore new recipes that contain tofu or tempeh.
- Enjoy edamame as a snack.
- Drink a glass of soymilk.
- Avoid foods with added sugars that lead to a sugar spike and potentially a hot flash.
- Limit saturated fat intake (from animal products).
- Consume an adequate amount of omega-three fatty acids (ground flaxseed, fish, seafood, nuts).
- Enjoy green leafy vegetables.
- Eat several servings of fruit each day.
- Eat whole grains and avoid refined grains.
- Incorporate nuts and beans in your diet.
- Enjoy extra virgin olive oil in moderation.

The literature supports an anti-inflammatory, nutrient-rich diet for decreasing hot flashes and night sweats. A Mediterranean diet, which is rich in fruits, vegetables, whole grains, nuts, extra virgin olive oil, legumes, fish a few times a week, and some dairy, may reduce hot flashes and night sweats. This dietary pattern also limits meat and sweet consumption. It is antioxidant-rich, anti-inflammatory, and filled with whole, plant foods.

Sexual Health and Nutrition

Nutrition and sexual health are rarely discussed together though they are both essential components of overall health. What women eat impacts their sexual health and well-being as middle-aged and more mature women.

Decreased sexual activity and sexual dysfunction are associated with a dietary pattern that includes many ultra-processed foods, added sugar and salt, and foods high in saturated fat, such as red and processed meat. Heavy alcohol use is also detrimental to sexual health. Furthermore, sexual dysfunction is more common in women with lifestyle-related chronic conditions, such as metabolic syndrome, type 2 diabetes, hypertension, high cholesterol, or cardiovascular disease.

An anti-inflammatory, antioxidant-rich diet, such as a whole-food plant-predominant diet or a Mediterranean diet, is associated with increased sexual activity and sexual well-being. Researchers have even studied specific foods, including watermelon, pistachios, apples, cacao beans, pomegranates, beets, and green tea, which support sexual health in women.

Since inflammation negatively impacts vessels throughout the body, including vessels in the pelvis and genitals, eating an anti-inflammatory diet helps to keep these vessels healthy. Having healthy genital-tissue blood vessels allows women to have a healthy sexual response, which is vital for sexual arousal, engorgement of the genital tissues, and vaginal lubrication. Without healthy pelvic blood vessels, painful vaginal intercourse is more common due to dryness. There are other causes of vaginal dryness after menopause too. See the chapter on social connection for more information.

Brain Health and Nutrition

Your daily meals impact your memory and mood. Eating foods that support brain health becomes increasingly important throughout and beyond the menopausal transition. The gut microbiome, the trillions of microorganisms that live in your intestines and help digest your food, impacts hormones that control the brain. If you want your brain to be healthy, you need to eat health-promoting foods.

In that regard, eating adequate fiber (think plant foods) is essential for gut microbiome health. Too often, midlife and more mature women are starving their gut microorganisms due to a lack of fiber. Eating a diet rich in fiber from whole or minimally processed plant foods will make your gut microbiome healthier, thus supporting your mood and mental well-being.

Limiting inflammation is vital for mood and decreasing the risk of dementia. Eating an anti-inflammatory diet rich in nutrients from whole foods is best. If these are unavailable, minimally processed foods (e.g., pre-cut broccoli, carrots, celery, packaged sugar-free steel-cut oatmeal, canned unsalted beans, frozen fruits, and vegetables with no added sugar and salt) can also decrease inflammation throughout your body. Accordingly, you should try to eat a rainbow of fruits and vegetables each day (or at least each week): red apples, orange sweet potatoes, yellow peppers, green spinach, blueberries, purple eggplant, and white cauliflower. Eating several cups of leafy greens each day provides your brain with adequate folate, essential for brain function. Berries, especially blueberries, are also great for brain health, as are spices, such as turmeric, cinnamon, and pepper which also decrease inflammation throughout your brain and body.

FOODS THAT SHOULD BE EMPHASIZED FOR BRAIN HEALTH:

- Rainbow of fruits and vegetables
- Leafy green vegetables
- Berries (especially blueberries)
- Walnuts and almonds
- Extra virgin olive oil
- Omega 3 fatty acids (ground flax seeds, oily fish)
- Spices
- Whole grains
- Beans, peas, and lentils

It is also important to remember that foods that increase inflammation throughout the body negatively impact your mood and brain health, thereby increasing the risk of mood disorders and dementia. Many women experience mood fluctuations and increased sadness or anxiety during menopause. While dietary changes should not substitute for mental health care or prescription medications that are essential for women with a mental illness, they can positively impact the mental health of many menopausal women. Limiting or avoiding inflammation-promoting foods, such as the following support mood and memory for menopausal women and decrease the risk of dementia.

FOODS THAT SHOULD BE AVOIDED OR LIMITED FOR BRAIN HEALTH:

- Ultra-processed foods (such as candy, chips, and fast food)
- Foods with added sugar or salt
- Red and processed meats (including bacon, hot dogs, and lunchmeat)
- Cheese
- Fried food
- Fast food
- Sugar-sweetened beverages
- Candy, cookies, and pastries
- Butter and margarine
- Corn, soybean, canola, and grapeseed oils
- Refined grains (like white bread, white rice, and pasta)

Another diet that is well known for its positive impact on brain health is the MIND diet. MIND stands for Mediterranean-DASH Intervention for Neurodegenerative Delay and is a hybrid of the Mediterranean diet and the DASH diet (Dietary Approaches to Stop Hypertension). It has most of the components of foods to emphasize and limits those that should be generally avoided, with a few other modifications. For more information on the MIND diet, talk to your healthcare provider or a dietitian, or do initial research on reputable websites.

At this point, you should go back to the two lists of foods and circle the changes that you would like to make to address hot flashes, bone health, sexual health, or brain health.

❑ What foods do you want to increase or add to your diet?

____

____

____

❑ What foods do you currently eat that you would like to decrease or eliminate?

____

____

____

❏ What were you most surprised to learn?

____

____

____

❏ What are you inspired to do differently?

____

____

____

Culture and Nutrition

What you eat is influenced by many factors, including your culture. Oldways (https://oldwayspt.org) is a non-profit organization that has wonderful nutrition resources that embrace the impact of culture on food and way of life. Consider visiting their website to learn more. Figures 6-2 to 6-6 feature the Mediterranean, Latin American, Asian, African Heritage, and vegetarian & vegan diet pyramids. Although all of the pyramids, except for the vegan pyramid, contain animal products, these pyramids are all plant-forward, emphasizing the benefits of a whole-food, plant predominant diet.

Suggestions for Healthy Eating

Even if you know what to eat to support your health, it can still be challenging to implement your plan. Obstacles, such as the cost of healthy food or not knowing how to prepare food to taste good, can all get in the way of healthy eating. The following are some suggestions to help you tackle common obstacles (e.g., cost, preparation and convenience, and taste) that women in midlife often have when trying to eat healthier.

COST:

- Purchase healthy foods in bulk to save money.
- Compare costs of foods within stores or between stores.
- Look for healthy, inexpensive food options, such as beans.
- Prepare food yourself, rather than buying it prepared (e.g., cook your beans rather than buying them pre-cooked).
- Look for affordable healthy food recipes on the Internet.
- Use canned or frozen fruits and vegetables.
- Cook in bulk and freeze food for later use.
- Shop for what you need from a list or recipe so you're not as tempted to buy things that you don't really need.
- Check to see if you qualify for SNAP benefits (Supplemental Nutrition Assistance Program).
- Look for sales or use coupons.

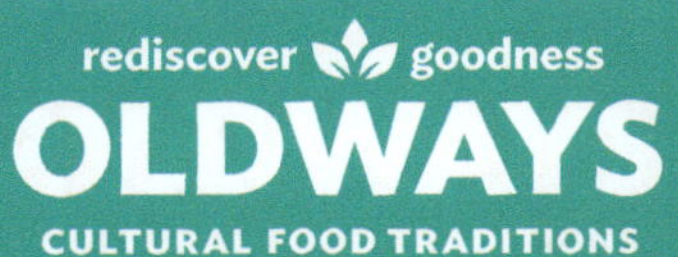

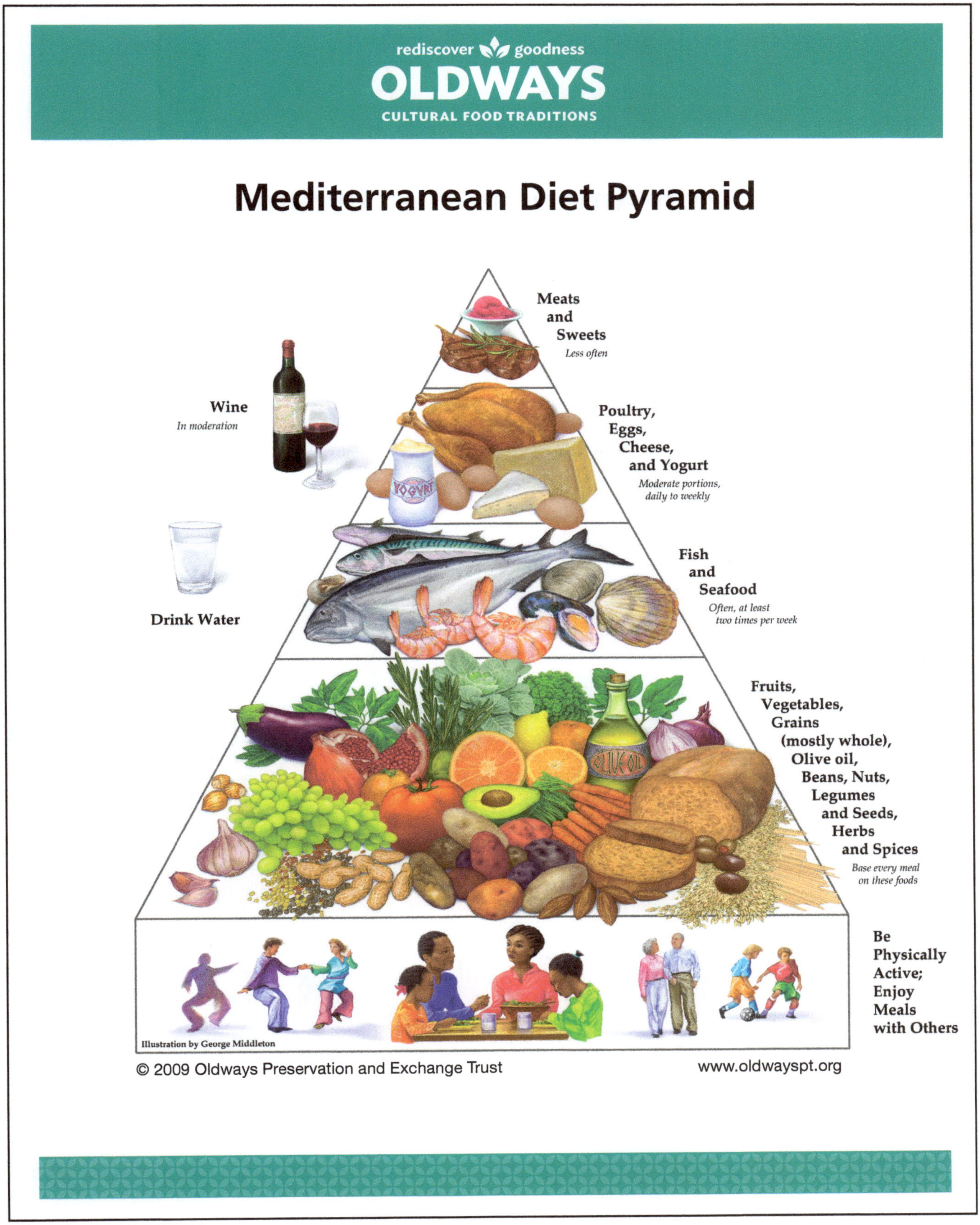
rediscover goodness
OLDWAYS
CULTURAL FOOD TRADITIONS
Mediterranean Diet Pyramid
Meats and Sweets
Less often
Wine
In moderation
Poultry, Eggs, Cheese, and Yogurt
Moderate portions, daily to weekly
YOGURT
Drink Water
Fish and Seafood
Often, at least two times per week
Fruits, Vegetables, Grains (mostly whole), Olive oil, Beans, Nuts, Legumes and Seeds, Herbs and Spices
Base every meal on these foods
OLIVE OIL
Be Physically Active; Enjoy Meals with Others
Illustration by George Middleton
© 2009 Oldways Preservation and Exchange Trust
www.oldwayspt.org

Figure 6-2. Mediterranean diet pyramid

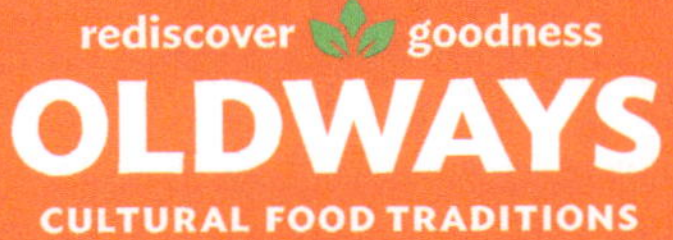

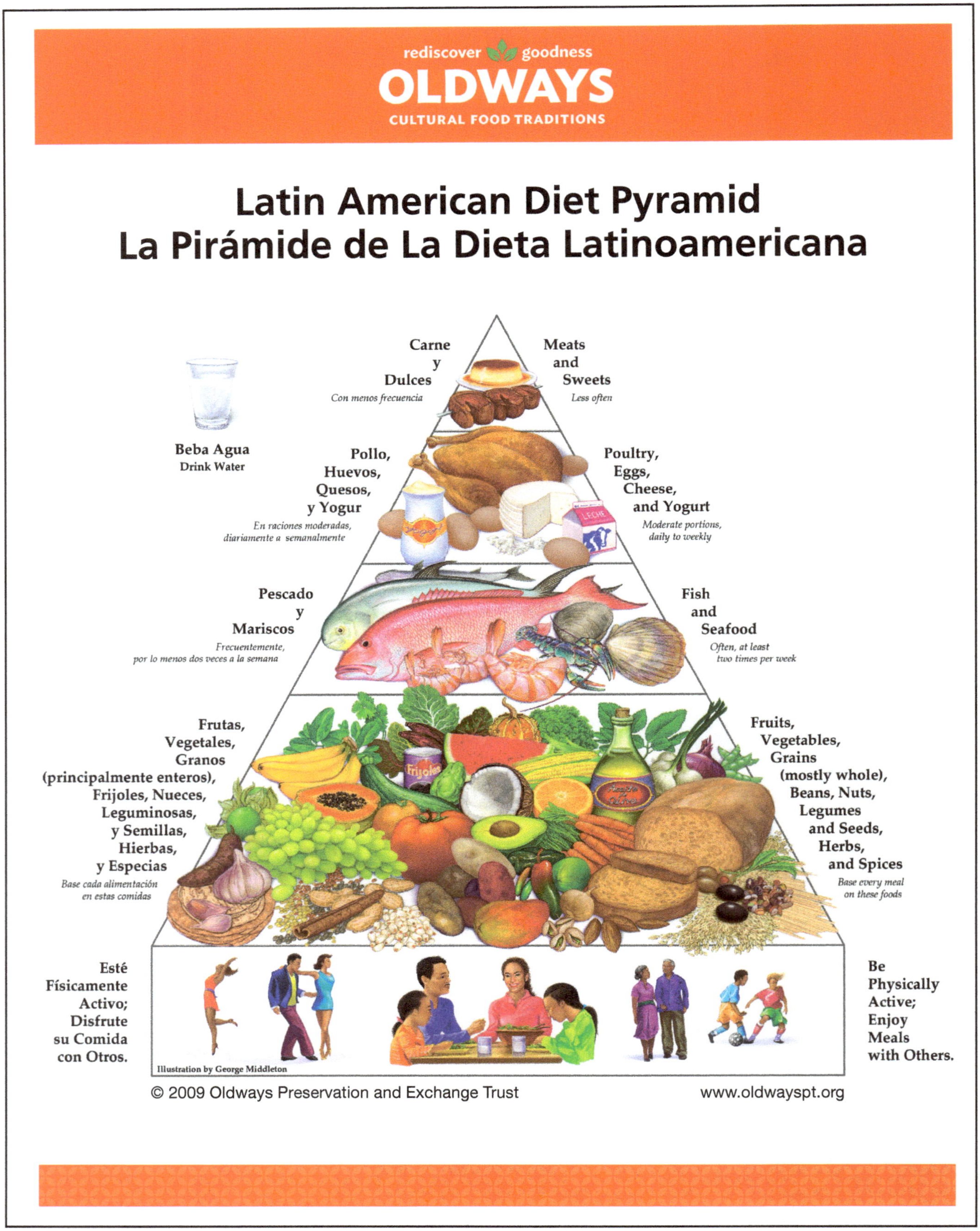
rediscover goodness
OLDWAYS
CULTURAL FOOD TRADITIONS
Latin American Diet Pyramid
La Pirámide de La Dieta Latinoamericana
Carne y Dulces
Con menos frecuencia
Meats and Sweets
Less often
Beba Agua
Drink Water
Pollo, Huevos, Quesos, y Yogur
En raciones moderadas, diariamente a semanalmente
Poultry, Eggs, Cheese, and Yogurt
Moderate portions, daily to weekly
Pescado y Mariscos
Frecuentemente, por lo menos dos veces a la semana
Fish and Seafood
Often, at least two times per week
Frutas, Vegetales, Granos (principalmente enteros), Frijoles, Nueces, Leguminosas, y Semillas, Hierbas, y Especias
Base cada alimentación en estas comidas
Fruits, Vegetables, Grains (mostly whole), Beans, Nuts, Legumes and Seeds, Herbs, and Spices
Base every meal on these foods
Esté Físicamente Activo; Disfrute su Comida con Otros.
Be Physically Active; Enjoy Meals with Others.
Illustration by George Middleton
© 2009 Oldways Preservation and Exchange Trust
www.oldwayspt.org

Figure 6-3. Latin American diet pyramid

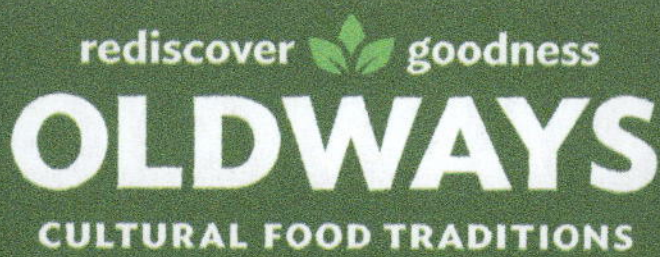

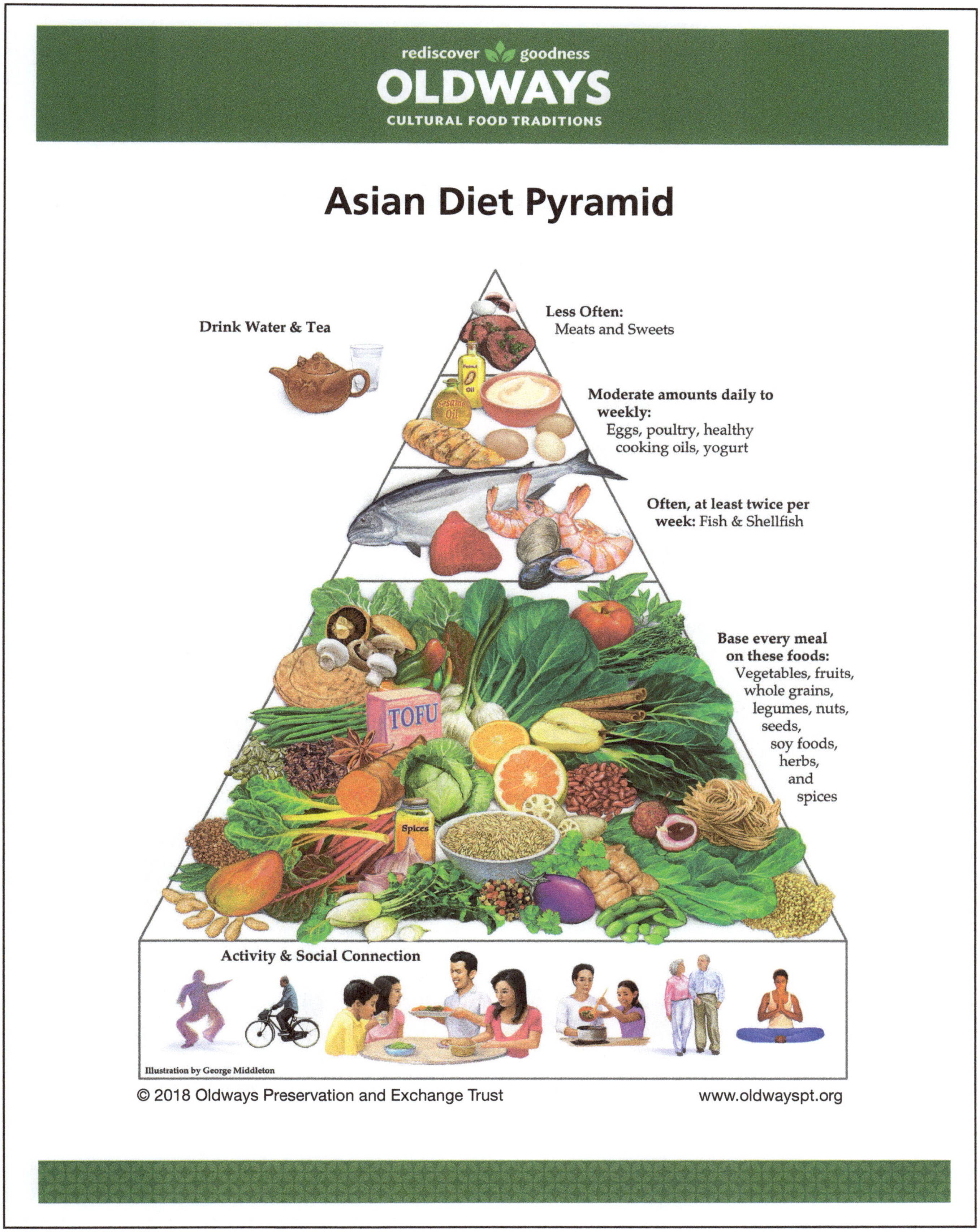
rediscover goodness
OLDWAYS
CULTURAL FOOD TRADITIONS
Asian Diet Pyramid
Drink Water & Tea
Less Often: Meats and Sweets
Moderate amounts daily to weekly: Eggs, poultry, healthy cooking oils, yogurt
Often, at least twice per week: Fish & Shellfish
Base every meal on these foods: Vegetables, fruits, whole grains, legumes, nuts, seeds, soy foods, herbs, and spices
TOFU
Spices
Sesame Oil
Activity & Social Connection
Illustration by George Middleton
© 2018 Oldways Preservation and Exchange Trust
www.oldwayspt.org

Figure 6-4. Asian diet pyramid

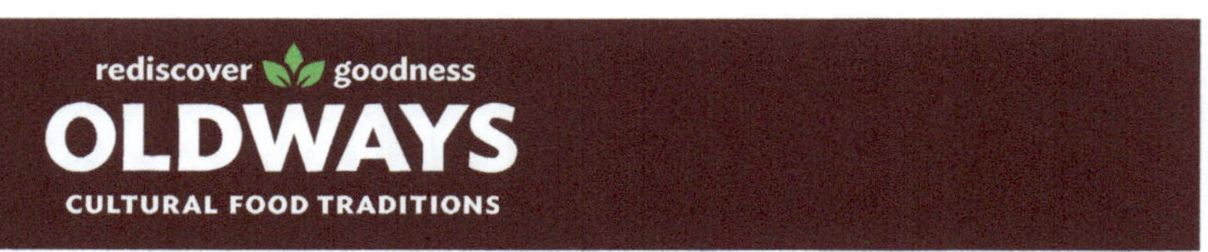

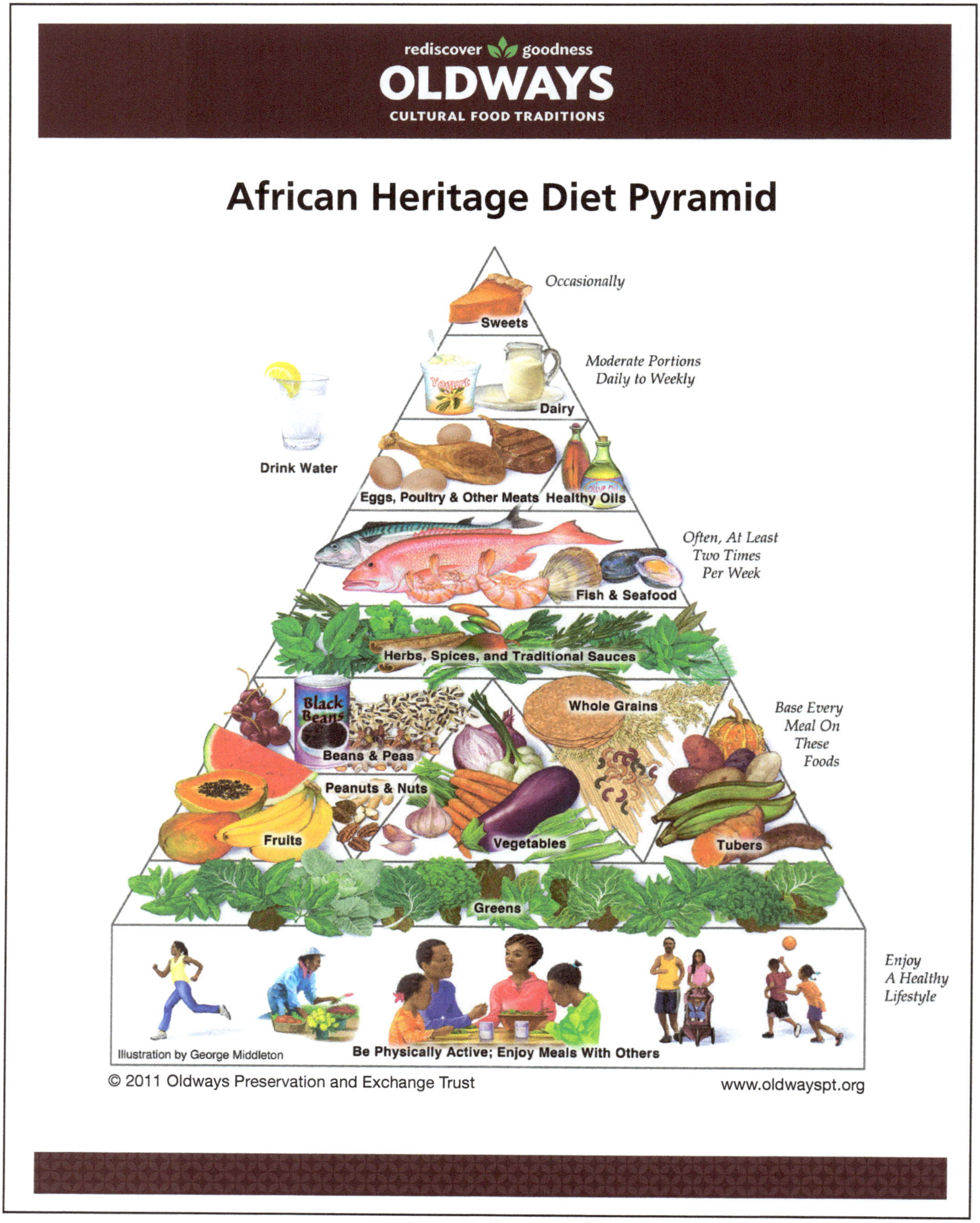
rediscover goodness
OLDWAYS
CULTURAL FOOD TRADITIONS
African Heritage Diet Pyramid
Occasionally
Sweets
Moderate Portions
Daily to Weekly
Dairy
Drink Water
Eggs, Poultry & Other Meats
Healthy Oils
Often, At Least
Two Times
Per Week
Fish & Seafood
Herbs, Spices, and Traditional Sauces
Black Beans
Beans & Peas
Whole Grains
Base Every
Meal On
These
Foods
Peanuts & Nuts
Fruits
Vegetables
Tubers
Greens
Enjoy
A Healthy
Lifestyle
Illustration by George Middleton
Be Physically Active; Enjoy Meals With Others
© 2011 Oldways Preservation and Exchange Trust
www.oldwayspt.org

Figure 6-5. African heritage diet pyramid

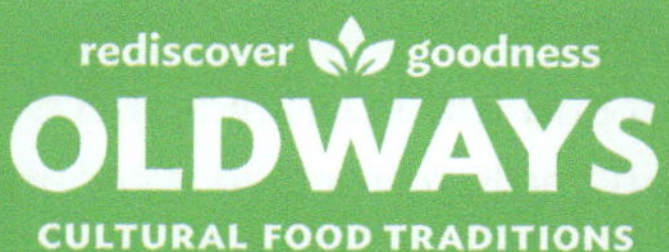

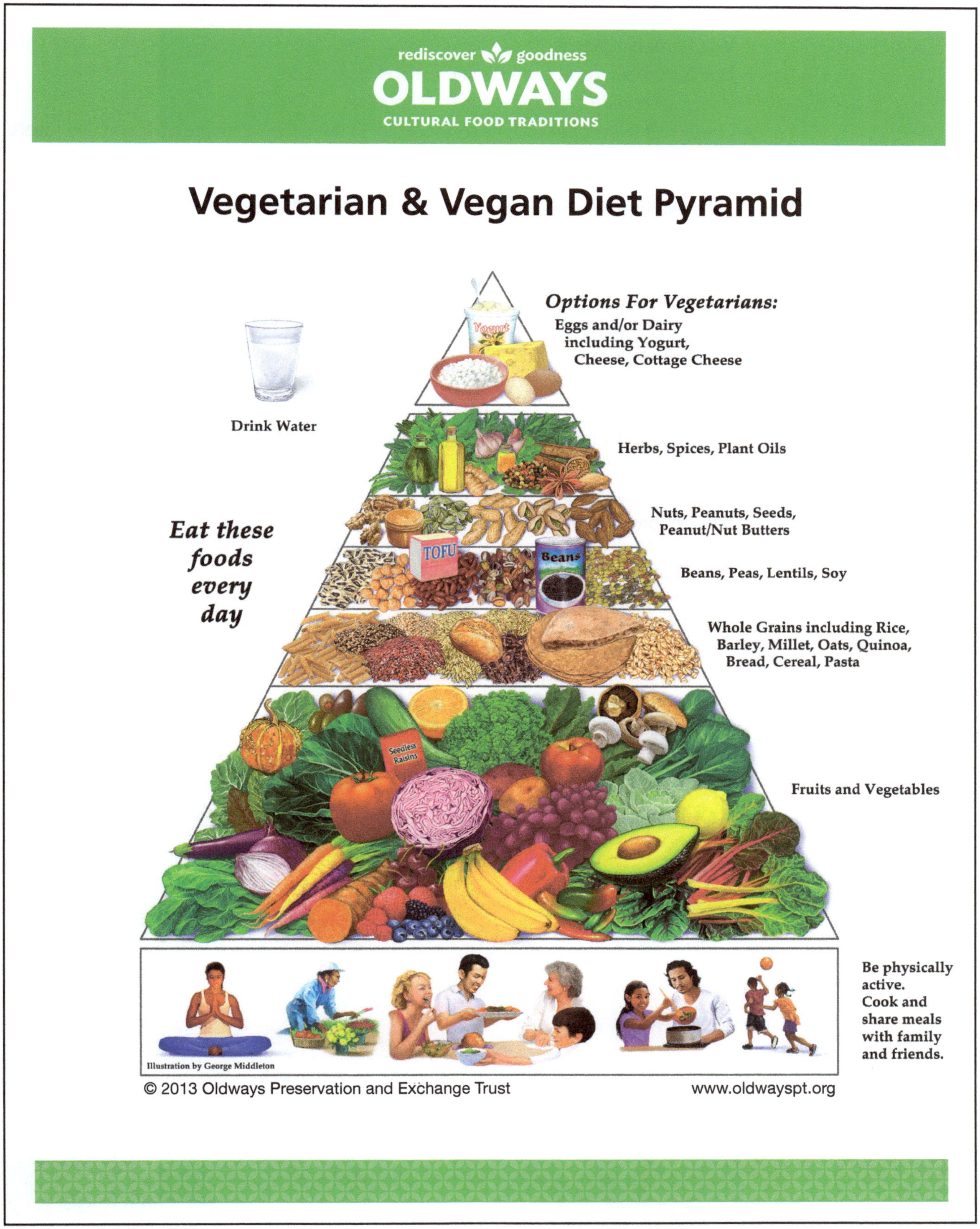
rediscover goodness
OLDWAYS
CULTURAL FOOD TRADITIONS
Vegetarian & Vegan Diet Pyramid
Options For Vegetarians:
Eggs and/or Dairy including Yogurt, Cheese, Cottage Cheese
Yogurt
Drink Water
Herbs, Spices, Plant Oils
Nuts, Peanuts, Seeds, Peanut/Nut Butters
Eat these foods every day
TOFU
Beans
Beans, Peas, Lentils, Soy
Whole Grains including Rice, Barley, Millet, Oats, Quinoa, Bread, Cereal, Pasta
Seedless Raisins
Fruits and Vegetables
Be physically active.
Cook and share meals with family and friends.
Illustration by George Middleton
© 2013 Oldways Preservation and Exchange Trust
www.oldwayspt.org

Figure 6-6. Vegetarian & Vegan diet pyramid

- Grow a garden or join a community-sponsored agriculture group.
- Visit farmers markets.
- Use food banks and food pantries, if cost is an issue.
- Use your reward cards to receive discounts.
- Check with your community or senior center to see if they offer free or discounted meals.
- A common concern when changing eating habits is whether the new way of eating will cost more. Many foods included in plant-predominant eating are relatively inexpensive (such as rice and beans). For more information about how to eat Whole-Food, Plant-Based on a budget, visit the American College of Lifestyle Medicine's resources at https://lifestylemedicine.org/project/patient-resources.

PREPARATION AND CONVENIENCE:

- Create a community of people in your neighborhood or nearby who are looking to eat healthy meals and organize a schedule, such that you can share the workload and cost.
- If not cost-prohibitive, buy pre-cut produce.
- Choose healthy meals that only need to be heated, rather than prepared from scratch.
- Look for easy meals or recipes when searching for recipes.
- Prepare meals for several days during the week when you have extra time.
- If food preparation is difficult, look for food assistance through meal delivery services, Meals on Wheels, or other community resources (a local dietitian or social worker should be able to direct you to resources).
- Explore companies that ship food to your home. You choose what you want to eat, how frequently you want to receive shipments, and the food arrives cold and at your door. Some companies send food that just needs to be heated, while others deliver the ingredients for you to cook.
- Order online and have groceries delivered to your home or brought to your car.
- Rather than cooking, enjoy a group meal at a community center.
- Look for recipes for just one or two people rather than typical-size recipes for a larger group.
- Look for healthy meals that can be microwaved or eaten with little preparation.

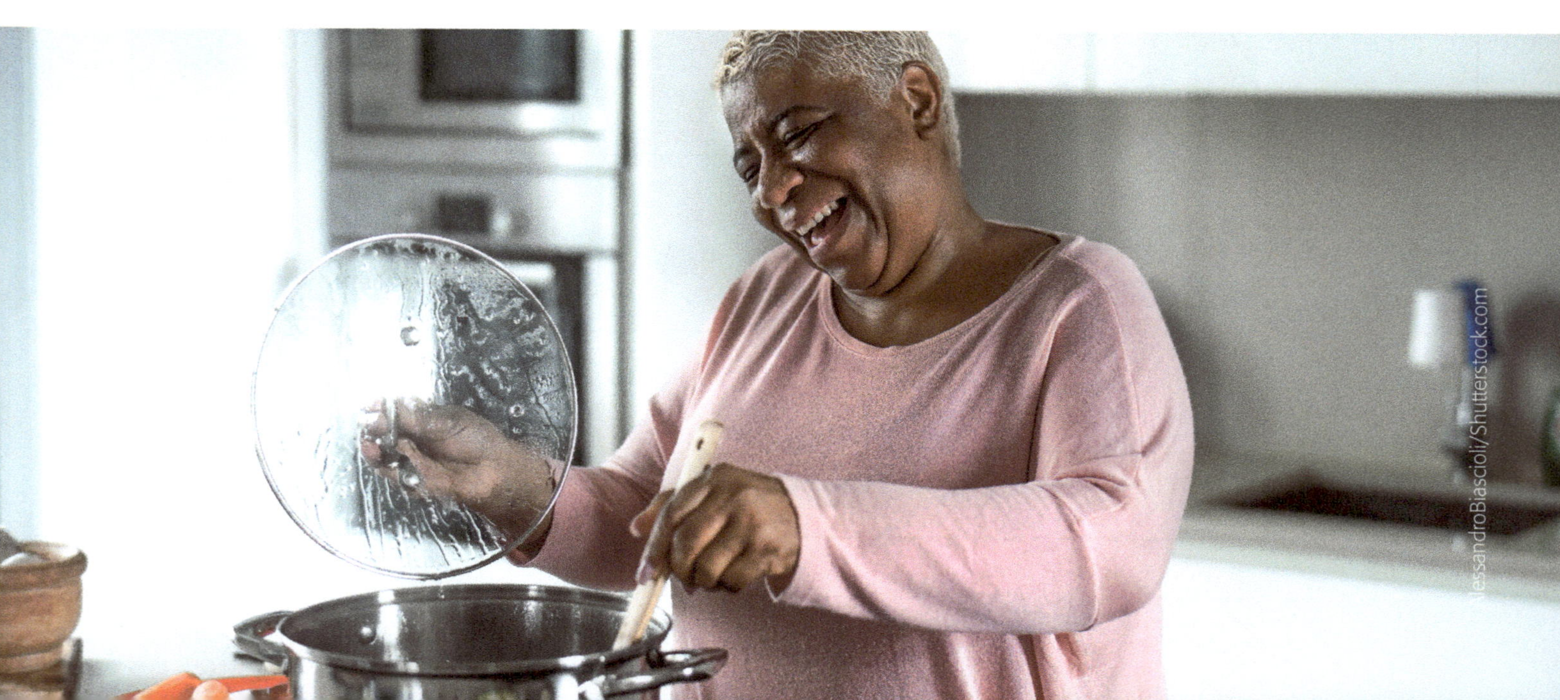
AlessandroBiascioli/Shutterstock.com

TASTE:

- Go to a bookstore or library and look at healthy cookbooks to get inspiration. The more you plan for and contemplate healthy meals, the more likely you are to follow through.
- Experiment with different recipes to see what you like.
- Be patient with yourself as it takes time to adjust to new tastes.
- Talk to your dietitian if you can't find tasty foods that meet your nutritional needs.
- If medications are altering the taste of food, talk to your healthcare provider about options.
- Try herbs and spices to flavor food as taste and smell decline with age.
- Invest in spices if you can afford it.
- Explore healthier ways to prepare your traditional foods.
- Make small changes.

Coaching Yourself on Nutrition With the COACH Approach

CURIOSITY

Before making your diet healthier, you need to understand how what you currently eat impacts your health. Get curious. For some women, keeping a food diary for a couple of days is beneficial. You can do this with a notepad and pen or a phone app.

❏ What parts of your current diet are health-promoting?

____

____

____

❏ What parts of your current diet are not health-promoting (such as too much soda or fast food, or too few vegetables or beans)?

____

____

____

____

OPENNESS

Discussing food can be a sensitive topic. Many people are resistant to even hearing about improving their health through nutrition, if it involves a behavior change. Thank you for being open to exploring this change.

- ❑ After reflecting on your responses to the questions in the previously noted curiosity section, what diet component do you want to change?

  ____

  ____

  ____

- ❑ What is holding you back from making the changes—perhaps not knowing how to prepare legumes or a concern that your spouse will not like the taste of new foods?

  ____

  ____

  ____

APPRECIATION

When making nutrition changes, it is beneficial to appreciate what resources or people can support you, as you make this journey to increase your chances of success.

- ❑ Think about a time when you enjoyed a really healthy meal. What was it about that experience that sticks in your mind? Sit back and appreciate that.

  ____

  ____

  ____

- ❑ What was a time in your life when you enjoyed healthy eating? What was going on then, and how can you replicate this?

  ____

  ____

  ____

- ❑ How can you address what is holding you back from making the healthy nutrition changes you identified in the aforementioned openness section?

  ____

  ____

  ____

❑ Is there additional information or education that would help you make the changes? Explain.

___

___

___

❑ Are there resources or experts you could connect with to help you make these changes (e.g. dietitians, your doctor, a wellness coach, trying a health app on your phone)? Elaborate.

___

___

___

COMPASSION

Be compassionate with yourself when trying to change how you eat. Behavior change is difficult. By the time you reach menopause, you have a half-century of eating patterns that are very ingrained in your daily life.

❑ Have you tried to make healthy nutrition changes that were unsuccessful or that you did not maintain? If so, what obstacles kept you from being successful?

___

___

___

In our culture, women's nutrition is often linked with body image. If you judge yourself based on what you eat, what number is on the scale, or what size you wear, it's time to abandon that thinking pattern.

❑ How can you alter your thinking around food and body image to be more self-compassionate?

___

___

___

___

HONESTY

Be honest with yourself. It's only through honestly considering where you are now and where you want to go that you'll make healthy changes.

- ❑ Do you think you will successfully make your desired nutrition changes? Why or why not?

  ____

  ____

  ____

  ____

- ❑ Is there anything you can do, people you can contact, or information you can learn that could make it more likely that you'll be successful?

  ____

  ____

  ____

- ❑ What nutrition changes will you make this week? Write your goal.

  ____

  ____

  ____

Whole-Food, Plant-Predominant Eating Pattern

The blue zones are the five places on earth where the oldest, healthiest people live. Dan Buettner, author of *The Blue Zones: 9 Lessons for Living Longer From the People Who've Lived the Longest*, as well as other books on the blue zones, helps people understand how they can modify their environment in order to optimize their health. Making healthier choices, easier choices, is a core component of Dan Buettner's message. The following are 10 food guidelines based upon the Blue Zones™ program and research. Although people eat differently in all five of the blue zones, a number of similarities exist in their eating patterns.

- Retreat from meat—People in the blue zones do not eat very much meat. When they do eat it, they only eat small portions.
- Reduce dairy—Dairy does not play a large role in the diets of people who live in the blue zones.

- Slash sugar—People in the blue zones consume much less added sugar than Americans typically consume. The Blue Zones™ guidelines encourage you to try to limit your added sugar intake to seven teaspoons of added sugar a day or less.
- Eliminate eggs—The Blue Zones™ food guidelines suggest eating, at most, three eggs per week, or eliminating them completely.
- Go easy on fish—Eating fish is not required for a healthy blue zones diet. The guidelines recommend that you eat fewer than three oz of fish, a few times a week or less.
- Snack on nuts—People in the blue zones typically enjoy a handful or two of nuts daily.
- Drink mostly water—Drinking adequate water (rather than dairy or sugar sweetened beverages) is encouraged. In the blue zones, water, coffee, tea, and sometimes wine in moderation are the core beverages.
- Daily dose of beans—Beans are a core part of the diet of many people in the blue zones. The food guidelines of the Blue Zones™ encourage you to have a half-cup to one cup each day.
- Go wholly whole—People in the blue zones eat a lot of whole foods. Sometimes they are enjoyed raw, and at other times, they are cooked. They also eat fermented food regularly. They avoid highly processed foods.
- 95–100 percent plant-based—Although most of the people in the blue zones don't exclude animal food products completely, the majority of what they eat each day comes from plants. The guidelines encourage you to prioritize a wide variety of plants and limit animal food products (meat, poultry, fish, dairy, and cheese). For more information on the Blue Zones™ and tasty recipes, visit www.bluezones.com.

There is a large gap between what Americans typically eat (also called the Standard American Diet—SAD) and the nutrition north star, a whole-food, plant-predominant eating pattern. Look at the Dietary Spectrum graphic detailed in Figure 6-7. Put an X where you think you are at on the spectrum. Next, put a star where you would like to be a year from now.

If your star is further along the spectrum than your X, you are wanting to move toward a more whole-food, plant-predominant way of eating. It can be confusing knowing where to start. The American College of Lifestyle Medicine has some wonderful resources for you.

Some people make a rapid, large switch when they start to eat healthier. The benefit of this type of switch is that you will likely notice that you feel better more quickly than if you take it slowly. However, some people do best when they make small changes and continue to move toward their goal. The right way to eat healthier is whatever way works best for you. Remember that it's a lifestyle and not a diet.

If you're moving toward a more plant-forward way of eating, look at Figure 6-9 and think about how you can move toward making your typical plate closer to what is shown on this graphic.

---

*For more information about lifestyle medicine and whole food, plant-based eating from the American College of Lifestyle Medicine, visit https://lifestylemedicine.org/project/patient-resources/ to get access to free resources including the Food as Medicine Jumpstart. Full Plate Living also has free resources for women who want to eat healthier. Visit https://www.fullplateliving.org/ to view their resources and recipes.

DIETARY SPECTRUM

AMERICAN COLLEGE OF Lifestyle Medicine

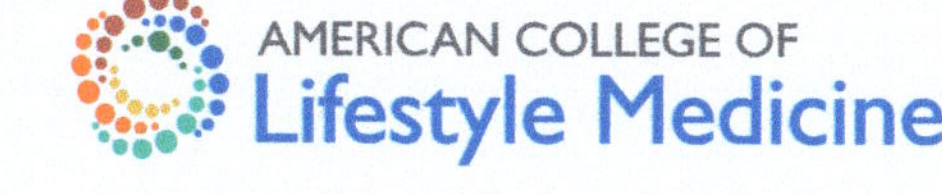

THE AMERICAN COLLEGE OF LIFESTYLE MEDICINE DIETARY POSITION STATEMENT

ACLM recommends an eating plan based predominantly on a variety of minimally processed vegetables, fruits, whole grains, legumes, nuts and seeds.

WHAT AMERICA EATS

WHOLE FOOD PLANT-BASED EATING PLAN

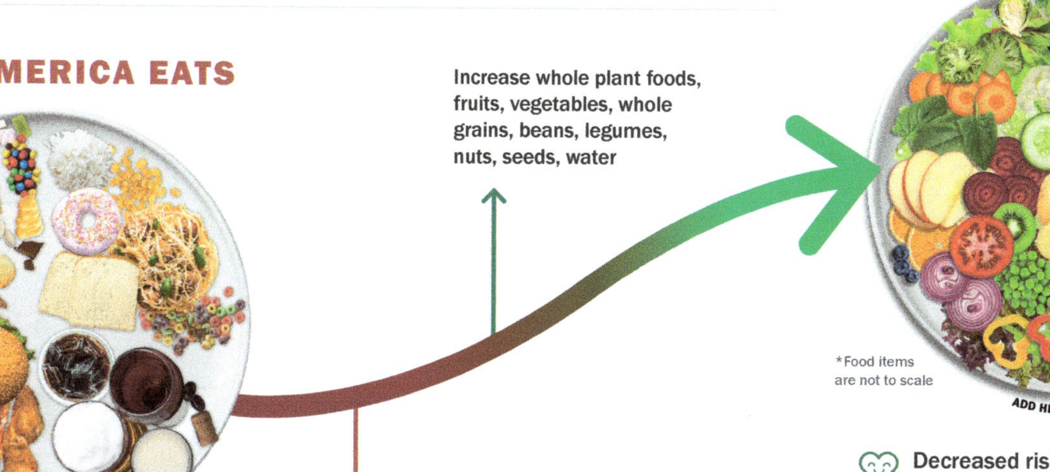

- Increased risk for Obesity, T2Diabetes, Heart Disease, and some Cancers
- Poor nutrition is the leading cause of death globally.

- Decreased risk for Obesity, T2Diabetes, Heart Disease, and some Cancers
- Chronic disease treatment and potential reversal

TIPS FOR IMPROVED NUTRITION AND HEALTH

- Any movement toward WFPB eating is positive
- More movement toward a WFPB eating plan increases impact
- Tailored and sustainable approaches are recommended

What We Eat in America (WWEIA) Food Category analyses for the 2015 Dietary Guidelines Advisory Committee. Estimates based on day 1 dietary recalls from WWEIA, NHANES 2009 2010.

Tuso PJ, Ismail MH, Ha BP, Bartolotto C. Nutritional update for physicians: plant-based diets. Perm J. 2013;17(2):61-66.

Food Planet Health. Eatforum.org. Published 2020. Accessed June 4, 2020

Figure 6-7. ACLM's dietary spectrum

GETTING STARTED

WHAT IS A WHOLE FOOD, PLANT-BASED DIET?

A whole food, plant-based diet is an eating pattern that emphasizes a variety of nutrient-dense, minimally processed vegetables, fruits, whole grains, beans and legumes, and nuts and seeds.

½ Fruits & Vegetables
¼ Plant Proteins
Drink Water
¼ Whole Grains
ADD HERBS & SPICES

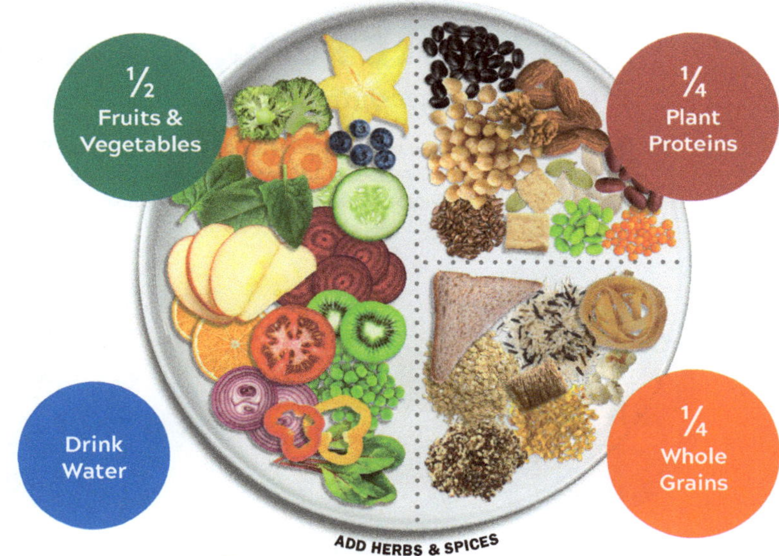

Focus on whole fruits and vegetables and eat a rainbow of color.

Vegetables: Dark leafy greens (spinach, kale, arugula, etc.), broccoli, squash, zucchini, carrots, tomatoes, beets, peppers, mushrooms, onions, celery, cauliflower, cucumbers, white & sweet potatoes, green peas, cabbage, whole plant fats (avocados, olives), and more.

Fruits: Apples, bananas, grapes, citrus fruit, berries, peaches, pears, pineapple, kiwi, plums, watermelon, starfruit, mangoes, just to name a few.

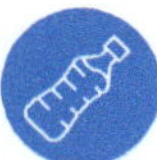

Drink water for hydration.

Add herbs and spices for flavor and antioxidant power.

Basil, cilantro, rosemary, parsley, thyme, dill, cumin, chili powder, pepper, turmeric, ginger, cinnamon, fennel, paprika, and many more.

Eat a variety of plant protein.

Legumes: Peas and beans, including kidney beans, pinto beans, white beans, black beans, lima beans, black-eyed peas, garbanzo beans (chickpeas), split peas and lentils, edamame, tofu.

Nuts and seeds: Almonds, pistachios, walnuts, pecans, nut butters, pumpkin/sunflower/chia/flax seeds, and more.

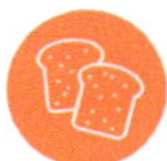

Choose whole grains.

Amaranth, barley, brown rice, buckwheat, bulgur, millet, popcorn, rye, quinoa, whole oats, whole grain bread/tortillas/cereals/flours, to name a few.

From *Food as Medicine Jumpstart* (Kayli Anderson, MS, RDN, ACSM-EP). © American College of Lifestyle Medicine; 2022. https://www.lifestylemedicine.org/

Figure 6-8. What is a whole food, plant-based diet?

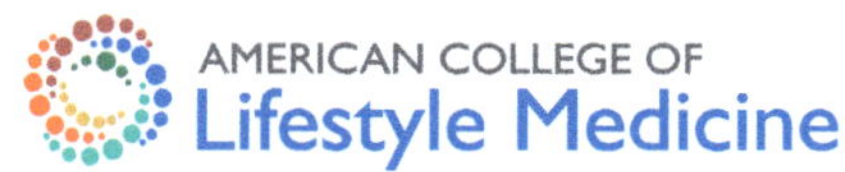

A WHOLE FOOD, PLANT-BASED PLATE

Nutrition Prescription for Treating & Reversing Chronic Disease

The American College of Lifestyle Medicine Dietary Lifestyle Position Statement for Treatment and Potential Reversal of Disease: ACLM recommends an eating plan based predominantly on a variety of minimally processed vegetables, fruits, whole grains, legumes, nuts and seeds.

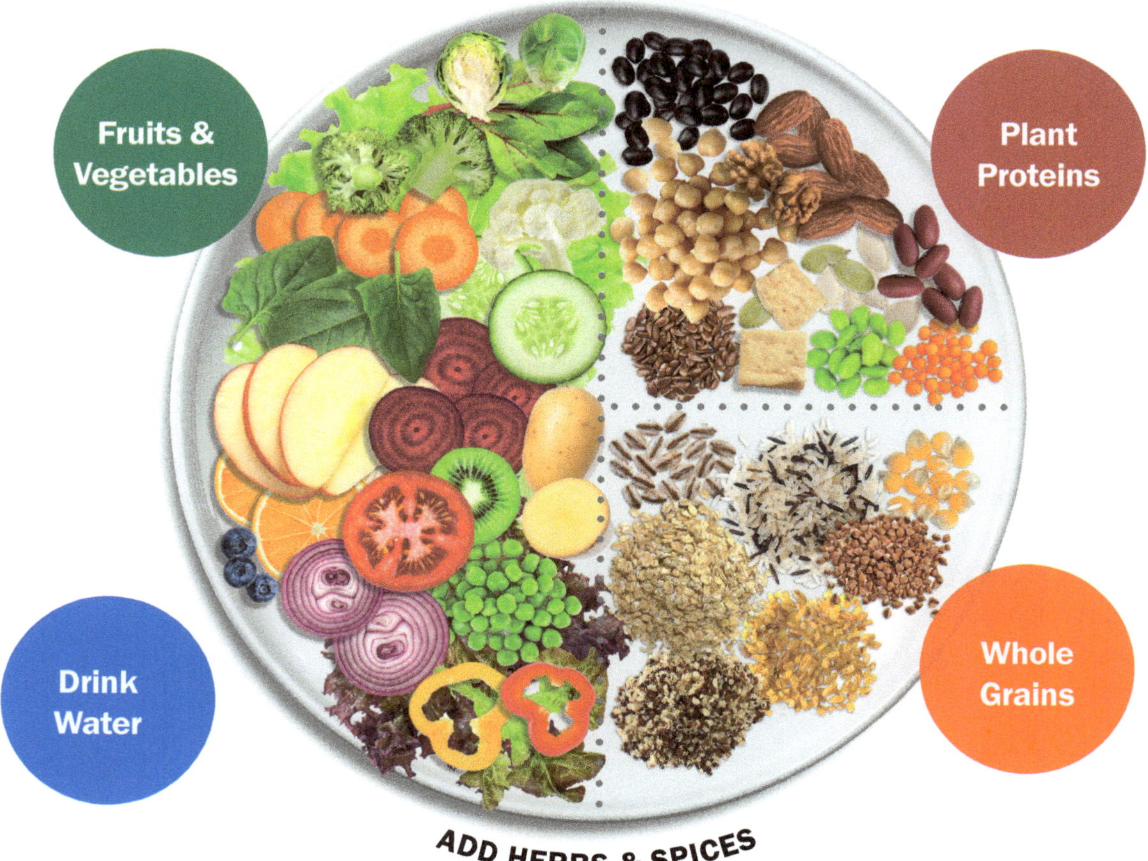

Include a wide array of fiber-filled, nutrient-dense, and antioxidant-rich whole plant foods at every meal. Use a variety of herbs and spices to enhance flavors.

lifestylemedicine.org

- **Focus on whole fruits and vegetables and eat a rainbow of color.**

Vegetables: Dark leafy greens (spinach, kale, arugula, etc.), broccoli, squash, zucchini, carrots, tomatoes, beets, peppers, mushrooms, onions, celery, cauliflower, cucumbers, white & sweet potatoes, green peas, cabbage, whole plant fats (avocados, olives), and more.

Fruits: Apples, bananas, grapes, citrus fruit, berries, peaches, pears, pineapple, kiwi, plums, watermelon, starfruit, mangoes, just to name a few.

- **Drink water for hydration.**

- **Eat a variety of plant protein.**

Legumes: Peas and beans, including kidney beans, pinto beans, white beans, black beans, lima beans, black-eyed peas, garbanzo beans (chickpeas), split peas and lentils, edamame, tofu.

Nuts and seeds: Almonds, pistachios, walnuts, pecans, nut butters, pumpkin/sunflower/chia/flax seeds, and more.

- **Choose whole grains.**

Amaranth, barley, brown rice, buckwheat, bulgur, millet, popcorn, rye, quinoa, whole oats, whole grain bread/tortillas/cereals/flours, to name a few.

Figure 6-9. ACLM's whole-food, plant-based plate graphic

AMERICAN COLLEGE OF
Lifestyle Medicine

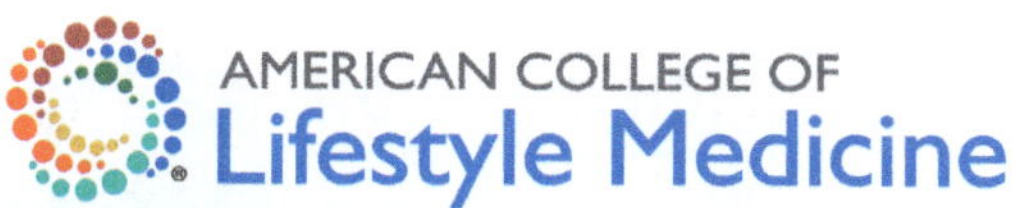

NUTRITION IN ACTION

Beans & Peas • Frijoles & Legumbres

- ☐ Black Beans / Frijoles Negros
- ☐ Black-eyed Peas / Frijoles de Ojo Negro
- ☐ Edamame / Haba de Soja
- ☐ Chickpeas / Garbanzo
- ☐ Kidney Beans / Habichuelas Rojas
- ☐ Lentils / Lentejas
- ☐ Lima Beans / Habas
- ☐ Navy Beans / Frijoles Blancos
- ☐ Peas / Chicharo
- ☐ Pigeon Peas / Guandules
- ☐ Pinto Beans / Frijoles Pintos

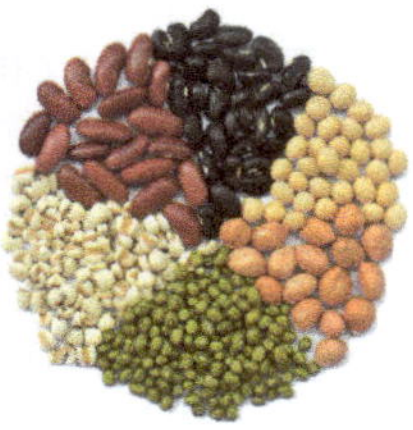

Nuts & Seeds • Nueces & Semillas

- ☐ Almonds / Almendras
- ☐ Brazil Nuts / Nueces de Brasil
- ☐ Chia Seeds / Servillas de Chia
- ☐ Flaxseeds / Linaza
- ☐ Hazelnuts / Avellanas
- ☐ Peanuts / Cacahuates
- ☐ Pecans / Nuez Pecana
- ☐ Pumpkin Seeds / Semillas de Calabaza
- ☐ Sunflower Seeds / Semillas de Girasol
- ☐ Walnuts / Nueces

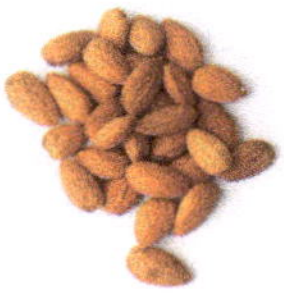

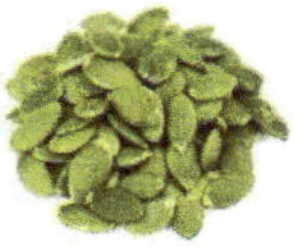

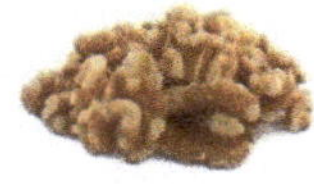

Grains • Granos

- ☐ Barley / Cebada
- ☐ Brown Rice / Arooz Integral
- ☐ Buckwheat / Alforfon
- ☐ Millet / Mijo
- ☐ Oats / Avena
- ☐ Quinoa / Quinoa
- ☐ Rye / Centeno
- ☐ Whole wheat / Trigo
- ☐ Whole grain Cornmeal / Harina de maiz de grano
- ☐ Whole wheat pasta / Pasta de trigo integral
- ☐ Wild Rice / Arroz Silvestre

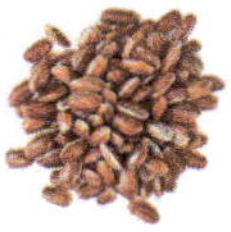

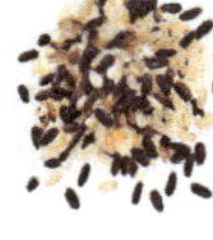

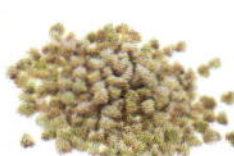

Notes

Figure 6-10. ACLM's nutrition in action

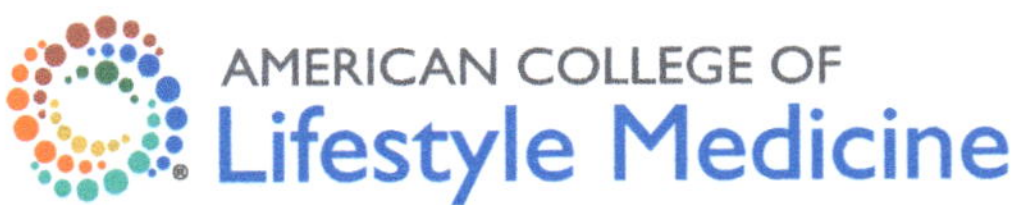

NUTRITION IN ACTION

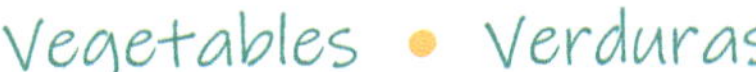

Super Foods Shopping List

Fruits • Frutas

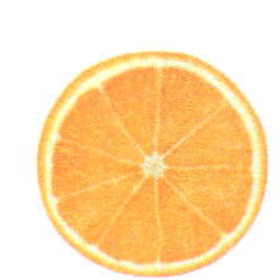

- ☐ Apples / Manzanas
- ☐ Apricots / Albaricoques
- ☐ Bananas / Platanos
- ☐ Blackberries / Frambuesas
- ☐ Blueberries / Zarzamoras
- ☐ Boysenberries / Moras
- ☐ Cantaloupe / Melon
- ☐ Cherimoya / Chirimoyas
- ☐ Cherries / Cerezas
- ☐ Tangerines / Mandarinas
- ☐ Cranberries / Arandanos
- ☐ Currants / Grosellas
- ☐ Figs / Higos
- ☐ Grapefruit / Toronja
- ☐ Grapes / Uvas
- ☐ Guava / Guayaba
- ☐ Honeydew Melon / Melon Verde
- ☐ Kiwi / Kiwi
- ☐ Lime / Lima
- ☐ Mango / Mango
- ☐ Nectarine / Chabacano
- ☐ Oranges / Naranjas
- ☐ Papaya / Papaya
- ☐ Passion Fruit / Fruta de la Pasion
- ☐ Peaches / Duraznos
- ☐ Pears / Peras
- ☐ Persimmons / Persimmons
- ☐ Pineapple / Pina
- ☐ Plantain / Plantano macho
- ☐ Plums / Ciruelas
- ☐ Pomegranate / Granada
- ☐ Quince / Membrillo
- ☐ Raspberries / Franbuesas
- ☐ Rhubarb / Ruibarbo
- ☐ Strawberries / Fresas
- ☐ Tamarind / Tamarindo
- ☐ Watermelon / Sandia

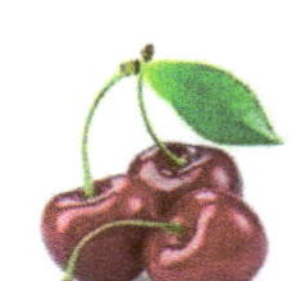

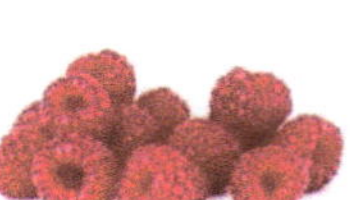

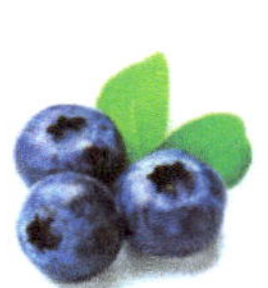

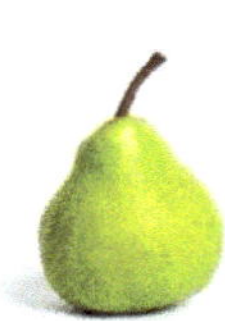

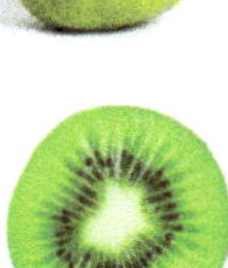

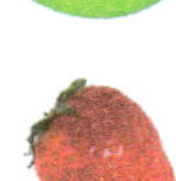

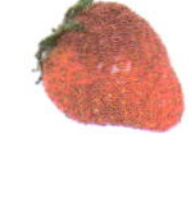

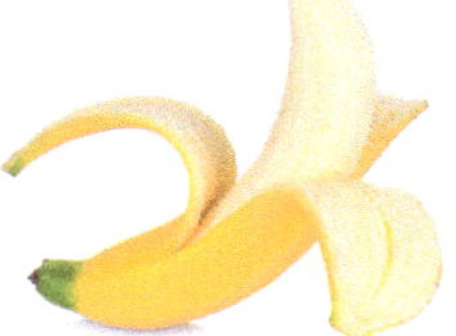

Vegetables • Verduras

- ☐ Artichokes / Alcachofa
- ☐ Asparagus / Esparragos
- ☐ Beet Greens / Hojas de Remolacha
- ☐ Beets / Betabel - Remolacha
- ☐ Bell Peppers / Pimentos
- ☐ Bok Choy / Col china
- ☐ Broccoli / Brocoli
- ☐ Broccoli Rabe / Brocoli de rabe
- ☐ Brussel Sprouts / Coles de bruselas
- ☐ Butterhead Lettuce / Lechuga manterquilla
- ☐ Watercress / Berros
- ☐ Carrots / Zanahorias
- ☐ Collard Greens / Berza
- ☐ Cauliflower / Coliflor
- ☐ Celery / Apio
- ☐ Chayote /Chayote
- ☐ Chili Peppers / Chiles
- ☐ Coriander / Cilantro
- ☐ Corn / Elote
- ☐ Cucumbers / Pepino
- ☐ Dandelion Greens / Dientes de leon
- ☐ Eggplant / Berenjena
- ☐ Endive Greens / Endivias
- ☐ Green Beans / Ejotes
- ☐ Green Cabbage / Col Verde
- ☐ Green Onions / Cebolla Verde
- ☐ Iceberg Lettuce / Lechuga repollada
- ☐ Jicama / Jicama
- ☐ Kale / Col rizada
- ☐ Kohlrabi / Colibano
- ☐ Leeks / Poro
- ☐ Mushrooms / Setas
- ☐ Mustard Greens / Hojas de Mostaza
- ☐ Nopales / Nopales
- ☐ Okra / Okra
- ☐ Onions / Cebollas
- ☐ Parsley / Perejil
- ☐ Parsnips / Chirivia
- ☐ Portobella Mushrooms / Hongos portobello
- ☐ Red Cabbage / Col Roja
- ☐ Romaine / Lechuga Romana
- ☐ Snow peas / Tirabeques
- ☐ Spinach / Espinaca
- ☐ Swiss Chard / Acelga
- ☐ Tomato / Tomate
- ☐ Zucchini / Calabaza

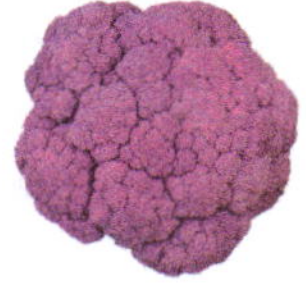

Figure 6-10. ACLM's nutrition in action (cont.)

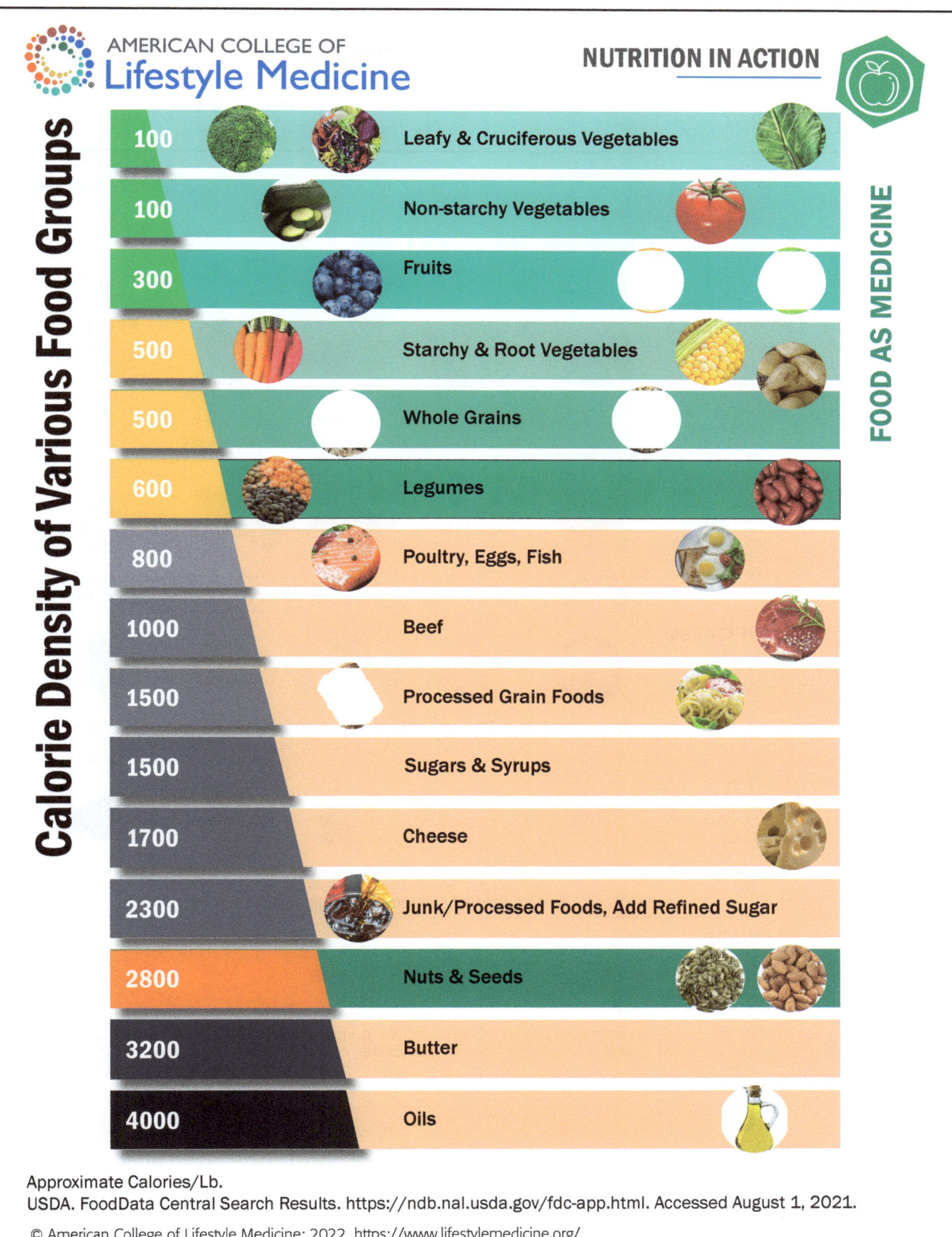

Figure 6-11. The calorie density of selected food groups

Whole-Food, Plant Predominant Recipes*

*From the American College of Lifestyle Medicine's Jumpstart Guide

Figures 6-12 to 6-14 provide examples of whole-food, plant-predominant recipes.

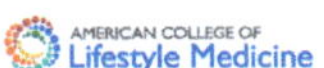

HOW TO MAKE A FILLING SALAD

1 LEAFY GREENS
Start with a hefty base of leafy greens, 2 to 3 cups

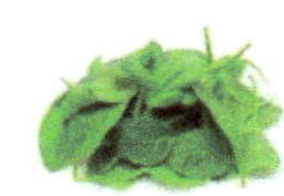
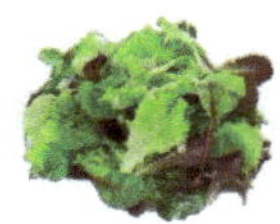
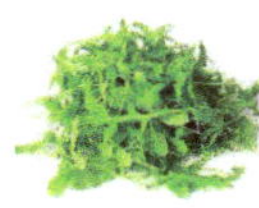
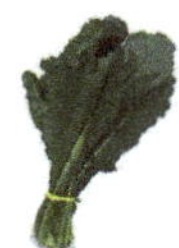
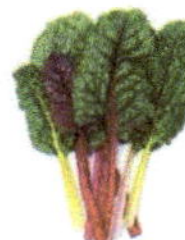

Baby spinach, chopped kale, Swiss chard, arugula, shredded cabbage, lettuce, spring mix, shaved Brussels sprouts, etc.

2 VEGETABLES
Add texture and color with a variety of vegetables, raw, steamed or roasted, unlimited

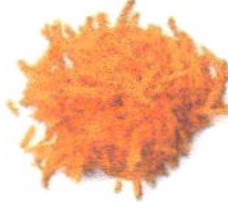
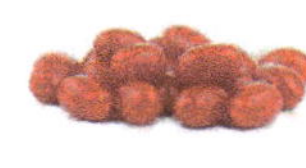
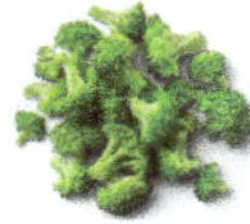
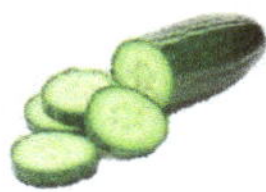
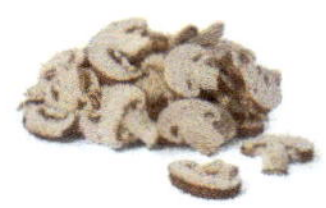

Artichoke hearts, asparagus, bell peppers, broccoli, carrots, cauliflower, cucumber, microgreens, mushrooms, onion, snap peas, summer squash, tomatoes, etc.

3 SMART CARBS
Add filling fiber with whole grains, starchy vegetables, and/or fruit, ½ cup

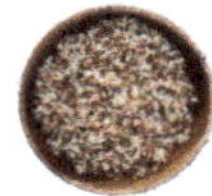
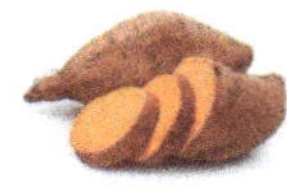
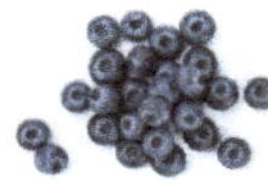
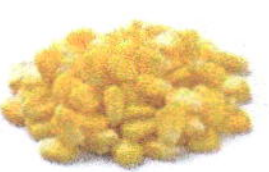
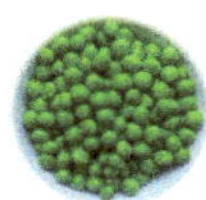

Quinoa, brown or wild rice, farro, barley, potatoes, yams, winter squash, corn, peas, mango, apples, berries, citrus segments, pomegranate seeds

4 PROTEIN
Add hearty plant protein with beans and legumes, ½ cup

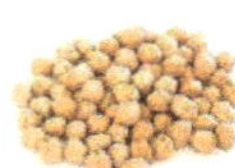
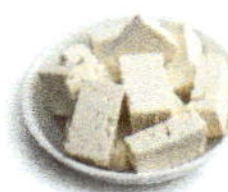
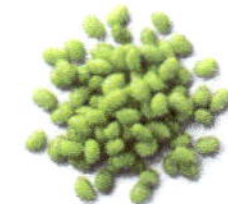
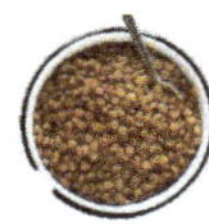
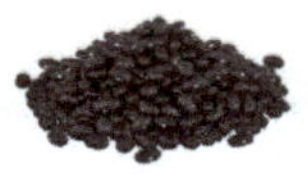

Chickpeas, black beans, kidney beans, white beans, green peas, lentils, edamame, organic tofu, organic tempeh

5 TOPPINGS
Add crunch & flavor with nuts, seeds, fresh herbs, and/or fermented foods, 1-2 tbsp

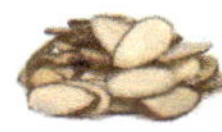
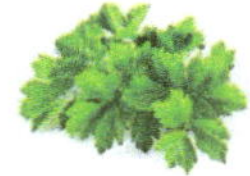
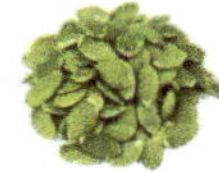
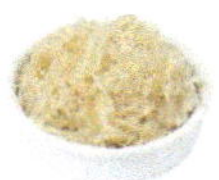
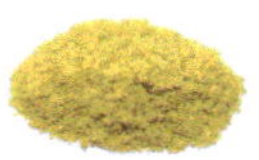

Almonds, walnuts, pistachios, pecans, pumpkin seeds, hemp seeds, nutritional yeast, sundried tomatoes, olives, basil, chives, cilantro, parsley, sauerkraut, kimchi, etc.

6 DRESSING
Add flavor with a squeeze of citrus, a dollop of dip, or a drizzle of dressing

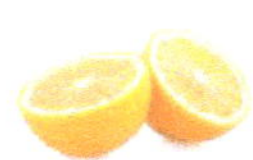
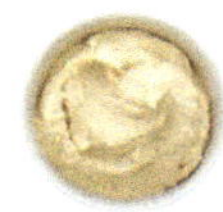
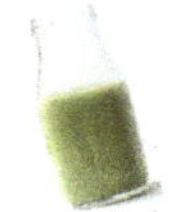
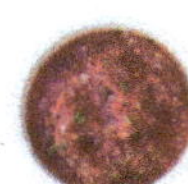
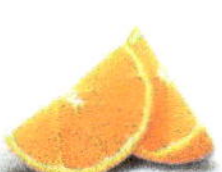

A squeeze of lemon, lime or orange juice, guacamole, balsamic vinegar, white wine vinegar, salsa, hummus, oil-free dressing

Figure 6-12. How to make a filling salad

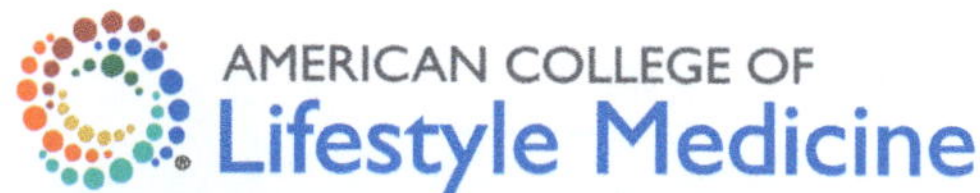

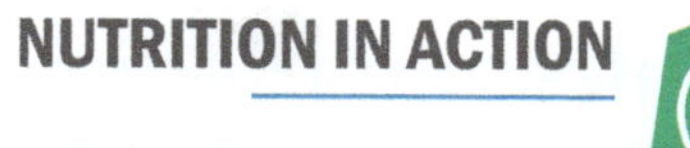

Green Smoothie Guide

1 LEAFY GREENS
Choose 1-2 cups, fresh or frozen

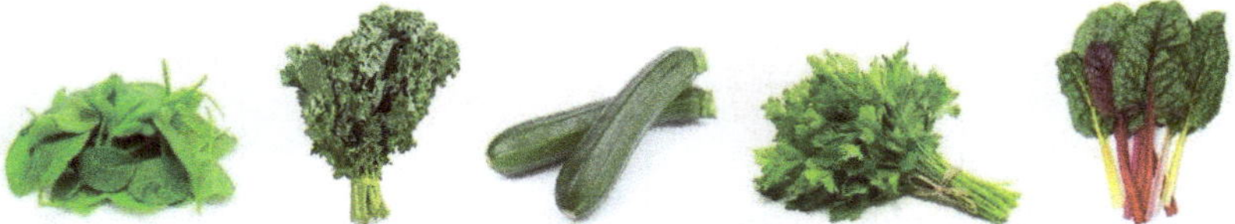

Spinach, kale, Swiss chard, arugula, parsley, cilantro (free to add other veggies like cauliflower, zucchini, carrots, beets or pumpkin)

2 FRUIT
Choose 1-2 cups, fresh or frozen

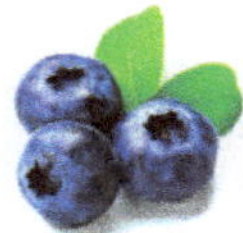
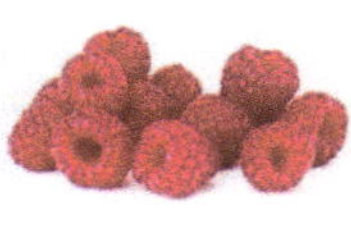
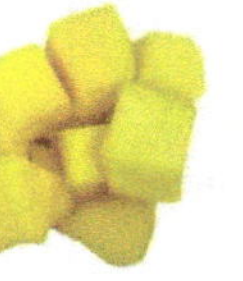
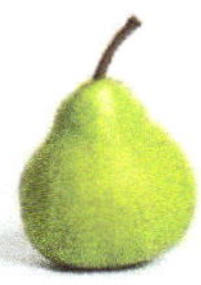
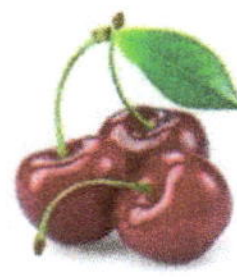

Blueberry, strawberry, raspberry, pear, pineapple, banana, apple, mango, cherries, peaches, etc.

3 PROTEIN
Choose 1 serving

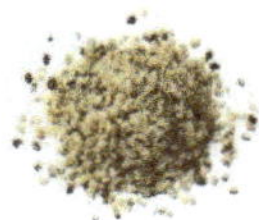
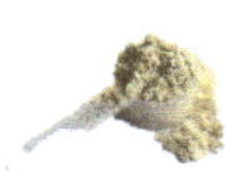
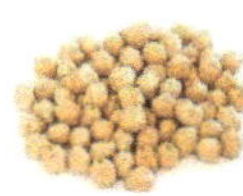
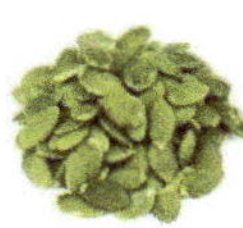
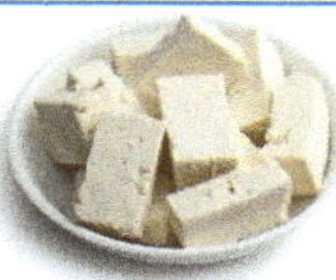

Hemp seeds (2-3 Tbsp), plant-based protein powder (½-1 scoop) organic silken tofu (1/2 cup), white beans or chickpeas (1/2 cup), unsweetened soy or pea milk (1 cup, counts as liquid too)

4 FAT & FIBER
Choose 1-2 tablespoons

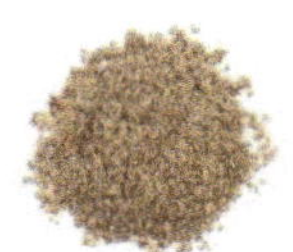
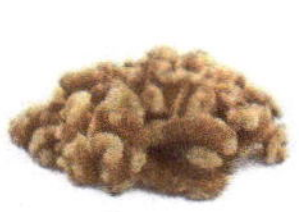
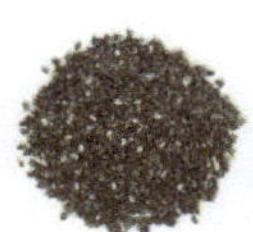
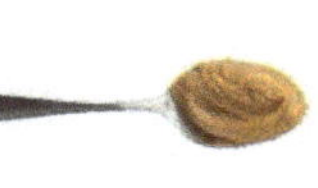
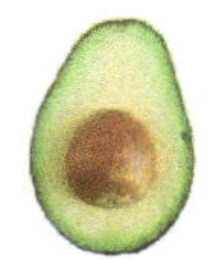

Flax meal, chia seeds, walnuts, avocado, nut butter

5 BOOSTERS
Optional, Choose ¼ - 1 teaspoon

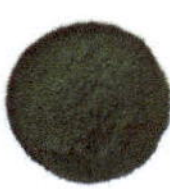
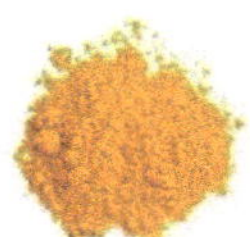
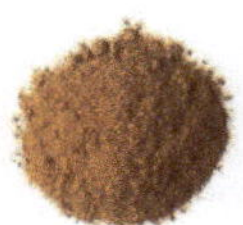
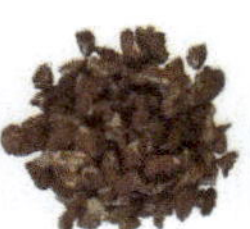
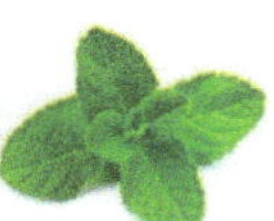

Spirulina, cinnamon, turmeric (+ black pepper), nutmeg, vanilla extract, Medjool date, ginger, cayenne, cacao powder, cacao nibs, mint

6 LIQUID
Choose 1-2 cups

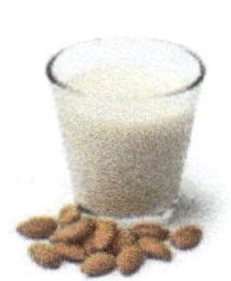
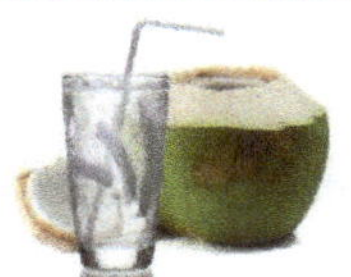
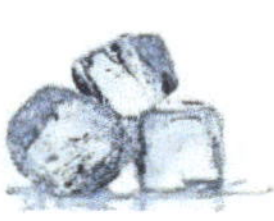
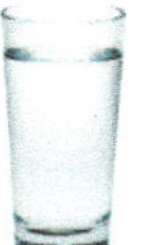
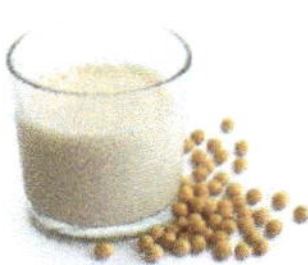

Filtered water, unsweetened plant milk (soy, pea, almond, cashew, oat, rice), unsweetened coconut water, green tea, ice for thickness

Figure 6-13. Green smoothie guide

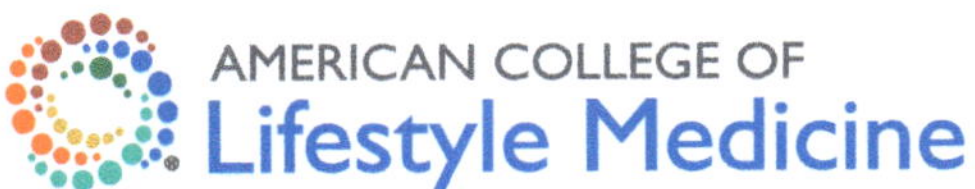

NUTRITION IN ACTION

HOW TO MAKE A NOURISH BOWL

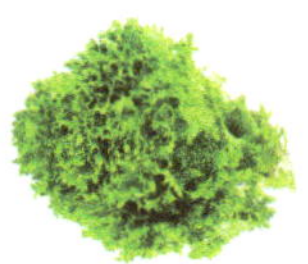 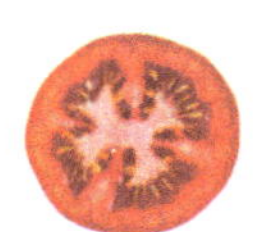 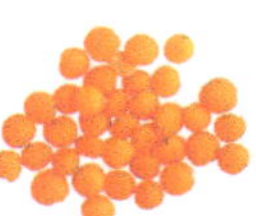 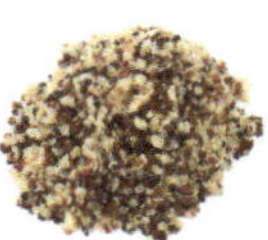 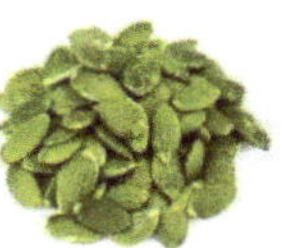 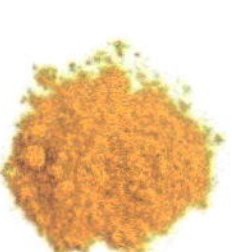

LEAFY GREENS *2-3 handfuls, raw or lightly cooked*	**OTHER VEGGIES** *1 cup, raw, steamed or roasted*	**PROTEIN** *½ - 1 cup*	**FIBER-RICH CARBS** *½ - 1 cup*	**HEALTHY FATS** *limit 1-2 to toppings*	**TOPPERS** *flavor elements*
arugula	artichoke hearts	beans: garbanzo, black, kidney	whole grains: quinoa, brown rice, millet, farro	avocado (¼)	lemon/lime juice
spinach	broccoli	lentils	sweet potato	olives (5)	fresh herbs: mint, parsley, cilantro, chives
kale	cauliflower	edamame	winter squash	nuts: walnuts, almonds, pistachio (1 Tbl.)	nutritional yeast
lettuce	carrots	organic tofu	corn	seeds: pumpkin, hemp, sesame (1 Tbl.)	vinegar: balsamic, apple cider, white
Swiss chard	bell pepper	organic tempeh	peas	hummus (2 Tbl.)	spice blends
shaved brussel sprouts	cucumber		fruit: berries, apples, oranges	dressing (1 Tbl.)	salsa
spring mix	green beans				
shredded cabbage	red onion				
	zucchini				
	summer squash				
	snap peas				
	tomatoes				

Nourish bowls are a simple way to assemble a meal utilizing already prepared food or ingredients you have in your pantry. A mix of dark leafy greens, protein, complex carbohydrates, vegetables, and healthy fats will provide you with energy and help you feel fuller for longer. Try different herbs, spices and sauces to add variety throughout the week.

Burrito Bowl
Romaine + grilled peppers + roasted sweet potato + black beans + salsa, cilantro, & lime juice

Mediterranean Bowl
Arugula + chopped tomato, cucumber, & red onion + garbanzo beans + quinoa + avacado + lemon juice

Asian Peanut Bowl
Massaged kale (with lime juice) + sliced cucumber & shredded carrots + edamame + brown rice + chopped peanuts + lime juice

Tofu Nicoise
Bibb lettuce + steamed green beans & sliced tomato + baked tofu + steamed new potatoes + sliced olives + Dijon dressing

Tahini Bowl
Spring mix + roasted broccoli & cauliflower + farro + lentils + mint & lemon tahini dressing

Figure 6-14. How to make a nourish bowl

Also keep in mind calorie density, especially if you are working on attaining a healthier weight. The calorie density graphic shown in Figure 6-11 will help you to understand that caloric density does not necessarily equal nutrient density. In fact, many of the lowest calorie-density foods are the most nutritious, such as leafy and cruciferous vegetables, non-starchy vegetables, and fruit. Just because a food has a very high-calorie density does not mean that you should avoid it. For example, nuts and seeds have a high-caloric density, however, they are very nutrient-rich and part of a healthy way of eating. If you are trying to maintain or lose weight, it's important to be mindful of your portion sizes, when you are eating calorie-dense foods, so that you don't regularly consume too many calories, causing unwanted weight gain.

A common concern when changing eating habits is whether the new way of eating will cost more. Many foods included in plant-predominant eating are relatively inexpensive (such as rice and beans).

The shopping list from the American College of Lifestyle Medicine, shown in Figure 6-10, is a great tool to use if you want to incorporate more plants in what you eat.

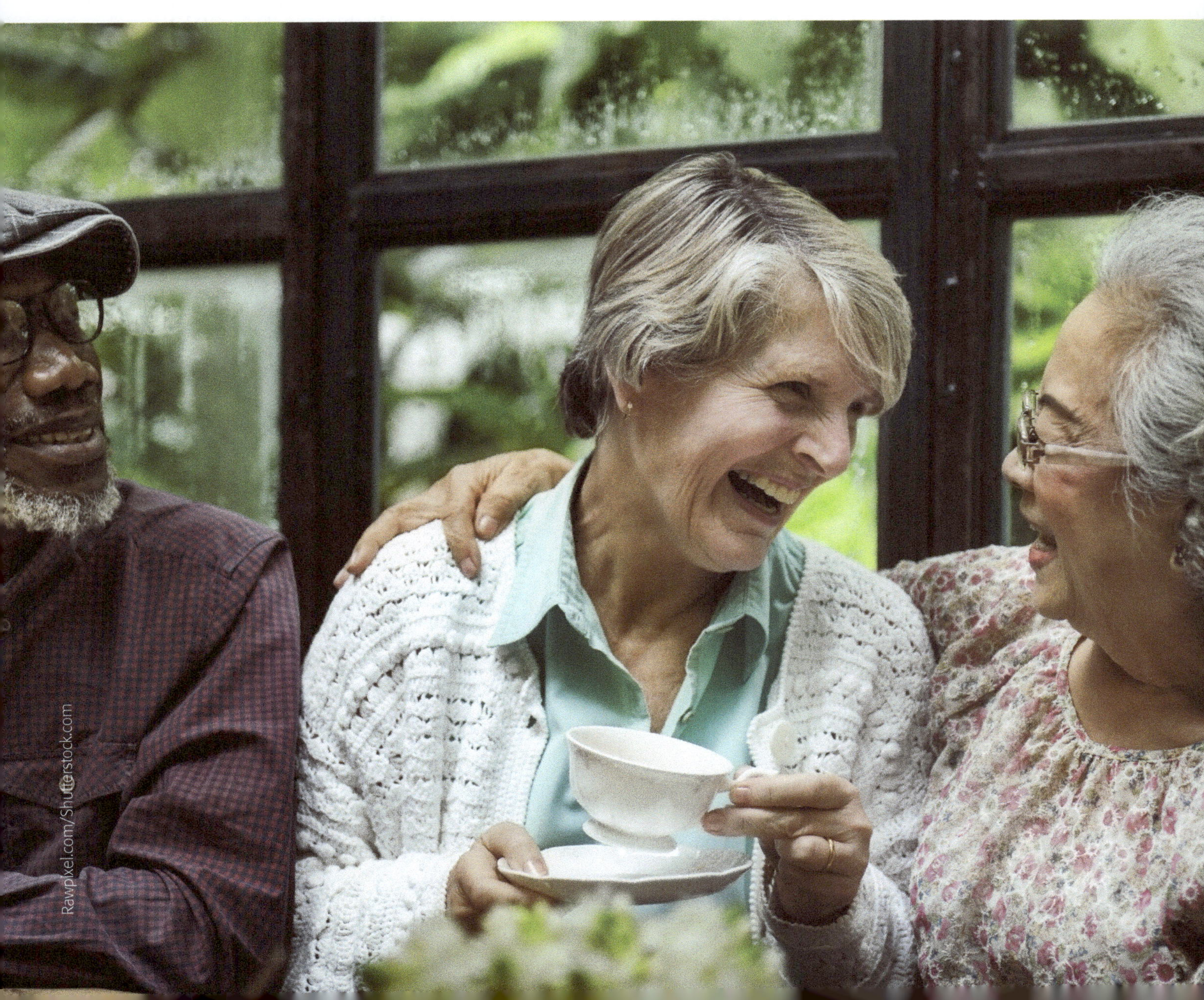

Rawpixel.com/Shutterstock.com

Nutrition Wrap-Up

Exploring your eating patterns and working towards a nutrient-dense eating style will help your overall health, especially during menopause and beyond. Being compassionate with yourself around diets and striving toward non-judgmental language supports a positive relationship with food. Choosing nourishing food helps your body, mind, and spirit.

For more information on whole-food, plant-based eating as well as healthy eating on a budget, visit the American College of Lifestyle Medicine's website at https://lifestylemedicine.org/project/patient-resources/ to access free resources.

References

1. U.S. Department of Agriculture and U.S. Department of Health and Human Services. Dietary Guidelines for Americans, 2020-2025. 9th Edition. December 2020. Available at DietaryGuidelines.gov.
2. Buettner D. *The Blue Zones: 9 Lessons for Living Longer From the People Who've Lived the Longest.* National Geographic Books: Washington, D.C.; 2012.

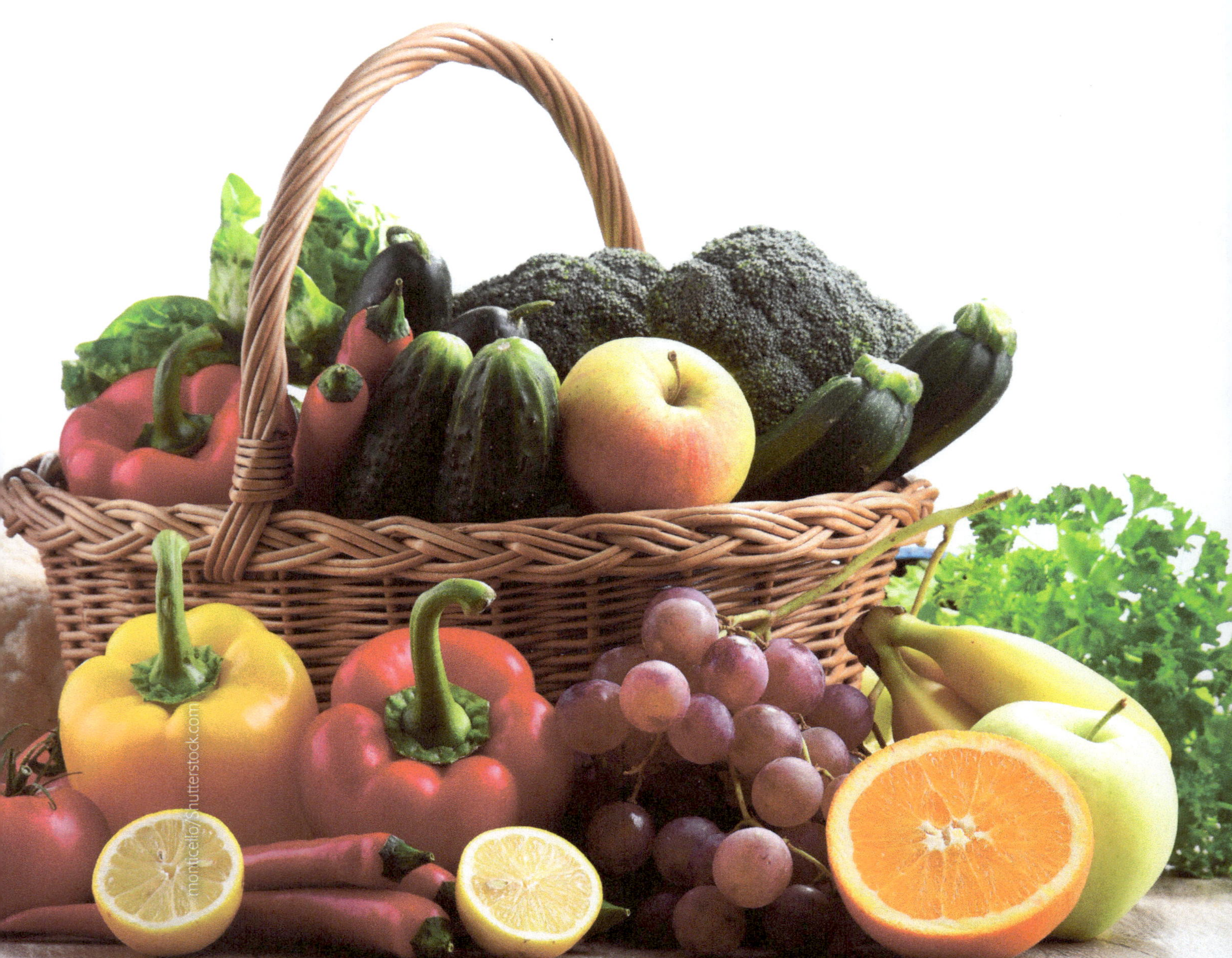

CHAPTER 7
GOALS

Goals Throughout Menopause, Midlife, and Beyond

Acronym—GOALS

Greatness
Opportunities
Attitude
Learn
Smart

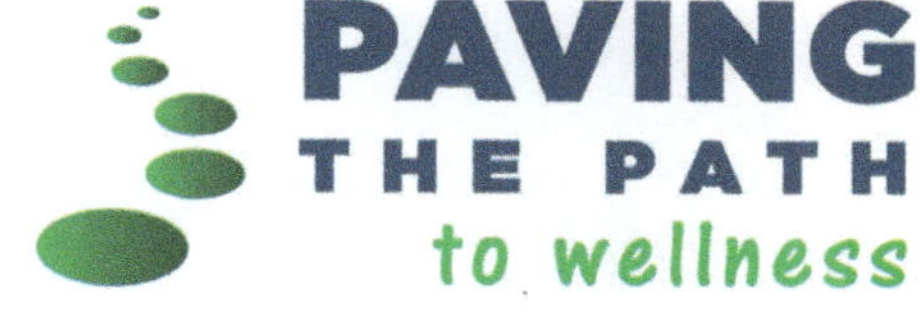

- *GREATNESS:* Goal-setting can help you attain greatness. Setting goals increases your likelihood of success when trying to reach new heights. So, don't be afraid to reach for the stars and work toward goals that connect with your purpose.
- *OPPORTUNITIES:* Look for opportunities to set goals. Anytime you want to change a behavior, set a goal. No behavior change is too big or too small.
- *ATTITUDE:* Having a positive attitude toward behavior change increases your chances of successfully achieving your goals. Engaging in positive self-talk and embracing a growth mindset will help you have an attitude that supports your well-being.
- *LEARN:* Whether or not you reach your goal, you can learn from the experience. If you attain your goal, consider what helped you succeed. If you are unsuccessful, learn from the obstacles you faced and brainstorm how you might overcome similar challenges in the future.
- *SMART:* When you commit to a goal, make sure it follows the SMART goal format. Your goals should be specific, measurable, action-oriented, realistic, and time-sensitive. Follow this format, and you'll increase your chances of success.

Having goals allows you to focus your energy and live a more purpose-filled life. Without goals, you may put energy into various activities that pull you in multiple directions, like wandering off and getting lost in the woods. Goals point you in the right direction and keep you moving along a path. Even if you don't succeed in reaching a particular goal, you direct your energy toward forward movement along your path. You need a north star and a guiding light which is often a vision for your future. Vision casting is a prerequisite in many ways to goal-setting.

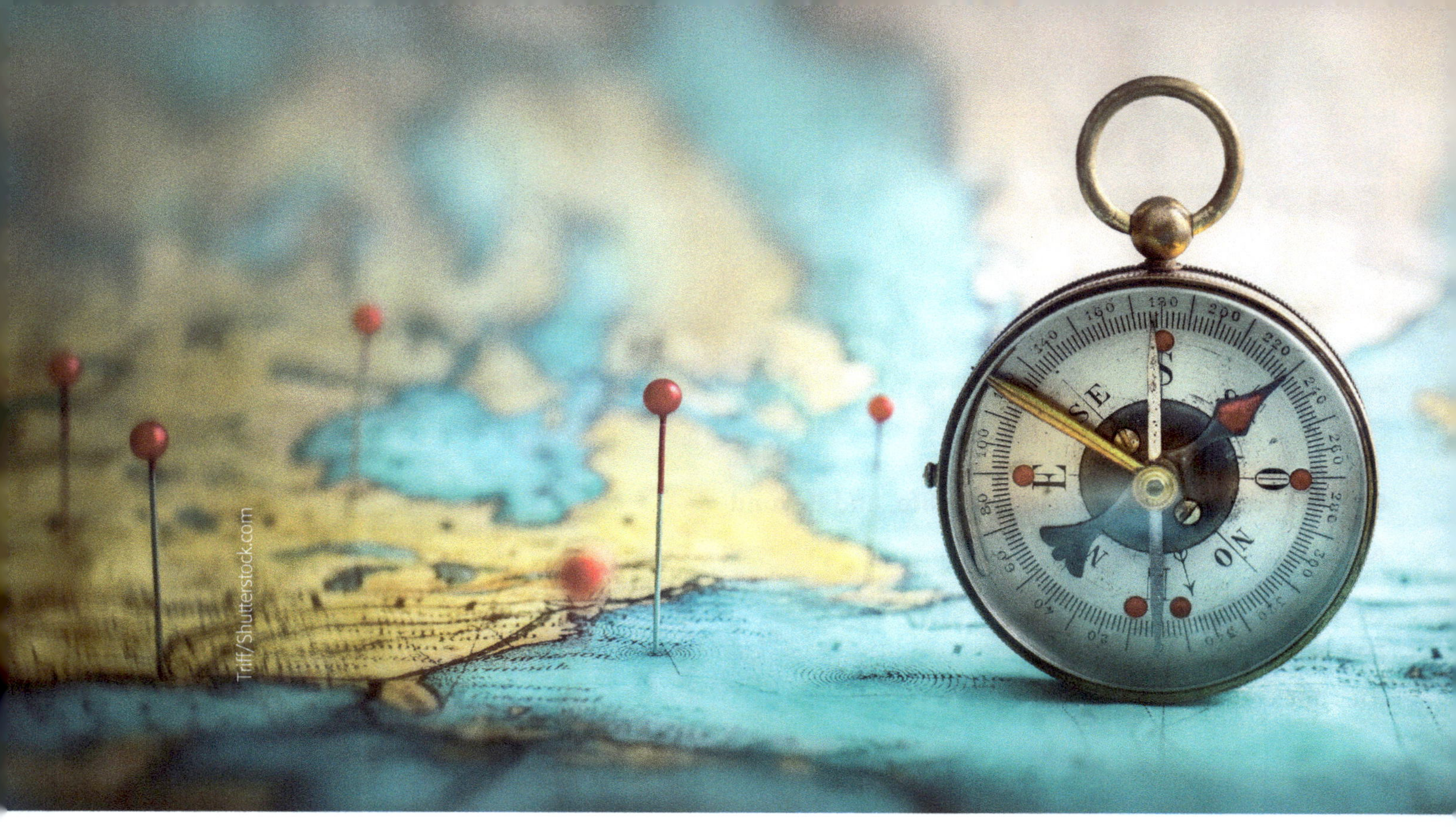

Triff/Shutterstock.com

Vision Casting and Your North Star

Vision casting invites you to consider what life will be like for you in 5, 10, or 20 years. The choice is yours. Then, use all of your senses to visualize yourself at that time. Think about what you are doing, what projects you are pursuing, the emotions that you are feeling around the relationships you are in, the way that your body is moving, the foods you are nourishing yourself with, the sleep that is restoring your energy levels, and especially, the things that excite you the most. When asked to think about their futures this way, some people are immediately drawn to titles and labels and maybe even weight and dress size, but this is, hopefully, not your focus. Envision how you want to BE in this world 5, 10, or 20 years from now.

❑ Describe your future vision of yourself.

____

____

____

❑ What steps do you need to take along your path to BE that person?

____

____

____

This is your north star, BEing the person you want to be, talking about things that interest you, moving comfortably through the physical world, loving the people in your life wholeheartedly, having a practice that brings you peace, and mindfully walking step-by-step to reach higher ground, striving to make the world a better place.

What is YOUR north star? By the time you reach midlife, most likely you have spent considerable time and energy helping others achieve their goals. If you are a parent, you've likely helped your children attain many goals, from learning to walk to graduating from high school. If you've been an employee, you've likely helped your company achieve annual goals that they would not have been able to reach without your support. Society even places goal expectations upon women, such as being cheerful, looking feminine, and having dinner ready for your family every night. Unfortunately, you may have lost yourself in all of this. Vision casting and goal-setting will help you find your way again.

Breaking Free From Boredom During Midlife and Beyond

Wake, eat, sleep, repeat. If you can relate to this, you may be caught in a monotonous cycle of repeating the same activities daily. This can lead to apathy, boredom, and "going through the motions" of life, which is not what anyone wants. Occasional boredom is usual, but you don't want it to permeate every aspect of your life. Although you likely do some non-glamorous activities daily (such as flossing your teeth and washing the dishes), even these activities can become more engaging through goal-setting. For example, you could set a goal to practice mindfulness while doing the dishes this week or think of three things you are grateful for while flossing. You can break free from boredom through goal-setting and re-energize your life.

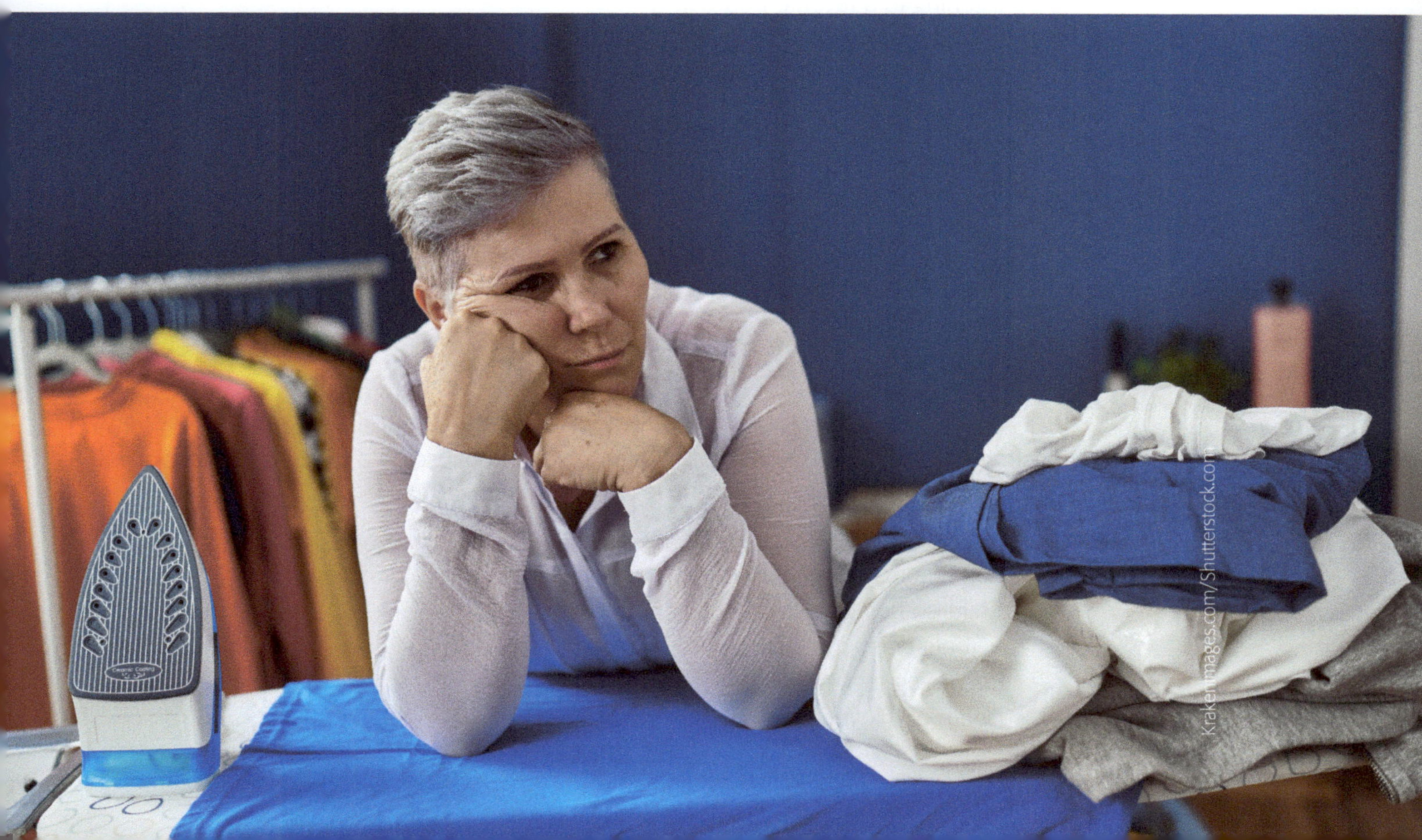

- [ ] What areas of your life do you find boring? These may be activities that seem monotonous or that you avoid doing because they do not currently bring you joy.

____

____

____

BREAKING FREE

- [ ] Evaluate whether the areas you noted in the previous question are worth your energy investment. For example, maybe there is a task that you no longer need to do or that you can delegate to someone else. If these are essential tasks or areas of your life that need attention, are they worth putting energy into through goal-setting to make them more enjoyable? Explain.

____

____

____

- [ ] Write down a goal that addresses one of these areas listed above that will help you break free from boredom in that area of your life. It can be a small goal, such as working on cleaning out your closet for five minutes every day this week while listening to a favorite podcast.

____

____

____

Although cleaning your closet or flossing your teeth may never be your favorite activities, goal-setting can energize how you accomplish these tasks and add joy to your life.

Midlife Transitions and Goals

From a medical point of view, menopause is a time of transition from higher to lower estrogen levels. For many midlife women, menopause is a time of transition that extends far beyond their hormone levels.

Among the common midlife transitions that occur in a woman's life are the following:

- Caring for children at home to children leaving home for college
- Children being single to children getting married
- Parents being independent to helping care for aging parents
- Becoming a grandparent
- Death of a loved one

- Death of a pet
- Enjoying relative health then managing chronic health conditions or getting an unexpected medical diagnosis
- Losing a job
- Changing place or type of career
- Suddenly reentering the workforce after more than two decades of parenting
- Marriage to a partner
- Separation or divorce from a life partner
- Being single for a long time or newly single—looking for a life partner
- Having regular periods to periods stopping and experiencing menopausal symptoms, such as hot flashes
- Living in a home independently to moving to a different living environment

Although uncertainty and anxiety can fill transitions, they can also be times of great potential. It's easy to remain passive or feel like a victim when moving from one stage in life to another, especially if it's not a desired transition. However, goal-setting during changes allows you to determine the direction of your future path. Time will march forward, and your journey will continue, but you have some control over your path, what you will do along your path, and how much joy you will experience.

❑ What transitions are you going through right now? Think beyond those that were detailed in the previous list. Your changes may not be as prominent as those listed. For example, adopting a new pet, getting a new certification in fitness training, downsizing your home, or renovating your house.

____

____

____

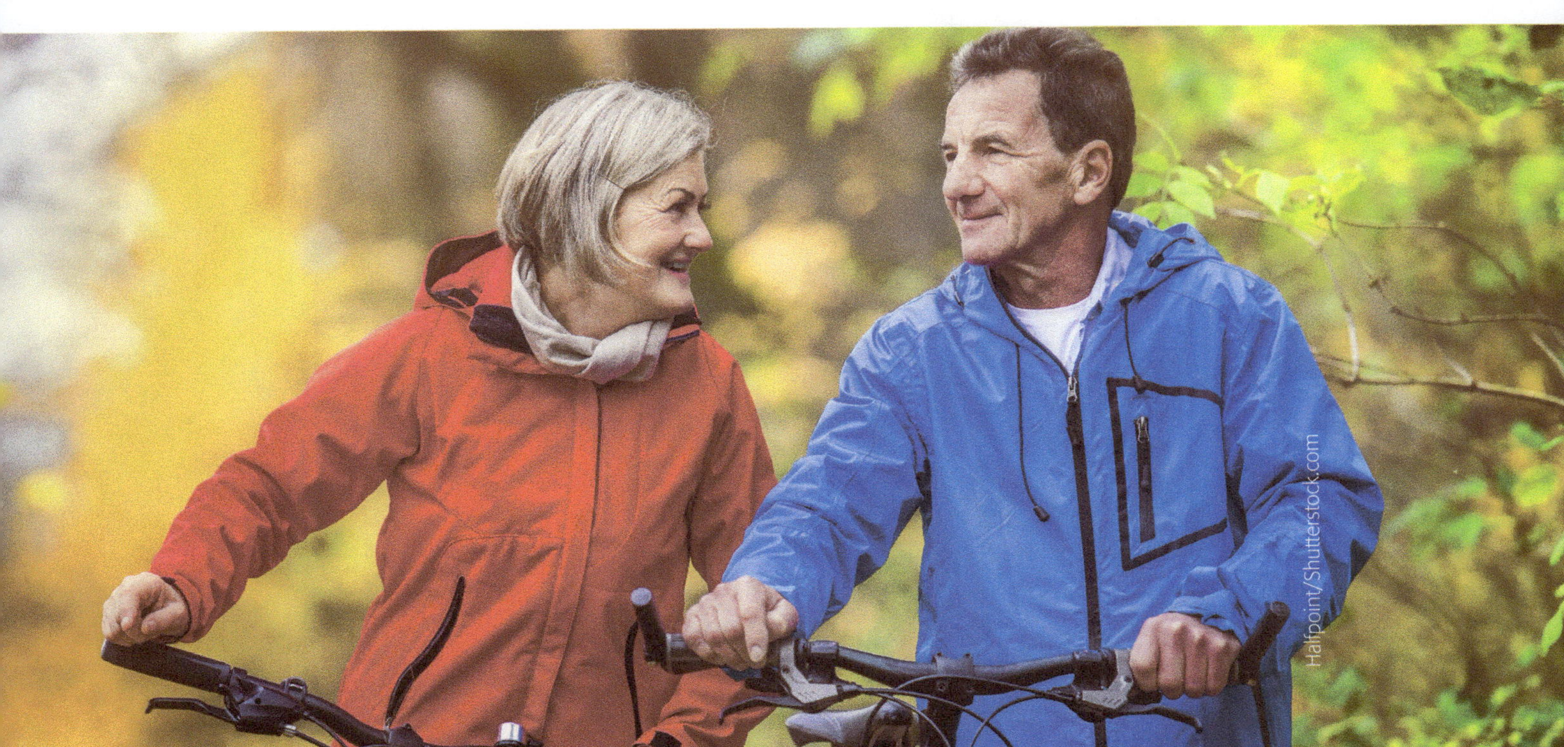
Halfpoint/Shutterstock.com

- ❑ Could you become more active in this transition process by setting a goal? Is there a goal that you could set that would help you with this transition? If so, describe the goal.

____

____

____

Fun Through Goal-Setting

You're never too old to have fun or start a new adventure. You deserve to have joy, excitement, and fun in your life. Goal-setting can help you achieve this. Women tend to set goals in areas where they already have some expertise. Midlife goal-setting is a great time to set goals in places where you have no expertise. For example, suppose you've never ridden a horse, spoken a second language, played a particular instrument, taken a stained glass-making class, or have any expertise in these areas. In that case, these could be excellent areas in which to set a goal (if they sound fun to you, too).

- ❑ What words come to mind when you think of fun, joy, and excitement? Brainstorm, and don't censor yourself. Write as many words as you can think of as quickly as possible.

____

____

____

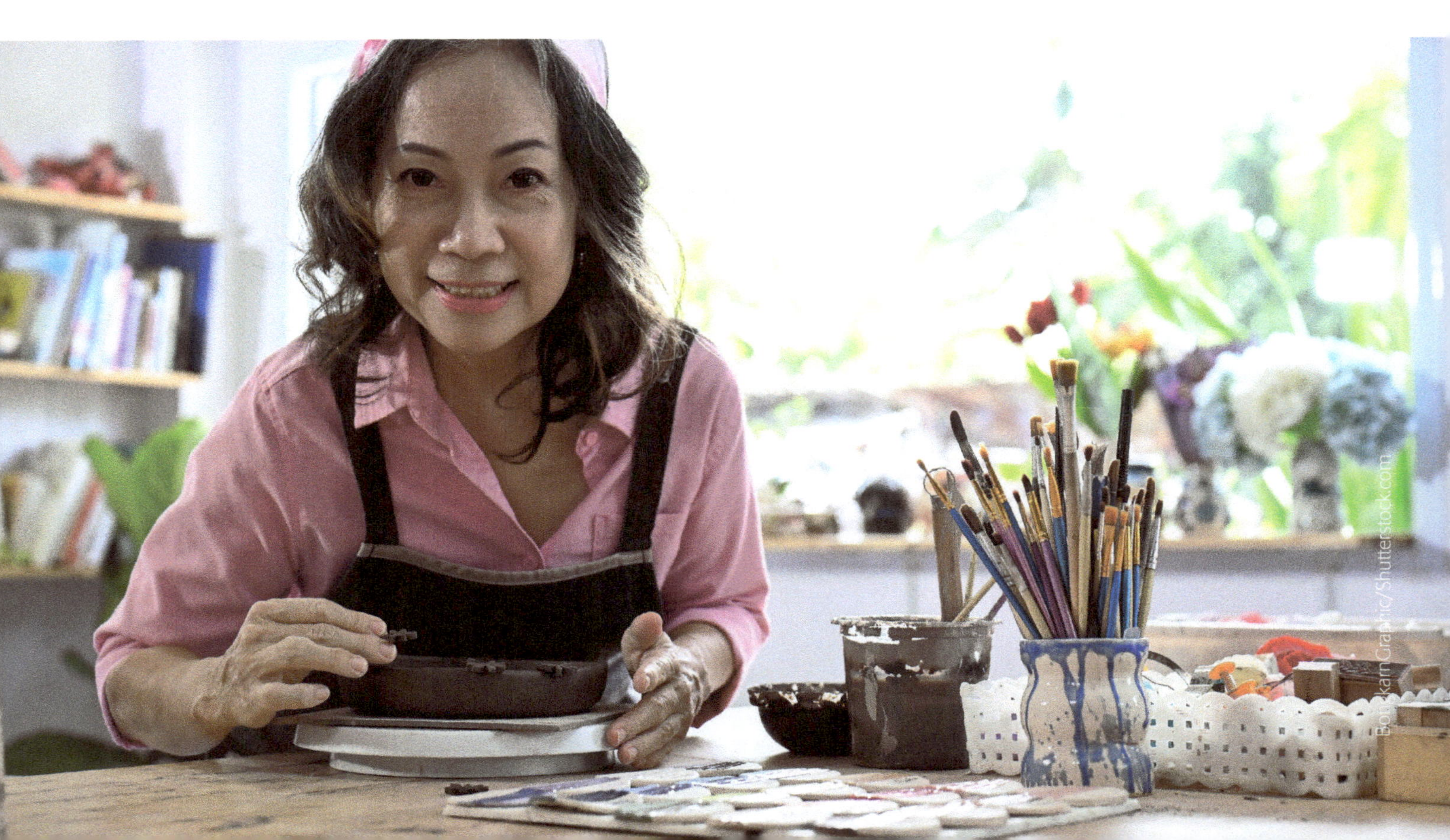

Boonkarn Graphic/Shutterstock.com

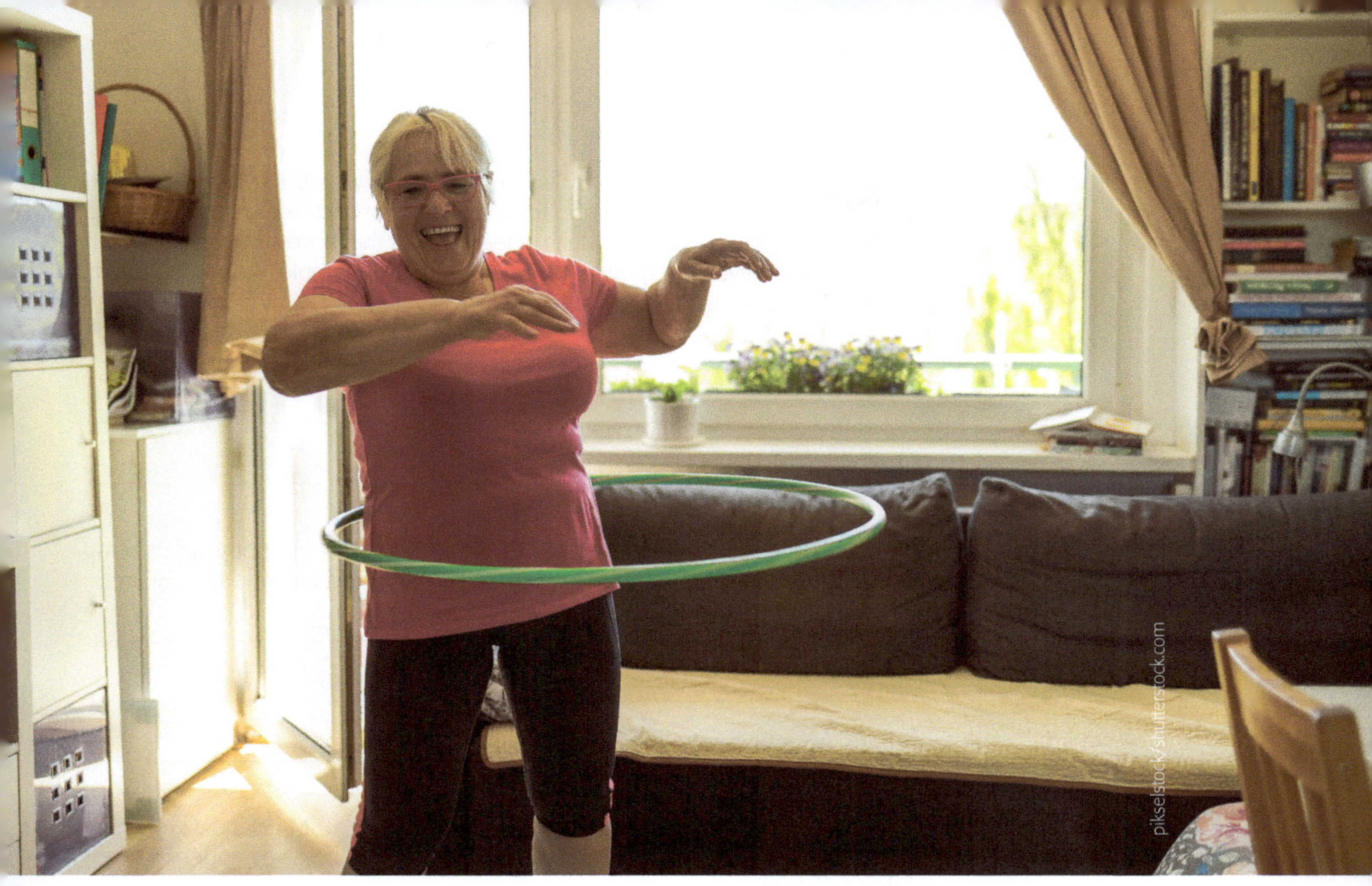
pikselstock/shutterstock.com

You may also want to set goals in areas that you don't have expertise. You can think of others, but some ideas to get you started include: travel, visiting parks, blowing bubbles, hula hooping, taking naps, reading historical fiction books, listening to a favorite podcast, going to the movies with friends, walking in a park, playing with grandkids, having tea with your partner, visiting animals at the zoo, going to the theater, skydiving, roller skating, eating chocolate, playing scrabble, glass blowing classes, shopping at your favorite store, savoring some herbal tea with a friend, hiking a mountain, making sandcastles, snowshoeing, playing with children at a playground, taking photographs of flowers, going for a walk with a dog, watching fish at a pet store, trying a new recipe, organizing your closet, volunteering at a local library, or donating your old clothes to a non-profit organization.

❑ List your top three options from this list or add your own ideas.

____

____

____

Remember, the journey is just as important (and sometimes more important) than achieving the goal. For example, even if you make a vase that won't stand up straight while taking a glass-blowing lesson, you can still have fun, enjoying the experience of learning a new skill.

- ❑ After looking at the aforementioned list, choose three words that inspire you to create a goal that would be fun for you to work toward or that would add adventure to your life, and write them below. Make at least one of these words be related to an area in which you have no expertise or experience. For example, your three words could be creativity, family, and the outdoors.

  ____

  ____

  ____

- ❑ Write three initial goals (one for each word) that excite you. Don't worry about being successful at this time. Just think of having fun and adding adventure to your life.

  ____

  ____

  ____

- ❑ Now, pick at least one of these three goals and make it a SMART goal. You may have chosen a very large or long-term plan. If so, consider breaking your significant goal into smaller pieces.

  ____

  ____

  ____

As noted previously, making your goals SMART goals will increase your chances of success. Smart goals are specific, measurable, action-oriented, realistic, and time-sensitive. For example, a SMART goal could be that you will visit the local botanical gardens with your friend next Tuesday morning.

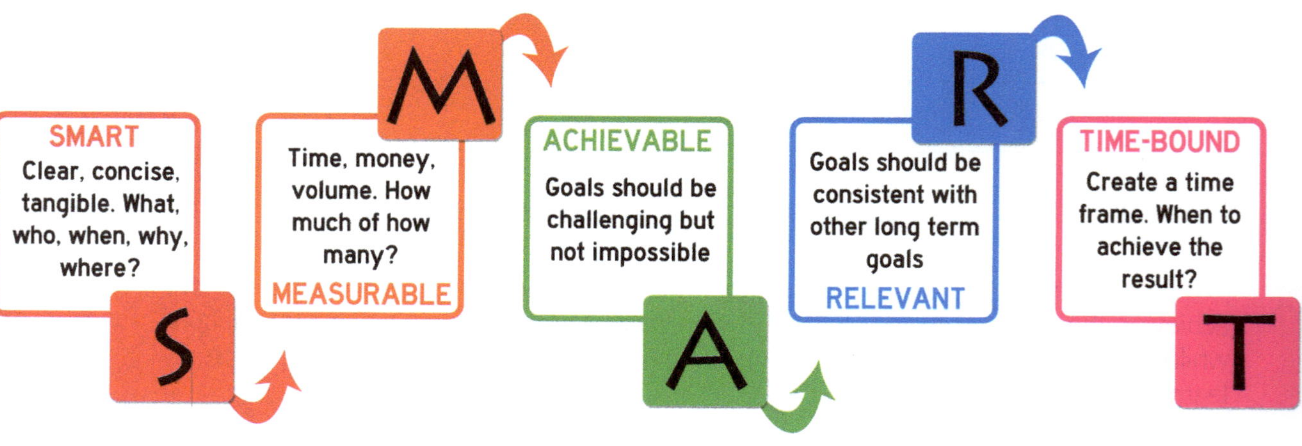

desdemona72/Shutterstock.com

The Goal-Purpose Connection

Later in this book, you'll focus on purpose in-depth, and you'll have a chance to explore areas of purpose in your life. Discussing purpose in this chapter is essential, since goals allow you to achieve your purpose. Knowing your purpose without having goals is like knowing the end destination of your journey but not having a map to help you get from where you are now to where you want to end. Goals help point you in the right direction and encourage you to take steps to move you closer to your purpose. Even if you aren't successful in achieving a planned goal, you will typically have moved closer to your desired destination and learned valuable information along the way.

❑ Circle the following phrases that resonate the most with you, or write other statements that connect with your sense of purpose. You may find that several of these ideas align with your purpose:

- Connecting deeply with your family or others
- Serving others in your community or elsewhere
- Standing up for those who are less fortunate
- Fighting for justice in a certain area
- Aligning your actions with your spiritual beliefs
- Being successful in __________
- Experiencing joy
- Loving others deeply
- Living into your full potential
- Making the world a better place
- Sharing your creative gifts with others
- Using your creativity with music or art to beautify the world
- Providing healing to others
- Being an example of integrity, compassion, and love
- Mentoring younger generations
- Finding ways to supply healthy foods to food deserts
- Gardening to provide fresh produce for your family and others
- Cooking nutritious meals for yourself, your family, and others
- Connecting with other people in your community while engaging in spiritual or religious activities
- Sharing your journey with others to help empower them along their way
- Learning from your past struggles and finding ways to help others, based on what you have learned
- Raising your children to contribute to society in a positive way
- Taking care of your pets and enjoying their companionship
- Staying healthy with an active body, peaceful mind, and joyful heart so that you can continue to contribute in your unique way
- Learning about the world around you, experiencing new cultures, speaking new languages, and connecting with people from all over the world to unite everyone as one

Pick one of the areas you circled that you want to address through writing a goal. Although what you circled may feel too ambitious or lofty to align with a realistic goal for you, remember that plans help you move in your desired direction. For example, if you circled "making the world a better place," you may want to call a friend who cannot get out of their home or contact a local food pantry to see if you could volunteer some time with that individual.

❑ Write a goal that aligns with an area that you circled above. Make sure that it is a SMART goal.

____

____

____

Dimensions of Wellness

As a busy woman, it's easy to become so focused on one area of well-being that you neglect other important areas of wellness. For example, maybe you've been very focused on your physical and financial health but neglected your sexual and spiritual health. Goal-setting can help you mindfully address your well-being dimensions that could use some attention.

In reality, several dimensions of health and well-being exist, including the following:

- Physical health
- Emotional and mental health
- Spiritual health
- Occupational or vocational health
- Financial health
- Sexual health
- Environmental health
- Social health
- Intellectual health

Circle the area(s) on the aforementioned list that you may have neglected or want to focus on with a goal. Then, read the following list of other areas that you may want to address through goal-setting and circle any items you would like to focus on this month or year:

- Exercise
- Nutrition
- Sleep
- Stress
- Brain health (e.g., dementia prevention, mood, cognition, memory)
- Body composition or weight (e.g., maintaining or gaining more muscle through strength training)
- Symptoms of menopause (e.g., addressing hot flashes or vaginal dryness)

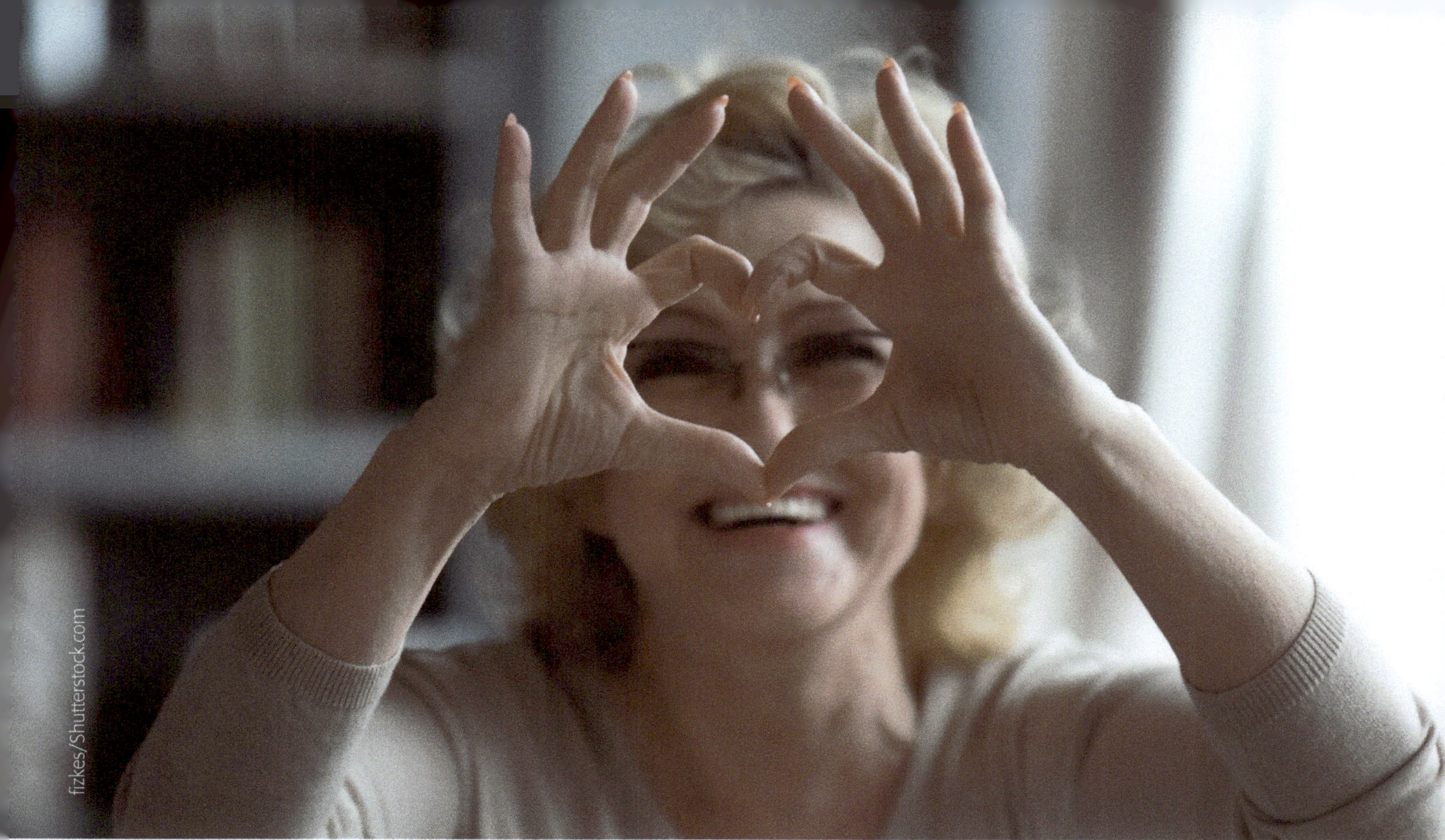
fizkes/Shutterstock.com

- Sexual health (e.g., addressing an issue with your gynecologist or reading a book to learn more)
- Confidence and pride in yourself as a middle-aged woman
- Prioritizing self-care time
- Social connection and network (e.g., connecting with others or creating a shared/team goal)
- Focus on family, marriage, partner, children, etc.
- Environment (e.g., cleaning an area of your home, making your bedroom more ideal for sleep, etc.)
- Making and honoring boundaries, and saying "no" when appropriate
- Cooking
- Gardening
- Making or listening to music
- Meditation and mindfulness
- Reading for pleasure
- Travel getaways by yourself or with a loved one

❑ Write three goals that connect with those areas that you circled in this list. Remember to make them SMART goals.

____

____

____

Habit Tracking

Tracking health habits that you are trying to change can increase your chances of success. You can use the Habit Tracker from the American College of Lifestyle Medicine to track your health habits (Figure 7-1). Also, there are numerous phone applications that can be used to track your health behaviors, such as the Daily Dozen application from Nutrition Facts.org.

Coaching Yourself on Goal-Setting With the COACH Approach

You can use the COACH Approach to help you create and be successful with your goals.

CURIOSITY

Throughout this chapter, you have explored areas you may want to focus on when creating goals. You've also written goals that align with these areas of importance in your life.

- ☐ Now is the time to get curious. Review the goals you have written and select three that you are excited about or feel called to address this week. Rewrite those goals in the following space provided.

  ____

  ____

  ____

- ☐ Why do you think these goals are exciting or are calling to you the most?

  ____

  ____

  ____

  ____

- ☐ What about these areas creates a childlike wonder for you and a desire to explore?

  ____

  ____

  ____

  ____

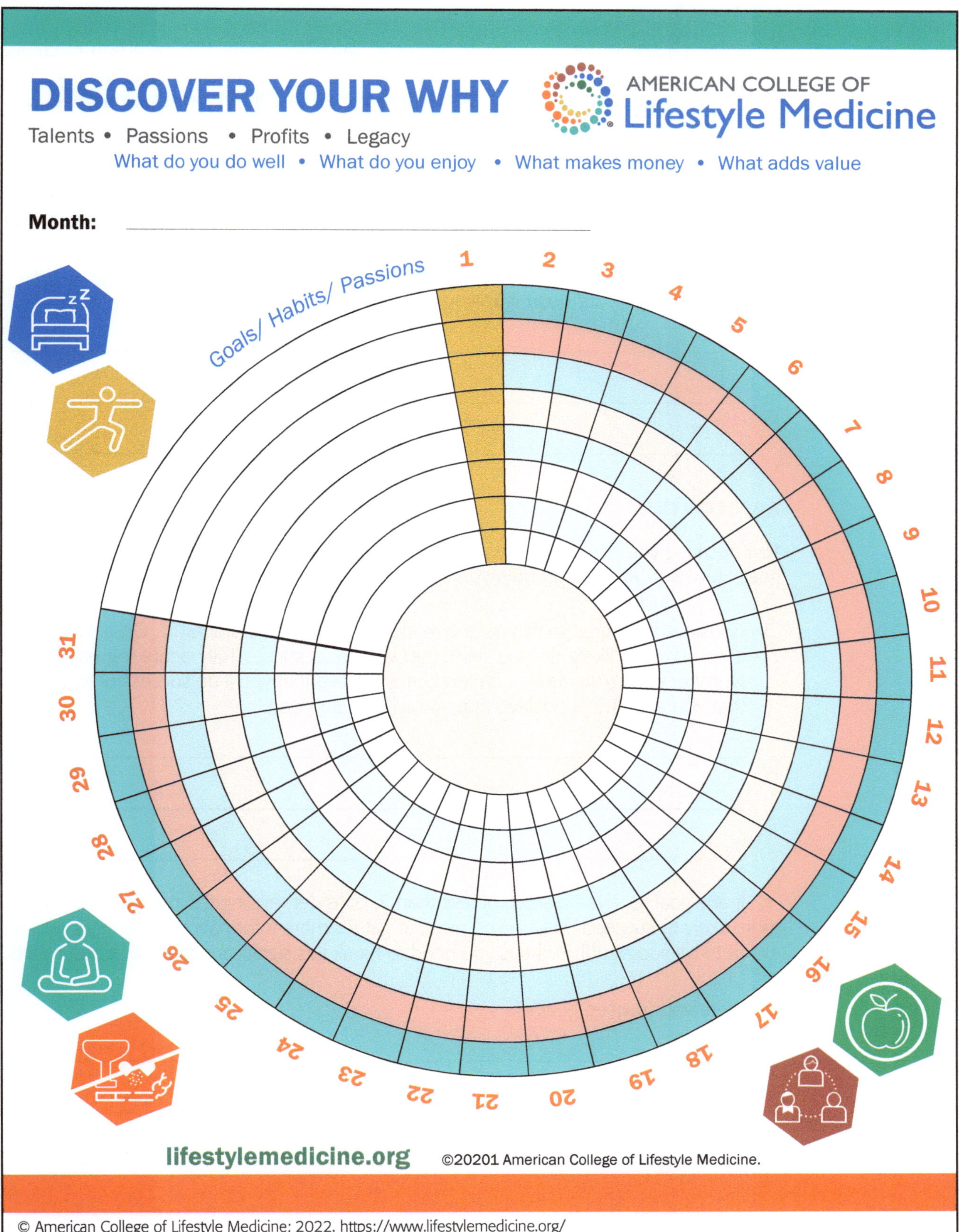

© American College of Lifestyle Medicine; 2022. https://www.lifestylemedicine.org/

Figure 7-1. The Health Tracker from the American College of Lifestyle Medicine

OPENNESS

As women, society gives you many "shoulds" regarding goals. It is common to create plans that align with the purpose of others or that you feel like you "should" do. You may be able to think of goals you have set in the past that were more aligned with what others wanted you to do than with your authentic self.

With openness, consider whether or not the three goals above are what you truly want to address. Then, after honest reflection, do you want to modify any of your three goals so that they truly align with what YOU want to do or what excites YOU? If so, adjust the goal(s) in the following space. Again, this is a place of no shame, blame, or guilt.

❏ What is it that your heart is calling you to do?

____

____

____

APPRECIATION

Just because you set a goal does not mean that you will be successful in achieving the goal. However, we want to help you be successful with achieving your goals.

❏ Consider the three goals you chose in the section on CURIOSITY. On a scale from 1 to 10, how likely do you think you will be at successfully achieving each goal? Number each separately, with ten being positive that you'll be successful to 1 being that you are almost positive that you will not succeed.

____

____

____

If any goal received a score of less than 7, consider revising the plan so that you are more likely to succeed. Maybe you need to gather more information or connect with an expert to be successful. Perhaps you need to break this significant goal into smaller parts.

❏ Write your revised goal(s).

____

____

____

____

- ❑ Think about a time when you were successful with a goal and identify the strengths you used to achieve it. Then, consider how you will use those strengths to achieve these goals and write about it below.

___

___

___

___

COMPASSION

By the time you reach midlife or beyond, you know that even if you have the perfect goal and the perfect plan, sometimes circumstances get in your way of success. Even when you try to consider the potential roadblocks that you may encounter, you cannot guarantee that you can avoid or overcome them. However, considering potential obstacles and possible ways to address them in advance increases your chances of success.

- ❑ What potential obstacles can you foresee preventing you from successfully achieving the goals you listed?

___

___

___

___

- ❑ How can you limit these potential obstacles or address them if they occur?

___

___

___

___

Be compassionate with yourself. There may be some obstacles that you can't overcome or that you may need the help of others to address. This is not a sign of weakness, that the goal was not a "good" goal, or that you failed. Instead, life sometimes has obstacles that are part of your life's journey that are like giant boulders along your path and are too heavy for you to move. Remember to be compassionate with yourself if you encounter such a boulder. In other words, remember to treat yourself the way you would treat a good friend and talk to yourself the way you speak to good friends. The words that you say to yourself are powerful, so be compassionate.

HONESTY

Everyone has areas of their life that they ignore, even though they could likely benefit from attention. Sometimes they are neglected due to shame, blame, or guilt. Other times, they are neglected, because they may bring up painful memories. Finally, areas may be ignored, because they feel too overwhelming to tackle, or you may be burnt out and feel like addressing them would likely not result in meaningful change.

- ❑ After honest reflection, are there any areas of your life that you neglect or ignore due to the reasons discussed above? If so, what are these areas?

  ____

  ____

  ____

- ❑ Would setting a goal around one of these areas that need attention support your overall health and well-being? Remember that you don't need to tackle the entire problem or reach a complete resolution. However, knowing that you are taking a step in the right direction by setting a goal may be necessary to get you started.

  ____

  ____

  ____

If you feel uncomfortable in any part of the journey, be honest with yourself and stop. Take a break and reflect. Identify what you need to put in place to feel comfortable moving forward. This might mean making an appointment with an addiction specialist and going to an intensive rehabilitation facility. It may mean making an appointment with a mental health professional because of the severe, prolonged sadness you've been experiencing yet avoiding. Consider making an appointment to evaluate the lump that seems to come and go in your right breast. Take stock, as well as the time, to address the things that you may have been putting off. Now is your time, and now is the time to be honest with yourself. Only you know the secrets you struggle with or torment you.

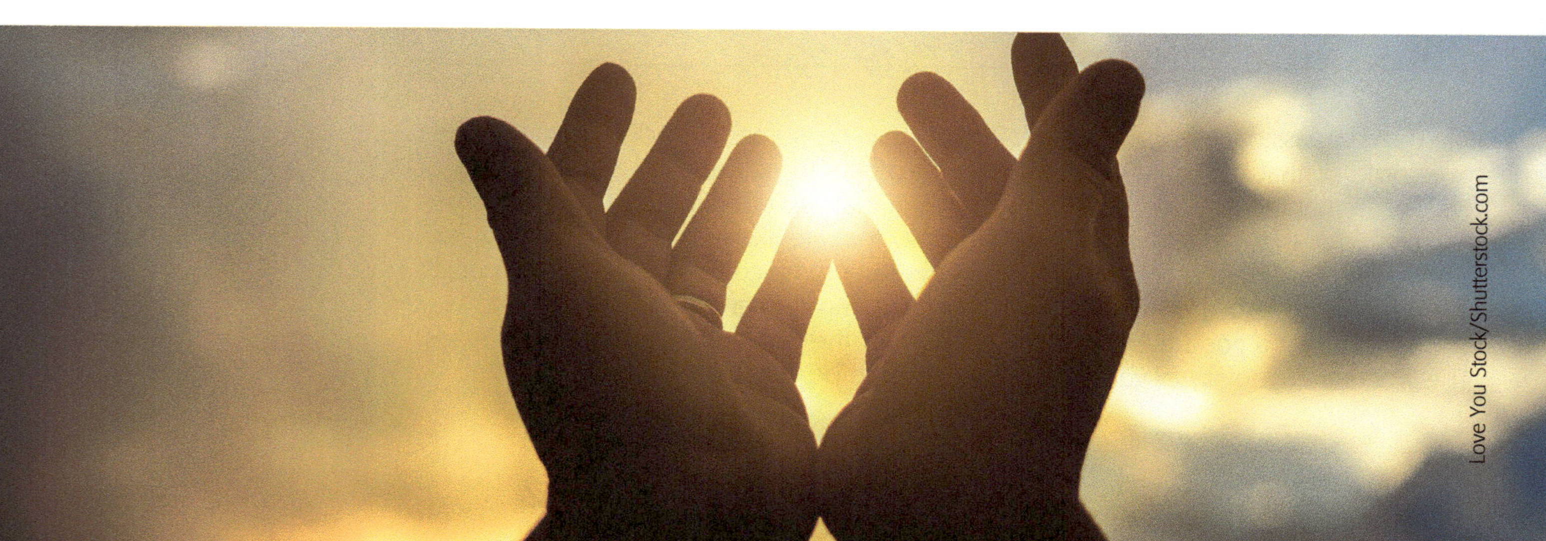

Love You Stock/Shutterstock.com

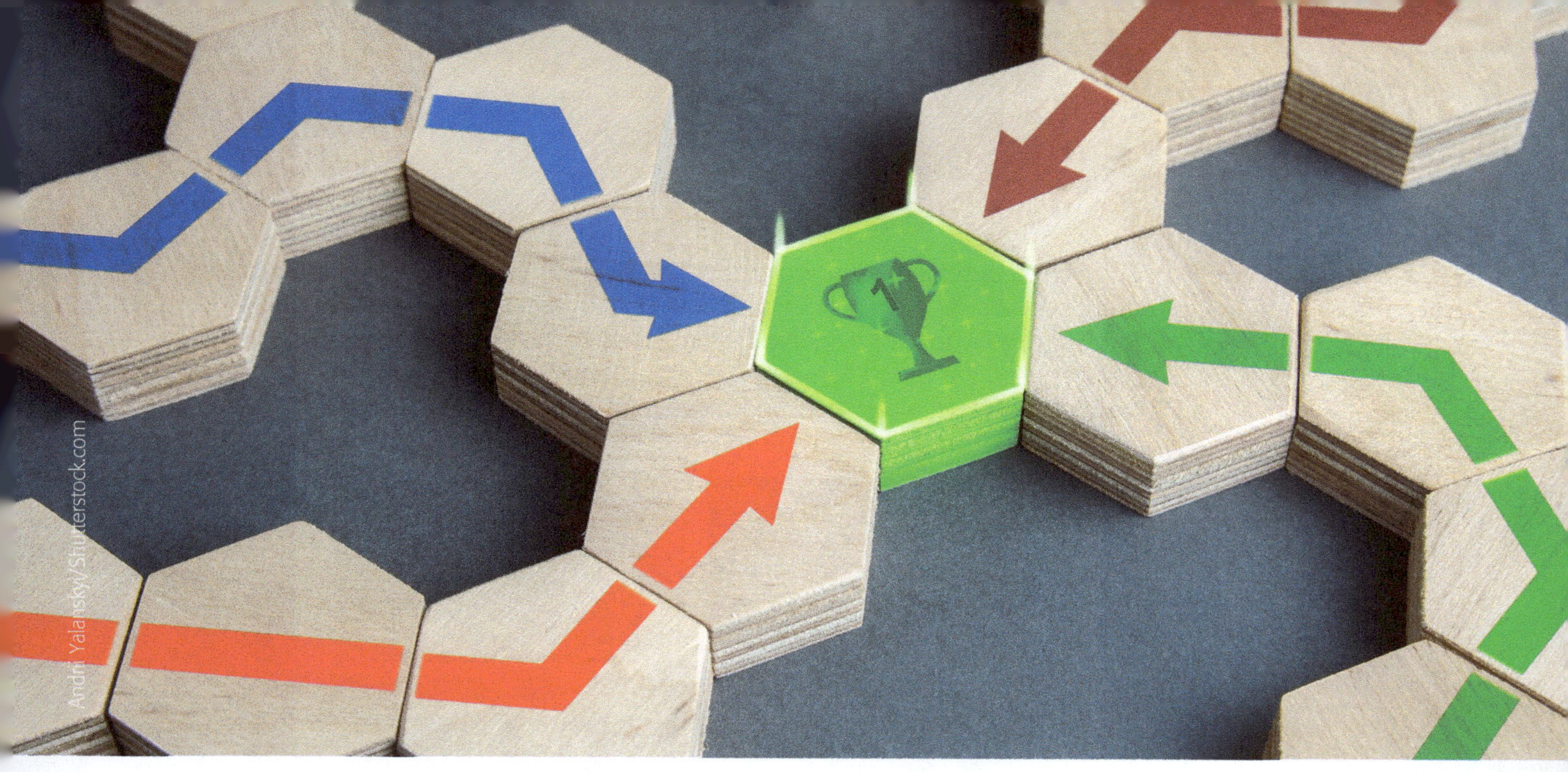
Andrii Yalanskyi/Shutterstock.com

Words of Wisdom From Dr. Michelle Tollefson

After working with many midlife and more mature women who have created and often achieved their goals, I have noticed a common theme when discussing their successes. Most women minimize the courage, perseverance, hard work, and determination that it took to work toward and often achieve their goals. When I acknowledge their hard work and congratulate them, they will typically share how it wasn't that hard (though often it was), that they should have done it long ago, or that it wasn't a large enough goal to be worthy of praise.

I think that society teaches women that we "should" naturally be eating healthy, exercising daily, juggling all of our responsibilities, and attending to the needs of others while maintaining a cheerful attitude and a smile on our faces. Societal expectations are impossible for anyone.

While working with midlife and more mature women, I encourage them to take pride in their accomplishments. Even if they haven't entirely achieved their goal, I work with them to explore how far they've come. I want my patients to celebrate the journey, the steps they are making along their paths, and every goal they reach. There is no accomplishment too small to celebrate and be proud of achieving.

As you create and set out to work toward achieving your goals, consider how you will celebrate the accomplishments that you make along the way. By highlighting and celebrating your success, you will help to teach other women that their achievements are worthy of praise.

- ☐ How will you celebrate achieving your goals?

  ____

  ____

  ____

Goals Wrap-Up

Through goal-setting, your words and actions will mindfully move you toward a more purpose-filled life. When your path seems too stressful or overwhelming to consider a long-term goal, focus on taking the next step in the right direction. Don't worry if you've wandered off the path. Every day, every hour, and every minute is another opportunity for a fresh start. Just set a new goal and move toward that north star…one small step at a time.

YES, I DID IT!
I WILL DO IT
I CAN DO IT
I'LL TRY TO DO IT
HOW DO I DO IT
I WANT TO DO IT
I CAN'T DO IT
I WON'T DO IT

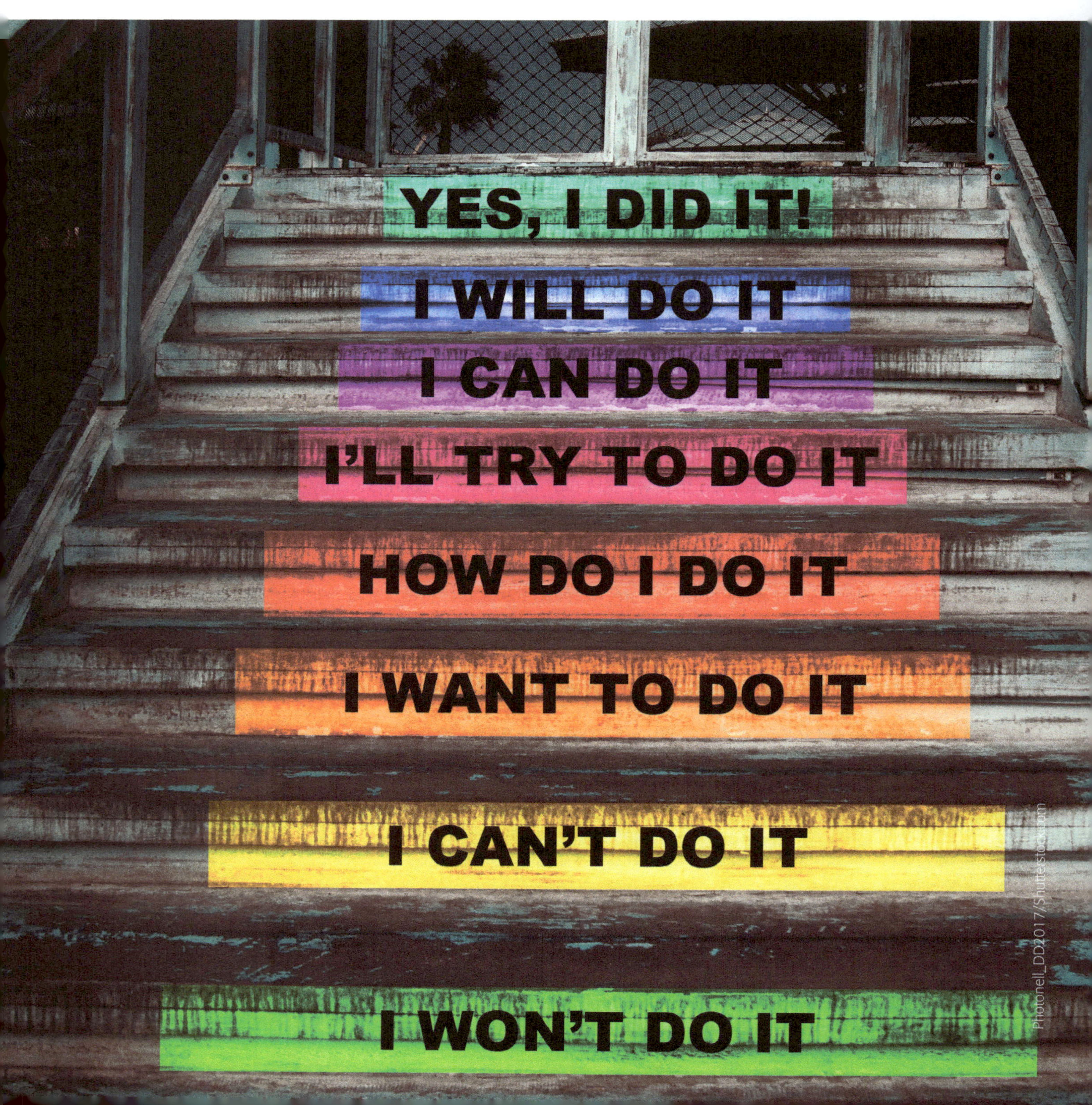

Photonell_DD2017/Shutterstock.com

CHAPTER 8
STRESS

Stress Throughout Menopause, Midlife, and Beyond

Acronym—STRESS

Savor	**Environment**
Talk	**Silly**
Reduce	**Spiritual**

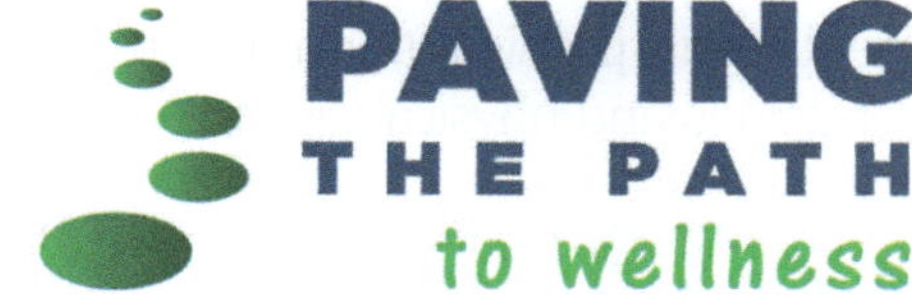

- *SAVOR:* Take time to savor precious moments. Practicing mindfulness decreases stress and helps you savor the beauty in and surrounding you.
- *TALK:* When you're stressed, pause, take a deep breath, and talk to someone. Whether you speak to a loved one, dear friend, or mental health specialist, your stress will likely decrease through connecting with another person and sharing your story.
- *REDUCE:* Reduce unnecessary commitments. Look at your calendar and schedule. Then reflect on what is stressing you out. If you can delegate items on your to-do list, do so. If you can shorten prolonged meetings, do this. When accepting engagements or new projects, check to see if they align with your priorities.
- *ENVIRONMENT:* Create a peaceful space in your home environment that supports your well-being. Consider incorporating elements of nature, calming lights, relaxing music, beautiful pictures, a journal, and anything else that helps you feel less stressed.
- *SILLY:* Incorporating opportunities to be silly and have fun throughout the day will decrease your stress. It's hard to be stressed when laughing and having fun with friends. Watch a funny video, hula hoop, blow bubbles, or see a comedy film. The options to incorporate fun in your life are endless.
- *SPIRITUAL:* Regularly engaging in spiritual practices that align with your beliefs can help you de-stress. Don't neglect your spiritual well-being. It is crucial for whole health.

As a midlife or more mature woman, you know that stress is a part of life and is here to stay. Unfortunately, there's no magic yoga pose, stress reduction ball, or pill that can make all of your stress go away. You've encountered stressors daily for at least half a century, providing you with knowledge that can help you confront stressful situations moving forward.

Menopause is a perfect time for examining how you view, experience, and deal with stress. Society teaches women that stress is something to be avoided and conquered. On the other hand, consider if this is always the case. In her book, *The Upside of Stress* (1), Dr. Kelly McGonigal writes that stress is "what arises when something you care about is at stake." If you embrace this view of stress, you can think about it differently. You can welcome its ability to signify that your body is getting ready for action, prepared to accomplish work, and ready to meet its demands.

Stress increases motivation, alertness, and performance, as long as it isn't beyond what is beneficial for your body and mind. Challenges can help your memory, immunity, attention, and productivity, if they're not excessive. They can make you more resilient so that you're better able to handle future sources of stress.

Experiencing stress also encourages you to reach out and connect with others due to the hormone oxytocin, which is sometimes called the "cuddle hormone." The next time you start to feel stressed, try to think of how it signals that you care about something, that change is happening, or that something is occurring that is part of the human experience, as opposed to something to be avoided at all costs.

Hopefully you'll focus on the upside of stress, as recommended by Dr. McGonigal. However, it's also essential to realize stress's downside. When anxiety levels remain high and become chronic, stress can be harmful to your health. A little pressure can increase mental and physical performance, but too much stress can also lead to mental health conditions and physical disease.

Before you explore strategies for managing stress to help you reach peak performance, rather than increase your chances for disease, it's beneficial to understand why being mindful of your stress level is vital as a midlife or more mature woman. Also, don't get discouraged while reviewing the downside of stress. After reviewing the negative impact of stress on health, you'll learn about evidence-based ways of addressing stress that you can start using today.

❏ What are the things that are causing you stress right now?

____

____

____

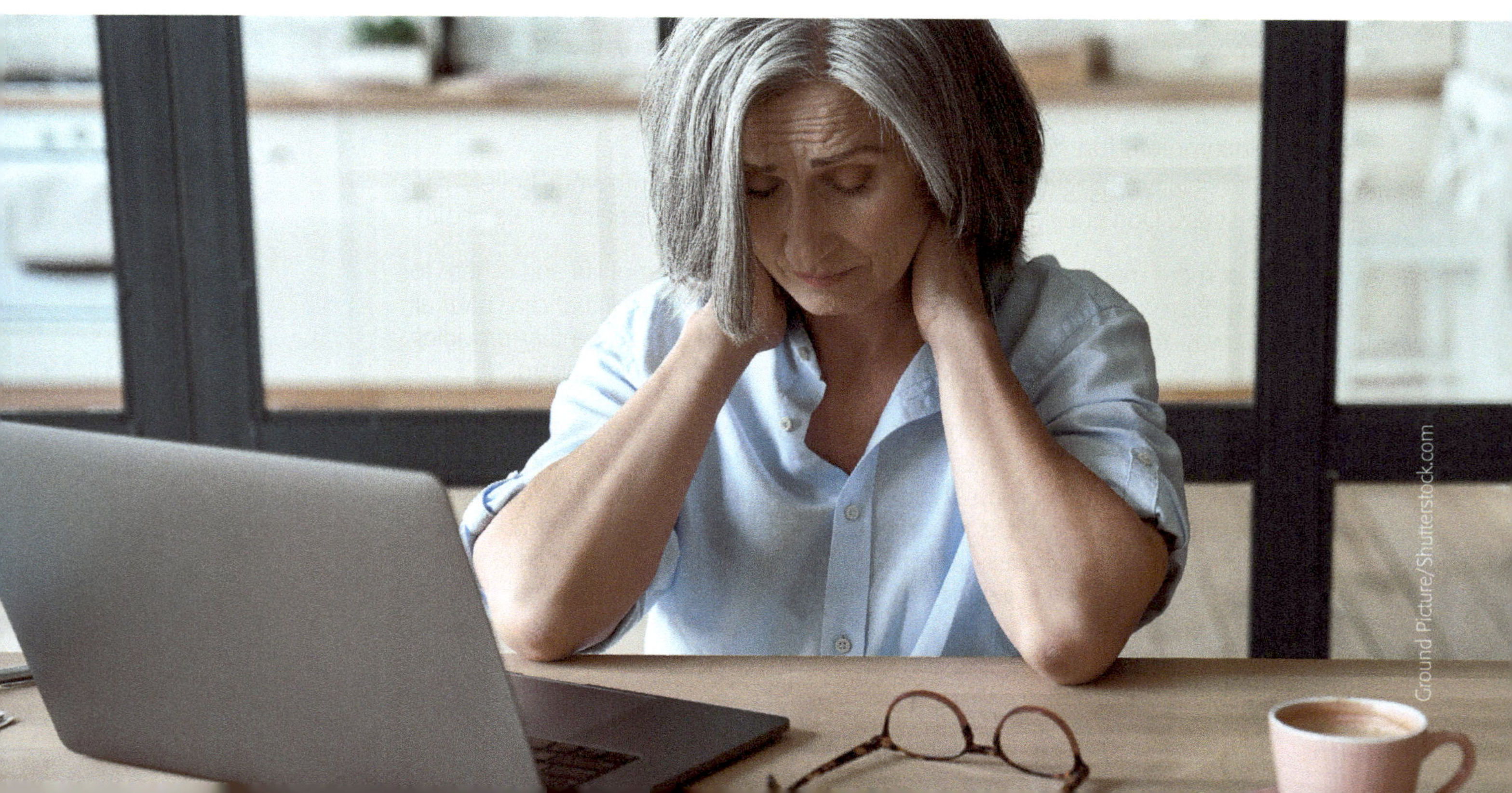

Ground Picture/Shutterstock.com

❏ Which of these things are in your control and are out of your control?

___

___

___

❏ Describe your current level of stress. Do you have too much, too little, or just the right amount of pressure to support your physical and mental well-being?

___

___

___

Stress During Menopause and Beyond

Even if you consider yourself a pro at dealing with stress, menopause can throw the calmest woman for a loop. Just because you are approaching menopause does not mean your other sources of stress disappear. Instead, menopause layers additional stressors on top of already busy lives. Menopause can feel like a time when everything changes and nothing stays the same, including your career, finances, family, relationships, mind, body, health, and hormones.

Many midlife and older women are caring for aging parents, raising grandchildren, supporting children still living at home, or are experiencing the loss of children leaving home for college. It's easy to feel overwhelmed, anxious, and burnt out. Ageism and sexism, experienced by post-menopausal women in many cultures, make this time of transition even more stressful.

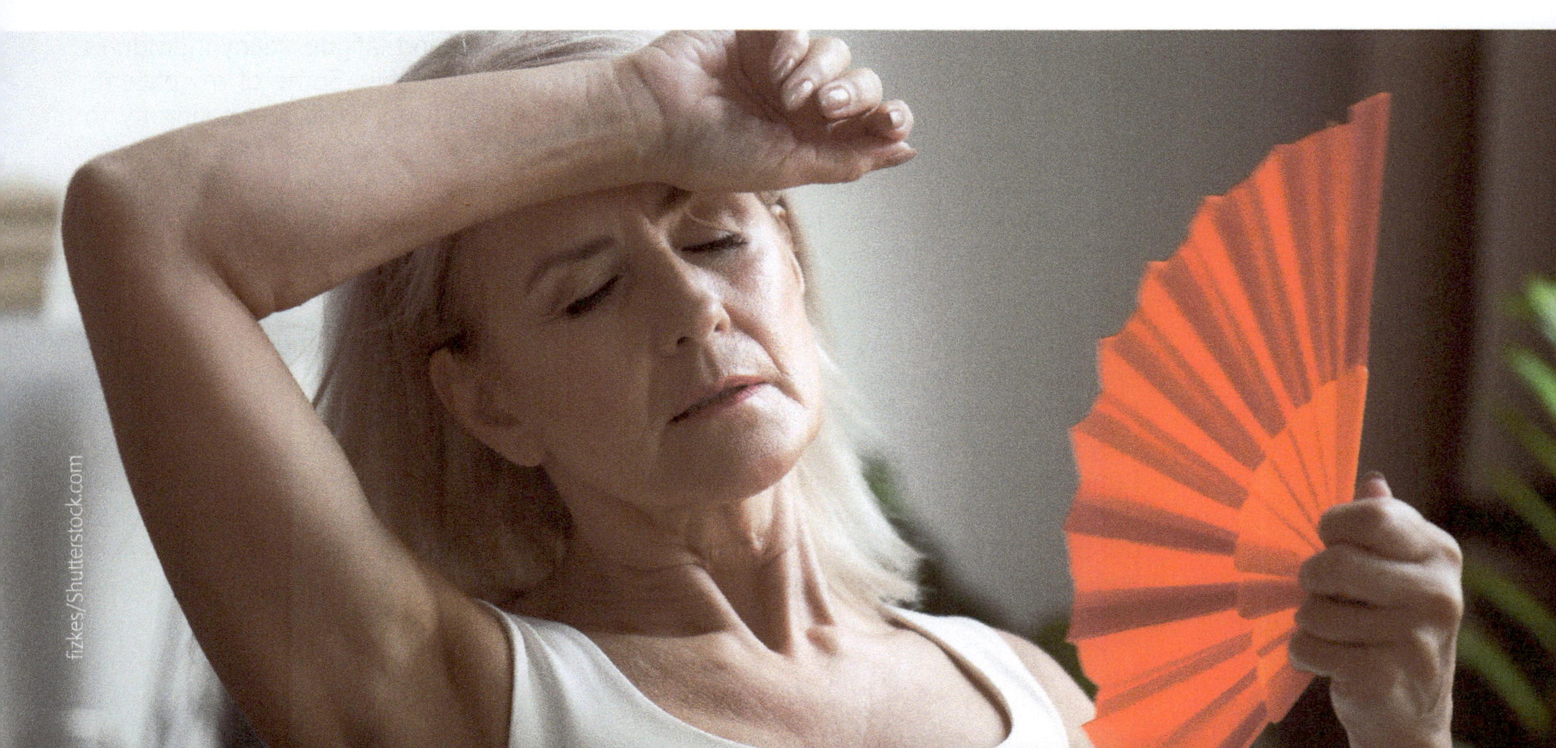
fizkes/Shutterstock.com

Menopause also brings welcomed changes. Many menopausal women are glad not to deal with monthly menstruation and to eventually not worry about contraception. Careers often flourish during midlife, but this may bring higher expectations, such as taking on leadership roles. Even if you are glad that your children are leaving for college, that you recently got a promotion at work, or that you have more time for yourself as a midlife or older woman, these are all changes, and even good stress is still stress.

Menopausal stress is real. Hormonal changes during menopause contribute to menopausal stress. During perimenopause (which can start several years before menstruation stops entirely), estrogen levels usually fluctuate widely. These estrogen level variations cause women to be more susceptible to the harmful effects of stress, especially since these hormonal changes lead to changes in hormone levels in the brain. During menopause, progesterone levels decrease (a hormone that supports calmness) and make it more difficult to handle stressful situations.

As if this isn't enough, when menopausal women get stressed, the adrenal gland diverts resources to produce cortisol (the stress hormone) that it would otherwise have used to make some estrogen and progesterone. This can worsen menopausal symptoms and mood symptoms too. Stress during menopause can increase hormonal problems, and hormonal changes in menopause can increase stress. This is why women need to optimize their stress resiliency during this transition.

Words of Wisdom From Dr. Michelle Tollefson

Women approaching menopause and women who have recently gone through menopause have visited my office with similar stories. What used to be minor sources of stress before menopause can sometimes make them feel like their world is falling apart. Women who described easily weathering daily stressors can feel like their mood is on a rollercoaster that feels out of control, when life gets incredibly turbulent.

My patients often report lying awake at night as daily stressors prevent them from drifting off to sleep. In addition, hot flashes may lead to nighttime awakenings, increasing their fatigue and susceptibility to the negative impacts of sleep deprivation the following morning.

In an attempt to combat late-night stress, insomnia, and fatigue, many individuals search for a midnight snack, which is rarely a fruit or vegetable. Some of my patients who are fatigued and stressed during the daily struggle with emotional eating try to increase their energy through sugar-rich food or get their minds off of their never-ending to-do list. This can lead to unwanted excess weight gain, another source of stress. They rarely have enough energy to exercise, even though this is one of the best ways to manage stress. Other women reach for a glass of wine to relax and help them fall asleep. This can also have negative impacts on sleep and overall health.

Menopausal stress has left many of them struggling with their physical and emotional health, wondering how to regain control of their lives. As my patients' hormones stabilize as they get further out from menopause, they often notice that they can weather the stressful storms of life without such drastic swings in their mood. I encourage them to be kind to themselves during this transition and remember that menopause and hormone changes are part of every woman's journey, if she lives into her 50s and beyond. They are not alone. They are not abnormal. What they are feeling and experiencing is not "all in their head." Menopausal stress is real!

Although I always advocate for healthy lifestyle behaviors, they are more important than ever for women experiencing stress while traversing menopause. I try to connect my patients with resources, referrals, and support to equip them to be successful in adopting healthy lifestyle behaviors. My patients who embrace healthy lifestyle behaviors during the menopause transition typically notice that eating healthy foods, exercising regularly, prioritizing sleep and social connections, avoiding risky substances, and regularly engaging in stress management activities improve their physical and emotional well-being. These activities are not a panacea for all menopausal symptoms, nor do they make life's stressors disappear, but they help make the journey a little easier, step by step and day by day.

Stress, Menopause, and Midlife Symptoms

High levels of chronic stress may cause or exacerbate many peri and post-menopausal symptoms, such as the following:

- Insomnia and other sleep problems
- Fatigue
- Weight gain, especially abdominal fat
- Decreased desire to have sex
- Mood swings and irritability
- Depression and anxiety
- Aches and pains
- Hot flashes and night sweats
- Difficulty concentrating
- Memory problems
- Decreased confidence
- Negative body image
- Relationship problems
- Risky substance use and relapse
- Risk-taking behaviors
- Tension in relationships due to ineffective communication (like passive-aggressive behavior, threatening, nitpicking behavior, yelling, avoiding, gossiping, or shutting down)
- Difficulty controlling blood sugar (increased risk of metabolic syndrome and type 2 diabetes)
- Heart disease and high blood pressure
- Irritable bowel syndrome
- Inflammation
- Damage to telomeres (the ends of chromosomes that help protect your DNA)

When you are experiencing extreme, prolonged stress, do you notice any of these symptoms? If so, circle them.

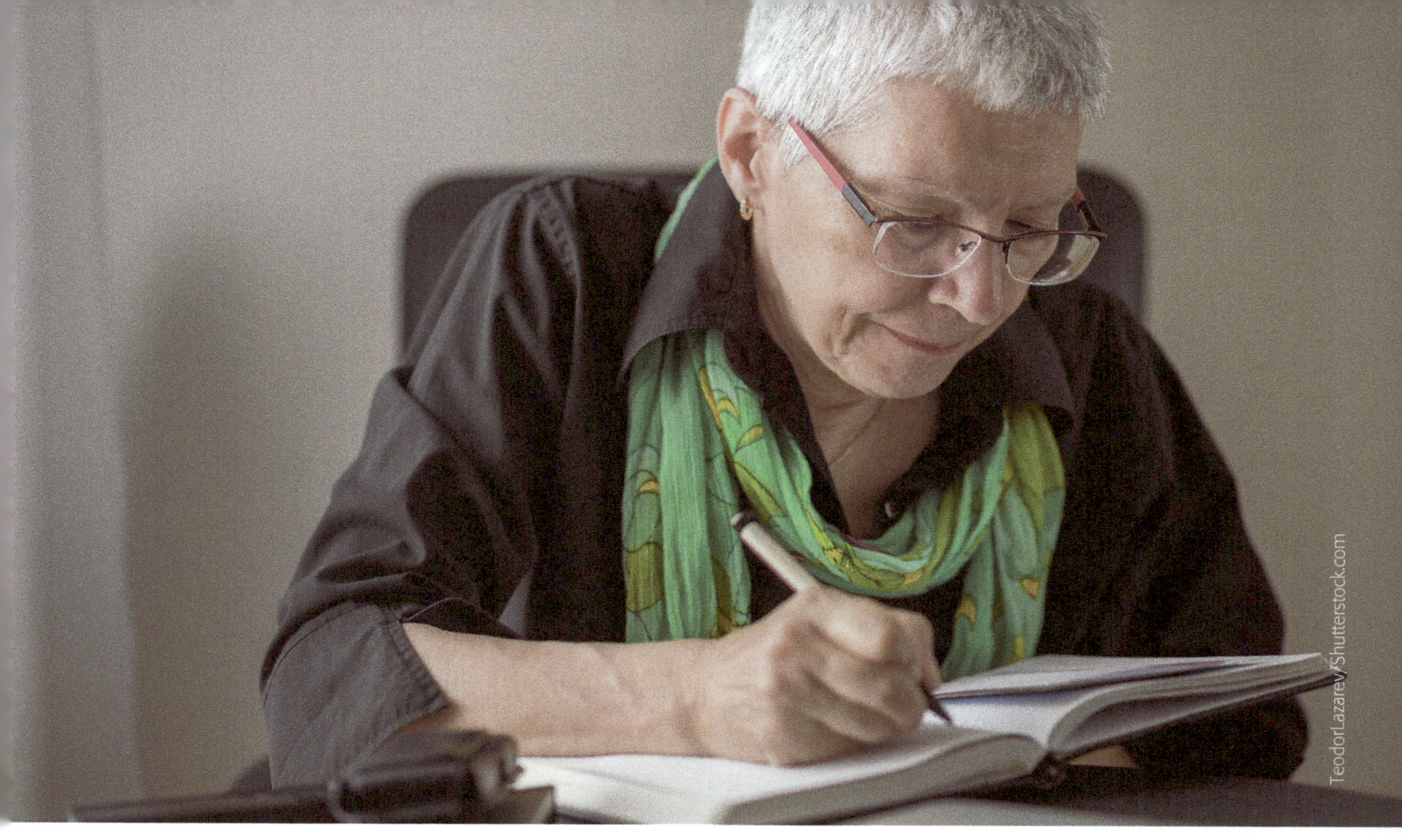
TeodorLazarev/Shutterstock.com

Stress Journal

For a few days to a week, practice being mindful of your sources of stress. These can be anything from minor annoyances (e.g., temporarily losing your keys) to significant sources of stress. Also, when you experience something stressful, write down anything you notice about your body (e.g., upset stomach, clenching your jaw, tight shoulders, a headache, etc.). In addition, please make a note of the thoughts that go through your mind and record them in your stress journal (Table 8-1), such as, you should not be feeling this way. You're so angry at ________ for making you feel this way. If you had done ________, then this wouldn't have happened. You're never going to learn how to deal with ________. You hate being rushed.

- ❑ What helped resolve the stress or helped you relax (if anything)?

  ____

  ____

  ____

- ❑ Review your stress journal. What insight did you gain from completing this journal?

  ____

  ____

  ____

Date and Time	Source of Stress	Body	Thoughts	Relaxation Method

Table 8-1. An example of a stress journal

When answering the following questions, use what you wrote in your journal while also considering other stressful experiences throughout your life.

❑ What are common sources of stress in your life now?

____

____

____

❑ What bodily symptoms do you feel when stressed?

____

____

____

❑ How can you be more aware of these symptoms to signal to yourself to engage in stress reduction/relaxation activities?

____

____

____

- ❑ Were the thoughts you thought when stressed helpful or harmful to you?

  ____

  ____

  ____

- ❑ What are some thoughts that you could replace these with to better serve your health and emotional well-being?

  ____

  ____

  ____

- ❑ What types of relaxation activities help you when you feel stressed? You can use what you wrote in your journal and expand upon it from what you remember using in the past.

  ____

  ____

  ____

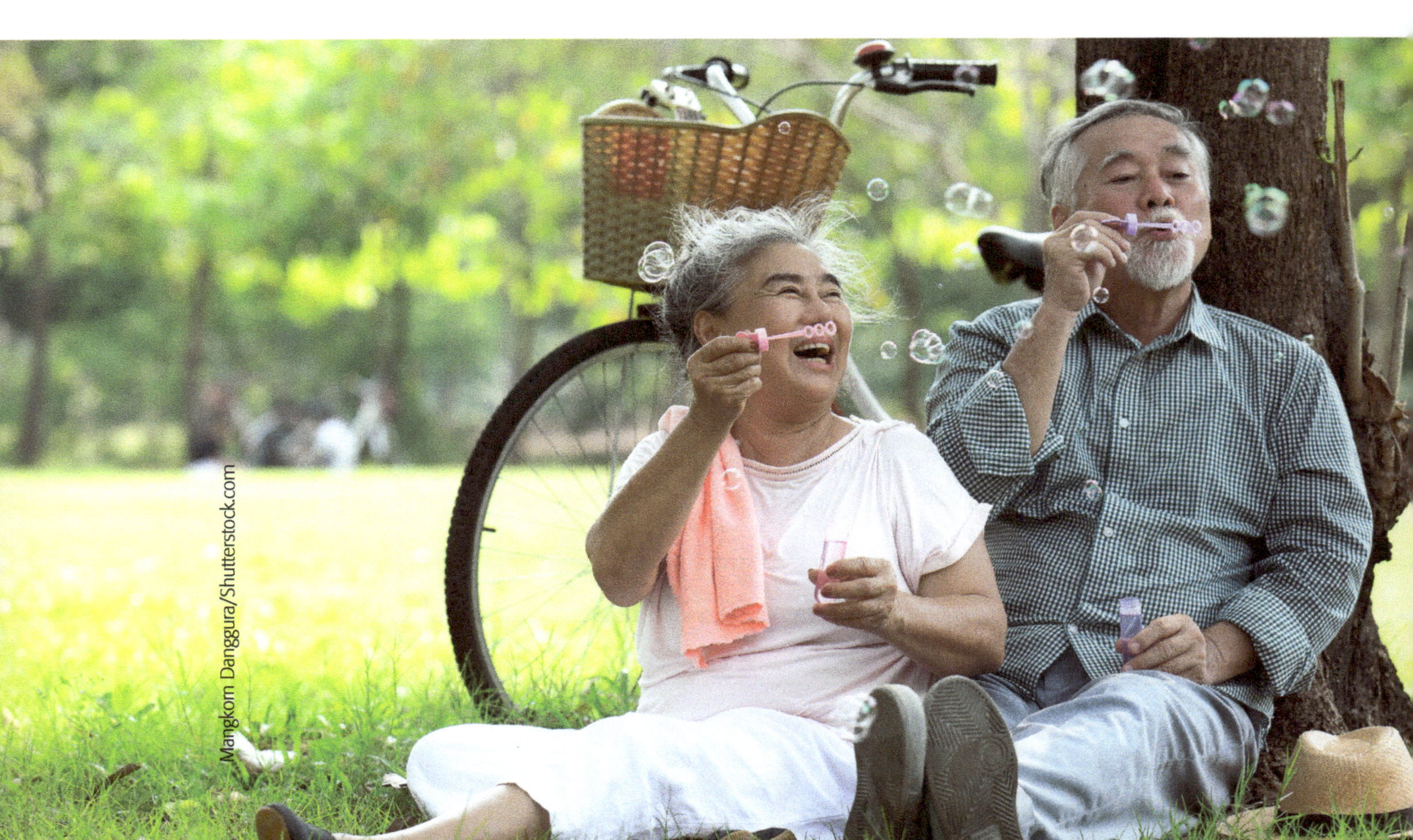

Mangkorn Danggura/Shutterstock.com

Sexual Health and Stress

Sexual health is a part of overall health for peri- and post-menopausal women. Since stress can negatively impact sexual health, it's essential to address it. Chronic stress decreases sexual thoughts, fantasies, and desires. It also reduces sexual arousal of the female genitals. Decreased arousal may result in decreased sexual pleasure and difficulty with having an orgasm. Women may have also been experiencing this during childrearing and other stressful times before menopause.

When you are stressed, you are more easily distracted. As distraction increases, sexual arousal decreases. With high levels of stress, your mood worsens, and anxiety increases. The vessels supplying blood to the female genitals can also be negatively impacted by chronic stress, decreasing vaginal lubrication and increasing vaginal dryness. It is important to note that vaginal dryness is often caused by reduced estrogen with menopause, regardless of stress levels. Stress that has negatively impacted vascular health in the pelvis can make this even worse.

When a woman is stressed, a part of her brain called the amygdala is activated. When the amygdala is activated, sexual desire decreases. Also, suppression of the amygdala (which occurs when relaxed) is necessary for women to orgasm. For this reason, researchers see stress, anxiety, anger, and fear associated with difficulty having an orgasm in women.

Although the research surrounding stress and sex may seem depressing, there is hope. Just as researchers know that distraction reduces sexual interest and pleasure, they've found that decreasing distraction and increasing mindful awareness can support sexual health. For example, engaging in mindfulness-based therapies has been shown to improve sexual arousal, desire, and sexual satisfaction. Research has also shown that progressive muscle relaxation, guided imagery, or diaphragmatic breathing can help. In addition, some women have experienced benefits from mindfulness-based cognitive behavioral sex therapy or mindfulness-based stress reduction for sexuality programs.

Regardless of whether you're struggling with your sexual health, or if you already are satisfied with your sexual health but want to improve it, reducing distraction, while increasing mindfulness and relaxation, is an excellent place to start.

Stress Management

Now that we've made you more stressed considering the potential negative impacts of chronic, high levels of stress, let's talk next about what you can do to be more resilient to stress, now and for decades to come.

EXPERIENCE

As a mature woman, you have many years of experience handling stressors that life throws your way each day. You've likely used some healthy behaviors to decrease stress (such as exercising or reading a relaxing book), as well as possibly some unhealthy behaviors (such as overeating or overconsuming alcohol). In addition, you typically learn new behaviors that help you navigate your stressful world as you age. You can also become better at healthily managing stress by learning new techniques from others or books such as this.

Consider your childhood and young adulthood and the stress management techniques you used during those periods of your life. What can you learn from how you previously dealt with stress that can help you better deal with stress now?

This is an excellent time to create a stress timeline (Table 8-2). Go from early childhood to now and indicate times in your life when there have been significant stressors.

When looking at these stressors, if there is something significant such as abuse or another trauma, now is the time to reach out to a mental health professional to work through these damaging events, if you haven't already done so or still need additional support.

- ❑ When considering the challenges you've experienced in the last year of your life, what has helped you best handle your stressors? For example, consider relaxation techniques, people in your life, how you think about the stressors, etc.

  ____

  ____

  ____

- ❑ In addition to learning from your experiences, you can learn from the experience of others. For example, consider friends and relatives and how they handle stress. Are there techniques that they've used that you would like to try? If so, which?

  ____

  ____

  ____

Childhood	**Adolescence**	**Young Adulthood**	**Now**

Table 8-2. An example of a stress timeline

- ❑ Consider female public figures who have been through stressful events and thrived despite their challenges. For example, Joan Lunden's breast cancer diagnosis, Oprah Winfrey's struggle with weight, Jennifer Hudson's tragic loss of family members, and others. How can you use their struggles or the struggles of others to inspire you to move forward beyond the mishaps that may have come your way?

___

___

___

___

- ❑ Are there people in your life who are your age or older who seem to handle stress well? List them in the space provided. Consider reaching out to them to learn more about their experiences of stress and how they learned to deal with it healthily.

___

___

___

___

- ❑ Are there people in your life who do not manage stress well? What can you learn from their behaviors?

___

___

___

___

- ❑ You can even learn from the experiences of others who you don't know personally. For example, have you seen others engaging in relaxation activities that seem exciting and fun, or that could work for you? If so, list them. What would you need to learn or do to be able to use these methods to help you manage stress?

___

___

___

___

THOUGHTS & BEHAVIORS

You've likely heard the serenity prayer: "God grant me the serenity to accept the things I cannot change, the courage to change the things I can, and the wisdom to know the difference." Theologian Reinhold Niebuhr (disputed)

Regardless of your spiritual and religious beliefs, this prayer can be helpful as you learn to handle stress better. There are obvious sources of stress that you cannot change in your life. For example, you may receive a medical diagnosis that you cannot change or learn that an upcoming show you were looking forward to was canceled due to circumstances beyond your control. Working to accept what you cannot change can decrease your stress and free your mental energy for addressing what can be changed. Sometimes it is beneficial to work with a mental health professional, if you feel stuck with being unable to accept circumstances that you cannot change (such as a history of trauma, the death of a loved one, or a recent divorce).

- ❑ What are sources of stress in your life that you cannot change but are struggling to accept?

  ____

  ____

  ____

  ____

- ❑ How can you work to address these sources? Would you benefit from connecting with others, possibly even a professional counselor?

  ____

  ____

  ____

  ____

The prayer asks for the "courage to change the things I can." Many women experience the same or similar sources of stress repeatedly without stopping to think about whether or not they can change this source of stress. For example, maybe you regularly misplace your keys, which leads to stress while searching for them. You could likely remove this source of stress by creating a place where you will always place your keys when you walk in the door. Or, maybe you feel stressed every year when your extended family comes to your home for Thanksgiving dinner. Perhaps, you could ask someone else to host the dinner the next time, or you could host the dinner but ask everyone to bring food to relieve the cooking burden that you've experienced in the past. You may feel uncomfortable at first about asking someone else to host or asking all of the guests to bring food, but relieving or decreasing the stress will likely be worth the effort.

- ❑ What are sources of stress in your life that you could change to decrease or eliminate the sources of stress? For example, consider delegation, removing the source of stress, or asking for help.

  ____

  ____

  ____

- ❑ How can you use delegating, removing the source of stress, or asking for help to address these stressors?

  ____

  ____

  ____

By this time in your life, you've hopefully learned to set boundaries and ask for help; however, many women still struggle with this. Setting boundaries and asking for help is not selfish. It does not mean that you are lazy or neglecting your duties. It does not make you less valuable of a person. It is okay to be assertive, ask for help, and protect your time and energy.

If you struggle with asking for help and creating boundaries, you're not alone. Usually, it becomes easier to do as you practice these behaviors. Remember, when you ask for help, and someone gives it to you, you allow them the opportunity to feel good. By not letting them help you, you are taking away this opportunity for joy inside them.

- ❑ Would setting boundaries to better protect your time or energy help your overall well-being and decrease stress? Explain.

  ____

  ____

  ____

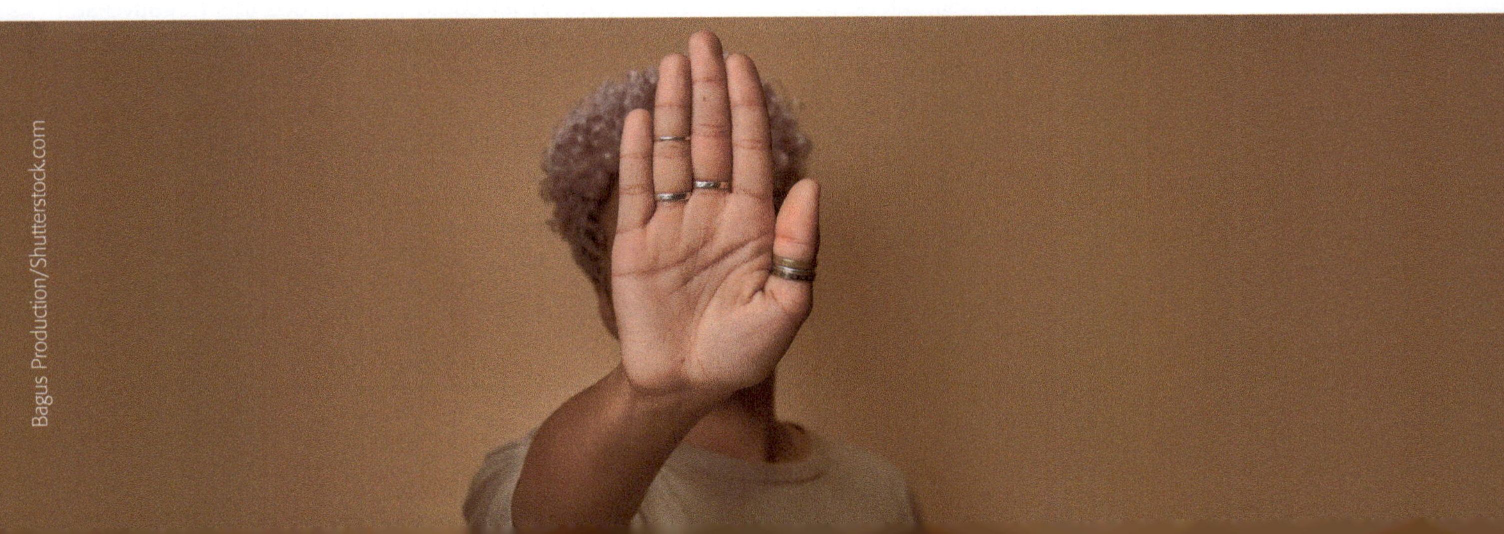
Bagus Production/Shutterstock.com

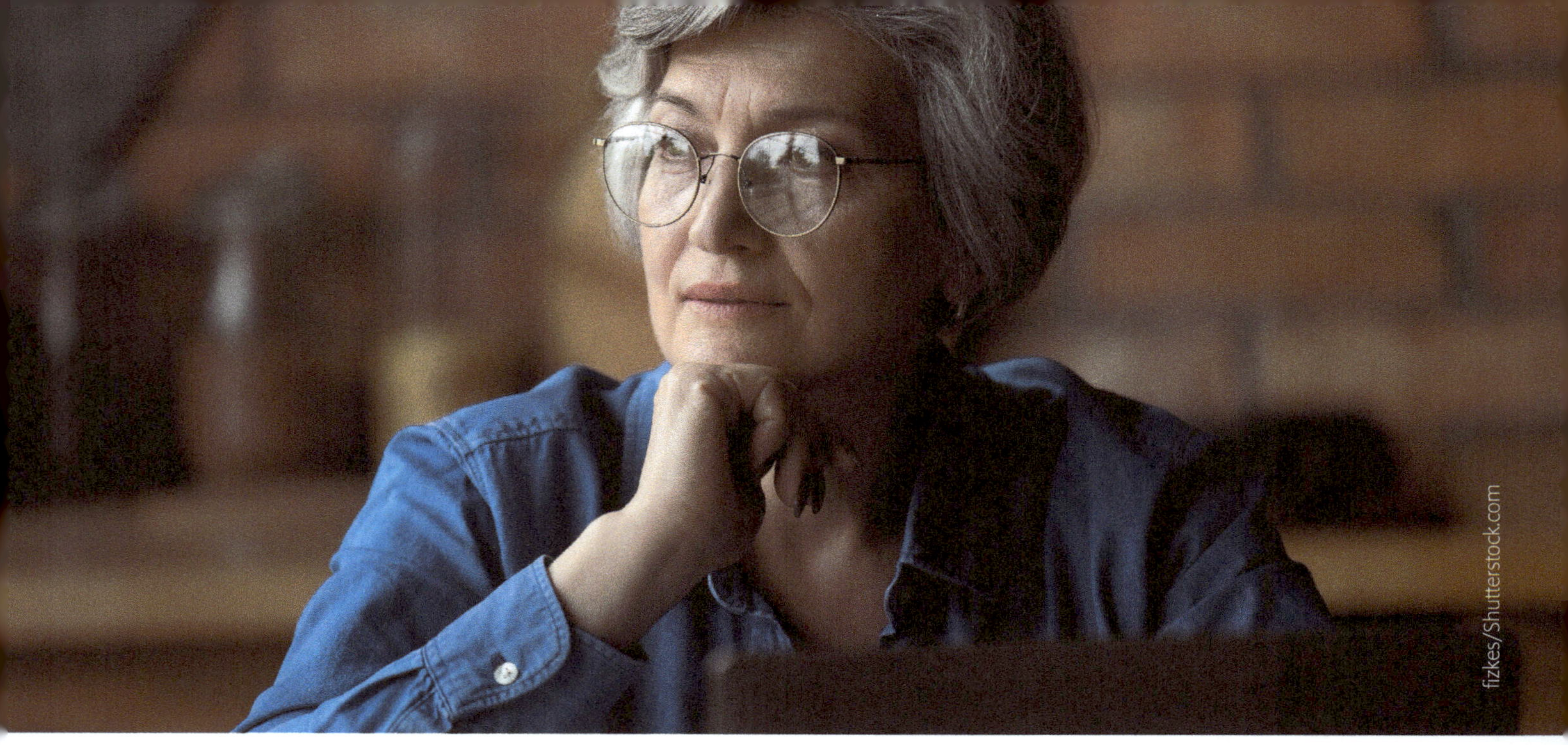

THOUGHTS

For most women, when they hear the word stress, they think of it as something to be avoided. But changing how you think about stress can support your health. As discussed earlier, Dr. Kelly McGonigal reminds individuals that having some (but not too much) stress can help them focus, motivate them, and help them understand what is most important in their lives.

You can't always change the situation, but you can change how you think about what you experience in life. As a midlife or older woman, you have decades of experience talking to yourself. Your self-talk impacts your mood, attitude, behaviors, and interactions with others.

❑ When you feel stressed, what types of thoughts typically come into your mind? What do you "say" to yourself?

____

____

____

❑ Is this self-talk helpful or harmful to you? What could you replace this negative self-talk with, if it is detrimental, to better support your health? For example, maybe you could remind yourself that this stressor is temporary. You could consider whether or not what you are dealing with will matter a few years from now. Maybe you could remind yourself that all humans experience stress, hurt, anger, sadness, and fear and that these are normal emotions.

____

____

____

Some women have experienced childhood or adult trauma. Other women may be experiencing such extreme stress levels that they need professional support. Still, others may be struggling with stressors, such as a negative body image, marital problems, or menopausal symptoms. If you are one of these women and haven't received the help you need to be the healthiest midlife or older woman you can be, please reach out for help.

The menopausal transition and beyond are ideal times for addressing mental health issues that may be holding you back from experiencing true health. Research has shown cognitive behavioral therapy (CBT) to be helpful for some of these issues. Mental health professionals are trained to help in situations like these. Ask your primary care provider for a referral or reach out directly to a mental health professional. Working with them and getting the resources you deserve can help you move forward with renewed strength, perspective, and health. Call 1-800-662-HELP (4357) for a free, confidential, 24/7, 365-day-a-year Mental Health and Substance Use hotline.

As a menopausal or more mature woman, perhaps you've had relationships that add negativity to your life. Luckily, you've likely also had connections with people who helped you weather life's stressful storms. Although we'll cover connections later in this book, it's essential to reflect upon the relationships in your life and how they help or hinder your health. Having a loved one or a trusted friend to freely express your feelings when worried, sad, or stressed allows you to process these emotions healthily. Rather than feeling alone, having a meaningful conversation about a source of stress can help put the matter in perspective and may help you consider ways to approach the issue that you wouldn't have thought of yourself. If you have people who add negative stress to you or make you feel worse when you discuss what's bothering you, it's important to consider how you relate with these people.

Never worry alone. Pull someone in whom you trust and respect when you feel your worrying has gone beyond five minutes. At that point, please reach out and talk to someone about it.

- ❑ List one or more people you can turn to when going through a very stressful time.

  ____

  ____

  ____

  ____

- ❑ How do they help you healthily handle your stress?

  ____

  ____

  ____

  ____

❑ Is there any issue causing you to stress and worry right now? Explain.

____

____

____

❑ Is there someone you want to reach out to discuss it?

____

____

____

❑ List one or more people who increase your level of negative stress or make it more difficult for you to handle stress.

____

____

____

❑ How can you change your interactions with them to protect your emotional health when stressed?

____

____

____

ENVIRONMENT

Your physical environment impacts your stress in positive or negative ways. As women age and since COVID has changed the work options to include working from home, at least a couple days a week, in many cases, women tend to spend more time in their homes. For this reason, it's essential to consider how your home environment causes or reduces stress.

You likely have some components of your environment that cause you stress, such as excessively loud noises, harshly bright lights, a temperature that is too hot or too cold, or uncomfortable seating. On the other hand, other parts of your environment may help you relax, such as dim lights, soft blankets, plants, and relaxing instrumental music. Although you likely cannot control all aspects of your environment, you can make some changes to help you relax.

- ❑ Think of the area in your home where you feel most relaxed. What aspects of your home environment help you to feel comfortable? Consider all of your senses.

___

___

___

- ❑ Is there a way to enhance these aspects or use them in other areas of your home or work to make these spaces even more relaxing? Explain.

___

___

___

- ❑ In what areas of your home do you feel the most stressed? What aspects of your home environment make you feel more negatively stressed? Once again, consider all of your senses.

___

___

___

___

- ❑ Is there anything you can do to address these stressful aspects of your home space?

___

___

___

___

- ❑ Do you have outdoor spaces like a patio that you can use more frequently?

___

___

___

___

SPIRITUAL HEALTH

Midlife and beyond is a typical time for women to assess their spiritual health. This connects with balance, as spiritual beliefs often help women handle stressful situations. A connection with a power greater than themselves impacts how many women relate to stressful situations and view them in the context of their lives. Viewing their life as part of something greater, of connecting with the past and what is to come in the future, can impact how women weather stressful times. Also, having a spiritual community that supports your well-being can help you handle stress more positively. Although someone can be spiritual without being religious, women often experience their spirituality through organized religion. Many religions involve song, movement, meditation, and prayer, which can help women manage stress.

❑ When considering your spiritual beliefs, how do they support you when you are experiencing high levels of stress?

____

____

____

❑ Is there anything you can do to increase how your spiritual health supports your ability to handle stress? For example, maybe when you feel overwhelmed, you want to try meditation or join a women's group at your church to support your well-being.

____

____

____

Many women feel that their spiritual leader (e.g., priest, rabbi, minister) can support them when they are going through challenging times and need to talk to someone. Consider the activities that nurture your spiritual well-being and leave you feeling more peaceful. Then commit to doing these activities regularly.

FOOD

Your food can negatively stress your body, or it can help your body handle stressors. For example, overindulging in ultra-processed foods (e.g., candy, cake, pastries, potato chips, ice cream, and processed meat) leads to increased inflammation and oxidative stress, negatively impacting your cells. Oxidative stress occurs when there are too many free radicals in the body and not enough antioxidants. This can adversely affect your heart, liver, gut, brain, and kidneys and increase your risk of lifestyle-related diseases (like type 2 diabetes, high cholesterol, and stroke). To combat oxidative stress, you can decrease your consumption of foods with added sugar and ultra-processed foods, including processed meat (bacon, ham, hot dogs).

A diet high in added sugars and saturated fat worsens stress and common menopausal symptoms. In addition, highly processed foods and simple carbohydrates (white bread, pasta, pastries, cake, pretzels) lead to blood sugar crashes and increase the release of cortisol (the stress hormone). Caffeine can also increase heart rate, make you hyperreactive, and make you more susceptible to the harmful effects of excessive stress.

In contrast, increasing your consumption of antioxidant-rich foods, including fruits and vegetables, helps your body deal with stress and enhances overall health. In addition, eating an anti-inflammatory diet, such as a whole-food and plant-rich, Mediterranean-style diet, decreases inflammation, decreases oxidative stress, and helps you to better handle the stress that you encounter in your daily life. Plus, you'll feel better and have more energy!

Consumption of adequate fiber and fermented foods (tempeh, kefir, yogurt, sauerkraut) supports gut microbiome health. This is important for mood regulation, as much of your body's serotonin is produced in the intestines and relies on a flourishing microbiome. In addition, serotonin impacts how your brain handles stress. So, enjoy fiber-rich foods and fermented foods regularly.

Adequate magnesium intake is also vital for cortisol metabolism. When you are feeling stressed and want to eat foods that support relaxation, reach for magnesium-rich foods, including leafy greens, salmon, avocados, bananas, and dark chocolate.

Some herbal teas, such as peppermint tea, chamomile tea, and green tea, contain L-theanine, supporting relaxation. In addition to the L-theanine in these teas, taking time to brew and sip tea can be a relaxing experience.

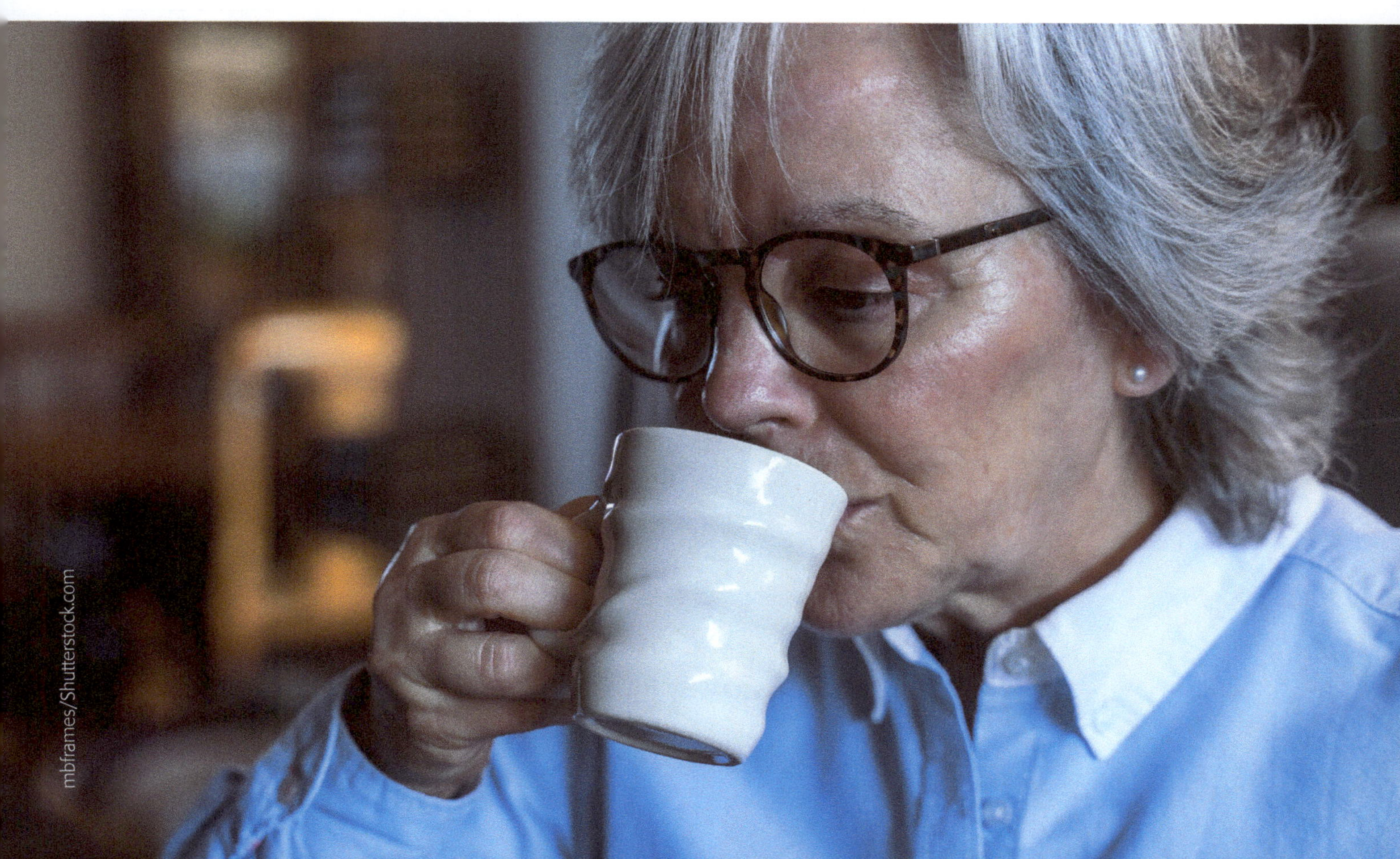
mbframes/Shutterstock.com

- ❑ How does what you eat support your body's ability to handle stress positively?

____

____

____

- ❑ How could you change what you eat to better support your body's ability to deal with daily stressors?

____

____

____

- ❑ We've mentioned many options for you to try and investigate that will help you handle stress. There are many more. Take this time to list some that are on your mind that haven't yet been covered.

____

____

____

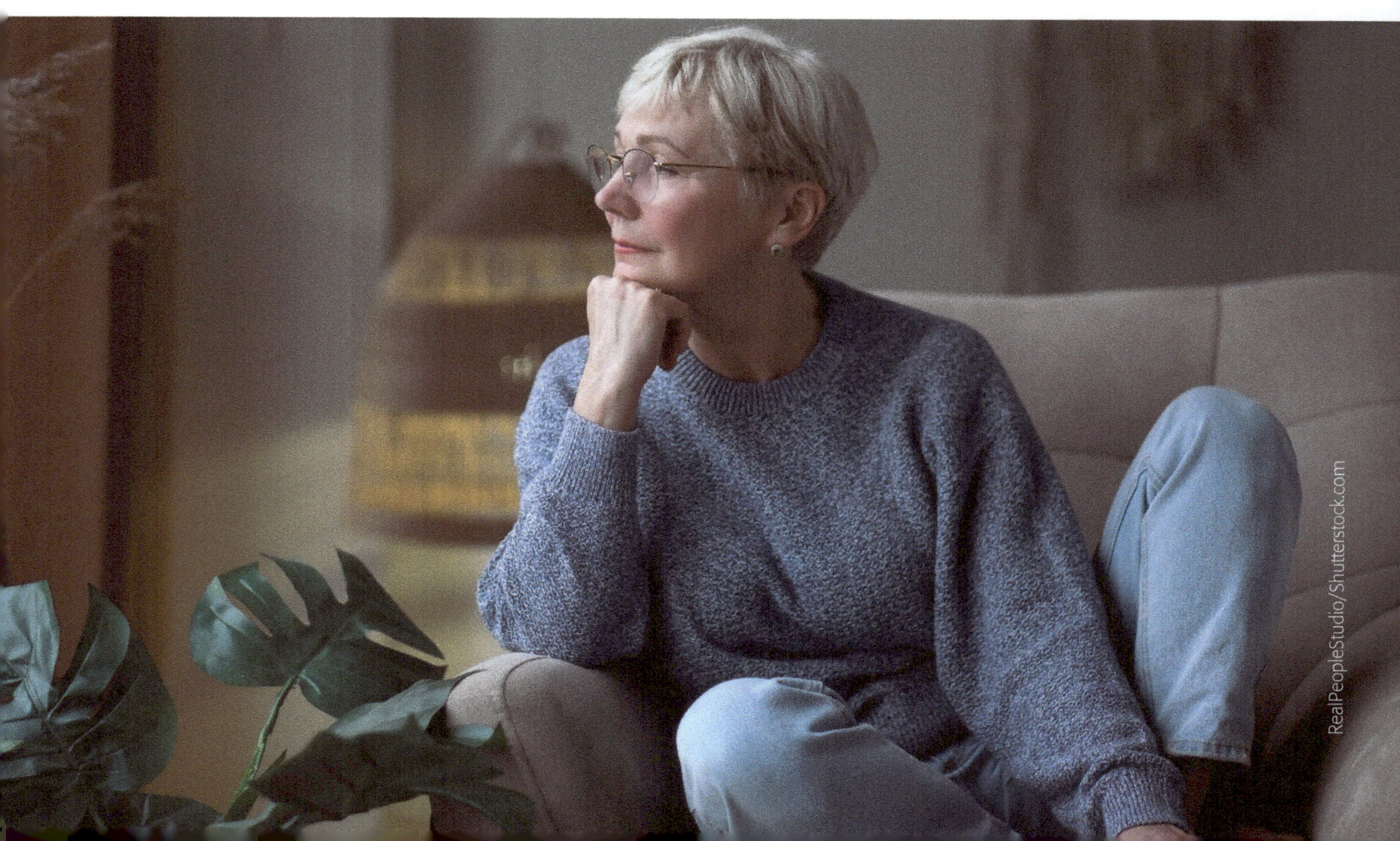

RealPeopleStudio/Shutterstock.com

In reality, there are a wide variety of other ideas for relaxation, including the following:

- 4, 7, 8 breathing
- Baking or cooking
- Bicycling
- Body scanning
- Dancing to music on the radio
- Decreasing interruptions (keep your cell phone away)
- Deep breathing
- Diaphragmatic breathing
- Doing art
- Engaging in self-talk that decreases stress
- Enjoying relaxing scents
- Exercising (aerobic and stretching)
- Focused relaxation activities
- Focusing on what you can control
- Forest bathing (spending time in nature)
- Gardening
- Hang a bird feeder outside your window
- Hula hooping
- Journaling
- Keeping a record of what is causing you stress
- Laughing and humor
- Limiting or being mindful of social media and news (TV, radio, etc.) overload
- Limiting technology
- Listening to relaxing music
- Massage
- Meditating (many different types exist, not all are spiritual)
- Paddleboarding
- Petting your dog or cat
- Playing an instrument (cello, piano, guitar, flute, drums)
- Playing with a fidget toy or playdough
- Practicing gratitude exercises
- Practicing mindfulness
- Progressive muscle relaxation
- Reading a book
- Singing
- Spending time in nature
- Spiritual health
- Stretching
- Taking a warm bath, sauna, or using a hot tub
- Talking to people who have expertise in areas that are causing you stress
- Walking
- Walking your dog or a friend's dog
- Working on time management
- Writing a book or your memoir (personal or to share with others)
- Yoga

Put a check next to the aforementioned activities that you currently use when you are stressed. At this point, can you think of anything else that might help you reduce stress? Circle the activities that you would like to try to help you manage your stress.

❑ Are there other activities not listed above that you would like to try to help you manage your stress?

____

____

____

____

- ❑ What goal can you set to support trying at least one of these new activities this week when you feel stressed?

____

____

____

Coaching Yourself on Stress With the COACH Approach

Throughout this chapter, you've explored healthy ways of reducing stress. However, as a midlife or more mature woman, you probably have developed some unhealthy coping behaviors that you engage in when experiencing negative stress. These behaviors can deter you from achieving health goals and prevent you from living a joy-filled life.

CURIOSITY

With a sense of curiosity and learning how to manage your stress in healthier ways, consider addictive behaviors (excessive alcohol use, smoking, or illicit drug use) that you may engage in to reduce your stress that are unhealthy. If needed, call the Substance Use National Hotline at 1-800-662-4357.

- ❑ Are there any behaviors you engage in when you are very stressed, which may be acceptable in moderation or at certain times, but are unhealthy when done in excess? For example, excessive alcohol use, gambling, overspending, excessive exercise, binge eating, or bulimic behavior?

____

____

____

____

- ❑ Who will you reach out to discuss this? Possibly your friend, a family member, therapist, physician, or healthcare provider? Now is the time.

____

____

____

____

❑ Do you engage in unhealthy self-talk, negativity, catastrophizing, or other ways of thinking that do not support your emotional health when stressed? Explain.

____

____

____

Remember, this PAVING program has no shame, blame, or guilt. Instead, take the cues you may be experiencing as signs to move forward in a more healthy direction.

OPENNESS

When people experience high levels of chronic stress, they may seek the use of addictive substances to "self-medicate." Unfortunately, repeated use of these addictive substances typically increases long-term stress.

At this moment, be open to acknowledging the sources of stress in your life, including people, projects, jobs, family members, and commitments. Be open to recognizing the issues and having conversations with the necessary people to create resolution in these various areas. Be open to help. You are not Wonder Woman, nor were you meant to be. This is the time to reach out for help if you are experiencing excessive stress or even a little anxiety that is disturbing.

❑ What source of stress will you address?

____

____

____

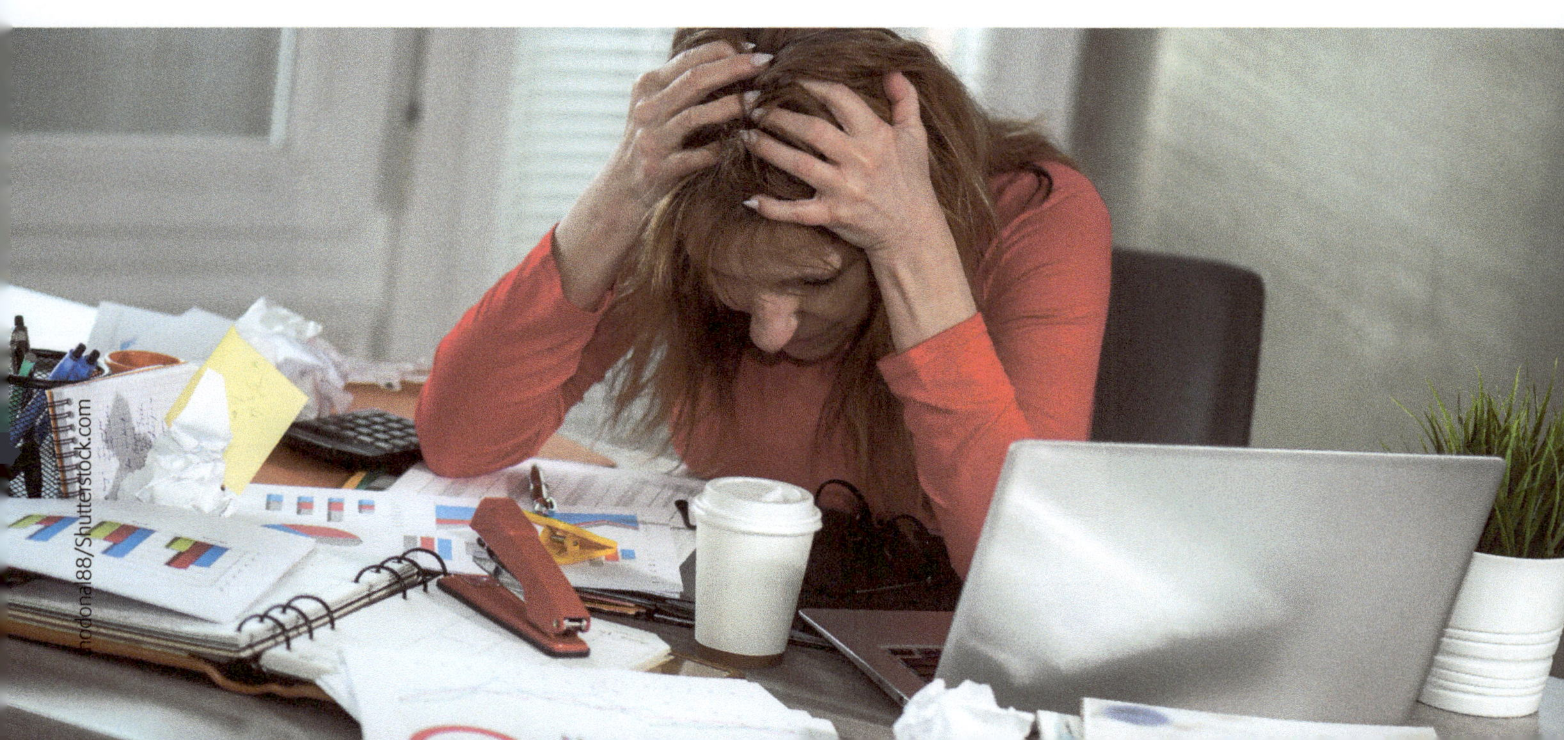

nodonal88/Shutterstock.com

- ❑ What are the next steps you will take to address it?

____

____

____

APPRECIATION

As a midlife or more mature woman, you've done many difficult things before. You've probably stopped unhealthy behaviors, started healthy behaviors, or changed ways of thinking to enhance your well-being. You also may have dealt with challenging situations, such as a medical diagnosis or the loss of a loved one.

- ❑ What qualities or traits do you possess that positively helped you handle challenges and stressors in the past?

____

____

____

- ❑ How can you use these qualities or traits to address the unhealthy behaviors or ways of thinking you've identified?

____

____

____

- ❑ Think about someone in your life who has gone through a chaotic time. How did they do it?

____

____

____

- ❑ What can you learn from their experience?

____

____

____

COMPASSION

When confronted with stress, thinking about addictive behaviors or unhealthy thoughts can be difficult. Also, changing these behaviors or patterns of thinking is often challenging and may require multiple attempts at change before being successful.

- ❑ What self-talk can you compassionately use to talk to yourself about how changing the behavior or negative self-talk could help your overall well-being?

  ____

  ____

  ____

  ____

- ❑ What are some healthier behaviors or ways of talking to yourself that you could use to replace the other behaviors?

  ____

  ____

  ____

  ____

- ❑ If your best friend were going through what you are currently going through, what would you say to them?

  ____

  ____

  ____

  ____

- ❑ List five ways to treat yourself compassionately in the next few days.

  ____

  ____

  ____

  ____

HONESTY

What support do you need to change your behaviors or negative thoughts and self-talk? Consider groups such as Alcoholics or Overeaters Anonymous, healthcare providers (for prescriptions for tobacco cessation), hotlines (tobacco cessation hotlines), books, websites, or professional organizations that address these issues.

Being honest with yourself and reaching out for help is not a weakness. However, you may feel weak in these difficult times, and you may need to rely on others to help give you the strength to move forward and get beyond the issues. Always remember that once you are on the other end, you will likely be able to be the strength that another person will need in a crisis or difficult time.

- ❑ Who can you open up to, honestly?

  ____

  ____

  ____

- ❑ What goal can you set to help you leave this negative behavior or way of thinking behind and handle stressful situations in a healthier manner moving forward?

  ____

  ____

  ____

Stress Wrap-Up

Although it can be stressful to learn about the negative health impacts of chronic stress during and after menopause, hopefully it motivates you to prioritize relaxation and healthy ways to manage stress in your life. Prioritizing your physical and mental health requires that you take time for yourself to pause and relax. Therefore, stress management activities are vital to optimizing your well-being as a woman, both now and for decades to come.

Reference

1. McGonigal K. *The Upside of Stress: Why Stress Is Good for You, and How to Get Good at It.* New York: Penguin; 2016.

CHAPTER 9
TIME-OUTS

Time-Outs Throughout Menopause, Midlife, and Beyond

Acronym—TIME-OUTS

Teach
Inward
Meaning
Energy
Others
Understanding
Turning down the noise
Spiritual

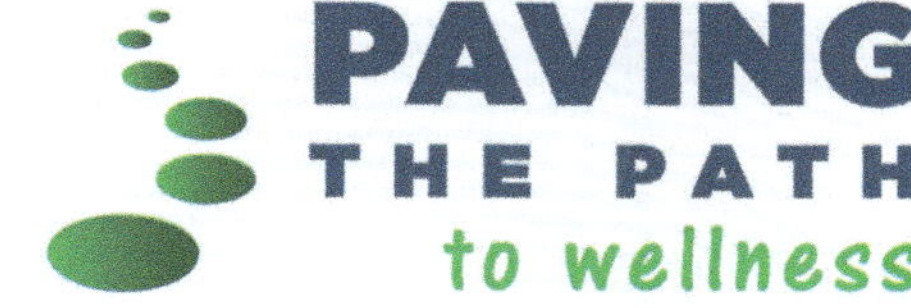

- *TEACH:* Time-outs are an ideal time to learn something new. Maybe you want someone to teach you to play a new instrument, speak a new language, or engage in a new activity. The possibilities are endless.
- *INWARD:* Time-outs allow you to turn your thoughts inward to learn more about yourself. Your life can get so busy that you don't allow yourself time for inward exploration. Time-outs provide the space for you to know more about yourself.
- *MEANING:* Time-outs bring greater meaning to your life. Rather than mindlessly spending the hours of your days, you can intentionally and mindfully use your time.
- *ENERGY:* Time-outs renew your energy. They allow you to recharge. They also give you time to mindfully decide where to put your time and energy.

- *OTHERS:* Time-outs can give you time to be alone, or they can happen when you are with others with whom you have meaningful relationships. Time-outs can help you connect with others on a deeper level, because you are mindfully pausing from the business of daily life.
- *UNDERSTANDING:* When you take a time-out, you can better understand what you need. Understanding what your physical body and emotional health need is an integral part of life.
- *TURNING DOWN THE NOISE:* It is beneficial to reduce the noise and spend time in silence when you take time-outs. This quiet pause can help you recharge, refresh, and then re-engage with the rest of your life.
- *SPIRITUAL:* It's easy to neglect your spiritual well-being when your schedules become busy. Use time-outs to support your spiritual well-being. Consider praying or reading a book that aligns with your spiritual beliefs. You can also use this time to meditate or spend time in nature.

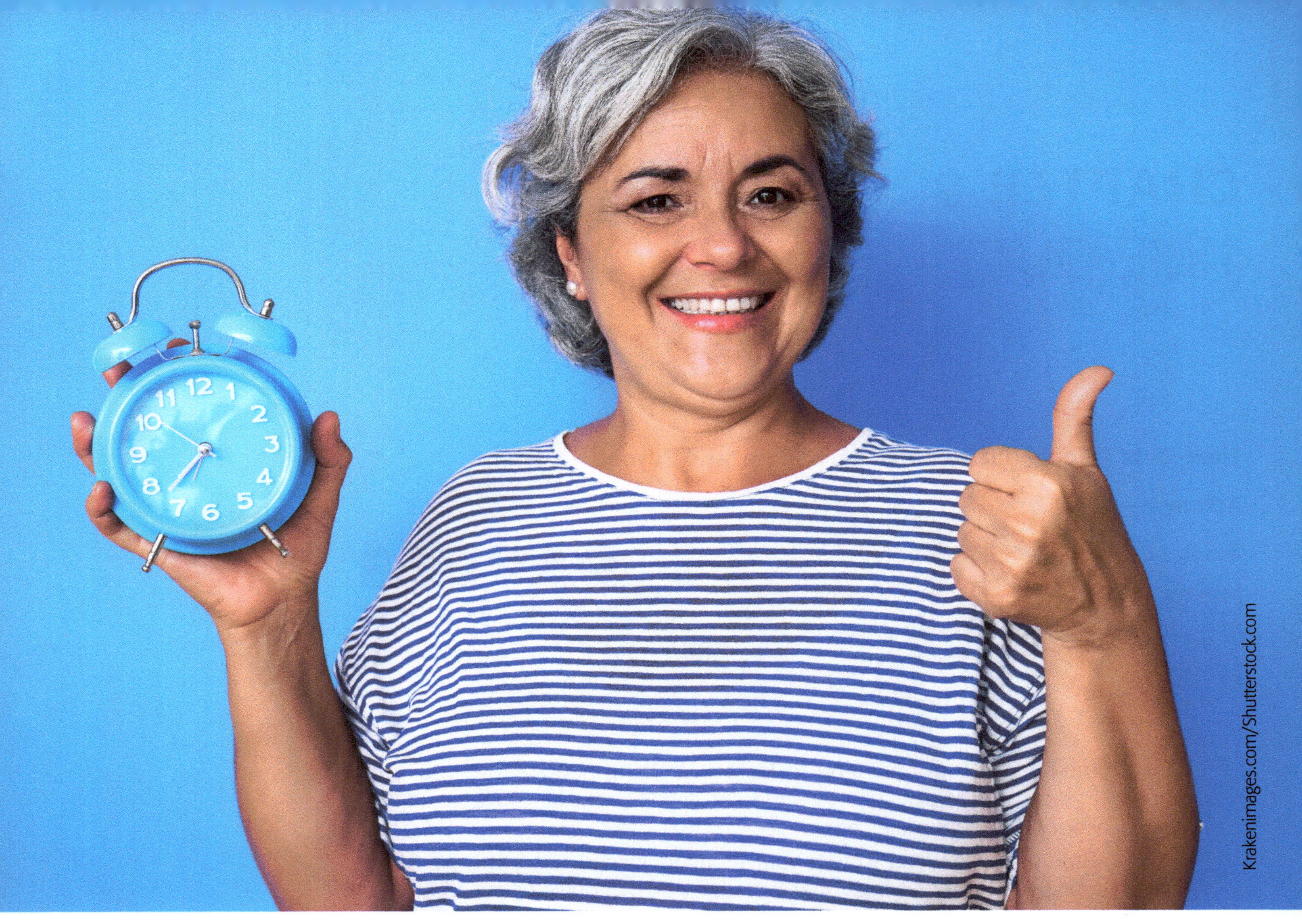

Time is your most precious gift. Unlike an adolescent who believes they are invincible, as a woman going through or who has gone through menopause, you know that your time on earth is finite. As you grow older, you want to wisely, thoughtfully, and mindfully spend your treasured time. Only through the intentional use of your time and taking time-outs for reflection and rejuvenation can you lead a purpose-filled life.

Time-outs in the PAVING program are synonymous with empowerment moments and empowerment tools. Don't think of time-outs as negative. Instead, reframe your concept of time-outs as a time for reflection, regrouping, reorganizing, and reenergizing. Time-outs help you tackle challenging situations and persevere to reach higher ground if and when chaos strikes.

- ❑ How has your view of time changed as you've aged? Does time seem to move faster? Do you value time with loved ones more?

  ____

  ____

  ____

❑ How intentional are you with the use of your time?

____

____

____

❑ How much time are you spending with your first, second, and third priorities?

____

____

____

Too Little Time

Many women feel like they never have enough time in this fast-paced, tech-filled, and information-overloaded society that values productivity. By the time women reach menopause, they have often been focusing on the needs of their children, partners, careers, and committees. As traditional caregivers in families and communities, women often become so accustomed to devoting their time to others that they don't even notice how little time they have dedicated to their own needs. If you don't take time-outs, you will get burnt out.

During or after menopause is an ideal time to pause and reflect upon how you are using your time. When you live moment to moment and day to day, allowing the world to fill your schedule, you can lose touch with yourself and stray from your purpose-filled path. Give yourself an opportunity to step back and see the larger picture. This will be empowering for you. If you feel yourself resisting taking time-out for reflection, it's probably even more critical for you to do so.

❑ What gets in the way of taking time-outs and using your time more intentionally?

____

____

____

❑ Is this something that you want to change? If so, what will be the next steps?

____

____

____

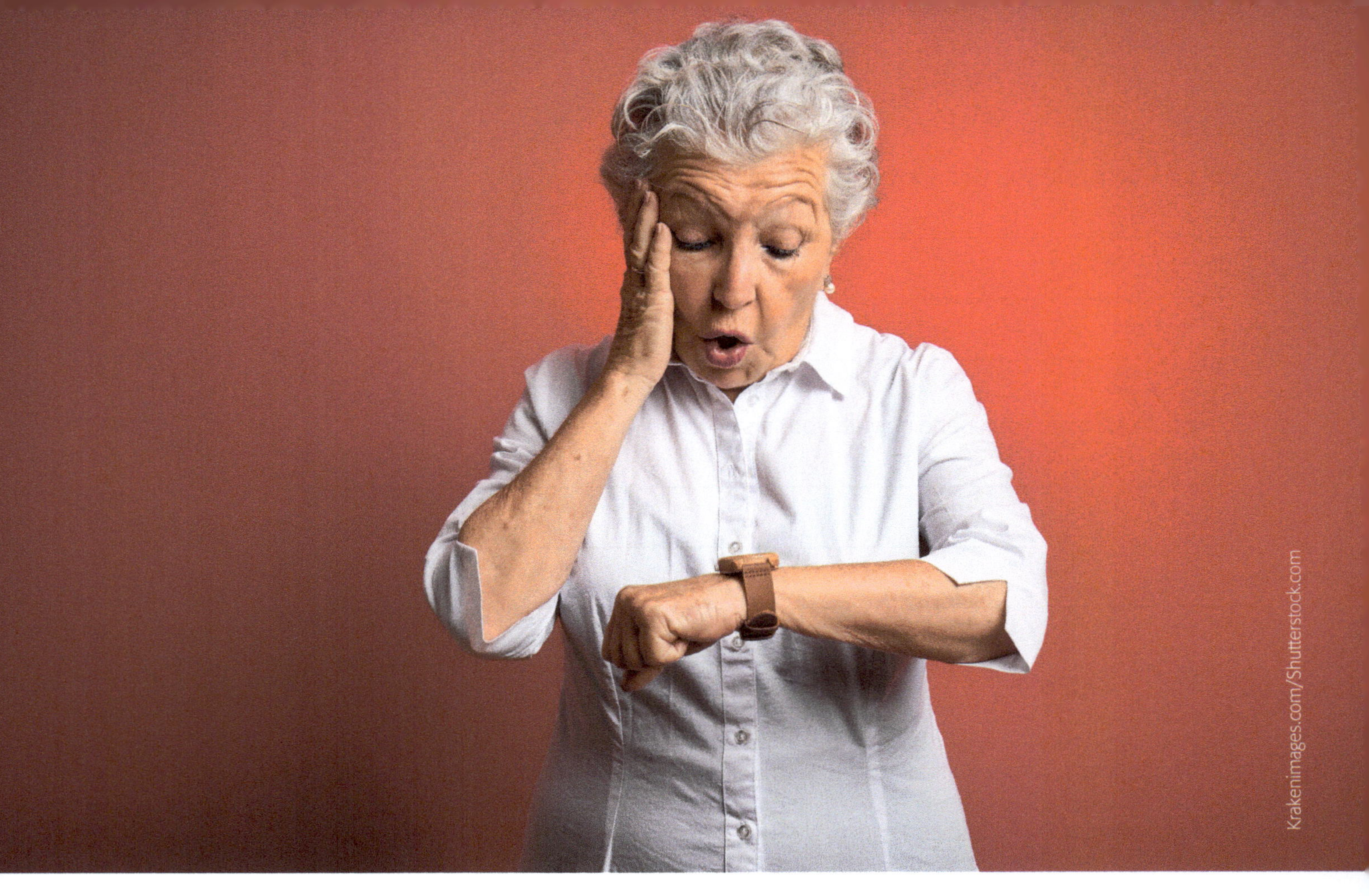

Krakenimages.com/Shutterstock.com

Time-outs allow you to pause from the craziness of life and be more present when you return from your rest.

- ❑ How do you feel when you return from a time-out and resume your activities? Consider energy level, mood, and attitude.

Too Much Time

Although many women, especially those going through menopause, feel like they don't have enough time to take time-outs and do all that is on their to-do list, others struggle with having too much time. After retirement, it is common for women to struggle with their sudden increase in free time, especially if their partner is at home or retired too, requiring the renegotiation of roles, space, and expectations. Having a sudden excess of free time can feel unsettling for women who worked full-time. Even if you have an abundance of unstructured time, you may benefit from taking a mindful time-out to reflect upon how you want to use your time more purposefully. Many purpose-filled paths that do not involve caring for children, a spouse, or a current career require time dedication.

- ❑ Do you struggle with having too much free time? If so, how can you use time-outs to reflect upon how to use your time more meaningfully to align with your purpose?

____

____

____

Some people associate time-outs with loneliness and boredom. You control what type of break supports your health and well-being. If you feel like you have too much alone time already, time-outs for you may involve taking time to connect with members of your community. If you already struggle with daily boredom, a time-out for you could be taking time to learn a new hobby. Time-outs should give you license for reflection to decide what you want to do with your time and then allow you to intentionally design your days to optimally use your precious hours in ways that support your unique needs and preferences.

Time Journal

It's easy to go from year to year, month to month, week to week, day to day, and appointment to appointment, without reflecting upon how you are spending your time. However, if you want to be mindful about how you are using your days and taking meaningful time-outs, you need to have a deeper understanding of what is filling your hours.

Open your calendar and review your last few weeks (or choose another few weeks if your past weeks have not been typical). After reviewing them, answer the following questions. Note that some activities may fit into multiple categories. For example, you may take a cooking class with your partner, which would fit into the appropriate food, connection, and learning categories.

- ❑ After reflecting on the use of your time, what insight did you gain? What surprised you?

____

____

____

- ❑ On average, how many hours per week do you spend:
  - Caring for your health through the healthcare system (e.g., doctor's visits, talking to your insurance company, driving to the pharmacy to pick up your prescriptions) __________
  - On food-related activities (e.g., meal planning, grocery shopping, cooking, eating, clean-up) __________
  - On planned physical activity (e.g., aerobic activity, resistance training, yoga classes, active leisure activities) __________

- Being inactive or sitting __________
- Sleeping __________
- Using social media or watching television __________
- On devices with screens __________
- Commuting __________
- Engaging in stress management/relaxation activities __________
- Doing activities that support your spiritual health __________
- Enjoying nature __________
- Having fun, experiencing joy, or laughing __________
- Learning new things __________
- Being creative __________
- Communicating or connecting with those whom you love or care about __________
- Worrying __________
- Shopping online or in stores __________
- Hobbies __________

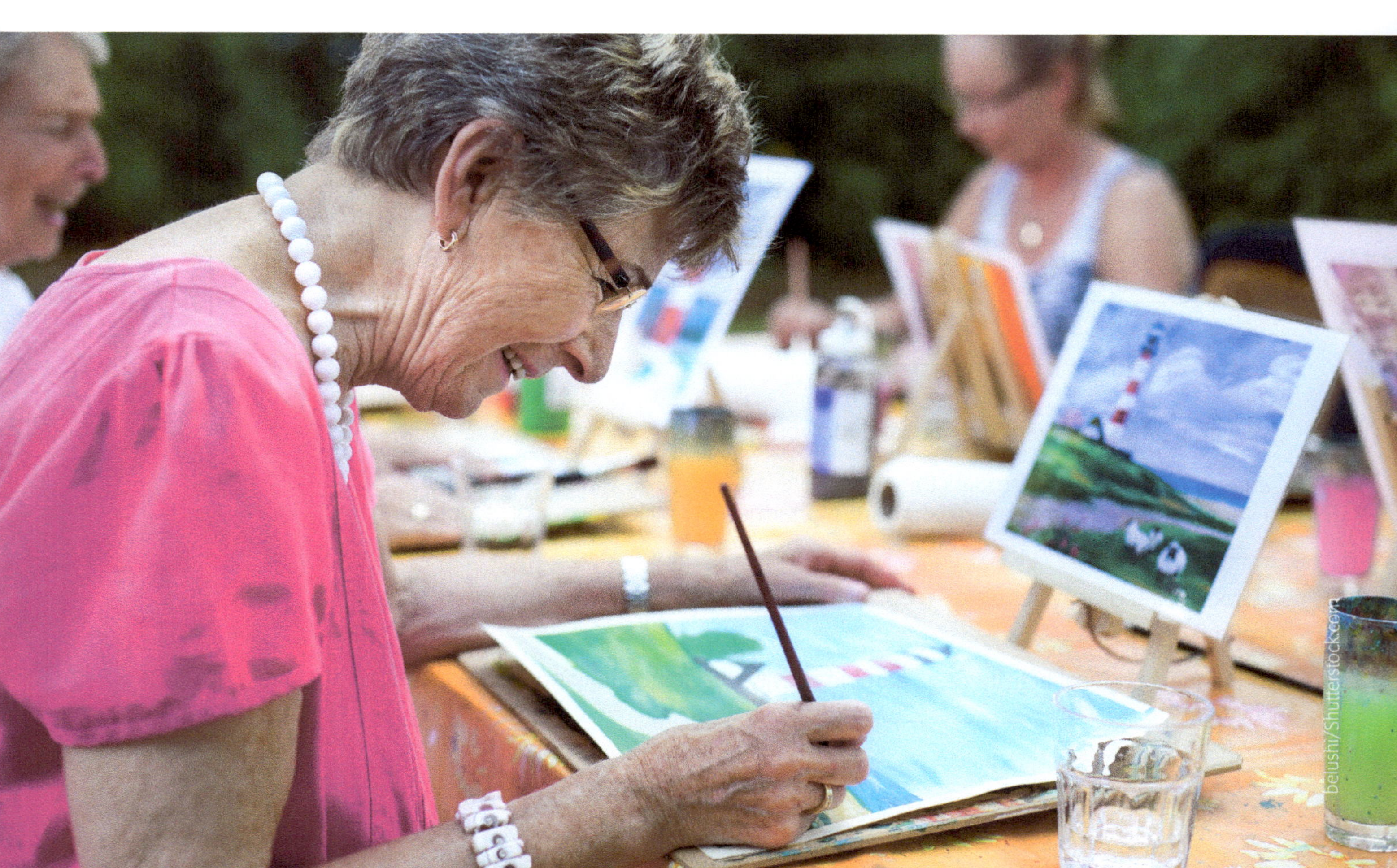
belushi/Shutterstock.com

By completing this activity, what did you learn?

- ❑ Are there areas that you want to spend more time on than you do currently?

____

____

____

- ❑ Are there areas that you want to spend less time on than you do currently?

____

____

____

- ❑ Do you want to make any changes to how you are using your time, and if so, what steps will you take next?

____

____

____

Time for Time-Outs

You don't need an entire free day to reap the benefits of time-outs. Even a few seconds can leave you more energized and ready to tackle the rest of your day. Look at the time-out spectrum detailed in Table 9-1 and consider what you currently use for time-outs.

Time-Out Spectrum							
Quick							**Longer**
10-seconds of deep breathing	Mantras	5-minutes of prayer	10-minute walk, jog, swim	20-minute conversation with friends	Massage	Half-day retreat	Vacation

Table 9-1. A sample time-out spectrum

- ❑ Do you need to take more mini time-outs? Do you need longer time-outs?

____

____

____

There is value in mini time-outs and having longer time-outs, such as a vacation. Ideally, you can enjoy short time-outs throughout each day while also planning for time-outs that require a more prolonged investment of your time.

It is best if you have various time-out options due to the complexity of your life. For example, when searching for a reprieve from a difficult conversation, a short time-out could involve deep breathing or a quick stretch. You can take longer time-outs, such as a staycation in your own home, working on relaxing and reorganizing for a few days, or a vacation where you go to the beach or spend time with family or friends. The point to remember is that time-outs can entail many different things.

Time-Out Timeline

What activities did you use to do for time-outs when you were in childhood, early adulthood, and last year? Consider what you used for very short time-outs, all the way through to longer time-outs, such as vacations. When considering childhood time-outs, the focus is not on time-outs as punishments but on things you enjoyed.

- ❑ List the activities you used for time-outs over the course of your early adulthood, adolescence, and early adulthood.

Childhood	**Adolescence**	**Young Adulthood**	**Now**

Table 9-2. Time-out timeline

- ❑ Are there any time-outs you used earlier in your life that you would like to incorporate into your life now? Explain.

____

____

____

Time for Health and the PAVING STEPSS

Taking time-outs will allow you to use your treasured time better. In doing so, you will increase your energy (which we will cover in the next chapter), better align your time with your life's purpose (also to be covered later in this book), and improve your social connections (the last of the twelve steps in the program). To obtain the full benefits from and have energy for the other PAVING STEPSS, you must take time out for yourself and be intentional with dedicating time to eating healthy foods, getting adequate physical activity, practicing stress reduction techniques, and sleeping. In addition, you are deserving of every minute you devote to self-care. As you hear on the airplane, in case of an emergency, you must put on your oxygen mask (i.e., take time for self-care), before you can care for others.

Look at several of the components of the PAVING STEPSS to better understand if you're devoting adequate time to each component or if there are areas that could benefit from increased attention and time. First, consider how much time you devote to these activities daily or weekly in these five areas.

❑ Do you feel like you are spending an adequate amount of time on these activities, or do you want to take time-out from your busy schedule to give these areas more time?

- Physical activity—

  ____

  ____

  ____

- Nutrition—

  ____

  ____

  ____

- Stress management—

  ____

  ____

  ____

- Sleep—

  ____

  ____

  ____

- Social connection—

____

____

____

The next chapter discusses energy. When you neglect taking time-outs for self-care, your energy level is affected. You can learn all the information in PAVING the Path to Wellness program, but if you don't take time-out from the rest of your life to implement the steps, you won't experience the program's full potential.

Take this moment to savor that you are reading this chapter right now. You have taken time-out to devote to your self-care. Acknowledge this, reflecting on any positive steps you've taken to make your life richer and more meaningful.

Some women are so busy that they don't even know what they would want to do if they genuinely took time out for self-care or reflection.

❑ What would you most enjoy doing, if you had an extra hour today with nothing scheduled and nothing on your to-do list?

____

____

____

❑ Consider your physical, emotional, mental health, and spiritual. What type of self-care are you most in need of now?

____

____

____

____

❑ What specific steps can you take to make time-outs for self-care a reality for you?

____

____

____

____

❑ What are your favorite self-care activities? List them.

____

____

____

Next to each one, put approximately how long it has been since you last experienced these activities.

Time for Fun

Do you remember your childhood when playing was your primary "job?" In childhood, play has a purpose. It teaches children how to interact with others, increases creativity, supports brain development, improves problem-solving abilities, and increases emotional well-being. As homework, chores, and responsibilities replace play, it is easy to forget what you gained from playing as a child. Reflecting upon what you enjoyed in your childhood and adolescence and then creating opportunities to experience play and joy supports well-being throughout midlife and beyond. Make a timeline depicting the types of play or fun activities you enjoyed during each period (Table 9-3).

Childhood	**Adolescence**	**Young Adulthood**	**Now**

Table 9-3. Timeline for the types of play and fun activities you enjoyed over your lifetime

❑ What was it about those activities that brought you joy?

____

____

____

❑ Do you still engage in similar experiences or activities that allow you to experience some of these same feelings? Explain.

____

____

____

As you get older and experience loss, it's easy for life to feel very serious and sad. Although taking time-outs to incorporate joy and fun in your life won't take away the loss, it can help you during these challenging times. Keep in mind that you are never too old to laugh, have fun, and be joyful. So, make it a priority to create and seek opportunities that bring you joy. These experiences, especially while connecting with others, support your mental, emotional, and physical well-being.

❑ What are some creative activities, hobbies, or recreational activities that you have done in the past, currently do, or would like to do in the future, that are fun? You may have already thought of and incorporated some of these in your workbook. Try to think of others you haven't listed, like board games, playing chess, playing cards, golf, gardening, hiking, cooking, scrapbooking, photography, painting, pottery, music, and bird watching.

____

____

____

❑ How can you create time in your life to experience these fun activities more frequently? Try to be specific with your plan.

____

____

____

____

❑ Are there people that could enjoy these activities with you? If so, list them here and consider inviting them to join you sometime soon.

____

____

____

____

Time for Spiritual Health

Spiritual health is a topic that is typically not addressed in books on health and wellness. However, most women consider spiritual health an essential part of their overall wellness. Although many women would agree that spiritual health is vital to well-being, what makes them feel "spiritually healthy" would likely vary significantly. For some women, their spirituality connects directly with a formal religious tradition. For many women, prayer is a beautiful way to take a step back from their everyday stress and dive into something comforting and empowering. For other women who do not identify with a religious tradition, spirituality may be a connection with something or someone greater than themselves. For those individuals, spiritual well-being may connect them with serving others or with nature. Regardless of your spiritual path, nourishing your spirituality supports wellness throughout the menopausal transition and the rest of your life.

Your spiritual well-being often connects with your purpose in life. For many women, it is an essential part of their identity. Spirituality can often help women through difficult times when dealing with health issues, unwanted significant life changes, and grief. It may help them make sense of a world that doesn't always seem to have answers and gives them hope for a brighter future. When you can't change your circumstances, your spiritual beliefs may help you find acceptance and process your feelings along life's journey.

- ❑ What does spiritual health mean to you?

  ____

  ____

  ____

- ❑ How do you feel about spiritual health, spirituality, and religion? Which one resonates with you?

  ____

  ____

  ____

  ____

- ❑ Why is your spirituality important to you? How does it help you through tricky times?

  ____

  ____

  ____

  ____

- ❑ Are you devoting as much time as you would like to nurture your spiritual health?

  ___

  ___

  ___

- ❑ How is your spirituality connected with your purpose in life?

  ___

  ___

  ___

  ___

Life can get so busy that you don't have time to examine your spiritual health. Unlike your physical health, you don't usually get a call from your doctor's office reminding you that it's time for your annual (spiritual) exam. However, your overall wellness may suffer without attention to your spiritual health.

For many people, finding time to be still and silent, to take time away from technology and social media, allows them to reflect on their spiritual well-being. Time spent in silence, prayer, or meditation is not wasted time. Instead, this quiet time may be what you need to better understand who you are, your place in the world, and connect with a significant part of yourself.

- ❑ What can you do to create time-outs that support your spiritual well-being, if you aren't already focusing on your spiritual health as much as desired?

  ___

  ___

  ___

  ___

- ❑ Who is someone in your life who is spiritual?

  ___

  ___

  ___

  ___

❑ Would it make sense for you to try to reach out to that person?

____

____

____

____

❑ What would you like to do during your spiritual time-outs? For some women, it may involve attending a religious service or reaching out to a spiritual leader; for others, it may include connecting with a group of spiritually like-minded women. Other options include quiet prayer or meditation time, listening to a podcast on spiritual health, reading the Bible, Torah, other Holy Book, or volunteering with a local non-profit. Still, other women may want to spend time hiking and enjoying nature.

____

____

____

____

Use this opportunity to write down and commit to a time when you will focus on your spiritual health (Table 9-4). Then, savor the moment and reflect upon how the activity enhances your overall sense of well-being.

Day and Time:	Activity:

Table 9-4. A timeline for focusing on your spiritual health

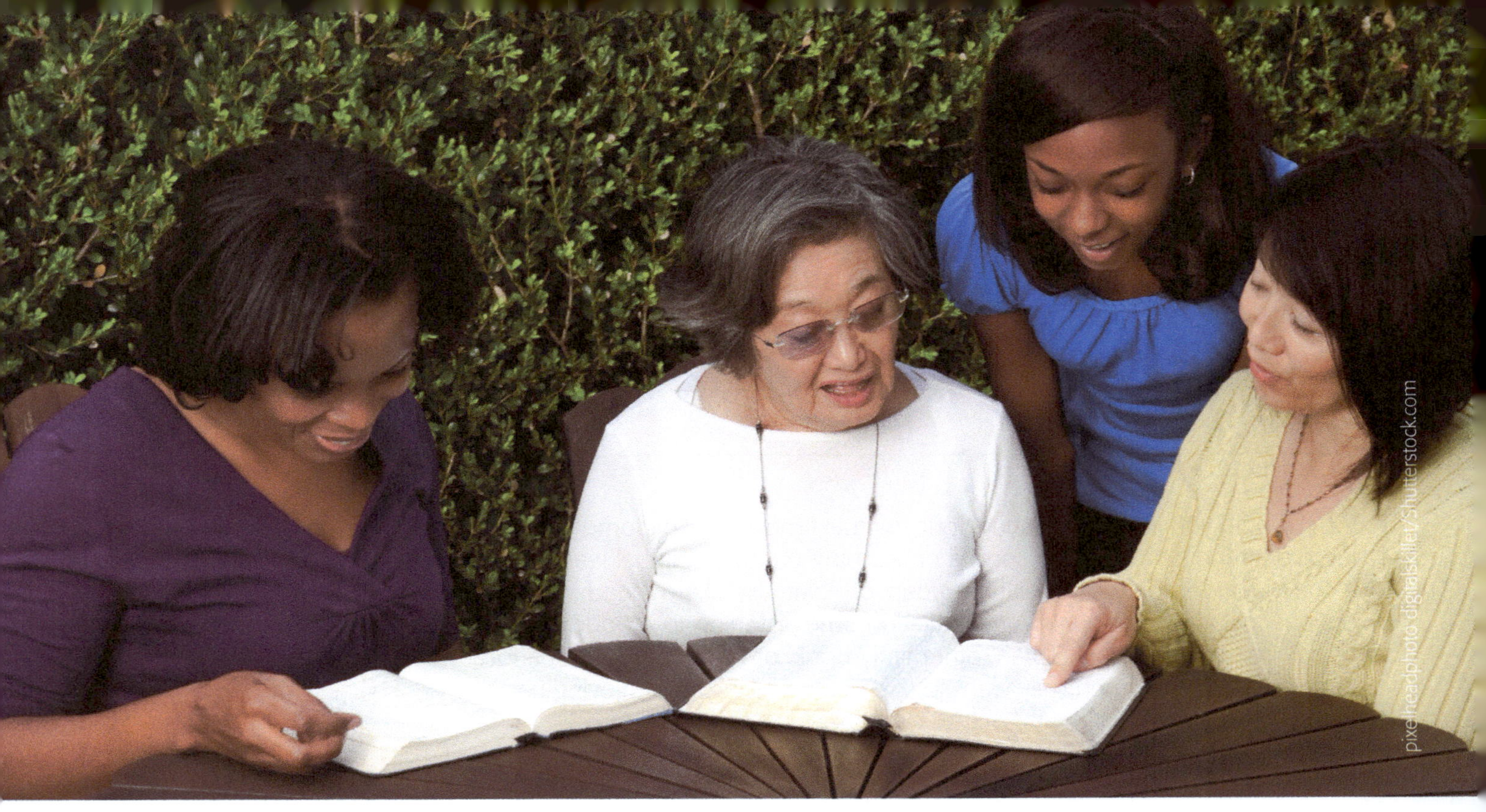
pixelheadphoto digitalskillet/Shutterstock.com

Avoiding the Multitasking Trap

Multitasking seems to be a way of life. As mothers, partners, business women, committee chairs, and activists, women wear various hats that require many tasks. When schedules get busy, it is common for women to try to do several things at once.

Now imagine wearing the hats representing six things you often do. It is ridiculous. Making dinner with your chef's hat while talking to a friend with your friend hat, while checking a text message with your work hat may seem like a reasonable way to prepare for an evening, until you see all of the hats you are trying to balance at one time.

Multitasking, as you commonly think of it, doesn't exist. Instead, your focus fluctuates between the various tasks, or you only give your full attention to certain aspects of each job, never giving your full attention to any of them. Rather than being more productive, you decrease your level of productivity and efficiency. Multitasking also decreases creativity and happiness while increasing stress, frustration, and anxiety. It requires multiple times to refocus, which drains your energy.

As you try to be more purposeful with how you spend your time, encourage yourself to try to limit multitasking. The first step in changing this unhealthy habit is becoming more aware of when you are trying to multitask. Then, consider what task is most important to focus on at this moment. Can one of the tasks wait, be delegated to someone else, or possibly be avoided altogether? For example, if you watch the news while making dinner, could you focus solely on cooking and watching the news later? Maybe you don't need to watch the news tonight at all.

Multitasking is also more common when you have multiple distractions surrounding you. For this reason, consider putting a "do not disturb" sign on your door while working, finding a quiet space to read, rather than a bustling coffee shop, where you'll overhear multiple conversations, or silencing your phone while focusing on a substantial project.

Once you become aware of your multitasking habits, you can choose to limit distractions and focus mindfully on one activity at a time. Then, hopefully, you'll be less stressed and happier too.

❑ When do you commonly multitask?

____

____

____

❑ How do you feel when you are multitasking or after you complete the tasks?

____

____

____

❑ Do you want to change your multitasking habits? If so, explain how.

____

____

____

IKO-studio/Shutterstock.com

Putting Time-Outs Into Action

Please be mindful of how you use your time while also taking time-outs to support your health. It's not about putting more things on your to-do list and packing more in less time. Instead, practice creating space in your life, in your daily schedule, to have time-outs that recharge you and allow you to flourish. The following are some suggestions for making time-outs a reality for you:

❑ Although you can take a time-out anywhere, create a unique space in your home to take time-outs. How can you make this place special, relaxing, and nurturing for you?

____

____

____

- ❑ It's easy to become so busy that you forget to take time-outs. Technology can assist you with this if you set alarms on your phone, watch, or another home smart device that reminds you to pause and take time for yourself. What can you do to remind yourself to take time-outs?

  ____

  ____

  ____

You can also schedule time on your calendar for time-outs. Just as you plan time for important meetings with others, it is equally important to schedule time-outs for you.

- ❑ Could you benefit from scheduling time-outs for self-care or spiritual well-being on your calendar? If so, how do you envision them?

  ____

  ____

  ____

When you try to take time-outs, time for self-care, or time to focus on your spiritual health, distractions can often get in the way of what you were hoping to experience during this time. However, if you are aware of the distractions that usually subvert your best intentions for time-outs, you can prepare in advance to avoid or limit these distractions.

- ❑ What distractions typically get in your way when you try to take time-outs? What can you do to remove or limit those distractions?

  ____

  ____

  ____

  ____

Remember, when you say yes to something that goes on your schedule, you are also saying no to something else that could have happened during that time. Maybe you can try to make your hour-long meeting 50 minutes instead, giving yourself 10 minutes of self-care time prior to your next appointment. When asked to take on a new commitment, mindfully consider the time and energy costs of this commitment and how it may impact your time-outs for self-care. You may need to work on being better at setting boundaries with others, creating a "no" list, instead of just having a "to-do" list, delegating, or outsourcing tasks (such as cleaning or food preparation if you are financially able to do so).

❑ What can you do to create adequate time in your schedule for time-outs? Remember, you deserve this.

____

____

____

____

❑ What is your "no" list? These are things that you will not agree to do under any circumstances, at least for the current time. Some examples include not taking on new projects, not agreeing to social engagements that you won't enjoy, not accepting invitations to meetings that you are not interested in or don't need to attend, and not saying yes to the neighbor that asks you to pick up their child for the fourth time this week.

____

____

____

____

Society expects women to be "people pleasers," For women who have taken on this role, sometimes for decades, taking time for themselves can be incredibly challenging. You may feel uncomfortable or guilty taking time-outs, or others may be judging you for doing so. If you think this way, remind yourself that you deserve time-out for self-care. No one needs to know your business or that you are taking a time-out. You are doing this for yourself. Taking time for yourself helps you return from the time-out with greater focus, energy, creativity, and clarity. Also, when you take time-outs, you are teaching others that taking time for themselves is essential.

For this reason, it may be good to share that you will be savoring some self-care. There should be no shame, blame, or guilt in taking time-outs for self-care. Just because you take time-outs does not mean that you neglect your duties. Instead, time-outs will help you with your to-do list when it is time to re-engage with it.

❑ Is it difficult for you to take time-outs because of how you feel about taking them? If so, why do you think you struggle with this?

____

____

____

____

❑ Is there anything you can do to change how you think about taking time for self-care? For example, use positive self-talk to remind yourself that you deserve to take time for self-care when you feel guilty.

____

____

____

Among the time-out favorites for women are the following:

- *Take a class:* Explore your local community center, online, and college courses. Many colleges offer non-credit, free, or reduced-cost courses for seniors. Also, you're never too old to go back to school. If you're interested in getting a degree, reach out to academic institutions to learn more. You may even qualify for significant financial aid.
- *Writing:* Consider journaling, writing your memoir, taking a writing class, writing poetry, or writing a book to publish. For many people, writing is very relaxing and can help you take a break from your other daily activities.
- *Musical instruments:* If you used to play an instrument or think it would be fun to try learning how to play a new instrument, this is an excellent opportunity to take musical time-outs. If you aren't sure you want to purchase an instrument, consider renting it initially. You can take classes in person or online. If you already play an instrument, consider how you could use playing the instrument for time-outs. If you don't play an instrument, maybe you want to sing or listen to music as your time-out.
- *Artistic expression:* Most women don't spend their days expressing themselves artistically. Taking time-outs to do something artistic, such as painting, drawing, doing stained glass, or pottery can be a creative way to break from your current routine. You don't need to be ready for a gallery show to benefit from artistic expressions as time-outs. Coloring in an adult coloring book or doodling can be a great time-out too.
- *Reading:* Whether it is reading for pleasure, to learn something new, or to finish a book for a book club, reading is a common way to take a time-out. Reading allows you to take your mind from what you were doing previously and go to another world. Experiment to see what type of books you enjoy the most and best support your time-outs.
- *Relaxation activities:* Meditation, mindfulness practices, progressive muscle relaxation, guided imagery, and focused breath work are all relaxation activities used for time-outs. If you are unfamiliar with these activities, consider taking a stress management class for relaxation or exploring reputable websites for guidance.
- *Movement:* If you spend much of your time sedentary, taking movement time-outs can benefit your physical and mental health. Take time to stretch, walk around your room or the block, lift some relatively small weights, or try a simple yoga pose. Also, consider taking a barre or Pilates class.
- *Hobbies:* Many women have hobbies that they've done or have wanted to do throughout the years. Whether it's doing a craft or gardening, hobbies help you get away from your to-do list and let you spend time doing something different. Some ideas are sewing, knitting, photography, scrapbooking, collage making, adult coloring books, word searches, crossword puzzles, and flower arranging.

- *Nature:* Most midlife and older women spend most of their time indoors. Consider getting outside and enjoying nature during a time-out. Whether going to a nature park for a hike, stepping outside your door for a quick stretch, or walking around your block, getting into nature helps you reset and recharge.
- *Pampering:* Taking time to get a massage, pedicure, or facial is a viable way to pamper yourself and take a time-out. Instead of going to a professional, you can also take a few minutes and give yourself a hand self-massage, paint your toes, or give yourself a facial. Pampering doesn't need to be expensive. Remember, you deserve it! What would feel good to you?
- *Traveling:* Plan a short trip to a mountain, beach, or another exciting location. Visit local historical sites that interest you, national parks, or hiking trails that you haven't yet explored. If you have the time and means, consider planning a vacation to another state or country.

What other ideas can you think of for time-outs? First, consider activities that you've seen others enjoy or that you enjoyed years ago. Then, push yourself to think of something new that is not on the list of favorite time-out activities and that you don't currently do.

❏ Which of the ideas on the list and those you just thought of do you want to try in the next month?

____

____

____

Words of Wisdom From Dr. Michelle Tollefson

When discussing menopausal symptoms with women, they frequently report feeling uncomfortable (both physically and emotionally) when they have a hot flash in a public environment. If they are alone during a hot flash, they can relax and allow the hot flash to pass without the additional anxiety that often accompanies hot flashes in an undesired location. However, they report feeling awkward, embarrassed, anxious, frustrated, and sometimes even nauseous in a social environment.

Our culture does not honor a woman's passage through menopause. Instead, society's ageism makes many women feel like they need to hide their menopausal transition and symptoms. Some of my patients have reported avoiding public meetings, social events, and even career promotions due to how uncomfortable having hot flashes in public makes them feel.

When I hear this from patients, I try to learn more about their underlying view of aging, menopause, and hot flashes. Some are worried that others will view them as less competent in the workplace or less valued as older women, if people know they have hot flashes. Others don't want to discuss their symptoms with other people besides me. I've been surprised at how many say they can't remember their peers discussing hot flashes.

My advice to my patients is to honor their feelings and take a time-out when they notice a hot flash starting. Rather than immediately trying to hide their hot flashes, I want them to take a mindful pause and decide what is best for them by asking themselves a few questions, such as the following, without feeling pressured to behave a certain way:

- Do I feel like sharing with those around me that I'm experiencing a hot flash, or would I prefer not to share this with others right now?
- Do I want to leave my current environment, or would I prefer to stay where I am now?
- What would help me feel the best, while I wait for this to pass (take a few slow deep breaths, remove my sweater, use a fan, get a cool drink, briefly walk outside, splash some water on my face in the restroom, etc.)?

There should be no shame or guilt for choosing what is best for you. Hot flashes can signal to take a time-out to consider what is best for you at the moment. Remind yourself that this hot flash is temporary, that it is an entirely normal part of being a woman, that you do not need to hide it, and that honoring what you want is a way to empower and care for yourself.

Although most of my patients don't report wanting to have hot flashes, they say that taking mindful time-outs to consider what is best for them when they have hot flashes has helped them feel more in control of their menopausal experience.

Coaching Yourself on Time-Outs With the COACH Approach

CURIOSITY

Most women rarely stop and pause to think about how they spend their time. Review the time journal that you completed earlier in this chapter.

❑ When could you benefit from taking time-outs in your typical days and weeks?

____

____

____

❑ What keeps you from taking time-outs or using your time like you want to use it?

____

____

____

❑ What do you see as the benefits of time-outs?

____

____

____

❑ What do you want out of the time you spend in these time-outs?

___

___

___

OPENNESS

To improve your well-being by taking time-outs, you have to be open to changing your schedule.

❑ Are you open to changing your current schedule, or are you intent on continuing your status quo? Explain.

___

___

___

❑ Are you open to spending time with yourself during a time-out, or does time alone make you feel uncomfortable or unproductive? Explain.

___

___

___

❑ Do you ever feel guilty about taking time-outs? If so, why do you think you feel this way?

___

___

___

___

❑ What self-talk could you use to replace the self-talk focused on guilt?

___

___

___

APPRECIATION

You can take time-outs without truly appreciating the gift you are giving to yourself by taking time to care for your well-being. Focus on appreciation and gratitude when you take a time-out.

- ❑ Reflect upon a recent time-out that you enjoyed. What did you enjoy the most about this time-out?

  ____

  ____

  ____

- ❑ How can you use mindful appreciation to enhance your time-outs?

  ____

  ____

  ____

Spending time today reading this book is an example of taking time-out for self-care. Acknowledge and savor this moment. We wish we were here to sit with you and share your gratitude for participating in the program and prioritizing you. Maybe one day we will all meet in person.

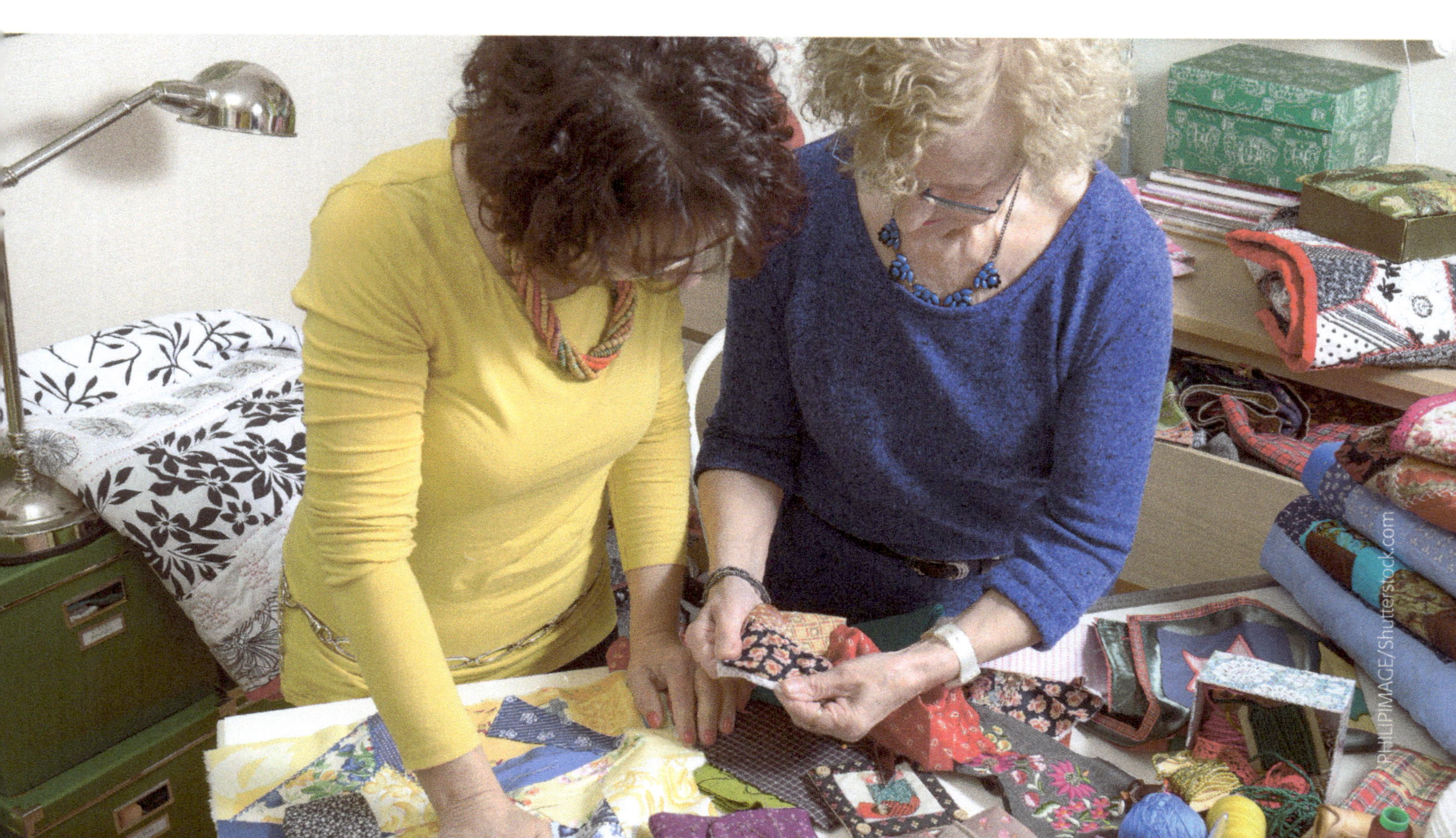
PHILIPIMAGE/Shutterstock.com

COMPASSION

Many women struggle with having so many things on their to-do lists that it seems impossible to take time for time-outs. Time-outs are probably the most important for those who are extremely busy, even if they are challenging to take. Even if you can't take an hour out of your schedule, you can still benefit from having mini time-outs of even a few minutes.

❑ If a friend of yours told you she was too busy to take time for herself, what would you say to her?

____

____

____

Many women feel loving-kindness and express it for others. Loving-kindness involves mindfully appreciating the inner beauty and true wisdom of those around you. Loving-kindness is expressed by listening to others, hugging others, accepting others for who they are- just as they are, and helping people to see and shine their light.

Sharing loving-kindness with yourself empowers you to thrive. You can do this by appreciating your inner wisdom and true beauty, which means listening to your body, honoring your feelings, savoring a moment in time, and celebrating your strengths.

❑ When was the last time you felt loving-kindness toward yourself? What were you doing?

____

____

____

❑ How can you replicate that feeling?

____

____

____

❑ Sharing loving kindness is sharing compassion. In what ways do (or can) you give yourself loving kindness daily?

____

____

____

HONESTY

Even if you start taking time-outs and honoring your need for self-care, it can be easy to slip back into old habits of packing your schedule so tightly that you don't have time for time-outs. Working with a trusted friend, family member, or mental health professional to help hold you accountable and be honest with yourself about your need for self-care can help you stay on track.

- ❑ Is there anyone who can help keep you accountable as you incorporate time-outs into your daily routine?

  ____

  ____

  ____

- ❑ How will you keep yourself accountable?

  ____

  ____

  ____

- ❑ Do you think you will take a time-out? Be honest. If so, why? If not, why not?

  ____

  ____

  ____

Time-Outs Wrap-Up

It is easy to become despondent when you think about how quickly time is passing. Rather than thinking about how you "should" have spent your past or what you "should" be doing in the future, try to be mindful of the minutes you have today. Focus on being grateful for the minutes, hours, and days you have before you, and try to align your time with what is most meaningful to you. Align your time with your purpose. Align your time with what your body and mind need and with what brings you joy. Align your time with what fulfills you spiritually. When you mindfully spend your time and use time-outs for self-care, you are genuinely PAVING your Path to Wellness.

CHAPTER 10
ENERGY

Energy Throughout Menopause, Midlife, and Beyond

Acronym—ENERGY

Environment	**Regulate**
Natural	**Generate**
Exercise	**You**

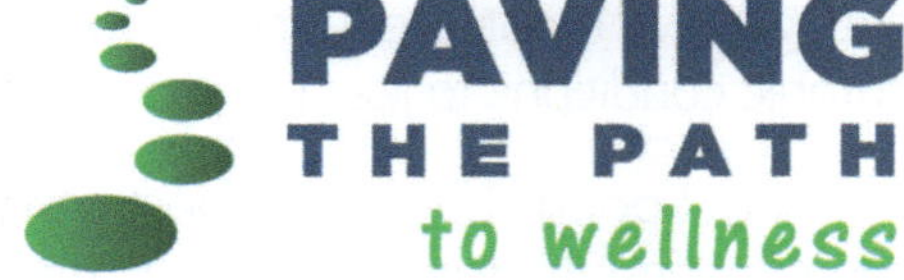

- *ENVIRONMENT*: Because your environment impacts your energy, surround yourself with uplifting people, an organized home, and stimulating activities. If your environment is draining your energy, take action and change it so that it energizes you.
- *NATURAL*: Use natural healthy energy boosters, such as nourishing foods, adequate hydration, getting restorative sleep, and spending time surrounded by nature, to boost your energy. Avoid addictive and risky substance use.
- *EXERCISE*: Exercise regularly. Engage in physical activity on a regular basis and decrease sedentary behavior to optimize your energy level. Try a variety of physical activities to see which you enjoy the most.
- *REGULATE*: Regulate your energy throughout the day by prioritizing activities and mindfully using time-outs for rest. Take breaks, as needed, so that you have the energy to make it through your day until bedtime.
- *GENERATE*: Engage in activities that create energy in your life and support your spiritual well-being. Certain activities generate more positivity for you, while others drain it. Try some energy-generating, fun activities, every day.
- *YOU*: Don't compare yourself to others. Instead, focus on your unique energy level, energy drainers, and energy boosters. Then, regularly check in with your energy level.

Increasing wisdom comes with age. Unfortunately, the same can't be said about energy. Fatigue is real and can make it challenging to engage in daily activities and get through the day without falling asleep. Fatigue can prevent you from flourishing. On the other hand, you don't have to settle for a life of fatigue. There is hope. This chapter will help you understand what gives you and drains your energy. Want to learn how to manage your energy to lead your life to the fullest? This chapter is for you. Read on.

Words of Wisdom From Dr. Michelle Tollefson

This isn't a typical live and learn, but it's a story that I believe is important to share. When I was diagnosed with breast cancer and undergoing chemotherapy, I was frustrated and saddened that I didn't have enough energy to engage with my children, especially after they returned home from school, until they went to bed. Even walking up the stairs to give them a goodnight kiss was sometimes impossible, as I was too exhausted to do the climb, even though I longed to kiss my precious children before they drifted off to sleep. Cancer had made me acutely aware, sometimes even painfully aware, of the fragility of life, time, and my energy limitations.

I met with an oncology counselor to discuss my lack of energy and stress. She told me about the Spoon Theory, which allowed me to understand better how to manage my energy during this challenging time. It also gave me a way to explain to those around me how I felt and why I was making changes with my activities and self-care to support my well-being.

Christine Miserandino coined the Spoon Theory. She used this concept to explain her struggles with limited energy due to chronic illness. She has helped others with and without chronic conditions to learn to manage their energy better to live their lives more fully.

The Spoon Theory suggests that everyone has a limited amount of "spoons," representing their limited energy each day. Those with chronic conditions or advanced age may have fewer "spoons" than others at the start of their day. Insufficient sleep, excessive stress, a lack of social support, unhealthy eating, or a lack of physical activity can also decrease a person's "spoon" reserve.

Your daily activities and stress use up your allotted spoons throughout each day. Even getting dressed, preparing meals, and visiting your doctor can use your spoons. If you don't manage your spoons adequately, you can get to the end of your day and be so spoon-depleted that you have no energy to finish your day. This is what was happening to me during chemotherapy. Although you may borrow spoons from the next day by pushing yourself hard, this will likely make tomorrow more challenging, with fewer spoons to begin that next day.

Just because you run out of spoons or energy at the end of the day does not mean that you are at fault or that your exhaustion could have been prevented through lifestyle modifications. There were days when I didn't think it would have mattered what I did. I just needed to care for myself with rest and was out of spoons by dinnertime, regardless of my daily activities. At those times, I just needed to give myself grace and permission to do what my body needed and not fight it.

However, there were other days when I could strategically use my spoons so that I could climb the stairs to kiss my kids goodnight, even while going through chemotherapy. My sister organized a sign-up for friends and family to bring me meals, so that I did not have to cook. My parents provided extra care for my children and were eager to help in any way possible. My husband, who was already extremely helpful, took on even more of our household duties to help me manage my spoons. He still reminds me to be thoughtful of using my spoons, especially when he offers to help me, and I decline his assistance, or I'm trying to push myself to keep going, even when I'm exhausted. It is essential to learn to ask for and receive help, which is a skill that I am still working on perfecting. Even though I'm grateful to have more energy than I did while undergoing chemotherapy, my energy is not as abundant as before. I still have to be thoughtful of using my spoons, especially if I get a cold, don't sleep well, or am going through a stressful time.

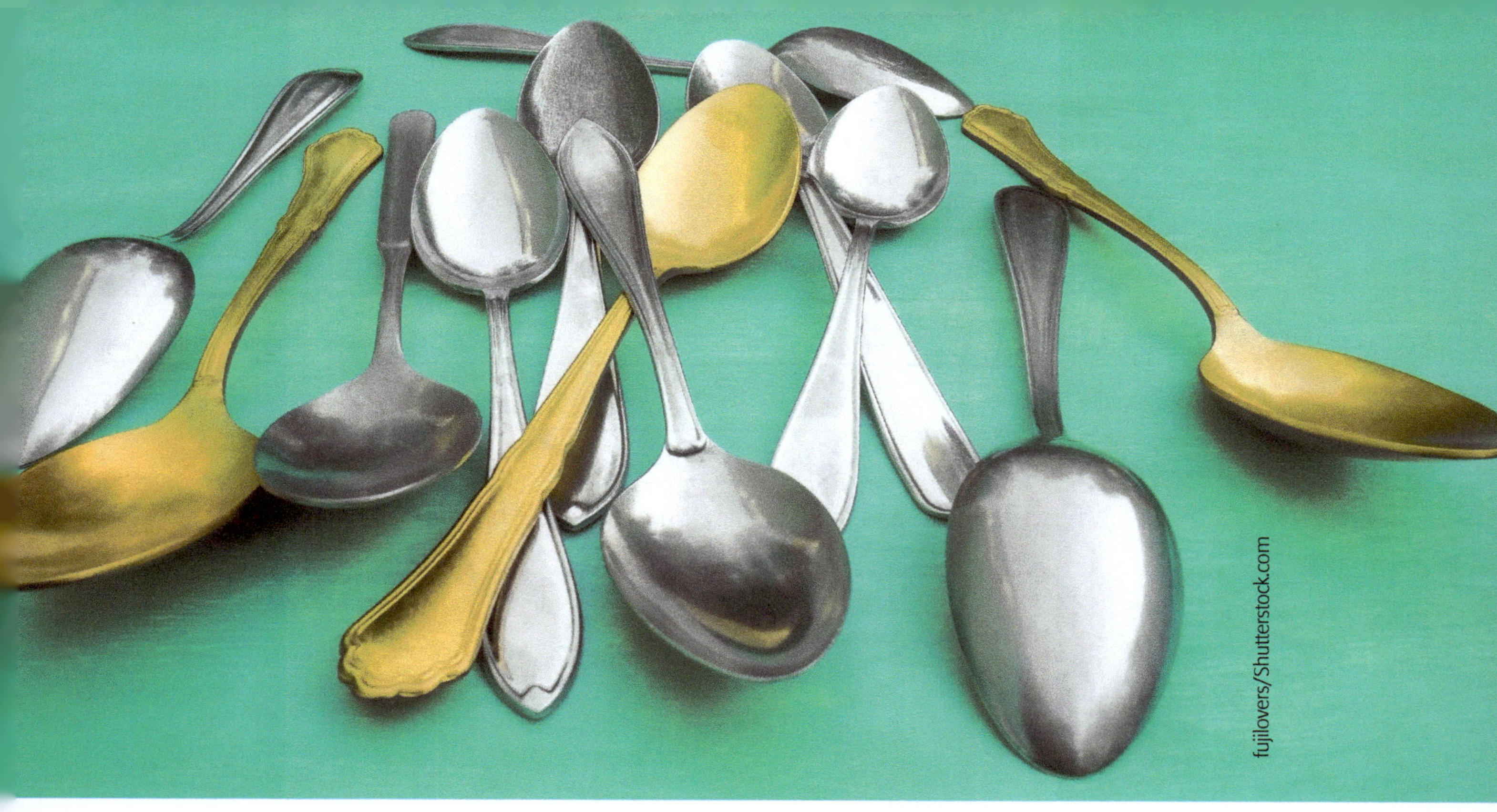
fujilovers/Shutterstock.com

We can care for our spoons and prevent them from being used so quickly by caring for ourselves through eating high-quality food, getting adequate (but not excessive) physical activity, being around people who support our well-being, getting sufficient restorative sleep, practicing stress management techniques, and avoiding risky substance use. We can also help ourselves by talking to ourselves like we would a friend.

I hope that learning about Miserandino's Spoon Theory will help you better manage your energy to fulfill your daily activities, desires, and purpose and walk up the stairs to kiss your kids goodnight, if that is your goal for the day.

Reflecting Back on Your Life

If you look back on your life, you may be able to think of a time when you were full of energy. This may be last month or five years ago, or even when you were a child. Think about what was fueling your enthusiasm. Was it simply curiosity about the world around you, as we experience in our childhood? Was it a new job or opportunity that excited you? Was it falling in love, or planning a vacation with a loved one? Was it learning new tips and strategies for healthy living from a book you were reading? Was it that you started a new exercise routine or tested out a Pilates class? Were you able to dive into your gardening hobby and watch your seeds grow? Was it taking a new class that connects you to exciting material and people?

❑ Describe the times in your life when you were full of energy.

____

____

____

- ❑ Write about a recent experience or the last time you felt like you were thriving with high energy levels.

____

____

____

Create an energy timeline (Table 10-1). Mark those times when you were the most energized and try to identify what was going on during that time.

Childhood	Adolescence	Young Adulthood	Now

Table 10-1. An example of an energy timeline

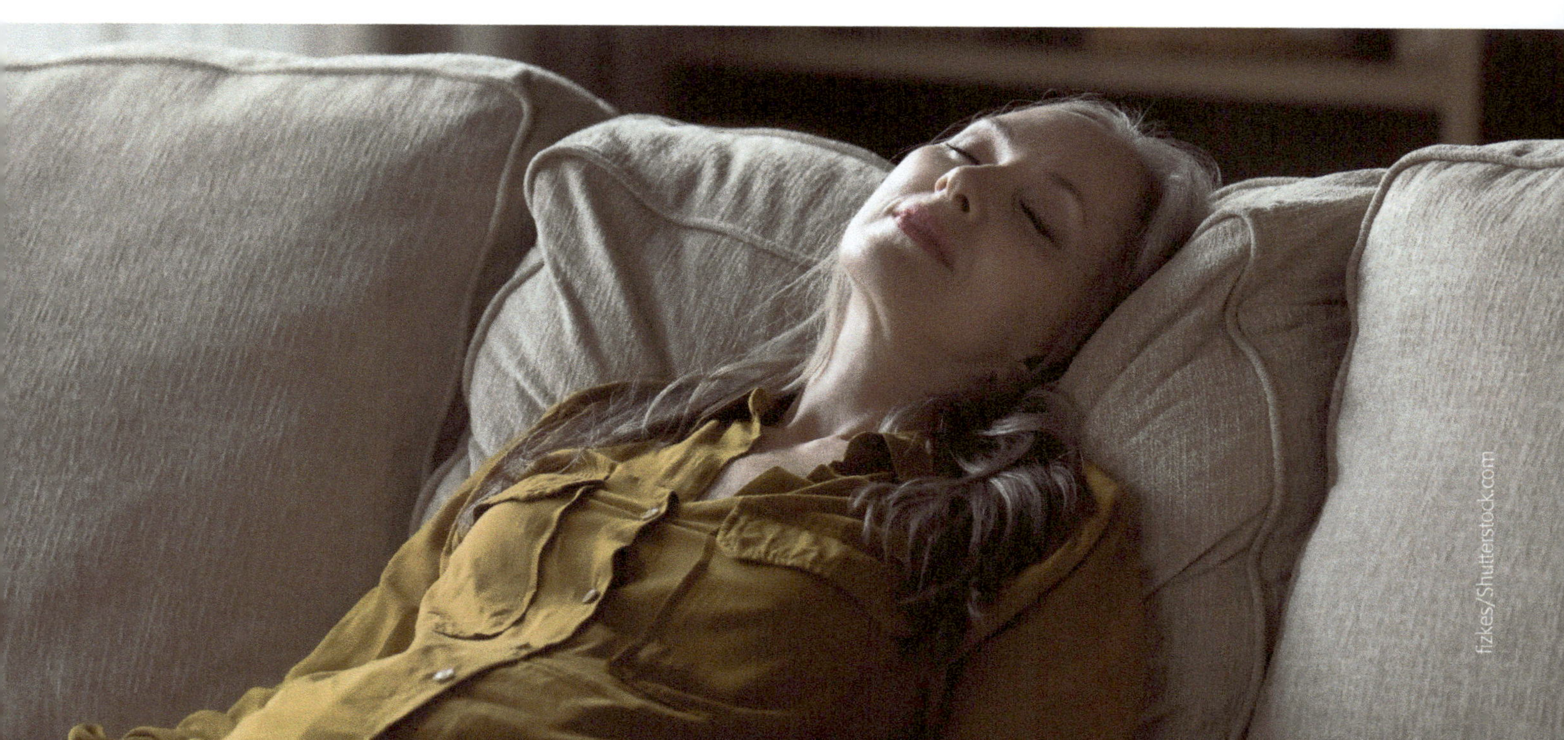

At some time, you've likely had very little energy, such as when you were nursing a newborn who frequently woke at night, were going through chemotherapy, or couldn't sleep due to anxiety about a loved one's illness. Many women during the menopause transition notice a decline in their energy and the "brain fog" that occurs when night sweats and hormone changes disrupt sleep. The good news is that the fatigue associated with the few years surrounding menopause often lifts, as night sweats stop and hormone levels stabilize. However, in other instances, an illness like COVID-19 or chemotherapy may leave you with chronically having less energy than you had previously. If something is taking your energy away, don't despair, there are still things you can do to maximize your energy each day and use it to the fullest.

If you're someone who had their energy abruptly decreased through a life event or illness, you likely have a new appreciation for how wonderful it feels to have adequate vigor to do what you want to do. When someone's energy status changes quickly, it often necessitates learning how to manage their energy. Even if you haven't had an illness or life event, energy management is still a valuable skill to learn. Throughout this chapter, you'll learn strategies to increase your power and wisely use the energy you have throughout your day.

Energy Journal

For the next several days, be mindful of your energy level throughout the day and fill out the timeline shown in Table 10-2. Make a note of your energy level when you wake up and progress throughout the day until you go to bed at night. Make a note of when you have the most energy and when you have the least. Try to notice how your strength ebbs and flows during the day. Also, pay attention to whether there are certain activities, places, or people who increase or decrease your stamina. For example, maybe you have more energy after eating breakfast or talking to your best friend but less energy after doing laundry or attending a stressful meeting.

❑ What did you learn from your energy journal?

____

____

____

____

❑ When do you typically have the most energy?

____

____

____

____

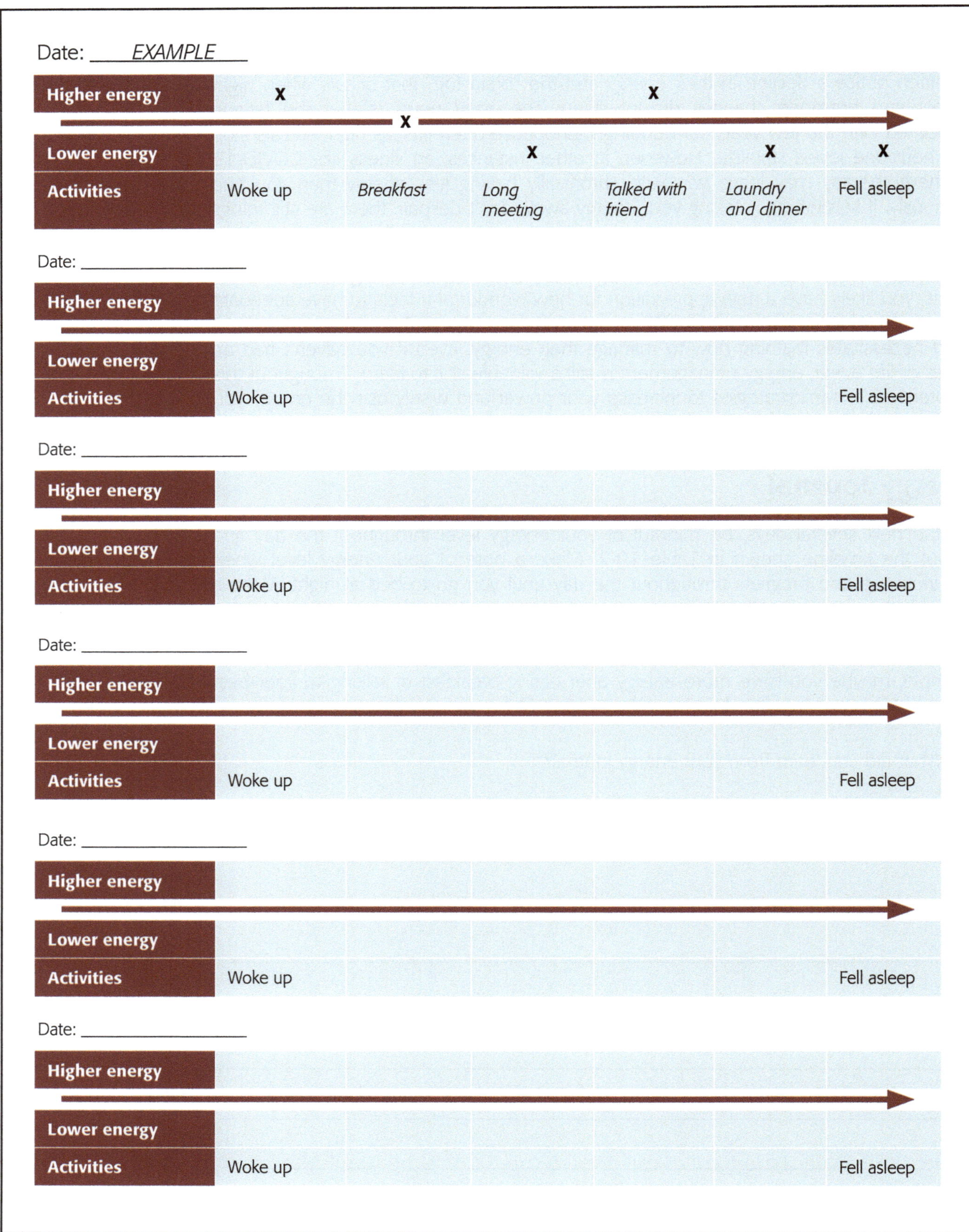

Table 10-2. An example of an energy journal

- [ ] When do you typically have the least energy?

____

____

____

- [ ] Energy boosters: What activities, places, and people increase your energy? Consider your timeline in Table 10-1, as well as other items not on your timeline.

____

____

____

- [ ] Energy drainers: What activities, places, and people decrease your energy? Consider your timeline in Table 10-1, as well as other times in your life, when your energy has been depleted.

____

____

____

The Energy-Purpose Connection

Having energy allows you to fulfill your purpose and to live life joyfully. Without adequate energy, even doing basic activities of daily living can be a struggle. A lack of vigor can leave you feeling like you can't accomplish what you want to in your life. Likewise, fatigue can prevent you from fulfilling your purpose in life. This book's next chapter covers purpose in further depth, but for now, it's beneficial to consider the connection between energy and purpose. When you do something that aligns with your purpose, you will likely feel energized and joyful. Likewise, having enough energy will support you in fulfilling your purpose. The two factors are beautifully intertwined, and alone neither can flourish. Examples of typical areas of purpose include the following:

- Helping make the world a better place
- Taking care of others
- Sharing your gifts with the world
- Practicing your spiritual beliefs
- Caring for your family or friends
- Creating works of art or beauty
- Volunteering
- Caring for pets
- Making your garden grow and supplying those in need with fresh produce
- Mentoring others who can learn from your experiences

- ❑ Think of times when you've engaged in activities that connect with these common areas of purpose and list a few examples.

- ❑ What is your energy level when preparing for these activities, engaging in them, and then after completing these activities?

Types of Energy

Not all energy is the same. For example, have you ever been physically exhausted from a long hike or from an intense workout but felt mentally and emotionally energized? Or, maybe you wake in the morning and are filled with physical energy. Still, immediately upon waking, you remember an argument you had with your friend last night and feel emotionally exhausted. Therefore, it is essential to be mindful of whether your energy tanks are empty or full regarding your physical, emotional, and spiritual energy.

- ❑ Where is your energy level right now with regard to the following areas?

Physical energy	Emotional energy	Spiritual energy

Table 10-3. Energy level assessment

- ❑ What is making your energy levels as high as they are currently reported?

- ❏ What is preventing your levels from being higher in each of these areas? You may want to consider what has drained your energy in each area, for example, situations, conflicts, people, places, responsibilities, and workload.

____

____

____

- ❏ What could increase your energy levels in each of these domains? You may want to consider what has increased your vitality level in the past, for example, supportive people in your life, activities, and places that may support your energy.

____

____

____

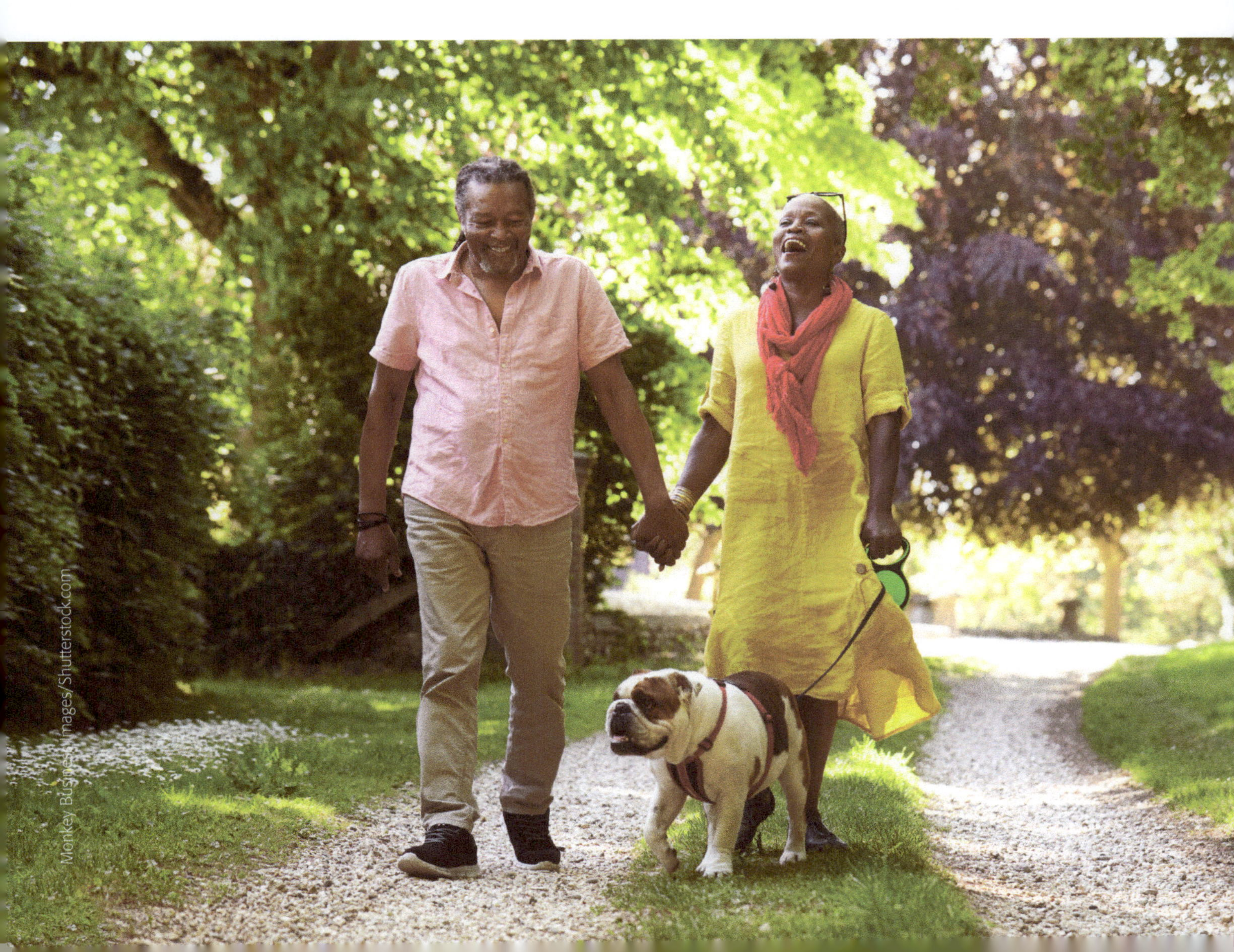

Monkey Business Images/Shutterstock.com

Emotional Energy

Certain activities, people, and places increase your positive emotional energy. For example, going to an amusement park or hiking may decrease your physical energy but be emotionally energizing. High levels of emotional exuberance may lead to positive emotions, such as joy and excitement.

You can also have high levels of negative emotional energy, such as fear, anger, and frustration. If these persist, they can drain your emotional and, eventually, your physical energy. Recognizing when you are experiencing strong negative emotions can allow you to pause and address the underlying problem or to support your well-being with self-care, as you weather life's storms. As discussed in the previous chapter, this would be a perfect time for a time-out or empowerment moment.

- ❑ What activities, people, and places increase your positive emotional energy?

  ____

  ____

  ____

  ____

  ____

- ❑ How can you increase these positive emotional vitality boosters in your life? Please identify a specific action, day, and time when you'll be able to participate in this activity.

  ____

  ____

  ____

  ____

  ____

- ❑ What drains your emotional energy or contributes to negative emotional energy? Please identify a specific step you can take to no longer engage in this behavior.

  ____

  ____

  ____

  ____

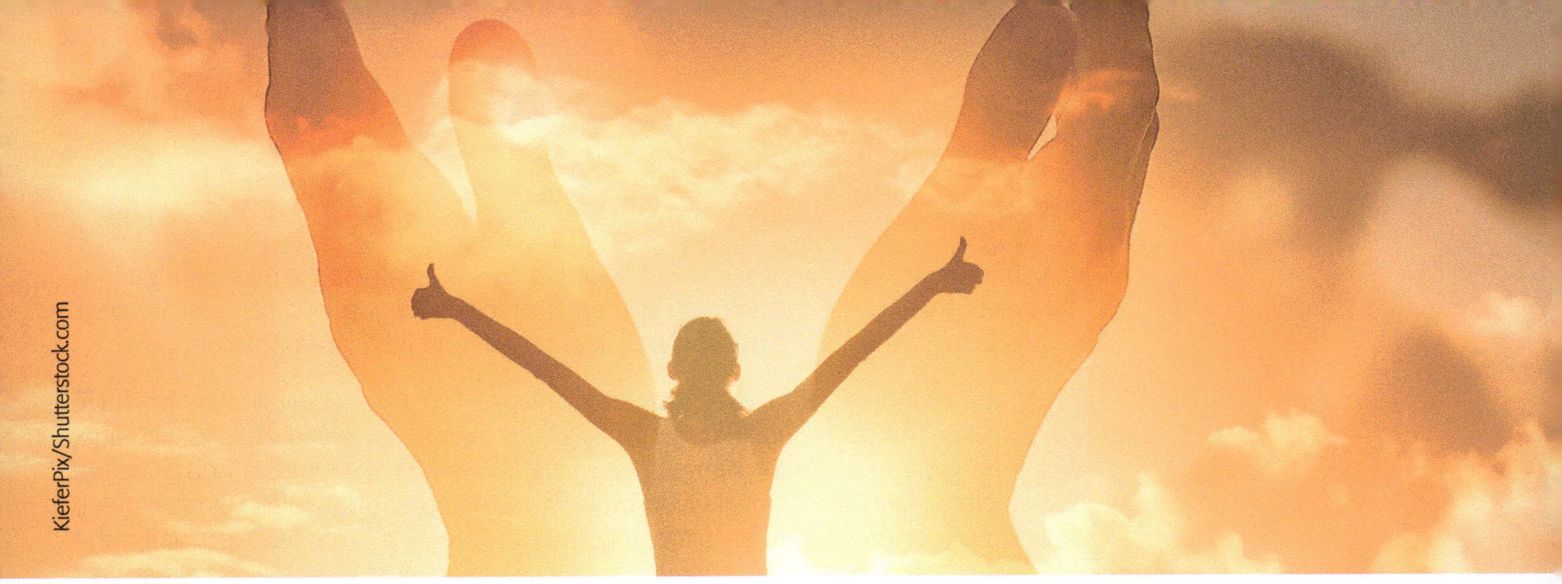
KieferPix/Shutterstock.com

Spiritual Energy

How you feel when you're spiritually passionate and what causes you to feel this way is as beautifully individualized as your fingerprint. When you feel spiritually energized, you may feel awe or wonder, as you connect with something greater than yourself. For example, you may feel spiritually energized from attending a religious service at your mosque, temple, church, or house of worship. Being surrounded by other believers and engaging in religious rituals, such as singing and praising, may increase your spiritual energy.

Some people become more spiritually energized when spending time alone in prayer or contemplative reflection. For others, being out in nature and looking up at the vastness of the stars in the night or contemplating the beauty of a leaf may increase their spiritual energy as they consider its origin. Looking into your grandchild's eyes or hugging a loved one may fuel your spiritual energy tank.

You can become so focused on the daily tasks that you neglect to support your spiritual energy. This program strives to support you in having a healthy body, peaceful mind, AND joyful spirit. Honoring what you need to have a joyful spirit will allow you to flourish and fulfill your purpose.

- ❑ When have you felt most spiritually energized?

  ____

  ____

  ____

- ❑ What can you do to support your spiritual vibrancy this coming week? Identify a specific action that you will complete on a particular day at a certain time this week. Remember, setting SMART goals, as we discussed earlier in this book, is essential in your wellness journey.

  ____

  ____

  ____

Energy Drainers

When your energy is low, it is customary to want to do something to increase your energy. Unfortunately, the world's demands on you don't typically stop just because you are tired. Stress and insufficient sleep are associated with fatigue and addictive behaviors.

They are also associated with increased relapse for those individuals who have stopped using addictive substances. In addition, people sometimes use caffeine, alcohol, tobacco, and drugs to change their energy levels. For example, although coffee or tea containing caffeine is not likely to be harmful, if you are not suffering from sleep difficulties, excessive caffeine can ultimately leave you feeling more fatigued, when the caffeine wears off. Likewise, alcohol, tobacco, and other drugs can negatively impact sleep, leaving people more exhausted the following day.

Using healthy energy boosters can sustain your energy and even increase it. However, before focusing on improving your energy, pausing to consider the cause and type of fatigue (physical, mental/emotional, or spiritual) that you are feeling can allow you to choose how to address this more mindfully.

Examples of common energy drainers include the following:

- Addiction
- Alcohol
- Arguments with anyone (loved ones, family, friends, or strangers)
- Being around negative people
- Betrayal of any kind
- Caffeine crash
- Caring for a sick or elderly loved one or child
- Dehydration
- Discrimination
- Disorganization
- Disrespect
- Excessive stress
- Feeling excluded
- Feeling like you are not enough
- Feeling like you can't live up to expectations
- Feeling misunderstood
- Feeling taken for granted or advantage of
- Hiding your true feelings or true self
- Illness, chemotherapy, or some medications
- Imposter syndrome
- Insufficient sleep
- Junk food
- Lack of exercise
- Lack of loyalty
- Lack of purpose
- Lack of time
- Loneliness
- Loss of a job
- Messy house or office
- Microaggressions
- Not having anyone to talk to
- Overscheduling
- Overwork
- Perfectionism
- Procrastination
- Sedentary behavior
- Sexual harassment
- Struggling with your identity
- Sugar crash
- The death of a loved one, pet, or relationship
- Tobacco
- Toxic relationships
- Witnessing or a history of trauma
- Witnessing or engaging in road rage

❏ After reading through this list, put a checkmark next to any example that resonates with you. The more checkmarks by an item, the more it resonates with you. Feel free to circle any items that have multiple checkmarks. Then, comment in the space provided on those items that resonate most with you. Share why you think these affect you.

If you realize that you've experienced trauma or events causing you mental anguish, this is an excellent time to reach out for help.

❏ Identify a supportive person you can talk to about any of the items you've circled.

The past influences you. The present is your gift. The future is your making. For the next few days, be mindful of when your energy level is low and then answer the following questions:

❏ Why is your energy low?

❏ What type of fatigue are you feeling? Note that it may involve more than one type of fatigue (physical, mental, or spiritual) at a time.

❏ What does your body, mind, or spirit want right now to increase your energy?

- [ ] What steps can you take to give your body, mind, or spirit what it needs?

____

____

____

Pay attention to how you feel after honoring what your body, mind, or spirit needs. So often, women push through their fatigue, trying to do everything without listening to their bodies, minds, and spirits. The PAVING the Path to Wellness program challenges you to be mindful of what you need to flourish. You deserve this.

Energy Boosters

There are many healthy ways to boost our energy. This chapter explores nutrition, physical activity, sleep, connection, schedule modifications, and recreational activities that can boost your energy when it is feeling low.

NUTRITION ENERGY BOOSTERS

When your body is well-hydrated and nourished, your cells have the fuel they need to perform. Without high-quality fuel, your energy level drops, and you feel fatigued. The following are some suggestions for boosting your stamina through nutrition:

- Avoid relying on artificial energy sources that can be unhealthy when used excessively, such as energy drinks or heavily caffeinated beverages. If you enjoy caffeinated tea or coffee, drink it earlier in the day.
- Avoid foods and drinks with added sugar. The natural sugar in fruits is healthy, but added sugar can cause your blood sugar to spike and eventually crash. Instead, try to eat smaller, more frequent meals that contain fiber and protein. Also, avoid ultra-processed foods with refined carbohydrates, such as white bread, pasta, rice, bagels, muffins, cakes, and cookies.
- Avoid excessive alcohol use. Alcohol can decrease your energy and interfere with sleep. If you don't drink, don't start. The American Heart Association recommends one drink maximum per day for women.
- Enjoy foods that support your energy, such as plant-based sources of protein and iron, fruits, vegetables, whole grains, beans, seeds, and nuts.
- Chew peppermint gum.
- Cook with spices.
- Don't skip meals. Doing so can cause your blood sugar to decrease, depleting your energy.
- Get adequate magnesium. Whole grains and nuts are magnesium-rich foods that are delicious and nutritious.
- Snack on carrots or blueberries.
- Maintain adequate hydration, as being dehydrated can lead to fatigue. Take your water bottle with you wherever you go.

❑ Explain what nutrition changes you could make to boost your energy.

____

____

____

MOVEMENT ENERGY BOOSTERS

Although it takes energy to move, engaging in regular physical activity typically leaves you feeling more energetic and boosts your vibrancy in the long run. As long as you don't exercise excessively, movement can be just what you need to optimize your energy each day. In that regard, consider the following suggestions:

- Exercise at a level that supports your energy throughout the rest of the day. Aerobic exercise increases your power, even if it seems counterintuitive. If you aren't already exercising regularly, talk to your healthcare provider for clearance. When you do start, work with a personal trainer or physical therapist, or start low and go slow, so as not to overexert yourself or become injured. Gradually, you can work up to more physical activity.
- Engage in tai chi, yoga, Pilates, or stretching.
- Engage in fun forms of movement that aren't traditional, such as skipping, playing on a playground, see-sawing, swinging on a swing, or hula hooping.
- Don't overexert yourself. Listen to your body, and when you need to rest or excuse yourself from an energy-draining activity, do so without shame, blame, or guilt.
- Take breaks often. If you are working on a project and find yourself sitting or working for hours, set the alarm to remind yourself to stand and stretch. Give yourself mental and physical breaks. Remember the importance of time-outs.
- If you do an activity that requires a lot of physical or emotional energy, plan time to recover fully. So often, we don't allow our bodies and minds a chance to recover from draining activities.
- Play with your pets.
- Find ways to move more throughout your day and decrease your sedentary behavior. For example, try running up the steps or doing a few jumping jacks while your tea is brewing.
- Play on a playground and express your inner child.
- Learn some new dance moves. Then, turn on the music and dance.
- Don't neglect physical symptoms that are draining your energy. Instead, see your primary care provider and reach out for help.
- Get on an exercise ball and move around.
- Do a plank.
- Stand on one leg and balance for as long as you can.
- Do a few push-ups or sit-ups.
- Jog in place.
- Take a walk around the block.
- Walk up and down the stairs.
- Walk with a friend for 10 minutes.
- Try a chair that moves, such as a "wobble chair" or ball chair.

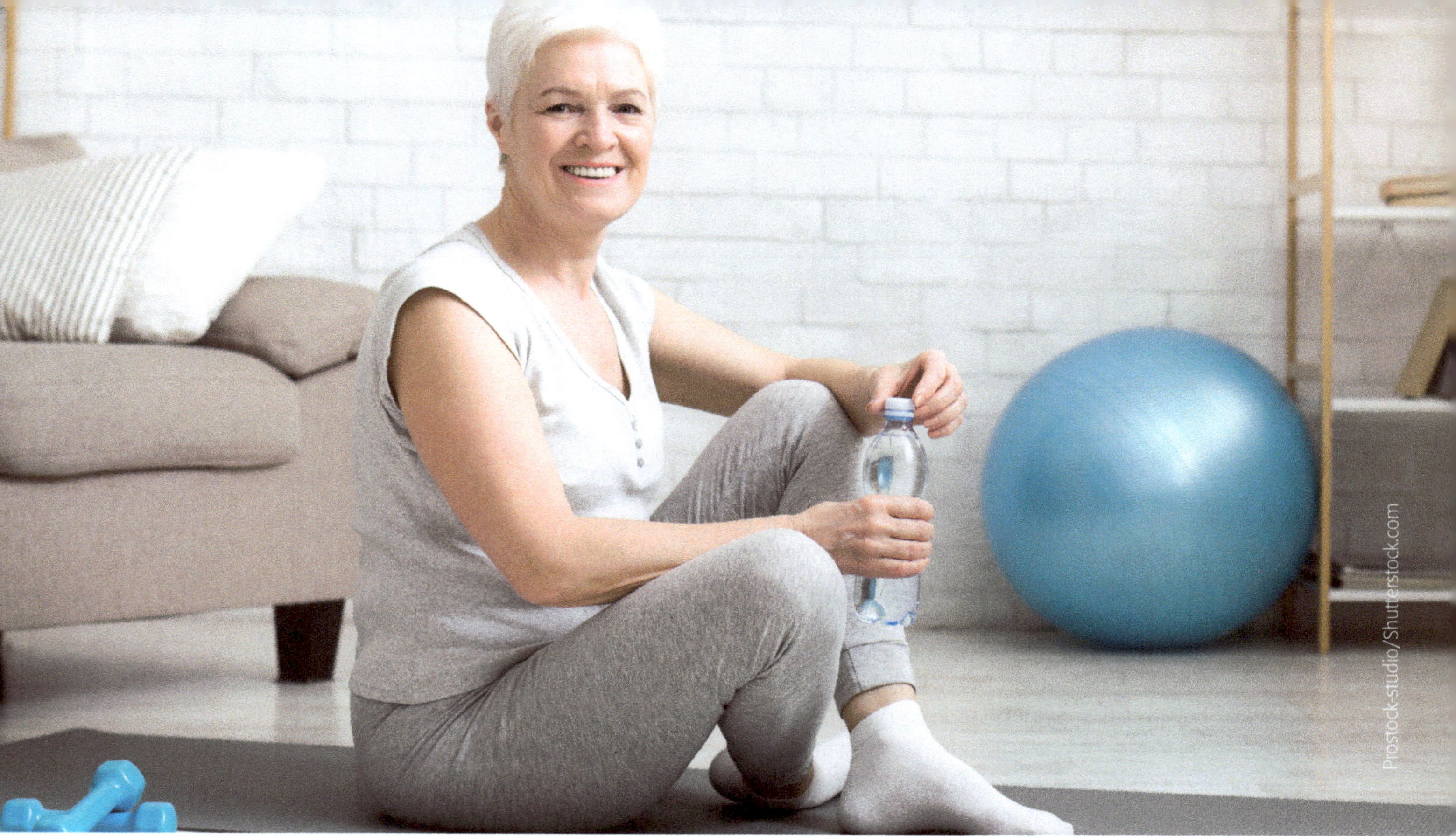
Prostock-studio/Shutterstock.com

❏ What are some physical activity energy boosters that you would like to try?

____

____

____

SCHEDULE TWEAKS FOR BOOSTING ENERGY

If you pack your schedule from sun-up to sun-down, you'll deplete your energy before it's time for bed. However, by mindfully scheduling time for rest and engagement, you can keep your energy flowing from morning to night. In that regard, the following suggestions can help:

- Create a routine that works for you and your energy levels. Look for patterns when you feel the most and the least energy. For example, if you have the most energy in the morning, schedule your most physically or emotionally demanding work then. Be mindful of how you use your energy "spoons."
- Prioritize your projects. Do those that are most important when you have the most energy or earlier in the day.
- Pace yourself to have enough energy to finish the day feeling good.
- Make sure to schedule mealtimes and time for exercise.
- Ask for help. Allowing others to support you is a gift to them. Don't try to do everything by yourself. There is strength in asking for assistance.
- If you are a caregiver, take breaks.
- Don't pack your day with too many commitments, excluding time for yourself, thereby draining your energy before you reach the end of your day.

- Schedule free time, or alone time, on your calendar every day, if you find it challenging to prioritize self-care and time-outs.
- Modify your lifestyle and schedule to support your energy level.
- Plan ahead. Consider planning, for example, your menu for the week, a trip, or how you will tackle cleaning your closet.
- Don't schedule meetings back-to-back. Instead, allow time between them to stretch, take a bathroom break, if needed, and get a glass of water.
- Break up your tasks into manageable chunks. Remember that you don't have to finish it all in one session.
- Make a to-do list.
- Tackle the small things on your to-do list until you feel energized to tackle something more extensive.
- Limit your time on tasks or with people who deplete your energy. On occasion, they are unavoidable, but do what you can to limit interactions or tasks that drain your energy while practicing self-care.
- Set boundaries.
- Use a calendar (paper, online, or your phone) to schedule your activities and stick with it.
- Engage in activities that boost how you feel about yourself. For example, try a new haircut or get a manicure.

❑ What are some ways that you could change your schedule to support your energy?

____

____

____

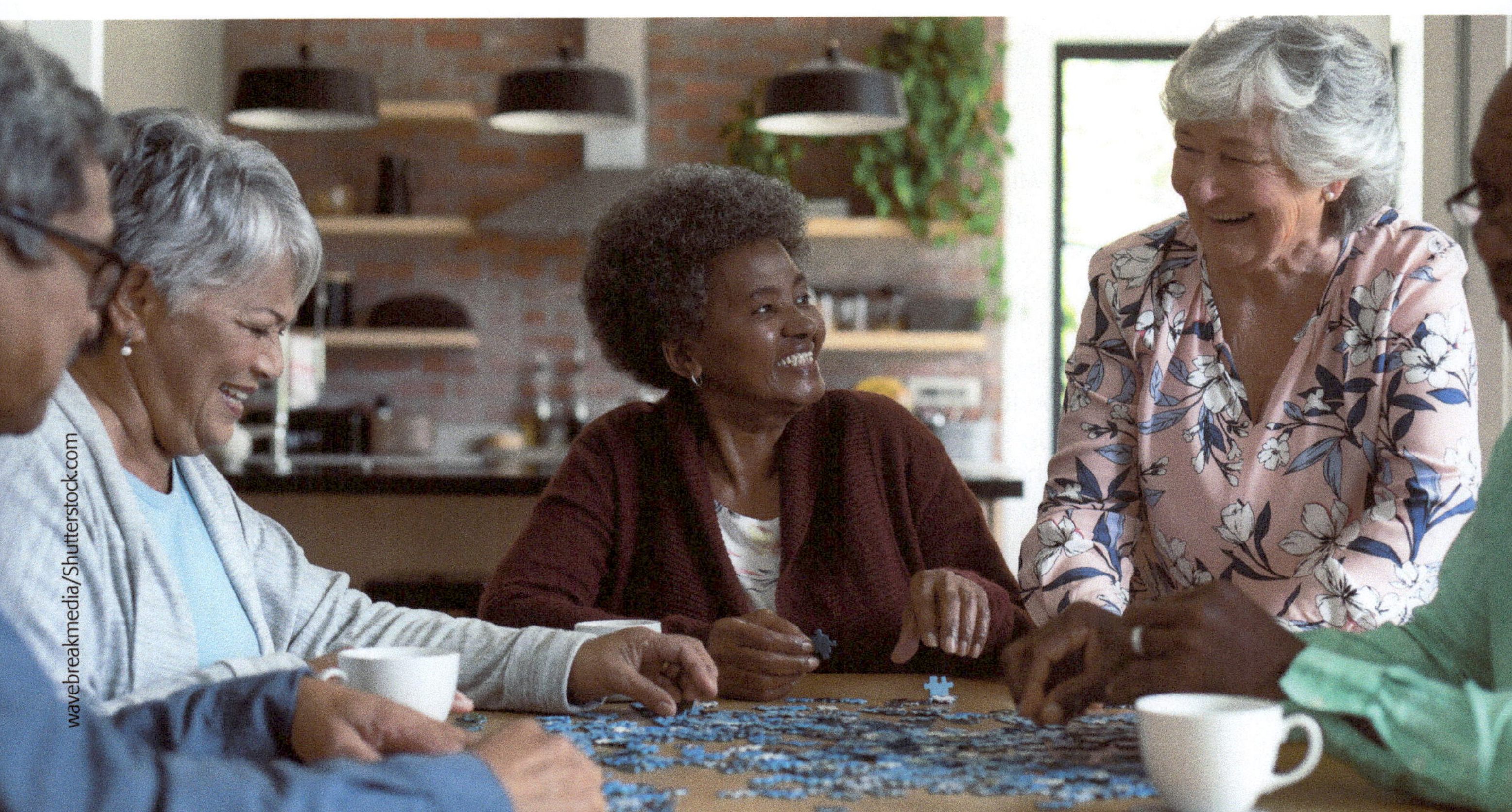

wavebreakmedia/Shutterstock.com

ACTIVITIES AND HOBBIES FOR BOOSTING ENERGY

Engaging in activities and hobbies can boost your energy and help you feel energized throughout the day. The following are some ideas for using recreational activities to support your energy:

- Spend time in nature every day. Also, look for ways to bring nature into your home, such as plants, rocks, flowers, and branches.
- Listen to uplifting music. Music can also support your spiritual energy level, if it is music that makes you feel connected spiritually.
- Get a massage or give yourself a hand massage.
- Practice stress management techniques, such as meditation, progressive muscle relaxation, mindfulness, and mindful breathing.
- Be mindful of your energy level throughout the day and look for opportunities to increase your energy naturally.
- Incorporate variety into your day. You can drain your energy from doing the same thing over and over.
- Regularly engage in hobbies that you enjoy alone and with others. Look for new hobbies to try.
- Do a body scan to look for places of tension in your body and then mindfully try to relax them.
- Investigate what energy boosters work best for you and do them regularly.
- Try to learn something new every day. For example, take a class, read a book, or watch an online video. Being a lifelong learner can boost your mental alertness.
- Don't engage in activities or interactions out of guilt or obligation. Instead, mindfully consider each invitation concerning the time and energy commitment involved.
- Keep your brain active and engaged. For example, try Sudoku or crossword puzzles.
- Play games with others. Community centers often have groups of people who play cards or other games that you can join.
- Do a jigsaw puzzle.
- Take breaks from screens (television, phone, computer, iPad).
- Limit social media time or take a social media "time-out" for an hour, day, week, or month.
- Watch a silly video on YouTube or a comedy movie.
- Find a new podcast that interests you and listen to it.
- Do something artistic, such as painting, drawing, doodling, singing, dancing, or playing a musical instrument.
- Write in a journal, or if you don't feel like writing, you can draw.
- Play with a fidget toy or use a de-stress ball. They aren't just for children. They can be fun for adults too.
- Do something creative. You could build a birdhouse, make a scrapbook, or take photos in your local park.
- Have fun cooking or baking something. You may even want to surprise a friend with what you have made, with a gift of food.
- Go shopping and have fun buying a new outfit.
- Write a poem.
- Visit the zoo or amusement park.

- Look in your newspaper to see what activities are going on in your city and try something new.
- Make something out of playdough, silly putty, or clay.
- Try a new app on your phone.
- Try a new hairstyle.
- Brush your teeth.
- Write with your non-dominant hand.

❑ How can you use recreational activities and hobbies to keep your energy boosted?

____

____

____

SLEEP AND REST ENERGY BOOSTERS

Suppose you feel fatigued; check in with your body to see what you need. If you need some sleep or even rest, don't fight it. Listen to your body. Among the sleep-and-energy-related suggestions that can be helpful are the following:

- Take a nap if you are tired. Remember to keep it less than 30 minutes and to finish before mid-afternoon.
- Get adequate sleep each night. Prioritizing your sleep is one of the best ways to boost your energy.
- Don't push yourself nonstop. Sometimes your body just wants to be still.
- Refer to the chapter on sleep for more details on this area.

❑ Do you want to change how you use sleep or rest to support your energy?

____

____

____

CONNECTION ENERGY BOOSTERS

You probably know people who energize you and others who drain your energy. Mindfully connecting with others allows you to keep your energy positive and boosted throughout the day. In that regard, consider the following suggestions:

- Remember that you are not a superwoman, nor were you designed to be a superhero. You must take care of yourself and your energy before you can care for anyone else.
- Connect with other women experiencing menopausal symptoms or other women who have experienced a similar condition (breast cancer or stroke) or situation (caregiver of someone with dementia or being single). Being around people who understand what you are going through can boost your spirit.
- Avoid gossip or engaging in negative self-talk, which can drain your energy. Instead, look for the good in others and engage in positive self-talk.

- Connect with people within your spiritual community, such as a community leader or other members.
- Worry and anxiety can drain you. Never worry alone. Reach out and share your concerns with someone else. Get professional help for anxiety if needed.
- Join a PAVING or peer support group.
- Call someone whom you know who will be supportive of you.
- Call a relative, childhood friend, or someone you haven't spoken with in a long time.
- Write an old-fashioned paper letter or send a card.
- Connect with others who support your well-being and make you feel good about yourself.
- Look for resources to support you in areas of your life, where your energy is low. Social workers, community organizations, friends, and professional healthcare providers may be able to help you.
- Volunteer regularly and serve others. Although it may seem like you're giving energy away, helping others can boost your vitality.

❏ How can you use connections to support your energy?

____

____

____

____

YOUR ENVIRONMENT ENERGY BOOSTERS

If you walk into a messy room, your anxiety level can increase, while your energy drains. In contrast, a tidy, bright, and engaging space can support you. The following are some ideas for using your environment to help your energy level:

- Tidy up your space. Disorder and clutter can drain your energy.
- Bring hand-picked flowers into your home.
- Get a plant to put in your office.
- Turn on some relaxing or uplifting music.
- Sit on or drape yourself with a soft blanket.
- Open your windows or doors to let fresh air inside.
- Find ways to brighten and beautify your home or apartment.
- Get some natural sunlight. In addition to getting exposure to the sun's rays, you'll also be spending time in nature and breathing the fresh air.
- Decrease the temperature of your room slightly, especially at night.
- Light a candle.
- Use aromatherapy or scents that invigorate you, such as orange, peppermint, rosemary, or cinnamon.
- Take a shower or a bath, or even splash some water on your face. The water can be energizing, especially if it is slightly cool.

❑ Is there anything you want to change about your environment to better support your energy?

____

____

____

SPIRITUAL-HEALTH ENERGY BOOSTERS

Don't forget your spiritual health. Neglecting your spiritual health can leave you feeling drained, even if you physically have enough energy. Boosting your spiritual energy depends greatly on what spirituality means to you. Consider the following ideas for increasing your spiritual energy, and then write in some other ways to boost your own:

- Attend a service at your synagogue, church, mosque, temple, or another place of worship.
- Read the Bible, Torah, Koran, devotional, or other Holy Book.
- Consider reading the works of spiritual leaders, such as the Dali Lama, Desmond Tutu, or Thich Nhat Hanh.
- Regularly engage in activities that resonate with your spirituality.
- Spend some time in silence.
- Participate in mantras or pray the rosary, if doing so aligns with your spiritual beliefs.
- Start a gratitude journal or practice thinking of what you are grateful for when you're driving in your car or brushing your teeth.
- Practice mindfulness throughout your day.
- Connect with a minister, rabbi, priest, or another spiritual leader.
- Pray.

❑ List several ways that you can boost your spiritual energy.

____

____

____

Fatigue

Although feeling fatigued is common during menopause, you should address any new fatigue or changes in energy level with your healthcare provider. Fatigue can be due to chronic fatigue syndrome, a low B12 level, a low iron level, hypothyroidism, illness, depression, and medications, as well as other medical problems. These are conditions that a medical professional can and should treat. Don't assume that all decreased energy is due to menopause or older age.

Furthermore, if you are struggling with fatigue after a prolonged illness, COVID, chemotherapy, surgery, or other significant life change, working with an exercise physiologist or physical therapist with expertise in rehabilitation can help you increase your stamina. Ask your physician or another healthcare provider for a referral if you want to have an exercise program designed just for you.

Coaching Yourself on Your Energy With the COACH Approach

CURIOSITY

Most midlife and older women want more energy, but many have not stopped to think of why they want more energy or what they would do with increased energy if they had it. Get curious and explore this.

❑ If you had more energy, what would you do with it?

___

___

___

❑ Would having more power allow you to better pursue your purposes?

___

___

___

❑ People can energize you or drain you. When you are thriving, you can help to energize others. Think of people who fill you with positive energy. What are some of their energizing characteristics (e.g., positivity, willingness to listen, empathy, openness to new ideas)?

___

___

___

OPENNESS

Most women want to be energy fillers and not drainers. To become more of an energy booster, you may need to be open to changing how you interact with others. Also, being an energy booster isn't about pretending to be happy or cheerful when you are sad. Sometimes, you need to have your energy boosted and can't necessarily help others. Being an energy booster is about being authentic with your emotions but avoiding gossip, negativity, or excessive competition that brings others down. You can actively look for ways to boost the energy of others and find opportunities to build others up.

- ❑ What can you do to be a positive energy booster for your friends, family, and those around you?

  ____

  ____

  ____

- ❑ When have you been an energy drainer, and why do you think it was that this happened?

  ____

  ____

  ____

  ____

- ❑ Is there anything you want to do differently to be less of an energy drainer in the future?

  ____

  ____

  ____

  ____

Remember, there is no shame, blame, or guilt in the PAVING program. If there are times that you need to take a time-out, you don't need to provide excuses, explanations, or reasons for this. Likewise, when you see others needing to take a time-out, you don't need to know why. It is important to honor everyone in the shape, space, or stage they are at in their lives, including yourself.

APPRECIATION

It's easy to feel like society expects you to be a superwoman. From careers to families, women are often expected to do it all, with a smile. However, it is essential to know your limits, set boundaries, and know when to stop, when managing your energy.

- ❑ How are you at appreciating your limits, knowing when to ask for help, delegate, or set boundaries to protect your time and energy?

  ____

  ____

  ____

- ❑ Are there changes that you want to make to protect your energy better? If so, what are they?

____

____

____

____

- ❑ If you put these changes into place, how would your life and energy level be different than they are now?

____

____

____

____

- ❑ Please share one positive affirmation you have about yourself here. What do you appreciate about yourself at this moment?

____

____

____

____

COMPASSION

Being fatigued is hard. When you are tired, even the most minor tasks can seem overwhelming. Most midlife and more mature women are not as energetic as they were during childhood, as the years, illnesses, and life circumstances take their toll.

- ❑ Are you compassionate with yourself when you are fatigued? What type of self-talk do you engage in when you are tired?

____

____

____

____

❑ How can you show more compassion to yourself and your energy limitations? Do you need to work on not overdoing it, not feeling guilty about your limits, and communicating with others more clearly about how you are feeling so they know if you need to change your activities to preserve your energy?

____

____

____

❑ Please complete this sentence. "I am compassionate with myself because…" There is no right or wrong answer to this. Just try to learn and grow from the questions in this book.

____

____

____

HONESTY

It is easy to turn to unhealthy energy sources to manage your fatigue. Some substances, like caffeine, are not dangerous when used in moderation but can be harmful when used in excess.

❑ Do you need to address any unhealthy or addictive forms of getting energy or unhealthy energy drainers (tobacco use, cannabis, alcohol use, prescription drug misuse, caffeine overuse, reliance on energy drinks)?

____

____

____

____

❑ Do you drink more than one alcoholic drink in a day? Do you smoke? Do you use opiates or other prescription medications without a prescription? If you answered yes to any of these, it's time to reach out for help.

____

____

____

____

Energy Wrap-Up

When it comes to fatigue during menopause and midlife, remember that you are not alone. Although about 20 percent of pre-menopausal women report physical and mental exhaustion symptoms, this doubles during perimenopause and rises to 85 percent of women after menopause (1). You are not a victim. You can mindfully manage your energy throughout the day and support your well-being through energy-boosting lifestyle behaviors. Through healthy lifestyle behaviors, you can have peaceful energy that gives you the ability to do what you want to do, even if you don't have the energy you did as a child.

When you commit to managing your energy, asking for help, being mindful of your commitments, eating nourishing foods, staying physically active, prioritizing sleep, and controlling your stress, you can end your day without using all your spoons. You can thrive with a peaceful energy that allows you to do what you want, be present in the moment, and live joyfully. Tomorrow is a new day.

The past influences us. The present is our gift. The future is our making.

Reference

1. Chedraui P, et al. Assessing Menopausal Symptoms Among Healthy Middle-Aged Women With the Menopause Rating Scale. *Maturitas*. 2007;57(3):271–278.

CHAPTER 11
PURPOSE

Purpose Throughout Menopause, Midlife, and Beyond

Acronym—PURPOSE

Personal
Understanding
Reflection
Potential
Others
Spirituality
Evolves

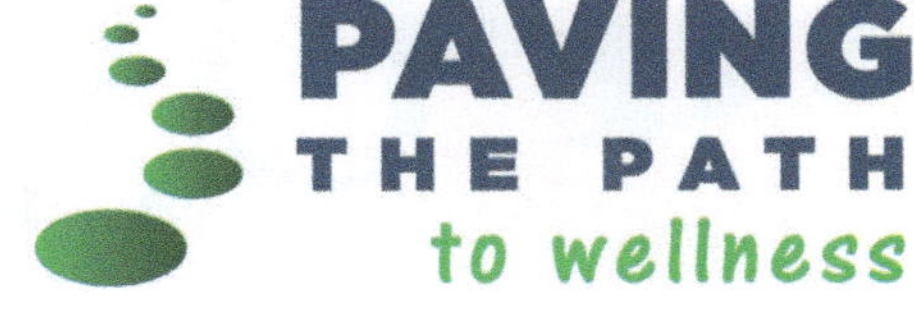

- *PERSONAL:* Purpose is individual. It is different for everyone, as all women have unique talents, gifts, values, expertise, passions, interests, and calling to live a meaningful, purpose-filled life in their unique way.
- *UNDERSTANDING:* Living a meaningful life means understanding how your purpose connects with opportunities for living it out. Look for ways to serve others, ask how you can help, and continue to grow in understanding your purpose's expression in the world.
- *REFLECTION:* Reflect upon your purpose and whether you are living it to the fullest. Take a time-out now. This is the perfect opportunity.
- *POTENTIAL:* Living a meaningful, purpose-filled life increases your potential for a vibrant, joy-filled, mentally and physically healthy life.
- *OTHERS:* Find ways to live out your purpose by connecting with others. Think of who you can serve and others you can partner with to accomplish this goal.
- *SPIRITUALITY:* Consider how your purpose in life and your spirituality are connected. Spirituality may or may not be religious, may or may not be practiced in a group, and may or may not involve meditation. Your spirituality is unique, just like you. Therefore, only you can define how your spirituality connects with your purpose.
- *EVOLVES:* Purpose usually evolves over time. As your life circumstances change or new opportunities arise, your purpose may change slightly or shift entirely. Being mindful of how your purpose has evolved will support your ability to live out your purpose fully in the future.

"Meaning cannot be given, it has to be found."

—Viktor Frankl, Austrian
Psychiatrist and
Holocaust Survivor

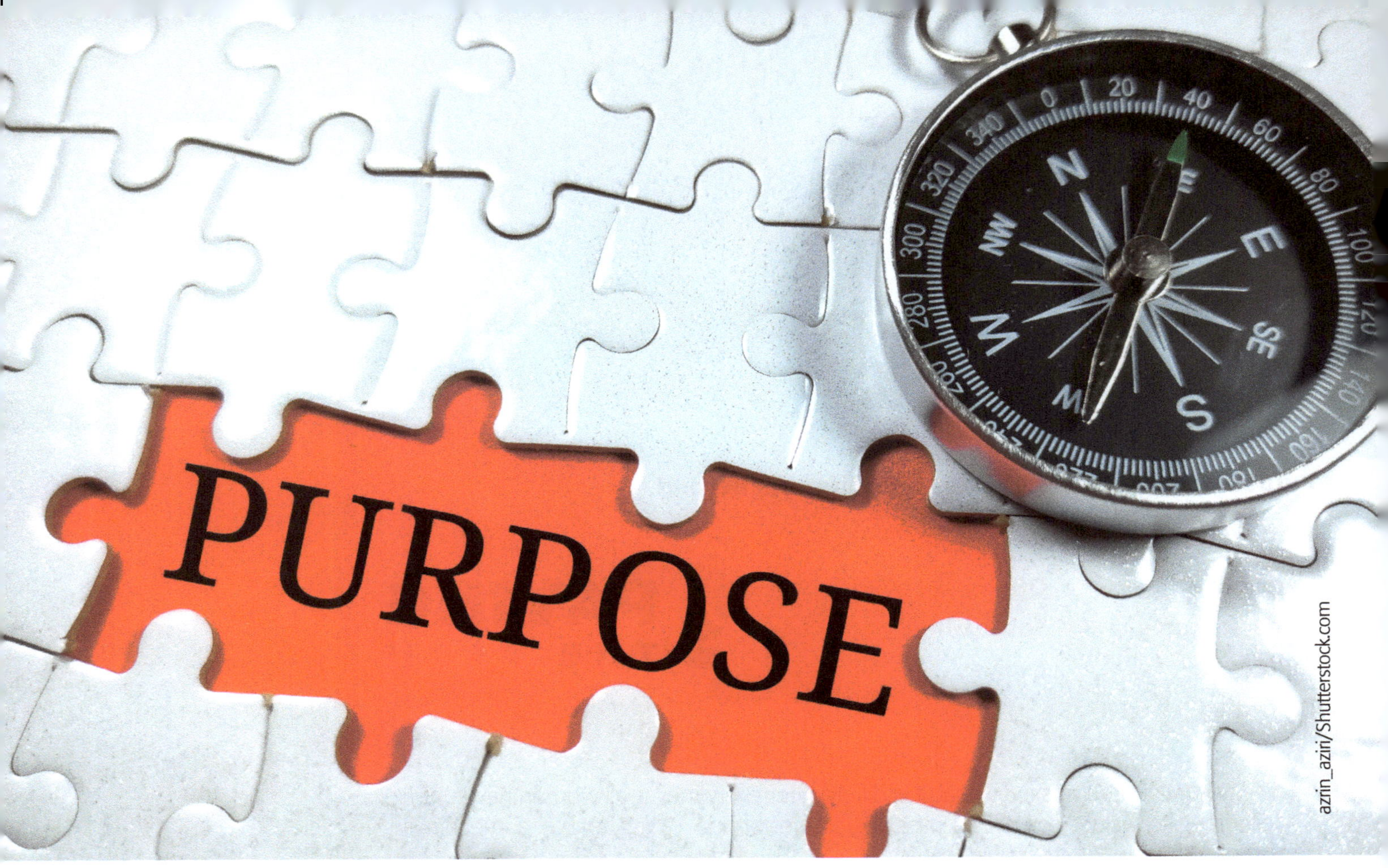

The Importance of Purpose

Everyone wants a purpose-filled life. Purpose energizes, activates, and inspires. It infuses life with meaning and helps people feel fully alive. Purpose guides behaviors and allows women to set meaningful goals. Research shows that a purpose-filled life increases longevity, improves outcomes for people struggling with chronic disease, and increases happiness. In addition, it improves brain and mental health, increases pain tolerance, and even decreases the risk of getting heart disease.

Purpose is one of the critical steps of the PAVING the Path to Wellness program, even though typical wellness programs rarely discuss it. Without purpose, you can eat healthy, exercise, manage stress, and get adequate sleep, but does it matter if you don't have a purpose? If engaging in these health-promoting behaviors aligns with your purpose, you are more likely to continue these healthy habits, as they have meaning in your life that extends beyond your body.

Reflecting on your life's purpose is beneficial for most people, but it is essential for midlife and more mature women. Menopausal and midlife women are part of the "sandwich generation," frequently caring for children and aging parents, with little time for self-care. Before midlife, many women's commitments align with raising their children, connecting with their spouses or partners, caring for elderly parents, and advancing their careers.

Around menopause and midlife, many of these responsibilities often shift drastically. Kids grow up and go to college and may move away from home. Changes occur in job responsibilities or career opportunities. Meaningful relationships shift, sometimes for the better and sometimes for the worse. Midlife may be a time of divorce. It's also a time when some people downsize their homes. If your purpose was to prepare your children for college, you might feel a void once they leave for college. Likewise, you will feel a void if your parents need regular support and pass away.

Change, especially if undesired, can lead to feelings of emptiness and even purposelessness. It creates a void. If not replaced with something meaningful, overworking, excessive shopping, gossiping, gambling, meaningless activities, drinking alcohol, emotional eating, tobacco use, illicit drug use, or other substance abuse may fill the void. A lack of purpose can feel lonely, unsettling, and boring. It may leave you feeling anxious, depressed, apathetic, or chaotic. A lack of peace prevails.

If you are someone who already has a deep understanding of your life's meaningful purpose, we encourage you to keep reading this chapter. You may want to consider if there are other areas of aspiration that you want to include in your overarching purpose or if there is something new that you want to embrace. This chapter may also help you understand the various facets of your purpose. You can choose how you want to live it out in your daily life, and this chapter will, hopefully, help you gain a deeper appreciation for how you can do this.

If you identify with these feelings associated with decreased motivation, know that you are not alone. This is unfortunately common. Don't despair; this void and emptiness create a space yearning to be filled with meaningful, purpose-filled activities. You deserve a beautiful life at every age and stage of your life. Throughout this chapter, you will explore your story, your uniqueness, and how you can use your journey to find your purpose (if you feel like you've lost it) or reenergize your purpose (if you already know what it is but want to work on it). Now is the time for a fresh start. You have the power to influence your legacy. Let's get started.

Purpose Timeline

Write or draw on the timeline (Table 11-1) what you considered your purpose to be at various times in your life.

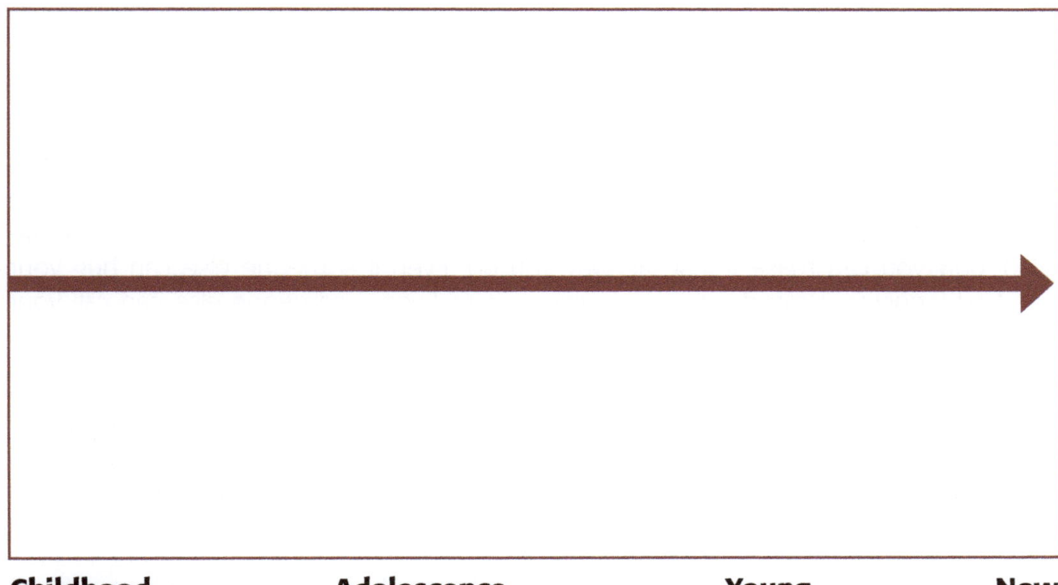

Table 11-1. An example of a purpose timeline

❑ How has your purpose changed over time?

___

___

___

❑ How has your purpose changed over the last few years?

___

___

___

❑ Are you feeling a purpose void in your life? Explain.

___

___

___

❑ What would you say to a dear friend who was feeling this way?

___

___

___

Your Uniqueness

You are unique. There is nobody with your experiences, interest, talents, values, strengths, and knowledge. You are one of a kind, as unique as a snowflake or a fingerprint. You were created for a purpose that only you can fill. Even if someone can make your signature salad, only you can make it just the way you do. Even if someone else can hug your grandchild, only you can do it in your unique way. Even if someone else can call your friend with an encouraging word, only you can encourage them the way you do it.

You aren't meant to accomplish someone else's purpose or what someone else thinks should be your purpose. Yet, the world needs YOU with every experience, talent, value, and strength you've gained throughout your life. Your purpose is a precious gem that shines brighter when shared. It will allow you to make your mark on the world as nobody else can do.

The following questions will help you to understand your uniqueness better. It will allow you to tell your story, define it more clearly, and execute your purpose.

- ❑ Whom do you love?

____

____

____

- ❑ What brings you joy?

____

____

____

- ❑ What values are most important to you? Typical values include kindness, honesty, compassion, spirituality, integrity, respect, responsibility, loyalty, generosity, empathy, and altruism, though you may have others.

____

____

____

- ❑ What are your strengths?

____

____

____

If you are unsure, consider asking others what they think are some of your strengths. Or, you may want to take the VIA Character Strengths survey at www.viacharacter.org. The three key features of signature strengths are that they are essential to who you are as an individual, that they feel effortless when using the strength, and that they positively energize you. The 24 strengths put forward by American psychologists Dr. Christopher Peterson and Dr. Martin Seligman in the book, *Character Strengths and Virtues* (1), include the following:

- Creativity
- Zest
- Fairness
- Self-regulation
- Curiosity
- Honesty
- Teamwork
- Humility
- Judgment
- Social intelligence
- Forgiveness
- Appreciation of beauty and excellence
- Perspective
- Kindness

- Love of learning
- Prudence
- Bravery
- Love
- Gratitude
- Hope
- Perseverance
- Leadership
- Spirituality
- Humor

❑ Which of the aforementioned strengths listed are your key strengths?

____

____

____

❑ What are some of your talents, hobbies, and things you enjoy? For example, gardening, telling stories, comforting those who are hurting, woodworking, listening, knitting, taking photos, teaching others, writing, cooking, playing pickleball, or traveling, are common areas of interest.

____

____

____

❑ What are areas and topics in which you have knowledge or expertise? For example, consider what you have learned during your career and formal academic education, as well as what you have learned informally over the years from your experiences.

____

____

____

❑ What are you passionate about? What issues do you feel called to address? Consider social justice issues and what you would change if you could change anything on the planet. They can be issues in your community, such as not having healthy food readily available in your neighborhood, or global issues such as world hunger or planetary health. Consider non-profit organizations you would like to connect with or are linked to already. You may also consider people or organizations you admire and want to join in their efforts or do something similar.

____

____

____

- ❑ What experiences or life highlights have you had that have helped you grow as a person, taught you life lessons, challenged you, inspired you, or made you proud?

____

____

____

Your strengths, talents, interests, experiences, blessings, and values are like a treasure box of gems. Share them with the world.

There are likely themes, threads, or areas of focus within these lists that you see throughout several areas of this book.

- ❑ What are some of your key themes?

____

____

____

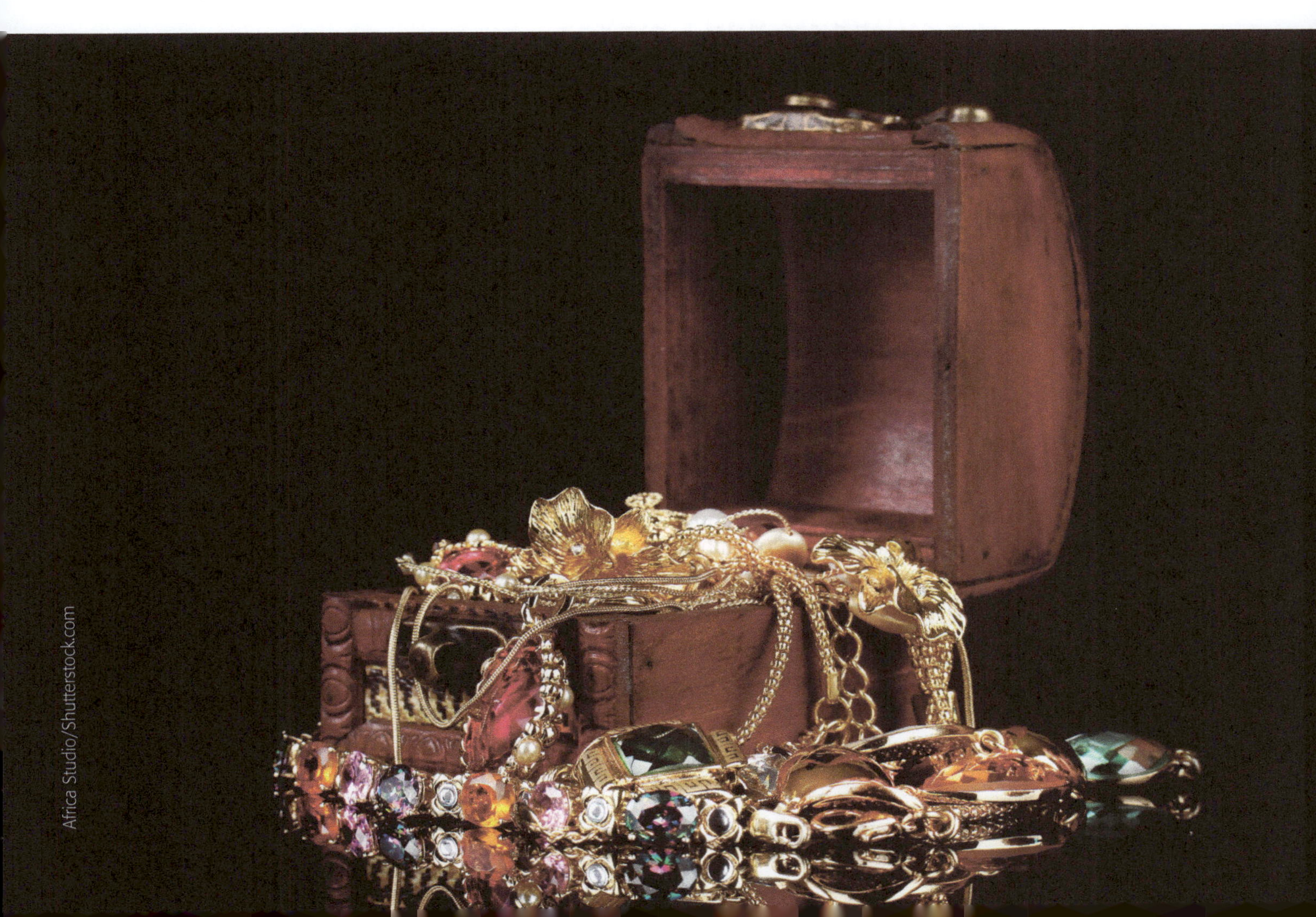

Africa Studio/Shutterstock.com

- ❑ After reviewing the words and ideas you've written in response to the aforementioned questions, is there anything you wrote about that you feel called to share with others that you're not already sharing?

  ____

  ____

  ____

- ❑ Were you surprised by anything that you learned from making these lists?

  ____

  ____

  ____

Whether or not you are already aware, your purpose connects with the words you wrote above. You will return to these lists as you craft a purpose statement later in this chapter.

Spirituality and Purpose

For many midlife and more mature women, their spiritual beliefs and values intricately connect with the purpose of their lives. As discussed previously in the book, spiritual health means different things for different women. Research has even shown spiritual development to decrease physical complaints of menopausal women. Having faith or spiritual beliefs also has been found to contribute to good mental health. Recognizing and fostering the link between your daily activities, spiritual development, and a meaningful purpose benefits your body, mind, and spirit.

Spiritual health often involves serving and loving others. Both spirituality and a meaningful purpose can add meaning to your life and strengthen connections with other people.

Think of the activities that you commonly do each day. If you are employed, consider your job. If you interact in your community, think of how you interact. Your daily actions can make the world a better place and align with your spiritual beliefs. For example, someone whose job is to greet people and prevent theft at a convenience store may connect their job to increase the happiness of others, make the world safer, and uphold the value of honesty. Someone who walks their dog daily and greets others on their path may connect this activity with a meaningful purpose of caring for their pet and adding joy to the lives of others as they see her smile and her dog's playfulness. A person who drives a delivery truck may brighten people's days through the packages she brings and even goes beyond that by saying a kind word to the people she sees while making her deliveries. Mindfully going throughout your day looking for ways to add joy to the lives of others or make the world a better place may connect with your spirituality and purpose.

- ❑ How can you connect the actions that you regularly do with meaningful purpose or your spiritual beliefs?

____

____

____

____

- ❑ How do your spiritual beliefs connect with a purpose for you (if at all)? Remember that you may have multiple purposes or facets of a primary life purpose.

____

____

____

____

Your Story and Purpose

As a woman going through or who has gone through menopause, you've lived enough years to have experienced suffering. Pain, sadness, grief, and struggles are part of the human experience. Although you don't want to be defined by your pain, your difficult times help shape your identity as a unique individual. Every woman has a story involving struggles, highs and lows, and challenges she's overcome. Struggles help women to become wiser and stronger. They help shape values and develop strengths. Your experiences, pleasant and unpleasant, have helped make you who you are today.

Reflecting upon and writing about your life's journey can help you make sense of the world, your struggles, and how they have shaped you as a unique individual. If the following prompts are not helping you, or you want to refine how you write your story, you may consider reading the biographies of others, watching movies of true personal stories, or asking people to share their accounts with you.

On the following timeline, mark the highs, the things you are most proud of, and your accomplishments (Table 11-2). Then, add critical milestones and significant life transitions to the timeline. These may be happy, such as a graduation or the birth of a child, or sad, like losing a parent, a pet, the beginning or end of a relationship, or a job.

Next, add other lows you haven't already put on the timeline. These are likely times of struggle, suffering, conflict, sickness, extreme stress, or sadness.

In reflecting on the lows in your life that bring up past trauma or any unresolved negative feelings you need help processing, please reach out to a mental health professional for support. This exercise can help you identify or refine your understanding of your purpose. However, it should not cause you additional pain.

Childhood	Adolescence	Young Adulthood	Now

Table 11-2. An example of a highs, most proud of, accomplishments, milestones, life transitions, and lows timeline

- ❑ When reflecting on your aforementioned timeline, what are the times you grew the most as an individual?

____

____

____

- ❑ What helped you become the unique person you are today on the timeline?

____

____

____

- ❑ Is there anything good that came from your struggles or suffering? Were you changed in any positive way from them? Indicate this area of growth with a flower of any kind.

____

____

____

____

- ❑ Did you learn any important life lessons? For example, maybe you realized that you were stronger than you thought when you went through chemotherapy or deepened your spirituality while grieving the loss of your mom.

____

____

____

- ❑ When you consider the timeline above, do you think of any important people in your life who helped you become who you are today? If so, list them here. How did they help shape you? When you think of them on the timeline, indicate their impact with a heart.

____

____

____

- ❑ What are you most proud about when reflecting on your timeline? Put a star by these on your timeline.

____

____

____

____

- ❑ Are there threads of meaning that you see when looking at your timeline?

____

____

____

Imagine writing about a close friend whose timeline and experiences mirror yours. How would you write about their life story? Try writing your life story using the third person's perspective. While some examples of what you may want to write about are detailed subsequently, please write about whatever you feel moved to express.

You can write as much or as little as you want. You may spend just a few minutes on this exercise, or this may inspire you to write your entire autobiography. Keep in mind that you are a gem. Like coal turned into a diamond through extreme pressure, the pressure you've experienced through life's challenges has made you into a diamond that can shine.

Writing your story can help you understand yourself better. This process can help you better appreciate the role of your times of suffering in your life's journey. If you look closely, you will find beauty in the challenges you've overcome, the scars you have, and the experiences that have made you wiser and stronger. There is beauty in imperfection and the lived journey. Viktor Frankl, psychiatrist and Holocaust survivor, describes despair as suffering without meaning. Everyone has suffered, but people can avoid despairing by trying to find meaning in the suffering.

CHILDHOOD

(Insert your name) was born in (insert year). Her childhood was ____. She enjoyed _____. Her childhood struggles involved ______. Some of her most significant lessons learned during childhood she learned from (insert name of someone), who taught her about ________ and to ________.

ADOLESCENCE

During her teen years, (insert your name) experienced _______. She had fun __________. She struggled with __________. During these challenging times, she became aware of her strengths such as _______. She also began to realize her passion for __________.

YOUNG ADULTHOOD

As a young adult, (insert your name) received training in __________ which aligned with her desire to be a (insert career if applicable). She experienced satisfaction in _________. She met ____________ who helped her to understand that ______________. It was during this time that she went through ___________ that helped her realize that life __________. It also helped her to refine her talent for _________. She struggled with _____________.

ADULTHOOD

Throughout adulthood, (insert your name) has been very involved in _____________. She has always felt called to care for ____________. The social injustice of ______________ is important to her because __________. During this time she developed a meaningful relationship with ____________ who helped her to realize _____________. Although she experienced extreme stress and pain during ____________, looking back on that time, she realizes that she learned the importance of __________ and that ____________.

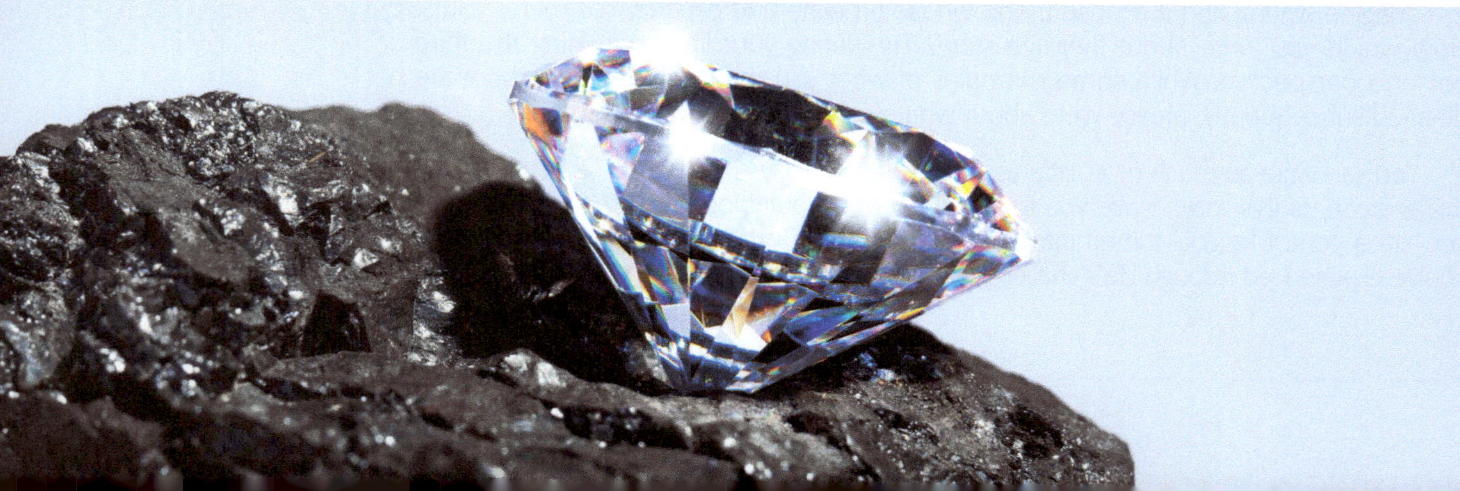
RTimages/Shutterstock.com

SUMMARY

In summary, (insert your name) is a woman of great strength because of the struggles that she experienced during ____________. She has deeper compassion for others because of _____________. She is grateful for the people in her life who taught her the importance of ______________. She has wisdom about _____________because of what she experienced during____________. She is proud of the knowledge that she has about ________________ and the skills that she possesses, such as _____________.

Moving forward, she hopes to share her gifts with others through __________________. She wants to connect with others who have struggled with _____________like her, in order to ________________. She can use her strengths and values to ______________________. She is grateful for_______________.

Think of ways that you can share your story (or part of it) with others. You may want to write your memoirs or autobiography. You could use your phone to record a video of you telling about your experiences and lessons learned. Although you can't avoid all suffering, you can help shape the narrative of your life and how you move forward. You can take pride in your story, and your journey, by embracing it and sharing it with those who may benefit from hearing it. You can reframe your adversity and use your account to propel you forward to greater heights. Storytelling has the potential to help you make meaning of your struggles and to drive how you live out your life's purpose.

Coaching Yourself on Your Purpose With the COACH Approach

Some people reflect upon their purpose daily, as they use it to guide their daily actions. Still, others go through life never considering their life's purpose. Most women are somewhere in between. If you struggle with thinking about this concept or don't know

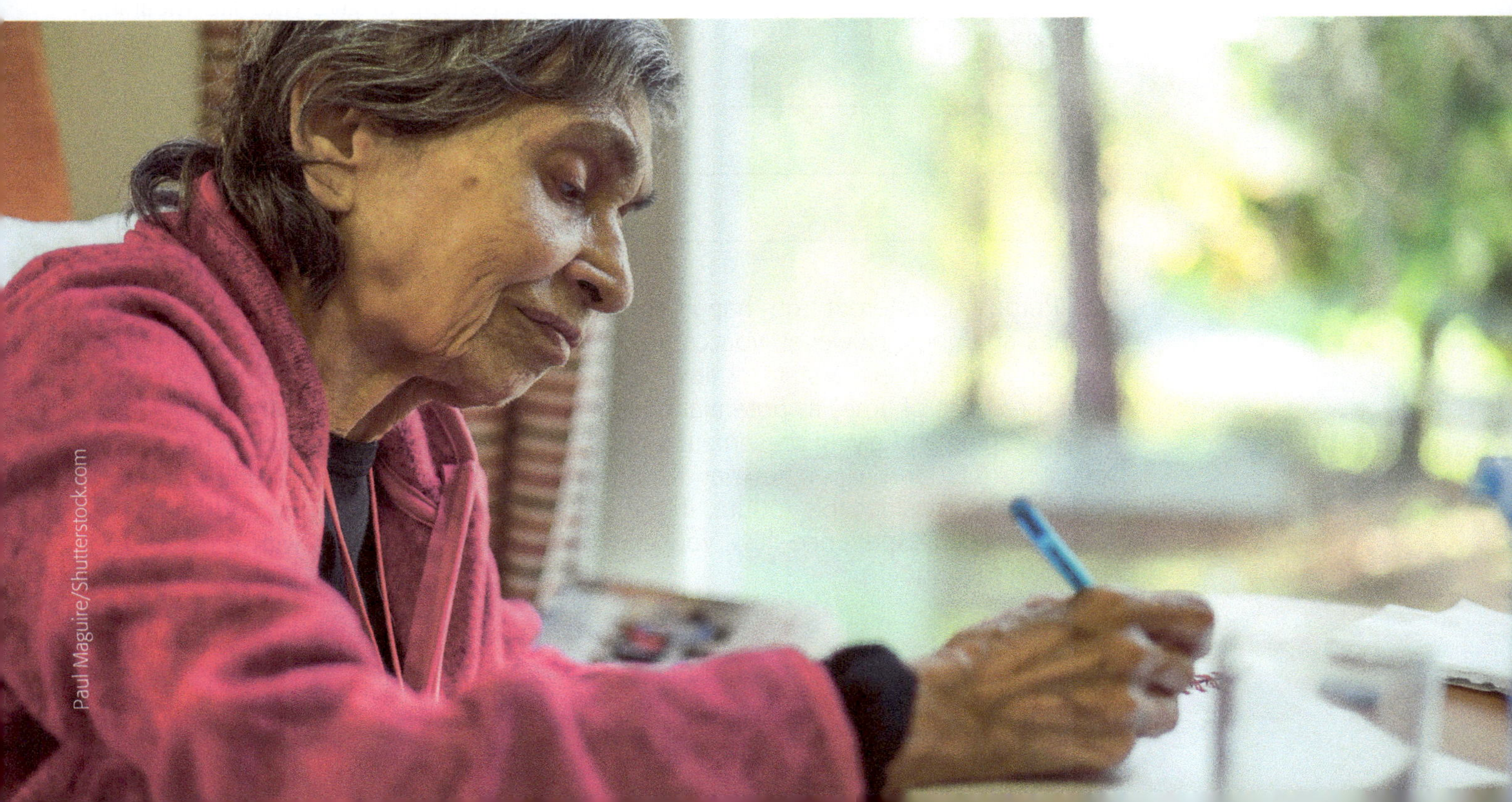

Paul Maguire/Shutterstock.com

what you would consider your purpose, you are not alone. Many midlife and more mature women are in the same place as you, searching for meaningfulness. This section will use the COACH approach to help you refine, clarify, or find your purpose or purposes.

A woman's purpose often changes or shifts with age. You may have more than one purpose or one significant purpose with multiple facets. One common thread seen when looking at everyday manifestations that women express is that they typically connect with others, someone, or something beyond themselves. They often involve high-quality connections, giving loving-kindness to others, belonging, or being part of something larger than oneself.

Since you are reading this book, you are part of something larger than yourself. You are part of the PAVING the Path to Wellness family. You belong. You are needed and wanted. You are part of OUR purpose, to help people have a healthy body, peaceful mind, and joyful heart. We invite you to become part of our larger purpose and join our non-profit organization to share the PAVING the Path to Wellness message with a world that needs more peace and joy. You can visit www.pavingwellness.org to connect with us.

CURIOSITY

- ❏ Part of your life's purpose often involves the people that women connect with regularly. What high-quality relationships do you currently have?

____

____

____

- ❏ Does what you contribute to these relationships help to give your life meaning? Explain.

____

____

____

Purpose is different from happiness. It is more constant, while happiness typically comes and goes. However, you can explore what makes you happy, brings you joy, or helps you achieve a state of flow (where you seem to be in the "zone" and may lose the sense of time) as potential clues to your purpose. For example, some people love teaching and giving presentations for large groups, while others may be terrified of doing this. Some people may experience flow when running marathons, while others may consider this torture. If you identify what brings you joy and happiness and helps you experience flow, you may be able to connect this with a meaningful purpose for your life.

- [ ] What activities energize you, are fun, and bring you joy and happiness?

____

____

____

- [ ] When do you lose track of time? For example, cooking, knitting, gardening, volunteering at a food pantry, engaging in environmental advocacy work, painting, playing with your grandchildren, or researching ways to prevent stroke.

____

____

____

- [ ] Is there a way that you could share these activities with others in a meaningful way?

____

____

____

You could be doing a million other things; instead, you are reading this book. You are working on having a healthier body, a more peaceful mind, and a more joyful heart. With curiosity, reflect upon why you want to have a healthy body, peaceful mind, and joyful heart to see if it aligns with your purpose. For example, you may be doing it so that you'll have more energy to play with children, so that you can experience a deeper connection with your creator (spiritual well-being), so that you can continue to work for several more years, or so that you are healthy enough to engage in activities that help make the world a better place.

- [ ] How does having a healthy body, peaceful mind, and joyful heart align with your purpose?

____

____

____

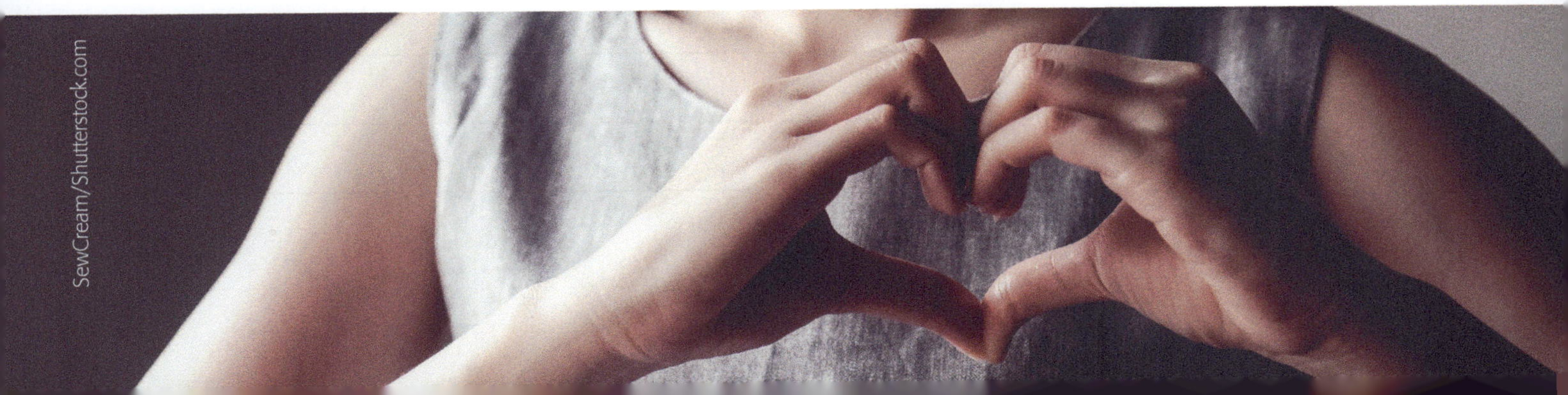

SewCream/Shutterstock.com

OPENNESS

You possess a particular mixture of values, strengths, talents, experiences, knowledge, and gifts that make you unique. Having these does not mean you will share them. You have the option of keeping them all for yourself. Aligning your gifts with your purpose often requires an openness to sharing them with others.

❑ Return to earlier in the chapter where you listed your values and strengths. Are you open to sharing your values, strengths, talents, experiences, knowledge, and gifts with others?

____

____

____

❑ Describe how you are currently sharing them and if there is anything that you want to do to share them more deeply, with a different group, or in another way? Explain.

____

____

____

❑ Do you want to do something to contribute your gifts, but you are hesitant due to how others may judge you?

____

____

____

Since there is no shame, blame, or judging in the PAVING Program, this is a safe place to explore this option. For example, maybe you're a doctor who would like to be a certified yoga teacher, or you're a lawyer who wants to learn to sing and play the guitar.

❑ What could help you move beyond that hesitancy? Remember, the world needs your unique gifts, and experimenting is part of the PAVING Program, as you learned in the chapter on investigations.

____

____

____

- ❑ Can you think of any other ways that you could share your strengths, talents, experience, knowledge, and gifts that you aren't already communicating or sharing with other individuals or groups? How could you do so in a way that feels meaningful to you?

___

___

___

- ❑ Think of someone who is sharing their unique abilities in a meaningful way. What can you learn from them?

___

___

___

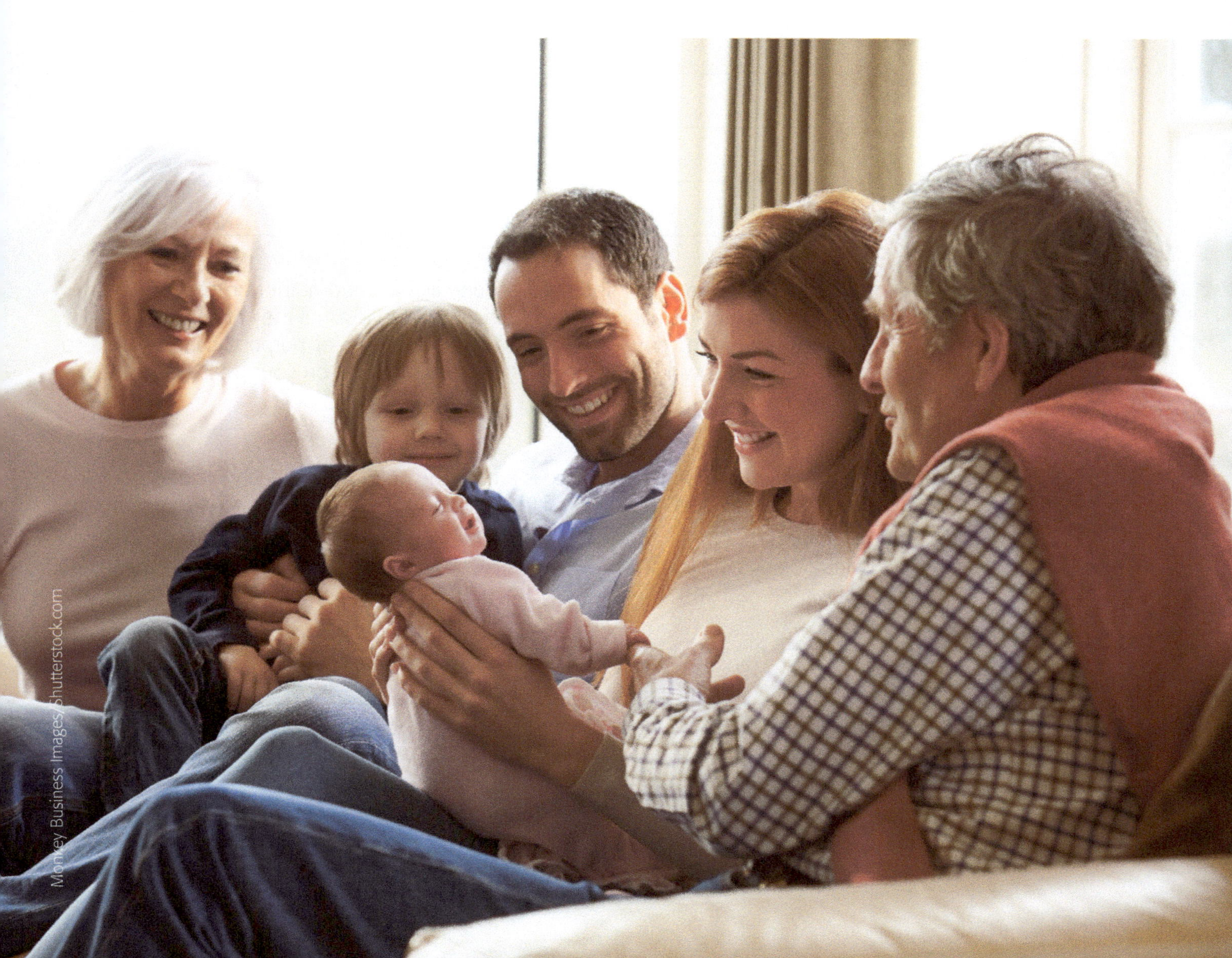

Monkey Business Images/Shutterstock.com

APPRECIATION

The people you love may be part of your purpose. For example, your children, grandchildren, nephews, nieces, spouse, partner, close friends, or colleagues may help give your life purpose.

- ❑ How could you share your gratitude with the people you love and help make your life more meaningful? First, consider telling them about their role in your purpose and life.

  ____

  ____

  ____

  ____

- ❑ Has someone influenced you positively, allowing you to pursue your purpose or hone your strengths? If so, now is a great time to appreciate them and express this appreciation by phone call, email, text, or whatever suits you.

  ____

  ____

  ____

  ____

In some cases, you may find it's someone like a grandmother or teacher who has since passed away. Spending time reflecting upon the lessons they taught you and the influence they've had on your current values and sense of purpose can continue to inspire you, thus allowing them to continue to be with you on your wellness journey.

COMPASSION

According to Viktor Frankl, "conscience is a meaning organ" (3). When you see something happen that doesn't feel right, and you feel called to address it, you follow your conscience.

- ❑ Is there anything your conscience leads you to do that could give your life meaning? Explain.

  ____

  ____

  ____

  ____

- ❏ Showing compassion for others, either a specific person or a group of people, often connects with a meaningful purpose. Is there a person you show compassion toward that helps to give your life meaning?

- ❏ Is there a group of people you show or feel called to show compassion for that is associated with meaning in your life?

- ❏ Who is someone you know or admire from history, past or present, who is an excellent example of living a life led by their conscience?

- ❏ What activities do you want to participate in that can help promote the cause, group of people, medical condition, or organization that aligns with what pulls at your heart?

HONESTY

Sometimes, women want to share something with others, but fear of rejection, uncertainty, or not knowing how to share leads them to keep their gifts to themselves. Reflect honestly upon what you wish you could be sharing with others but currently are not communicating.

- ❏ Are there ways in which you want to share your talents, knowledge, gifts, or expertise, but you are holding back? Why do you think this is so?

- ❏ Are there steps you want to take to share this with others, and if so, what will be your next step? If not, why do you not want to move forward at this time?

- ❏ Do you feel free to follow your purpose that gives your life meaning, or do you feel like you must conform to the expectations of others? Explain.

- ❏ It can be easy to go through life, filling your days with appointments and activities that don't align with your purpose in life. Does your calendar schedule reflect what is meaningful in your life and your true intention?

- ❏ If not, is there anything that you want to do to make a change toward aligning your daily activities with your purpose?

- ❑ Do you need to forgive yourself for something? Now is an excellent time to be honest with yourself and forgive.

  ____

  ____

  ____

- ❑ Do you need to forgive others for something? Now is a good time to give that forgiveness and free yourself.

  ____

  ____

  ____

Mission Statement

You've spent a considerable amount of time in this chapter reflecting upon your unique attributes and how they can add meaning to your life and the lives of others. Hopefully, you better understand your life's story and how your struggles have shaped the amazing woman you are today. Next, you'll clarify your purpose with a mission statement or vision statement.

Consider where you see yourself in one, five, and ten years. Think about where you are now and where you want to go. Think of others who are leading purpose and meaning-filled lives. Consider the legacy you want to leave. Finally, think about how you can make the world a better place. After spending at least five minutes reflecting on these prompts, write a mission or purpose statement in the space below. You are not limited to a single purpose. You may have several or many facets of one overarching goal.

My purpose is to ______________________________

____

____

If you're struggling with this prompt, you can continue thinking about it and return any time. You may also want to review some of the following examples. Remember that there is no purpose too big or too small. The main point is that it should be meaningful to you.

Your purpose may be to…

- Show kindness to others.
- Deepen your spirituality.
- Love your family and close friends.
- Make the world a better place.

- Work to make money to support an organization in which you believe.
- Work to make money for your children to go to college.
- Mentor those who are coming after you at your place of employment.
- Help reduce suffering in the world.
- Add joy to the life of others through your friendliness and humor.
- Help those who are lonely by expressing loving-kindness to those who are alone.
- Teach others to take photos since this is your hobby and where you have expertise, and you want to share this with others.
- Volunteer at the local food banks to help those who are hungry.
- Watch your grandchildren while your child works and help your grandchildren to grow up with strong values.
- Work for social justice with a non-profit organization.
- Help others in need by cleaning out your home and donating items to a charity.
- Work in your garden and share some of the produce and flowers with others.
- Support your spouse/partner so that the two of you can work together to have a loving home for your extended family.
- Write a book and share your story in hopes that it will inspire another.
- Join a march in support of a worthy cause.
- Run for local government.
- Sit on a town board, like education or transportation.
- Teach classes that inspire students to be lifelong learners.

"gifts + passions + values = purpose"
—Richard Leider (2), Best-Selling Author and Coach

Living Your Purpose

You can know your purpose without fully living your purpose. However, you are meant to live out your meaningful purpose. For example, a common goal is to make the world better. However, you can live this out in a multitude of ways. Even a more specific purpose, such as helping raise your grandchildren to be productive members of society, may be fulfilled through various activities. So, whether you've known your purpose for decades, have just realized your purpose, or have recently found a new one, it's time to get creative with determining how you want to live out your purpose.

Imagine yourself in the future when you are fully living out the purpose you have identified. This purpose you've identified may feel like it's calling you. Close your eyes and imagine how you would feel, what you would be saying and doing, who else would be around you, what you would see and hear, etc.

- [ ] What does it look like for you to fully live out your purpose? (If you have more than one purpose you've identified, pick one or more to explore).

____

____

____

- ❑ How can the PAVING principle of investigation help you to live your purpose more fully? For example, you may want to learn more about a non-profit organization, connect with a local theater troupe, ask your nephews and nieces how you could best support their academic growth, or ask your food bank if they are accepting new volunteers. What do you want to investigate now?

  ____

  ____

  ____

- ❑ How can the PAVING principle of variety help you live your purpose more fully? For example, maybe your purpose is to serve those in need, and you're already volunteering at a homeless shelter. However, you may want to incorporate variety by sponsoring a child in need or visiting someone who lives in a nursing home. Another idea is tutoring an adult who is working toward their GED exam.

  ____

  ____

  ____

- ❑ How can the PAVING principle of social connection help you to live your purpose more fully? Is there a way that you could connect with others who have a similar goals to yours? For example, are there organizations for grandparents helping raise their grandchildren, a non-profit organization addressing planetary health, a group of women at your church who regularly meet to support those experiencing domestic violence, or another organization that connects with your purpose that you could join?

  ____

  ____

  ____

- ❑ What other opportunities are there for you to fulfill your meaningful purpose? Think locally in your community, state, nationally, and even globally. Don't limit yourself. Remember, no purpose is too small nor too big.

  ____

  ____

  ____

It's easy to intend to prioritize your projects and commitments with your purpose in mind, but your schedule can quickly become overrun with your daily to-do tasks.

When someone asks you to be on a new committee, take on a new role, commit to an engagement, or schedule a meeting, ask yourself if it aligns with your purpose. Pass, if it does not align, and you are not required to do it. When you agree to something that takes time, you say no to something else that could fill that time. To live a mindful, purpose-filled life, you need time to fulfill your purpose.

- ❏ Do you currently have enough time and energy to devote to your purpose? If not, how can you take more time or increase your energy to fulfill your purpose?

  ____

  ____

  ____

If you don't make time for what is meaningful in life, your schedule will become filled with other tasks, and you will not live out your purpose. Try to prioritize projects that are in alignment with your purpose starting now. There is no time like the present.

- ❏ If you feel comfortable doing so, reach out to a loved one or friend and share your thoughts about your purpose. Consider discussing how you are already living out or plan to live out this purpose. Ask them about their purpose. Share valuable feedback you received.

  ____

  ____

  ____

- ❏ Are there others with whom you want to explore a common purpose? For example, if you are part of an organization or business or have a partner or spouse, consider asking them to join you in assessing your purpose as a couple or a group. This discussion may lead to a mission statement for your family, group of friends, or organization. A mission statement identifies the goals and values of a group, organization, family, or company. It is essential to have your purpose defined to create a meaningful mission statement. What are your thoughts about having a common purpose and mission statement for your group or partnership?

  ____

  ____

  ____

  ____

Some of the following questions you may be able to answer now, or you may want to return to them once your purpose is more solidified.

- ❑ What goal do you want to set for living out your purpose over the next 10 years?

____

____

____

- ❑ What goal do you want to set for living out your purpose over the next five years?

____

____

____

- ❑ What goal do you want to set for living out your purpose over the next year?

____

____

____

- ❑ What goal do you want to set for living out your purpose over the next month?

____

____

____

- ❑ What goal do you want to set for living out your purpose this next week? Make sure your goal is SMART (specific, measurable, action-oriented, realistic, and time-bound). For example, your goal could include researching current community service opportunities in your region or phoning a few friends to create a network.

____

____

____

Also, be on the lookout for opportunities for you to live out your purpose, serve others, and go beyond what you've already been doing to live your purpose-filled life. Don't limit yourself. Be creative. Have fun! You were born to live out your purpose! The world needs you!

Words of Wisdom From Dr. Michelle Tollefson

It happens time and time again. A midlife or more mature woman, typically having already been through menopause, comes into my office feeling tired, unmotivated, and disengaged. While discussing her symptoms, she mentions that her daughter left for college, her son moved out and has a new job, she recently retired from her career of 30 years, and she no longer wants to do the social activities she used to enjoy. She reports "feeling old" and doesn't feel like her usual self but doesn't know what is wrong. Instead of enjoying her additional free time, she is bored. She is happy that her children are thriving and independent, this is what she wanted for them, but she feels an emptiness that she wasn't expecting with them out of her home. She has her partner, but their relationship doesn't seem to have the "spark" she used to enjoy. Every day feels like it is similar to yesterday.

There are many reasons for fatigue and the symptoms mentioned above. However, after screening for and ruling out depression and other underlying physical causes of these symptoms, I often realize that it is a loss of her sense of purpose at the root of her problems. It's common for the purpose to shift during midlife when family and career responsibilities often change from how they've been for many years. Unfortunately, many women have never taken a time-out to reflect upon what they want their purpose to be now and in the future.

Once a woman understands why she feels the way she does now, she can decide how to move forward. This may involve reflecting, reading, connecting with friends or older women who have gone through similar experiences, praying, speaking with a counselor, journaling, or reading books about purpose. Through this process, which is sometimes very quick and sometimes lengthy, she hopefully emerges with a renewed passion for life, motivated to live her life purposefully.

It's often several months between visits, but when I see her next time, she typically walks into the office more enthusiastically, ready to share the insight she's gained and the changes made since we last met. Whether she's decided to use the skills that she learned during her career to help a new non-profit organization, volunteer with a local charity, or engage with her spiritual community, she's usually excited to share how she's fulfilling a meaningful purpose for the next part of her life's journey.

Purpose Wrap-Up

Never underestimate the power of living your purpose. We've seen it time and time again. With a renewed focus on meaningful purpose, women struggling with a spark that had become dim often realize that they are on fire for living a purposeful, passionate, and meaningful life.

References

1. Peterson, C., & Seligman, M. E. P. (2004). *Character Strengths and Virtues: A Handbook and Classification.* New York: Oxford University Press and Washington, DC: American Psychological Association.
2. Richard Leider, Three Steps to Unlocking Your Purpose, accessed 5/5/2022. https://richardleider.com/three-steps-to-unlocking-your-purpose/
3. Viktor Frankl America. Meaning from a Logotherapy Perspective. https://viktorfranklamerica.com/2021/03/03/meaning-from-a-logotherapy-perspective/, accessed 5/5/2022.

CHAPTER 12
SLEEP

Sleep Throughout Menopause, Midlife, and Beyond

Acronym—SLEEP

Silent	**Eight**
Lights	**Prepare**
Every day	

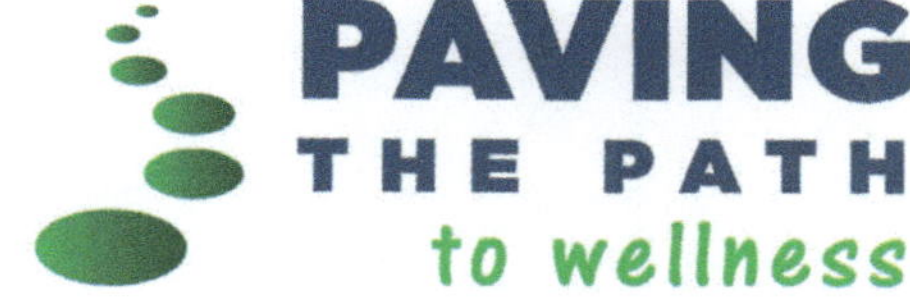

- *SILENT:* Keep your bedroom as quiet as possible. If you can't get rid of unwanted sounds, consider using a "white noise" machine or earplugs. Silence supports deeper sleep.
- *LIGHTS:* Get exposure to bright lights during the day and keep the lights dimmer late at night. Avoid looking at screens that emit blue wavelength light in the evening. Keep your bedroom as dark as possible, using an eye mask, blackout curtains or shades.
- *EVERY DAY:* Try to go to bed and wake up at around the same time every day. Don't try to skip out on sleep during the work week with a plan to sleep for longer on the weekend. Sticking to a regular schedule supports optimal sleep.
- *EIGHT:* Be aware, according to the Sleep Foundation, healthy adults need about seven to eight hours of sleep each night for optimal functioning. Prioritize sleep. Your body and mind will thank you.
- *PREPARE:* Prepare for getting a good night's sleep through your daytime behaviors. Don't take naps late in the day. Avoid large meals, alcohol, caffeinated beverages, and exercise close to bedtime. Get outside and enjoy the morning sunshine, engage in physical activity, and eat nourishing foods during the day.

You might take sleep for granted, until you struggle with it. When you get a "good night's sleep," you wake, feeling refreshed and ready to start your day. You don't even think about the high-quality sleep that supports your energy, mood, and learning ability throughout the day.

When you struggle with sleep, nights can seem endless, as the hours tick by, while you watch your clock, hoping to sleep again before morning arrives. Although sleeping may seem like a passive activity, while your body waits for the day, it is a very dynamic and essential behavior. Engaging in regular daily activities can be a struggle, when your sleep is of poor quality or insufficient duration. In addition, you may feel more emotional, and remembering well-known facts may be challenging. Unfortunately, inadequate sleep becomes so common for many women that they become accustomed to going

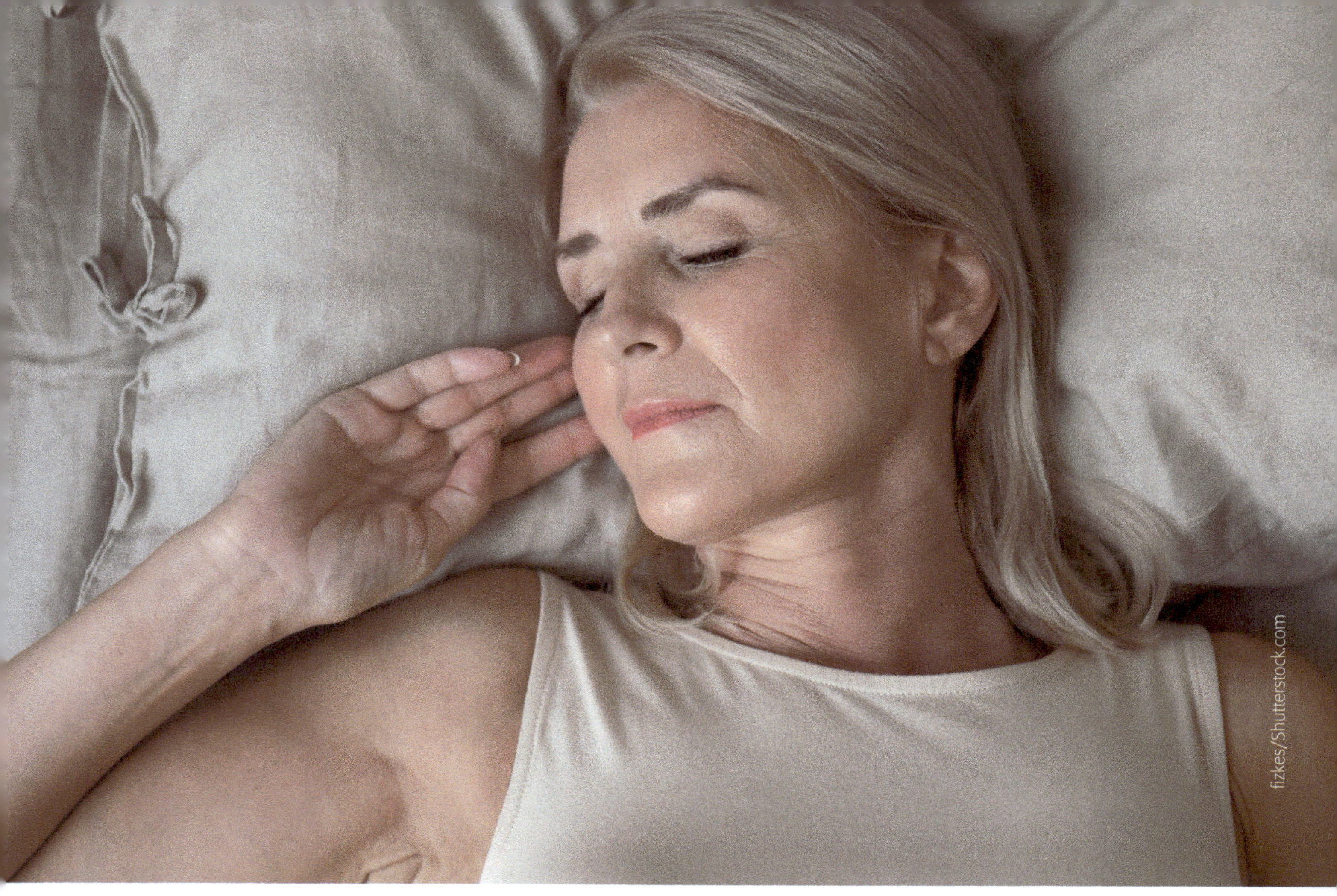

through life in a sleepy, low-energy state, not even realizing how their lack of sleep has negatively impacted their body and mind.

To optimize your health, you must prioritize sleep. As your estrogen levels decrease with menopause, it becomes increasingly difficult to fall asleep and stay asleep for many women. Although aging and menopause both make getting high-quality sleep more challenging due to increased night awakenings, decreased deep sleep, and increased time spent trying to fall asleep, your sleep requirements do not decline, when you are going through or went through menopause. The Centers for Disease Control recommends that menopausal, midlife, and more mature women get seven to eight hours of sleep each night. Getting restorative sleep is just as important, if not more important, as you age. Now is an ideal time to reflect upon your current sleep habits and make changes that will support your sleep for decades to come.

- ❑ How do you feel when you get a "good night's sleep"? Consider how your body feels as well as your mood and emotions.

  ____

  ____

  ____

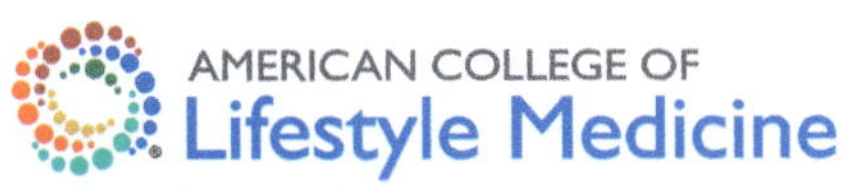

Menopause and Sleep

Vasomotor Symptoms (VMS): hot flases and night sweats. These are episodes of sweating, flushing, and heat in the head, neck, chest and upper back.

High FSH Levels

Abrupt Drop in Estradiol Levels

RESULTS

Difficulty falling asleep and staying asleep

How Does the Menopause Transition affect Sleep?

20% Experience Obstructive Sleep Apnea

40% Experience poor sleep and increased nightime awakenings

60% Experience Restless Leg Syndrome

80% Experience Vasomotor Symptoms (VMS)

What is the Menopause Transition

- Menopause is defined as 12 months after a woman's last menstrual period.
- The menopause transition inlcudes the years leading up to menopause when a woman may notice changes in her menstrual cycle, increased depression or anxiety, hot flashes, and more difficulty falling asleep or staying asleep.
- These symptoms are due to dramatic fluctuations in secual hormones such as estrogen and progesterone.

What Can You Do?

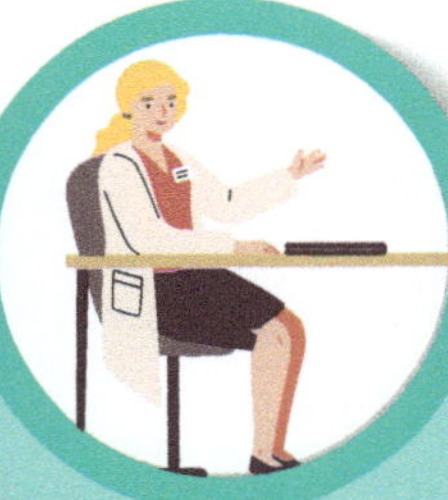

Talk to your Doctor

If you have concers or questions, visti your primary care provider to see what is best for your sleep during your menopause transition.

Nutrition

A whole food, plant-based diet can aid in giving you the proper amount of nutrition. Include a wide variety of colorful fruits, berries, green leafy vegetables, beans, and lentils to improve sleep.

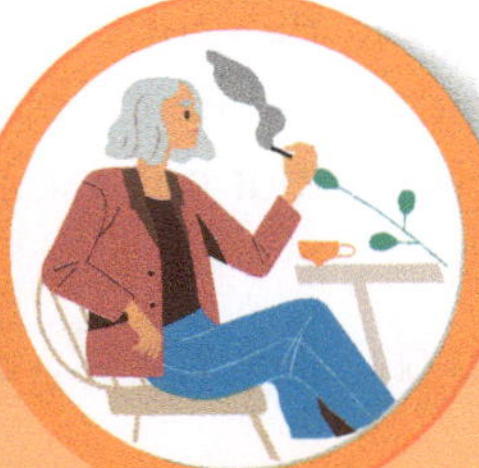

Avoid Risky Substances

Tobacco, caffeine, and alcohol are associated with more hot flashes and reduced sleep quality.

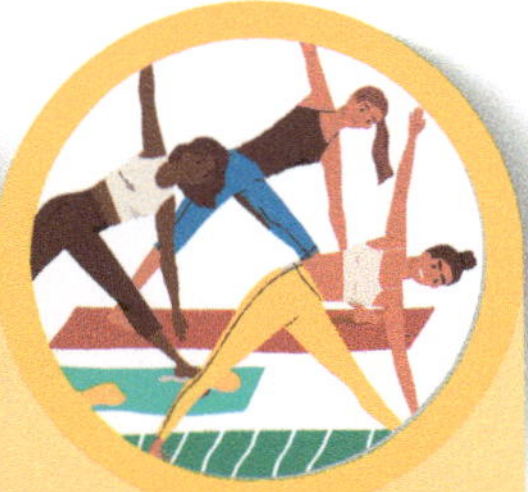

Exercise

Incorporate movement in your daily routine. Walking, running, and gardening can help reduce stress and improve sleep quality. Strecthing or gentle yoga before bed may help both VMS and sleep.

How Does Alcohol affect sleep during Menopause Transition?

- May worsen sleep apnea
- May worsen VMS
- Can cause urinary irritation
- More frequent awakenings
- Increased heartburn or reflux

Figure 12-1. Menopause and sleep

❑ How do you feel when you don't sleep seven to eight hours?

____

____

____

Why Sleep Is Important in Midlife and Beyond

Getting adequate sleep is important throughout a woman's lifespan, but it is even more essential as you age. During the menopausal transition and into menopause, women often struggle with weight gain, increased aches and pains, fatigue, mood changes, and problems with memory. Inadequate sleep can worsen each of these factors. The good news is that getting adequate sleep can help these symptoms too.

Your body loves adequate sleep because it:

- Improves your heart health and decreases your risk of a heart attack and stroke.
- Strengthens your immune system.
- Decreases your chances of getting diabetes, and if you have it, it makes it easier to control your blood sugar.
- Helps your body recover and repair faster from injuries.
- Decreases pain sensitivity which is beneficial if you experience aches and pains.
- Increases your energy and combats fatigue.
- Supports healthy blood pressure and cholesterol levels.
- Helps your gut bacteria (microbiome) be healthier.

Food, Weight, and Sleep

Getting adequate sleep helps menopausal women eat healthfully and maintain or attain a health-promoting weight. If you sleep less than seven to eight hours regularly, you are more likely to consume energy-dense, unhealthy foods high in added sugar and fat. It also becomes more challenging to make healthy food choices since emotional eating, impulsivity, night overeating, and cravings increase due to a rise in ghrelin (the hunger hormone). Also, even when you finish a large meal, you may not feel full or satisfied, if your sleep is inadequate due to decreased leptin (the hormone that makes you feel full) with sleep deprivation.

Many women struggle with unwanted weight gain during menopause. Insufficient sleep makes weight loss more challenging and weight gain more common due to increased intake of high-calorie, low-quality foods. Also, gaining fat rather than muscle is more common with insufficient sleep. Furthermore, if weight loss does occur, it is more likely to be muscle mass (lean mass) while retaining fat.

With sleep deprivation, the body does not process sugar optimally, increasing the risk of getting metabolic syndrome (overweight, high blood pressure, diabetes, and high cholesterol) and type 2 diabetes. It also makes controlling blood sugar more complex, when women are not getting adequate sleep.

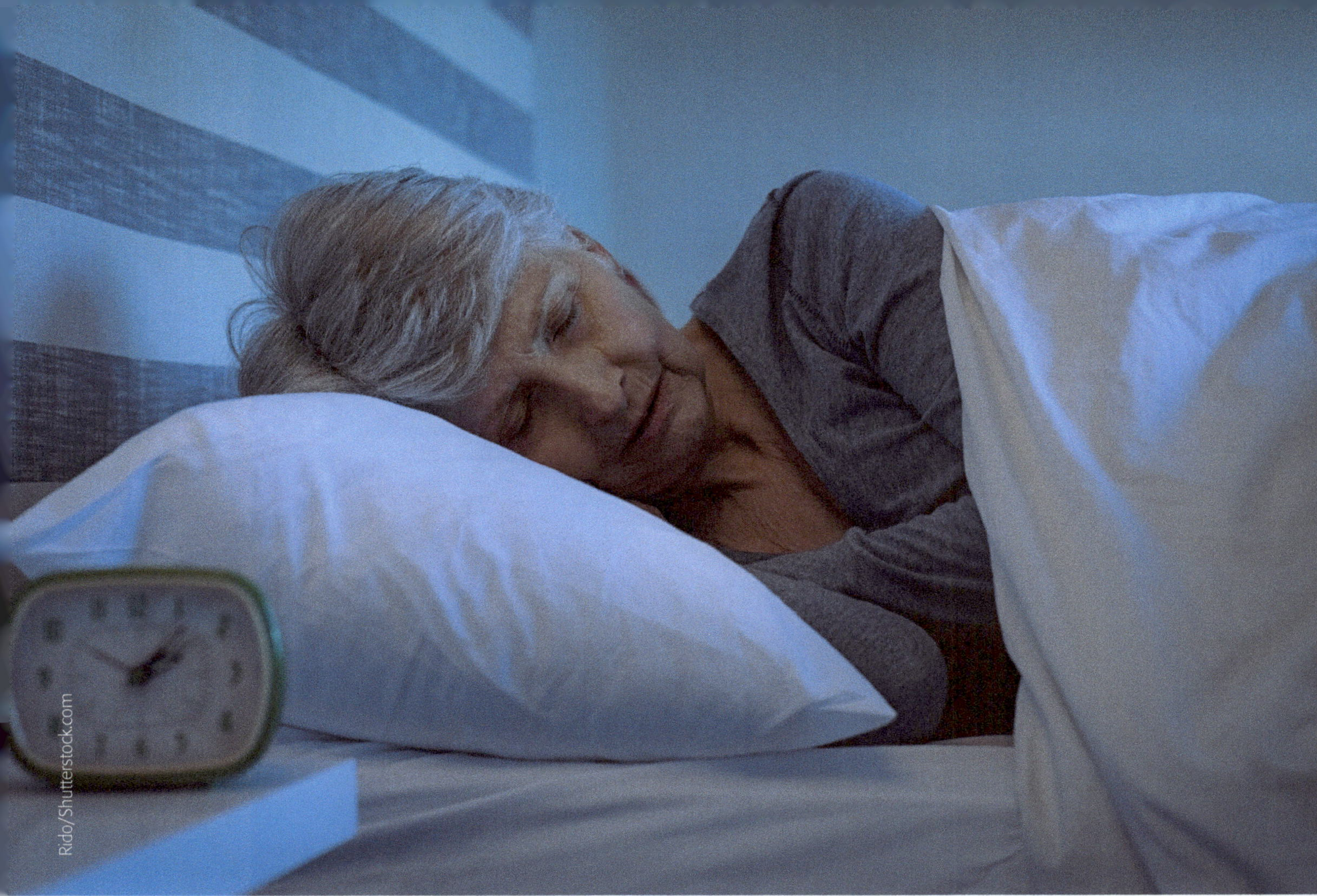
Rido/Shutterstock.com

Your brain loves adequate sleep because it:

- Helps you better manage stress.
- Decreases your risk of depression, anxiety, and other mental health problems.
- Decreases your risk of dementia, including Alzheimer's disease.
- Decreases your risk of having a stroke.
- Helps keep your memory sharp.
- Allows you to learn new skills and facts and then store those facts to use later.
- Helps you better remember facts and memories from long ago.
- Increases your chances of feeling good, more positive, and optimistic.
- Supports healthy relationships.
- Improves your creativity.
- Decreases impulsivity.
- Decreases addictive behavior and reduces chances of relapse.
- Improves your ability to control your emotions.
- Helps you with problem-solving.
- Improves your ability to communicate well with others.
- Decreases feelings of anger.
- Makes you a safer driver (because it decreases the likelihood of dangerous drowsy driving).

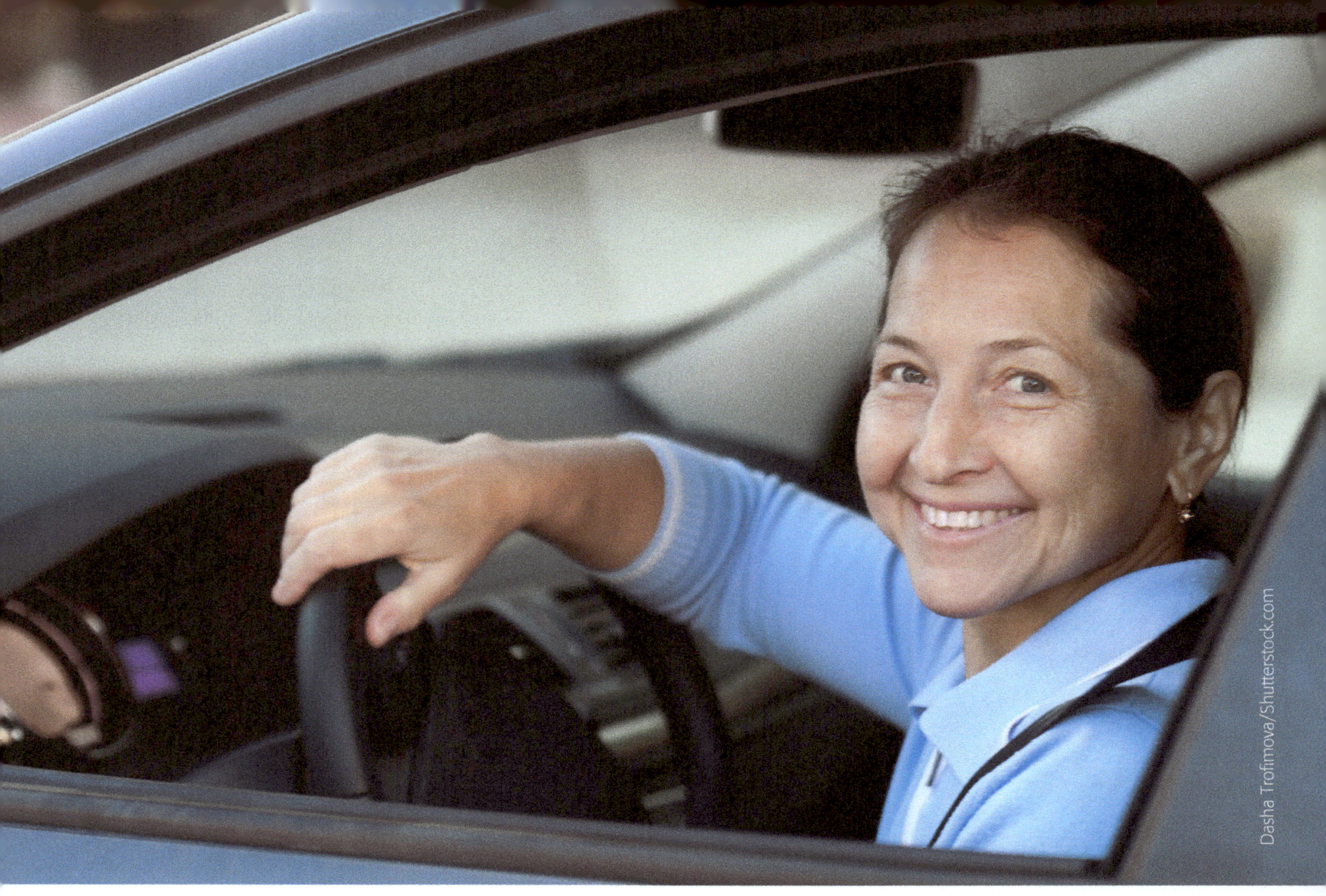
Dasha Trofimova/Shutterstock.com

Your brain is very active while you sleep. One of the most critical activities while sleeping is clearing out waste products that neurons (brain cells) make during the day. You can think of the glymphatic system as a waste disposal system for your brain. It removes products including amyloid, whose buildup is associated with Alzheimer's disease. Although scientists don't fully understand the complex causes of dementia, they know that optimizing sleep is vital for brain health and, as such, it decreases the risk of getting dementia.

Put a checkmark by the things on the previous list that are important to you. The more checkmarks on the list, the more important it is to you. Also, keep in mind that if you are like many menopausal or more mature women who struggle with sleep, you need to work on improving your sleep hygiene.

- ❑ After reading about the benefits of adequate sleep, why do you want to optimize your rest? Use ideas from the aforementioned list or think of your own. For example, maybe you want more energy to take your morning walk or have a better mood when interacting with your family.

  ____

  ____

  ____

The Challenges of Sleep During Midlife and Beyond

It's not your imagination. Sleep becomes more challenging during the menopausal transition for many women, which often persists beyond menopause. As you age, sleep becomes more fragmented with night awakenings. In general, during and after menopause, women often also struggle more with falling asleep, as well as then awakening very early, before their desired wake time. In addition to decreased sleep quantity (the number of hours spent sleeping), sleep quality also declines as deep sleep decreases.

Medical problems that become more common with age and the medications used to treat these conditions can also contribute to sleep challenges during menopause and beyond. Women who share a bed with their spouse or partner, who is also aging, experiencing medical problems of their own, and taking medications that may negatively impact their sleep, may struggle with sleep due to their partner's health challenges. A spouse or partner may be snoring, which is an indicator of sleep apnea, and is a risk factor for stroke. This is something that you should be aware of for your spouse or partner as well as yourself. Ask them if you snore. If you or your spouse or partner snore, you are encouraged to talk to a doctor about potential screening for sleep apnea. Many sleep disorders also increase in frequency or severity during menopause, including insomnia, obstructive sleep apnea, and restless leg syndrome.

During menopause, many women will notice that they start to fall asleep earlier in the evening and wake very early. Some women are bothered by this change, as they age, while others are not. If you fall asleep earlier in the evening and wake earlier in the morning, know that you are not alone, and that this is normal as you age.

Hot flashes that happen while trying to sleep are called night sweats. Some women wake shortly before a night sweat happens, while others wake during the night to find themselves sweaty and overheated. Although night sweats typically decrease after about five years for most women, the need to get up in the middle of the night to use the bathroom often does not decrease. These nighttime awakenings make getting adequate sleep a challenge. Don't despair however; this chapter provides evidence-based suggestions for improving your sleep shortly.

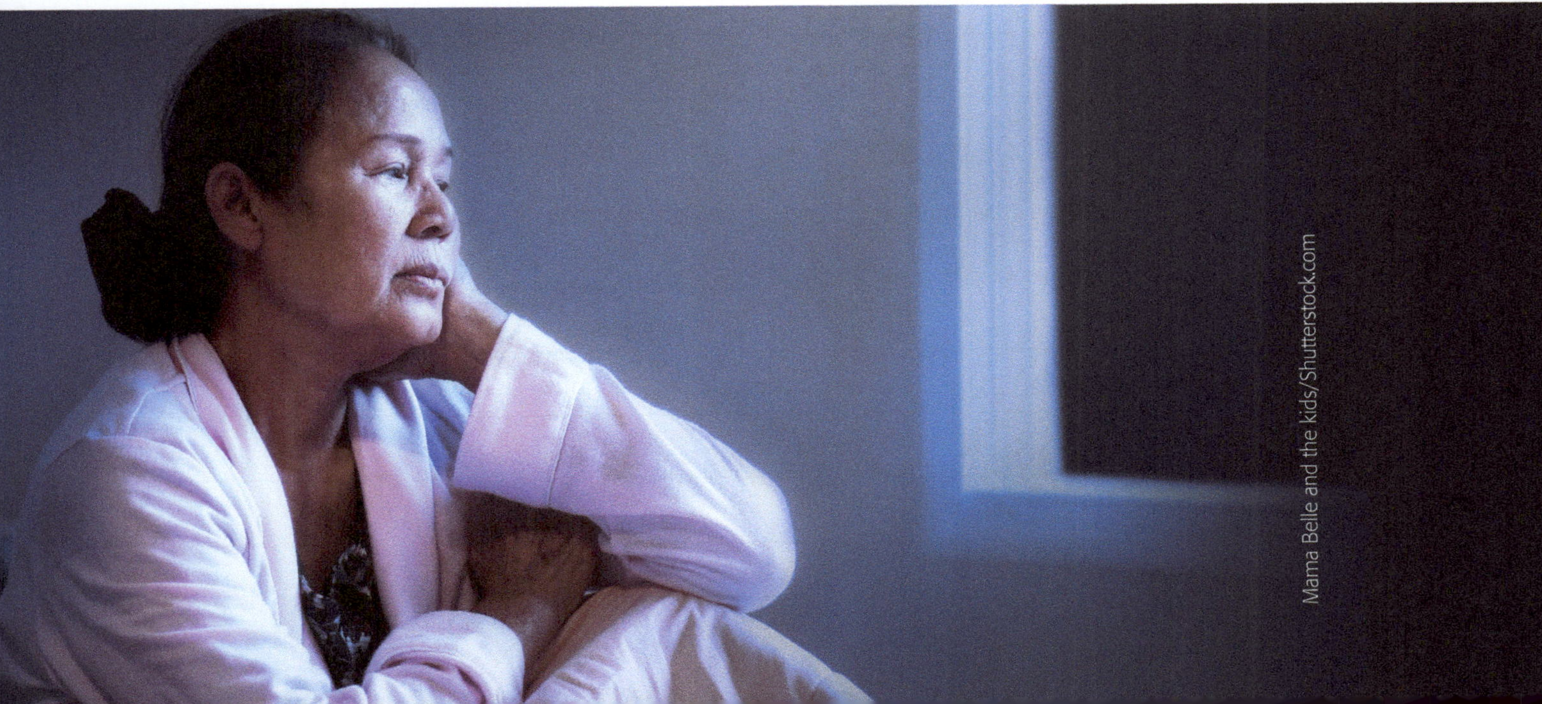
Mama Belle and the kids/Shutterstock.com

Sleep Journal

Keeping a sleep diary for a week can help you better understand your sleep habits, what enables you to sleep better, and potential causes for your disrupted sleep (Table 12-1). It can be helpful to know what you did during the day that might have contributed to how you slept on a particular day (e.g., time of exercise, time of outdoor light exposure, dim lights at night, warm shower before bed, when you shut off your phone, computer, TV, or an argument with a child or partner).

Date: ______________________________

Time you got into bed: ______________________________

Whether you had difficulty falling asleep: ______________________________

Estimated number and time of night awakenings: ______________________________

Reasons for night awakenings: ______________________________

____

____

____

Other sleep problems: ______________________________

Estimated number of hours spent sleeping: ______________________________

Time you woke and got out of bed: ______________________________

How you felt in the morning: ______________________________

____

____

____

On a scale from 1-10, how energized were you when you woke up? ______________

Other insights about last night: ______________________________

____

____

____

Table 12-1. A sample of a sleep journal

You will be asked to reflect on your journal and answer questions about it at the end of this chapter in the section on coaching yourself on sleep with the COACH approach.

Practical Advice for Improving Sleep

NIGHTTIME WAKENING TO URINATE

As you age, the likelihood of waking during the night to urinate increases. Many women over the age of 60 wake at least once a night to urinate. Bladder capacity also decreases with age. Night sweats are also associated with nighttime trips to the bathroom. Although waking once a night to use the bathroom is often expected, needing to urinate twice or more per night is called nocturia and deserves a discussion with your healthcare practitioner. It may be a normal part of aging for you. On the other hand, it could also be a sign of something more serious, especially if it is new for you, worsening, or is associated with other symptoms, such as painful urination (a sign of a urinary tract infection), leaking urine (incontinence), or swollen legs (edema).

In addition to regularly disrupting sleep, waking to urinate at night increases the risk of falls and injuries. For this reason, it's beneficial to explore lifestyle modifications that can decrease your need to urinate at night. It's also wise to make your environment safer, so that when you wake at night to use the bathroom, you are less likely to fall and get injured.

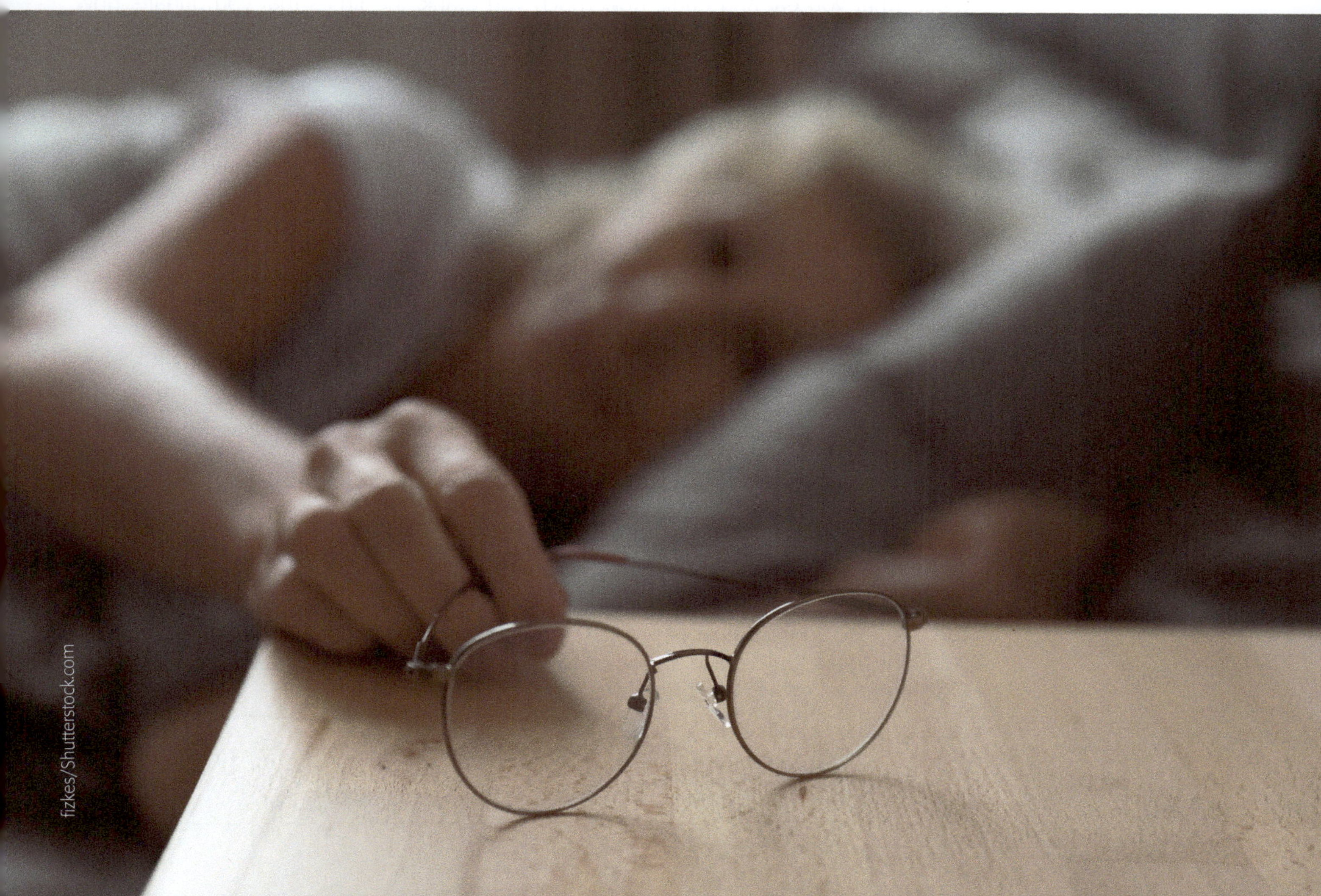

fizkes/Shutterstock.com

Among the suggestions for decreasing nighttime awakenings to urinate are the following:

- Stay well-hydrated during the day.
- Limit the amount of fluids that you drink starting about two to four hours before bedtime (remember to stay well-hydrated starting early in the day).
- Limit the amount of foods that you eat (e.g., watermelon, cucumbers, soup) that contain a lot of liquid as you get closer to bedtime.
- Urinate immediately before you go to bed.
- Talk to your physician to see if there are underlying causes (diabetes, obstructive sleep apnea, urinary tract infection) that should be treated.
- Avoid alcohol and caffeine, especially later in the day, as they are bladder stimulants.
- Avoid artificial sweeteners.
- Avoid acidic foods and drinks that can stimulate the bladder.
- Take measures to decrease hot flashes and night sweats.
- If your legs swell, use support hose and elevate your legs during the day (in addition to talking to your physician).
- Do pelvic floor muscle exercises (Kegels) to strengthen pelvic muscles (see the chapter on physical activity).

If you've started to wake more at night to urinate or are waking twice or more, make an appointment with your healthcare provider. While waiting to see your provider, you may want to keep a voiding (urinating) diary where you record: the times you eat and drink, what you eat and drink, how much you drank, the times that you urinate, how much you urinate, if you leak urine, and if you feel a strong urge to urinate, as well as any other symptoms.

One way to identify whether you are dehydrated is to notice the color of your urine. If your urine is dark yellow, you are likely dehydrated. It's important to stay hydrated during the day. There's no need to limit your water intake. Simply investigate your drinking and urinating patterns.

If you wake during the night to go to the bathroom, it's essential to make your home as safe as possible. Even if you don't wake up to urinate at night, the aforementioned suggestions can also make your home safer to reduce the risk of injury (to yourself and others).

❑ On average, how many times do you wake during the night to use the bathroom?

____

____

____

Circle the suggestions on the aforementioned list that you want to try to see if you can decrease your number of nighttime awakenings to use the bathroom. In addition, if you think you should make an appointment to talk with your healthcare provider about nighttime awakenings, call today and make an appointment.

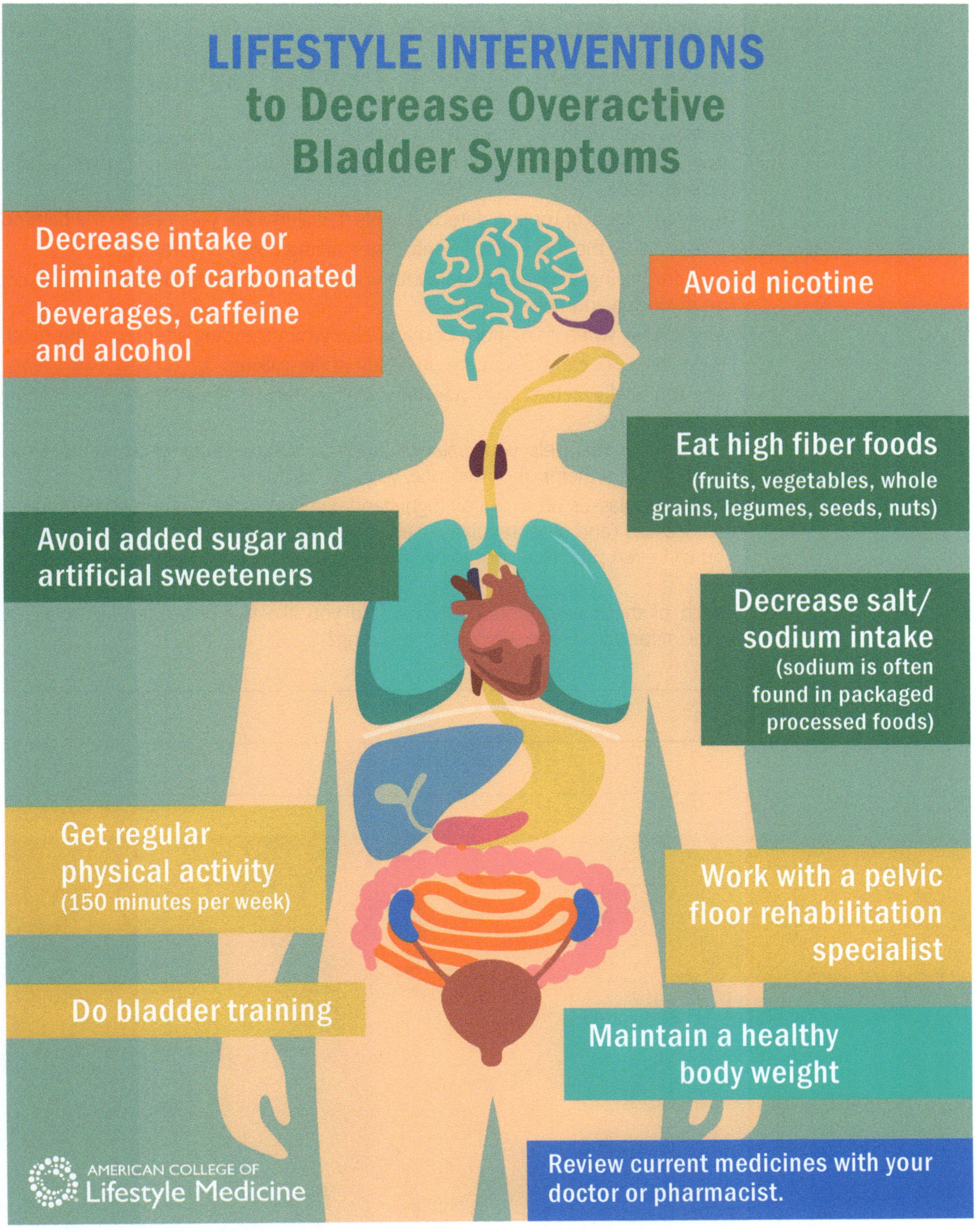

LIFESTYLE INTERVENTIONS to Decrease Overactive Bladder Symptoms

Decrease intake or eliminate of carbonated beverages, caffeine and alcohol

Avoid nicotine

Eat high fiber foods (fruits, vegetables, whole grains, legumes, seeds, nuts)

Avoid added sugar and artificial sweeteners

Decrease salt/ sodium intake (sodium is often found in packaged processed foods)

Get regular physical activity (150 minutes per week)

Work with a pelvic floor rehabilitation specialist

Do bladder training

Maintain a healthy body weight

AMERICAN COLLEGE OF Lifestyle Medicine

Review current medicines with your doctor or pharmacist.

Figure 12-2. Lifestyle interventions to decrease overactive bladder symptoms

Decreasing Fall Risk With Nighttime Wakening and in General

- Remove loose items that increase your risk of tripping (e.g., electrical cords, magazines, plants).
- Remove rugs, as they are a tripping hazard.
- Have a light by your bedside that you can quickly turn on when you get up to use the bathroom.
- Have night lights or motion-detecting lights that illuminate your path to the bathroom.
- Have a rail by the toilet to hold onto when sitting down or standing up.
- Consider having a mobile phone with you or an emergency device that you could use if you fell and needed help.
- Stand slowly when rising from bed and also when standing after using the toilet.
- Use a walker or cane, if you are unsteady while walking.
- Stay physically active with aerobic activities and resistance training activities during the day.
- Do exercises that help your balance (such as balance training programs, working with a physical therapist on balance, yoga, or tai chi).
- Have your glasses on a nearby nightstand. Everyone needs a designated place for their glasses (and other regularly used—and misplaced—items, including their keys). You can even purchase special eyeglass stands on which to place your eyeglasses.

❑ Which of these recommendations would you like to put in place to make your home safer and decrease your risk of falling?

____

____

____

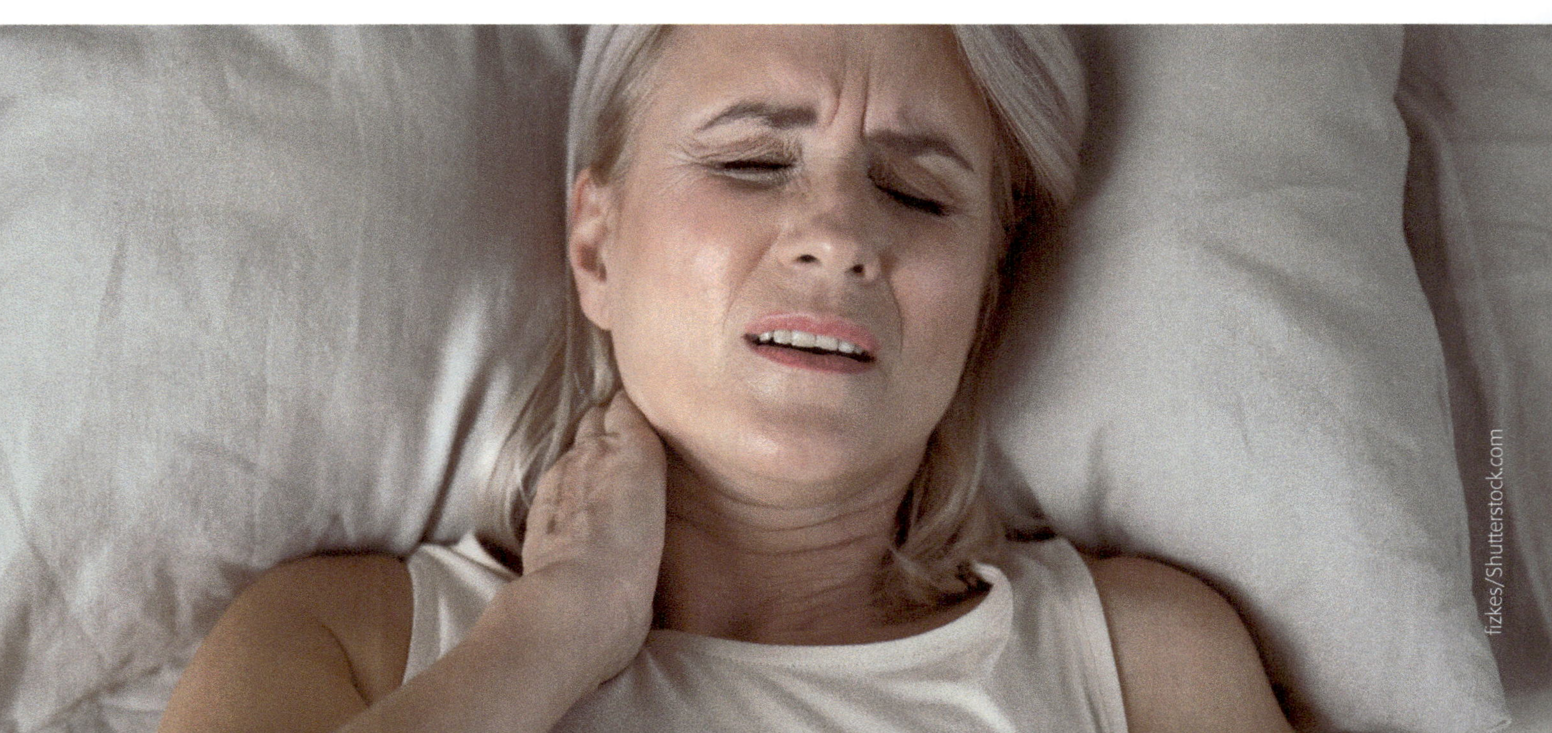

fizkes/Shutterstock.com

NIGHTTIME WAKENING DUE TO NIGHT SWEATS

Night sweats are often associated with nighttime awakenings for perimenopausal and menopausal women. The following are some suggestions that can help decrease night awakenings due to night sweats:

- Avoid alcohol, spicy foods, and caffeinated beverages, as well as other foods or beverages that trigger hot flashes and night sweats for you.
- Increase ventilation by opening a window or using a fan.
- Wear light and cool sleepwear that are moisture-wicking or made from natural fibers, such as cotton.
- Wear loose sleepwear that does not restrict movement.
- Have light sheets on your bed with a blanket on top, so that you can choose what covers you.
- Have a fan nearby that you can turn on during the night, if you get hot, or keep a fan on throughout the night.
- Have a water bottle nearby with cold water to drink, if you have a hot flash and this helps you.
- Keep your bedroom slightly cool.
- Engage in stress management techniques before bed to help you relax.
- Have a change of sleepwear nearby.

If you take the aforementioned precautions and still wake up with night sweats, remind yourself that these are a normal part of menopause that most women experience during this transition. Tell yourself, "this will pass." Take some slow, deep breaths and try to remain calm. Take off layers of bedding to cool yourself. If you feel like a drink of cold water and don't struggle with nighttime awakenings to use the bathroom, take a drink of water. You may also want to turn on a fan, turn down the temperature in your room, or open a window.

Some women keep a bottle of water with a mist nozzle that they can use to spray their face or chest with a cool mist. On occasion, it may help to change positions and flip over your pillow (it may feel cooler on the side you haven't used). You may also want to practice guided imagery, where you imagine that you are somewhere cool and refreshing. Ideally, these suggestions will help you get back to sleep momentarily.

Even though hot flashes and night sweats are typically due to the hormone changes of menopause, there can be other causes. Staying in close communication with your healthcare provider during this time is important so that any symptoms you are experiencing can be addressed.

❑ If you experience night sweats, what are some of the suggestions that you want to try?

____

____

____

____

❑ Is there anything else that helps you when you experience night sweats (or that used to help you if you used to experience night sweats but no longer do)?

____

____

____

PREPARING FOR A RESTFUL NIGHT THROUGHOUT THE DAY

What you do during the day has a tremendous impact on your ability to sleep well that coming night. If you are struggling with sleep or want to optimize your sleep, try the following suggestions for daytime activities that can increase your chances of refreshing sleep overnight.

NUTRITION:

- Do not eat a heavy meal or drink excessively within three hours of bedtime.
- Don't go to bed hungry.
- Eat a fiber, fruit, vegetable, and legume-rich diet (associated with improved sleep quality and fewer nighttime awakenings in menopausal women).
- Avoid a low-fiber, high-saturated (animal) fat diet, as it is associated with increased fatigue, insomnia, and worse sleep quality.
- Avoid foods with a lot of added sugar, as they can increase insomnia and decrease deep sleep.
- Enjoy foods that are rich in isoflavones and tryptophan (seeds, nuts, and beans).
- Eat a high-quality diet that supports your gut microbiome (associated with decreased night awakenings and falling asleep quicker).

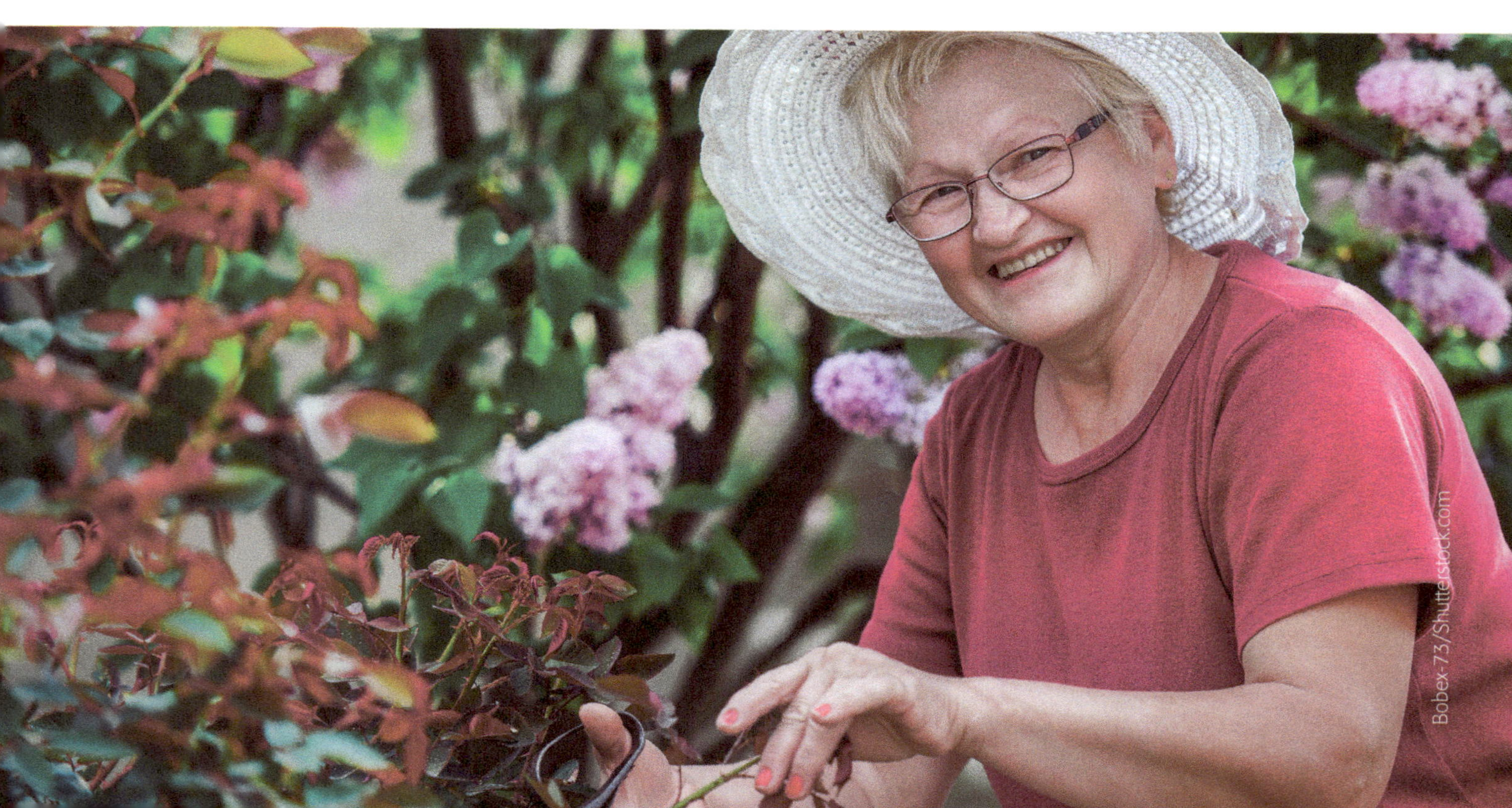
Bobex-73/Shutterstock.com

PHYSICAL ACTIVITY:

- Engage in regular aerobic exercise during the day.
- On the other hand, do not engage in aerobic activity within three hours of bedtime.

SUBSTANCE USE:

- Avoid nicotine.
- Limit or avoid caffeinated products (or use them only in the morning).
- Limit or even avoid alcohol, especially if struggling with sleep (decreases sleep quality and increases nighttime awakenings).

OTHER BEHAVIORS:

- Don't nap during the day, if you are struggling with nighttime sleep, and know that it's normal for your alertness to decrease a little in the mid-afternoon after lunch.
- Don't nap after 3 p.m.
- Don't fall asleep in the early evening.
- Don't fall asleep on your couch or other locations besides your bed.
- Go to sleep and wake at approximately the same time every day.
- Practice stress management techniques throughout the day.
- Get outdoor bright light exposure in the morning.
- Try not to fall asleep watching TV.
- Limit all screens one hour before bed.

Dr. Matthew Walker, the author of *Why We Sleep* (1), explores sleep science in depth and suggests modifying outdoor light exposure, if you desire to shift your sleep time. Bright outdoor light delays melatonin release. Melatonin signals your body to prepare for sleep.

If you want to go to sleep later than usual, avoid morning outdoor bright light exposure or go outside with sunglasses on in the morning. Try to go outside in the late afternoon (without sunglasses) to get some outdoor light exposure later in the day, delaying melatonin release. Menopausal women may find this beneficial. As you age, melatonin release happens earlier in the evening, resulting in typically earlier bedtimes and earlier morning awakenings. This is not necessarily bad. It may work well for your lifestyle. If this is bothersome, and you prefer to go to sleep later, try adjusting your outdoor light exposure. If you want to go to sleep earlier than your usual time or at the same time, get bright outdoor light exposure in the morning and keep your lights dimmer in the evening, or use sunglasses outside, as your bedtime approaches.

❑ Have you noticed that certain activities during the day help you sleep better at night? If so, what are they?

____

____

____

- ❑ Circle any of the aforementioned list of daytime suggestions that you want to try to improve your nighttime sleep.

- ❑ What recommendation will you try tonight?

  ____

  ____

  ____

  ____

BEDTIME ROUTINE

Having a bedtime routine isn't just important for children; it's also vital as you age. Again, use the principle of investigation to consider what works best for you, as you prepare for sleep. The following are some suggestions though you may have other routines that help you wind down in the evening:

- Go to bed around the same time every night. Consider setting the alarm, if you have trouble remembering to prepare for bed at a consistent time.
- Avoid bright indoor or outdoor light, fluorescent and LED lights, and digital screens such as cell phones, TVs, computers, tablets, and lights that emit blue-wavelength light and decrease the release of melatonin.
- Try to avoid the use of electronic devices close to bedtime. If you do use them, however, use the night settings that block some of the blue-wavelength light or wear glasses that block the blue-wavelength light.
- Use dim lights in the evening, especially, as you get closer to bedtime.
- Put on comfortable sleepwear that is not restrictive and that will keep you cool if you have a night sweat.
- Try to keep your environment (and yourself) calm, as stress and anxiety can make it harder to fall and stay asleep.
- Do some stretching exercises or relaxing yoga poses.
- Engage in other relaxing pre-bed activities, such as reading a calming book, praying, meditating, or writing in a gratitude journal.
- Take a warm bath or shower in the evening before bedtime (improves sleep quality and deep sleep).
- Keep your hands and feet warm (improves sleep, as dilated blood vessels in the hands and feet help release heat from your body and result in a lower core body temperature that increases melatonin).
- If you're not tired, can't fall asleep, or wake during the night and can't fall back asleep for about 20 minutes, get out of bed and do something relaxing and then return to bed when you are tired.

❑ Describe your typical pre-bedtime routine.

___

___

___

❑ Place a checkmark next to any of the aforementioned suggestions that you want to incorporate into your pre-bedtime routine in the future. Explain.

___

___

___

❑ What is one thing that you can do tonight to improve your sleep quality or quantity?

___

___

___

YOUR BEDROOM

Ideally, your bedroom should be a sleep sanctuary. When you enter your bedroom, it should cue your body and mind that it is time to relax and prepare for slumber. The following are some suggestions for preparing your bedroom to support sleep optimization:

- Put water, a fan, night light, glasses, or anything that you may need if you wake during the night, on a bedside table.
- Increase ventilation or turn on a fan if you typically get hot.
- Ensure that your room is a suitable temperature for sleep (65 degrees Fahrenheit is optimal for sleep, which generally is a little cooler than most peoples' homes but not cold).
- Try to keep electronic devices out of your bedroom.
- Keep your bedroom quiet and get earplugs, if you need them.
- Consider keeping your cell phone outside of your bedroom (unless you need it for safety when you wake during the night) or at least have it silenced.
- If you can't make your bedroom silent, consider "white-noise" devices to help block sounds.
- Keep your bedroom dark, with the use of room darkening shades or blackout curtains, if needed, but have lighting available (motion detected lights, night lights, a light by your bedside) for safely walking to the bathroom during the night.
- Remove distractions, keeping your bed only for sleep (and sex).
- Do not eat, work, or watch television in bed.
- Have a comfortable bed, pillow, and sheets.
- Consider turning your clock away from you so that you don't focus on the time if you awake.

- ❑ In what ways is your bedroom already a "sleep sanctuary?"

  ____

  ____

  ____

- ❑ Put a checkmark next to the aforementioned list of suggestions that you already utilize.

- ❑ Is there anything you want to change to make your bedroom even more supportive of high-quality sleep?

  ____

  ____

  ____

  ____

Sleep Help

Although the information we've covered will help many of you to get a better night's sleep, certain sleep conditions deserve the help of a sleep medicine specialist. If you struggle with getting regular high-quality sleep due to difficulty falling asleep, waking too early, waking during the night, snoring, or are often fatigued during the day, call your primary care provider or get an appointment with a sleep medicine specialist. Furthermore, menopausal women have an increased risk of several sleep disorders, such as obstructive sleep apnea, insomnia, and restless leg syndrome, which a health practitioner knowledgeable about these conditions should treat. There are physicians with expertise in helping people get a better night's sleep. Don't suffer in silence without trying to get help.

Although you may be tempted to use over-the-counter medications to help you sleep, reach out to your healthcare provider if you are struggling. These over-the-counter sleep aids can often have unwanted side effects, especially as you get older. In addition, there are risks of using over-the-counter and prescription sleep medications. Although sleep medications have a place, they are not a panacea, and you should not take them without discussing the risks and benefits with your healthcare provider.

Also, as you age, you release less melatonin. Many individuals use over-the-counter melatonin supplements for jet lag. For some of these individuals, it is effective for short-term use. On the other hand, people frequently take melatonin without discussing the risks and potential benefits with a member of their healthcare team. Rather than starting to take melatonin by yourself, talk to your primary care provider about whether or not this is right for you. There are potential side effects, as well as drug interactions, that many people who use it aren't aware of when they start it.

Cognitive-behavioral therapy for insomnia (CBT-i) helps many menopausal women with insomnia while also showing promise for decreasing night sweats. It helps women with their thoughts and behaviors surrounding sleep and has had significant success in helping midlife and more mature women who struggle with sleeping problems. For more information on cognitive behavioral therapy for insomnia and other sleep information, visit the National Sleep Foundation's (2) website at www.sleepfoundation.org.

Words of Wisdom From Dr. Michelle Tollefson

My patients usually expect me to ask about what they are eating and if they are physically active, but many are surprised to hear me ask about their sleep. I've been surprised throughout the years by how many women struggle in silence with sleep, assuming that trouble sleeping is part of aging and nothing can be done to help them. Although getting high-quality sleep becomes more challenging as women age, there is evidence-based help to support peri-menopausal and post-menopausal women with getting better sleep.

Many women struggle with night sweats during the peri-menopausal transition and often several years after having officially gone through menopause. Although some women use hormone replacement therapy, there are many women who use lifestyle modifications (such as those described earlier in this chapter), to deal with night sweats. Even though lifestyle modifications may not completely eliminate hot flashes, they usually help to a certain extent. Also, most women can benefit from sleep hygiene recommendations, as well as the recommendations given earlier to decrease hot flashes, whether or not they are using hormone replacement therapy.

Although I've prescribed sleeping medications in the past, I now use lifestyle recommendations to help women sleep, often referred to as sleep hygiene. Although the recommendations described throughout the chapter may not have the support of the pharmaceutical industries, they can often make significant changes to a woman's sleep and, therefore, her health. I think that my patients are often skeptical about whether or not simple suggestions, such as taking a warm shower before bed and staying on a regular sleep/wake schedule, can make a difference. However, when they implement these changes, they often return, sharing how surprised they were to find that these suggestions made a significant difference in their lives.

Although many of my patients still wake up once a night to use the bathroom or don't fall asleep as quickly as when they were in their teens, they usually notice significant improvement. They also commonly report that their mood has improved, that they feel more energetic, and that they feel better physically as their sleep improves.

Some women have sleep problems that deserve more than my sleep recommendations. In these cases, I refer them to a sleep medicine specialist, another physician with sleep expertise, or to a health professional trained to provide cognitive behavioral therapy for insomnia (CBT-i). Sometimes, these women require a sleep study, some are diagnosed with sleep apnea and receive treatment with CPAP or other devices, and some decide to use medication to manage their sleeping problems. Even for women who require more specialized treatment, many sleep hygiene techniques can still support their other therapies.

I've learned from treating many menopausal women with sleep challenges that sleep typically becomes more challenging as women age; however, through sleep hygiene and support from sleep medicine specialists or CBT-i, on occasion, most women see significant improvement in their sleep. In addition, they usually feel well-rested, happier, and healthier after prioritizing sleep.

Coaching Yourself on Sleep With the COACH Approach

CURIOSITY

Let's get curious and learn more about your sleep by reflecting on your sleep journal that you completed earlier in this chapter. Review it and then answer the following questions:

- ❑ About how many hours of sleep do you get each night? Does it fluctuate widely, or is it fairly consistent?

  ___

  ___

  ___

- ❑ How many hours of sleep did you get when you felt your best? Do you think this is the typical number of hours you need to sleep to feel your best? If you are getting adequate sleep, you should not feel tired mid-morning nor need caffeine to stay awake.

  ___

  ___

  ___

- ❑ How consistent are the times when you go to bed and get up in the morning?

  ___

  ___

  ___

- ❑ Do you take naps? If so, for how long and at what time of the day?

  ___

  ___

  ___

- ❑ What is disrupting your sleep (e.g., a pet, snoring of your partner, early sunrise, needing to use the bathroom, anxious thoughts)?

OPENNESS

- ❑ Do you believe that you only need less than seven (or even 6.5) hours of sleep? If you believe this, be open to the fact that you are perhaps not one of the 50 families ever identified, that have a genetic mutation allowing them to sleep less than 6.5 hours and still be productive and healthy with this little sleep. Be open to checking the NIH Research Matters for more information (3).

- ❑ After learning more about your sleep from your sleep journal and answering the aforementioned questions, are there any changes you want to make? Explain.

- ❑ What obstacles to making these changes, might you encounter?

- ❑ What are some ways that you can overcome these obstacles?

Be open to altering the amount of caffeine or alcohol that you consume. Also, be open to logging these behaviors to better understand how they may be negatively impacting your sleep. In addition, be open to discussing sleep with your healthcare provider, if you are taking sleep medications, over the counter sleeping aids, are snoring, or having other sleep difficulties.

Many people want to avoid medications (for sleep or night sweats), which is understandable. Be open, however, to having a discussion about hormone replacement therapy with your healthcare provider. It is not for everyone. Only you and your provider can determine if hormone replacement therapy or sleep medication is safe and appropriate for you.

APPRECIATION

Again, review your sleep journal and then answer the following questions.

- ❑ How do you typically feel when you wake in the morning (refreshed, tired, achy)?

____

____

____

- ❑ Do you have insight into what behaviors during the day contribute to sleep problems at night?

____

____

____

____

- ❑ What other insight did you gain from doing your sleep journal?

____

____

____

____

If you are a sound sleeper, it is time for you to cherish and savor this fact, realizing that many people suffer from inadequate sleep. If you are suffering from inadequate sleep, realize that help exists. Hopefully, this chapter has provided you some insight. Remember that your healthcare provider is a phone call away.

COMPASSION

Age brings challenges with getting a "good night's sleep" for most women, which can be frustrating, especially if you are someone who used to not have difficulties sleeping. It's normal for women to take something for granted (such as sleeping well) when they are not having problems with it.

❑ Consider how you feel about having more sleep challenges now that you are older. It's normal to feel frustrated, angry, confused, or sad. Imagine that you are speaking to a friend who has just shared these struggles with you. What would you say to that friend?

____

____

____

If you are having night sweats, realize that you are not alone, and this too shall pass. Practice self-compassionate self-talk, when you are struggling during the middle of the night. Consider trying the methods previously described to address night sweats or talk to your healthcare practitioner.

HONESTY

❑ Do you have trouble with sleep? There is no shame, blame, or guilt about it. If you have trouble with sleep, now is the time to address it.

____

____

____

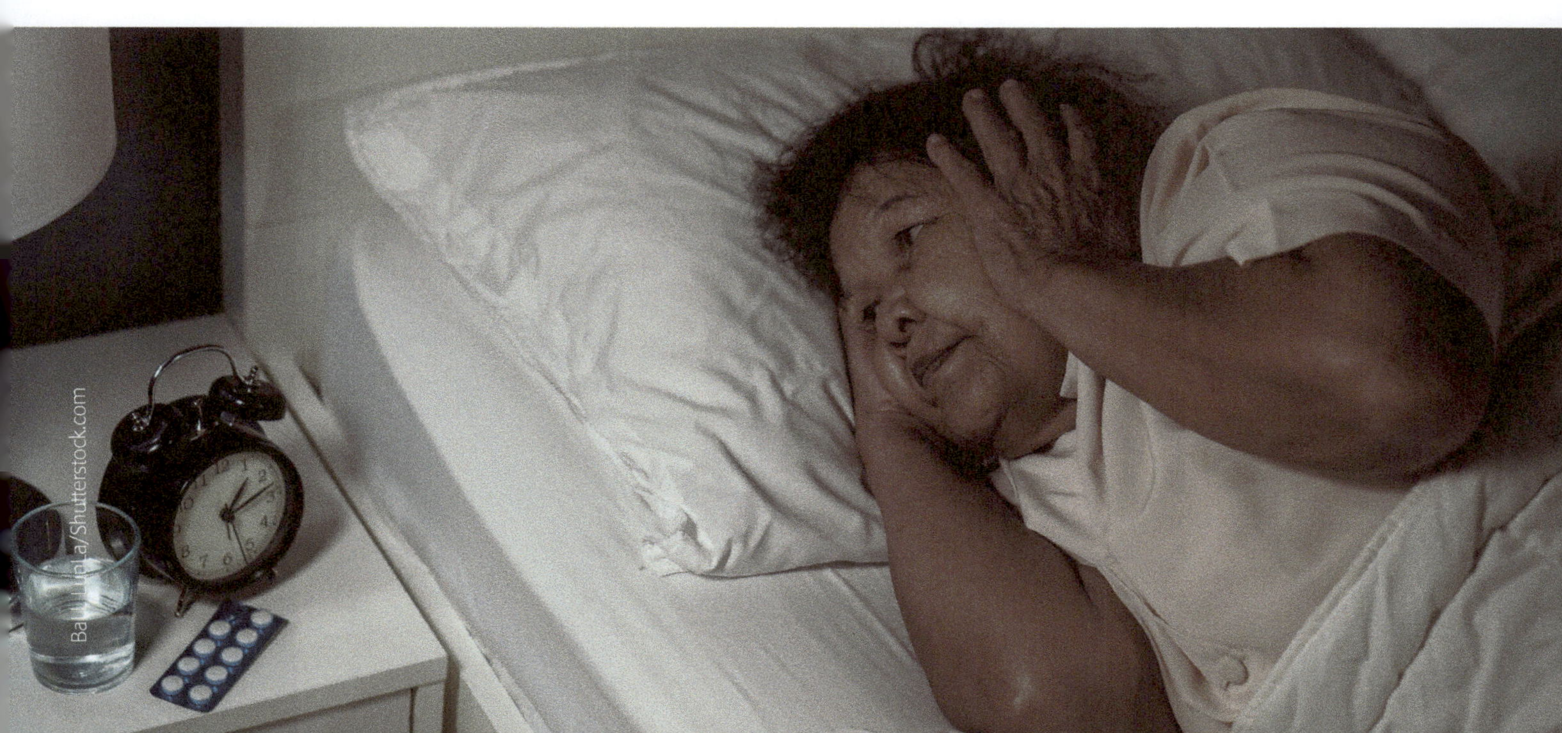

- ❑ Do you have trouble with sleeping pills or alcohol? If so, take this as a sign to address it? What is your next step? Will you call your healthcare provider or a hotline? Will you talk to a loved one? Do something to get help.

  ____

  ____

  ____

Hopefully, the information shared in this chapter will be sufficient to help you improve your sleep. However, some women will benefit from connecting with their primary care provider, a sleep medicine specialist, or a health professional, trained in CBT-i (cognitive behavioral therapy for insomnia).

- ❑ Do you think you could benefit from talking to your primary care provider, a sleep specialist, or receiving CBT-i? If so, when will you reach out to connect with them?

  ____

  ____

  ____

Sleep Wrap-Up

Although you may have hoped that we'd be sharing an over-the-counter remedy or a prescription that would return your sleep to how it used to be decades ago, we hope you'll put effort into trying some of the suggestions reviewed in this chapter. Although most women often take sleep for granted, this is an essential area of your health to prioritize. You may be reticent to try these sleep hygiene suggestions, but trust us, the effort is usually worth it. We hope that you'll feel well-rested soon.

References

1. Walker M. *Why We Sleep: Unlocking the Power of Sleep and Dreams.* New York: Simon and Schuster; 2017 Oct 3.
2. Sleep Foundation Website https://www.sleepfoundation.org/how-sleep-works/how-much-sleep-do-we-really-need
3. Shi G, et al. A rare mutation of β1-adrenergic receptor affects sleep/wake behaviors. *Neuron.* 2019 Sep 25;103(6):1044-55.

CHAPTER 13
SOCIAL CONNECTION

Social Connection Throughout Menopause, Midlife, and Beyond

Acronym—SOCIAL CONNECTION

PAVING THE PATH to wellness

Search
Opportunities
Community
Individuals
Activities
Love
Candid
Opinions

Need
Negativity
Energy
Compassion
Time
Interests
Options
Nourish

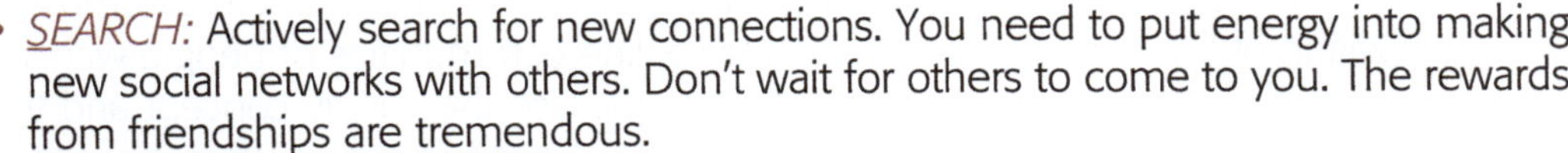

- *SEARCH:* Actively search for new connections. You need to put energy into making new social networks with others. Don't wait for others to come to you. The rewards from friendships are tremendous.
- *OPPORTUNITIES:* Look for opportunities to connect with others. Whether it's talking to the cashier at the grocery store, someone you pass while walking your dog, or talking on the phone with your sister, opportunities for connection abound.
- *COMMUNITY:* Identify what communities you are part of or can join. Consider your spiritual community, ethnic community, and neighborhood community. Reach out and connect. Join new communities or deepen your connection with your current communities.
- *INDIVIDUALS:* Dedicate time to maintaining your individual connections with family, friends, and acquaintances. For relationships to flourish, you need to get to know people as individuals and appreciate the inner beauty of each individual as well as their unique qualities.
- *ACTIVITIES:* Look for ways to enjoy social connections while engaging in activities. Whether walking with a friend, taking a group class, or playing a team sport, you get double the benefit of exercise and connection.
- *LOVE:* Share your love with others. Connecting with people on a deep and meaningful level is powerful. Cherish the people you love and let them know how deeply you value them.

- *CANDID:* People value relationships, where they can be candid and honest. Encourage others to be open with you. If you are in a relationship where you can't be candid and be yourself, consider temporarily removing yourself from the connection or work to make it a more honesty-filled relationship.
- *OPINIONS:* Share your opinions with others in a respectful manner. Also, listen to what other people say and honor their opinions. Even if you disagree with their views, you can at least learn more about their point of view.
- *NEED:* Don't be afraid to express your needs to others and ask what they need from you. Letting people know how they can help you is a gift to them.
- *NEGATIVITY:* If you are involved in relationships, where you feel negativity coming from the other person or that leave you feeling negative, stressed, or angry, consider separating yourself, at least temporarily, or work to address the negativity. Consider whether you bring negativity to any of your relationships and how you can alter this. Negativity is toxic to relationships and should be avoided or addressed.
- *ENERGY:* When you connect with others in meaningful relationships, it boosts your energy. Seek out relationships with positive, uplifting, and supportive people, and be mindful of your energy during and after the interaction. If your energy is being drained, it's time to address this. See the energy chapter for more information.
- *COMPASSION:* People are hurting and longing for someone to meet their pain with compassion. Even if you haven't experienced the same circumstances, you can feel compassion and empathy, as every person has experienced pain and suffering.
- *TIME:* For connections to flourish, you need to devote time to the relationships. Your time is precious. Time spent investing in relationships is well spent.
- *INTERESTS:* Look for other people who share your same interests. Join a community organization of like-minded people, look for online communities of people with your same passions, and explore social media groups. Use the variety concept and think about new activities and interests you can pursue. Have fun seeing what is out there!
- *OPTIONS:* When considering various options and you are unsure what to do, reach out to a trusted friend and ask for advice. Their words of wisdom may be just what you need to make the choices along your path a little clearer. If you're worried about something, don't worry alone. Talk to a friend.
- *NOURISH:* Nourish your body and mind by sharing a conversation, cup of tea, coffee, or a meal with someone. Spending time with others nourishes our souls and helps fuel us throughout our day.

Social Connection—Understanding the Basics

To pave your path to wellness, you must take time-outs. However, too much time alone, especially if you feel lonely, isolated, or disconnected from others, is dangerous for your well-being. Women are social beings, meant to flourish when connected in meaningful ways with others.

Menopause allows women to pause and reflect upon their social connections. With mindfulness, you can decide which connections need reestablishing, strengthening, or creating. You can foster meaningful social relationships that will support your health and the well-being of those you connect with for decades to come.

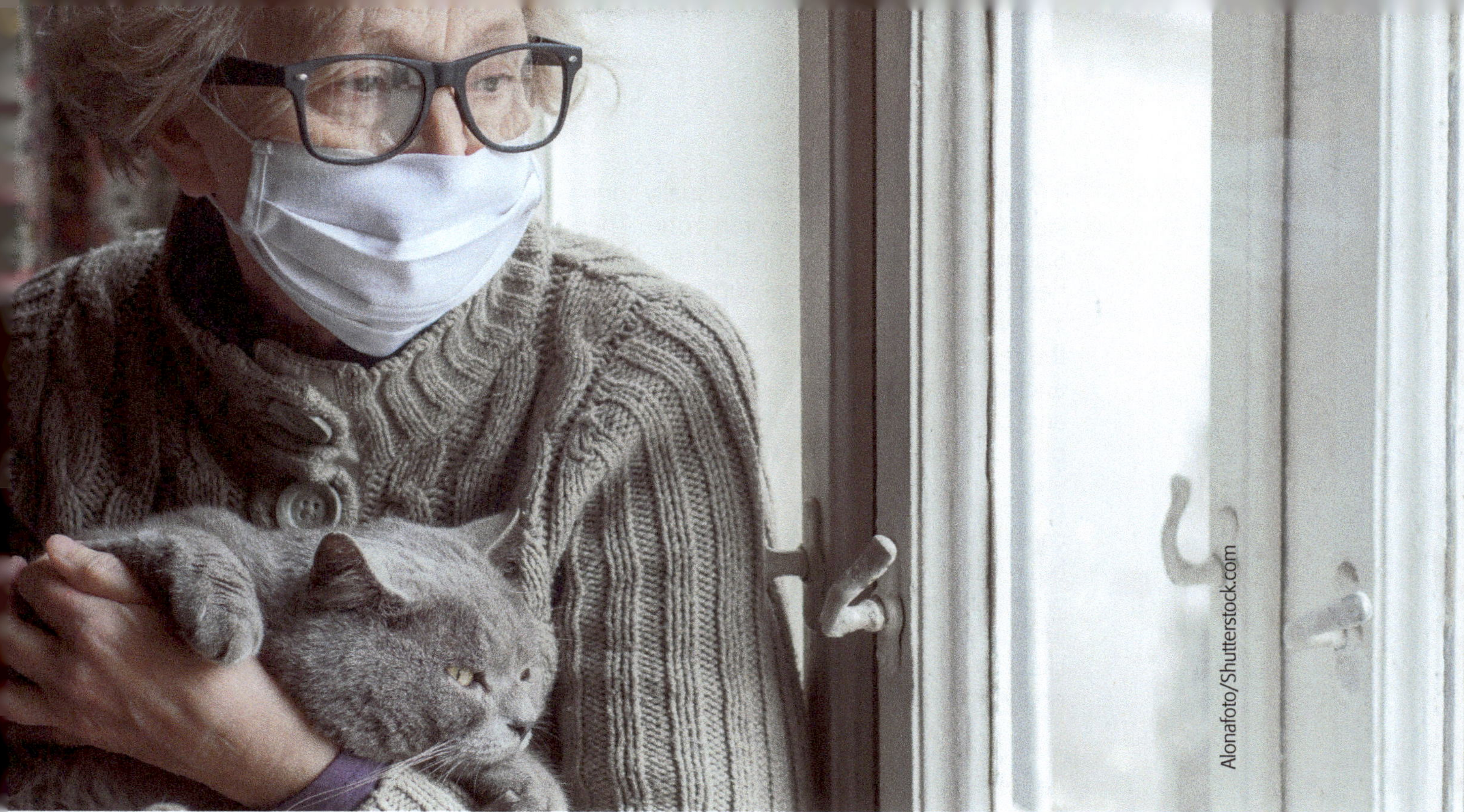
Alonafoto/Shutterstock.com

Unfortunately, loneliness is common. Even before the COVID-19 pandemic, 43 percent of people aged 60 and older reported feeling isolated (1). The pandemic made feelings of loneliness worse, as people stayed apart, socially distancing, to protect themselves and their loved ones. Several social factors contribute to midlife loneliness, including retirement, death or illness of parents, a spouse, or a partner, kids leaving home for college, marital problems or divorce, chronic illnesses that make connecting with others more challenging, and many other circumstances beyond your control.

Women often look back after menopause and realize that they've spent so much time on their career and family that they've neglected previous connections they once had. If this has happened, know that you are not alone. It is likely that women who you went to school with, who were in your wedding party, or who you knew from decades ago, also became busy with their careers and family over the years. As a result, they may long to reconnect too. For many women, midlife feels like a time when everything is changing, and not necessarily for the better. Even when you're active on social media, you can still long for meaningful, deep connections.

Women often struggle in silence, thinking that they are the only ones having trouble with creating and sustaining meaningful connections through menopause and beyond. However, it is a common challenge. Menopausal symptoms, such as mood changes, facial hair, anxiety, irritability, weight gain, difficulties with self-esteem, hot flashes, body aches, skin changes, dark spots, wrinkles, thinning hair, change in body shape, and decreased interest in sex, can make connecting even more difficult in this transition period.

During this time, it can be easy to decline invitations, spend more time at home, and withdraw inward. Unfortunately, this may start a downward spiral as you become more accustomed to spending time alone believing that others don't want to interact with you, leading to more withdrawal and isolating behavior. We do not want this for you. You are worthy of connecting in meaningful ways with others on various levels: with new people you meet, acquaintances, friends, family, and possibly an intimate partner.

Meaningful connections usually don't happen by accident and often involve stepping outside your comfort zone. They take effort to create, maintain, and foster. Science highlights the importance of social connection to your mental and physical health, as perceived social support increases the quality of life in menopausal women in several areas. It may help physical, psychosocial, and sexual quality of life. Although the research is mixed, some studies show that social connections decrease hot flashes and night sweats. Meaningful social connections also reduce menopausal anxiety and can support a positive mood. They help women when they need emotional and physical assistance and encourage them when life gets rough.

Having supportive social relationships is beneficial for your brain. Social connection can lift your mood, support your memory, and decrease your risk of dementia. Your brain truly wants you to interact with other people. Responding and reacting to the words and the body language of someone else requires multiple areas of the brain, not just the part of your brain involved in hearing, the auditory cortex. You are also more likely to be physically healthy if you connect with others. For example, many people enjoy walking and talking.

Loneliness is associated with an increased risk of high blood pressure, infections, depression, anxiety, cardiovascular disease, dementia, and even premature death. Connecting with other women going through menopause or who are in a similar phase in their life as you, can help you be your best self. In addition, connecting with older women who have already gone through this life phase can provide hope, reassurance, and guidance.

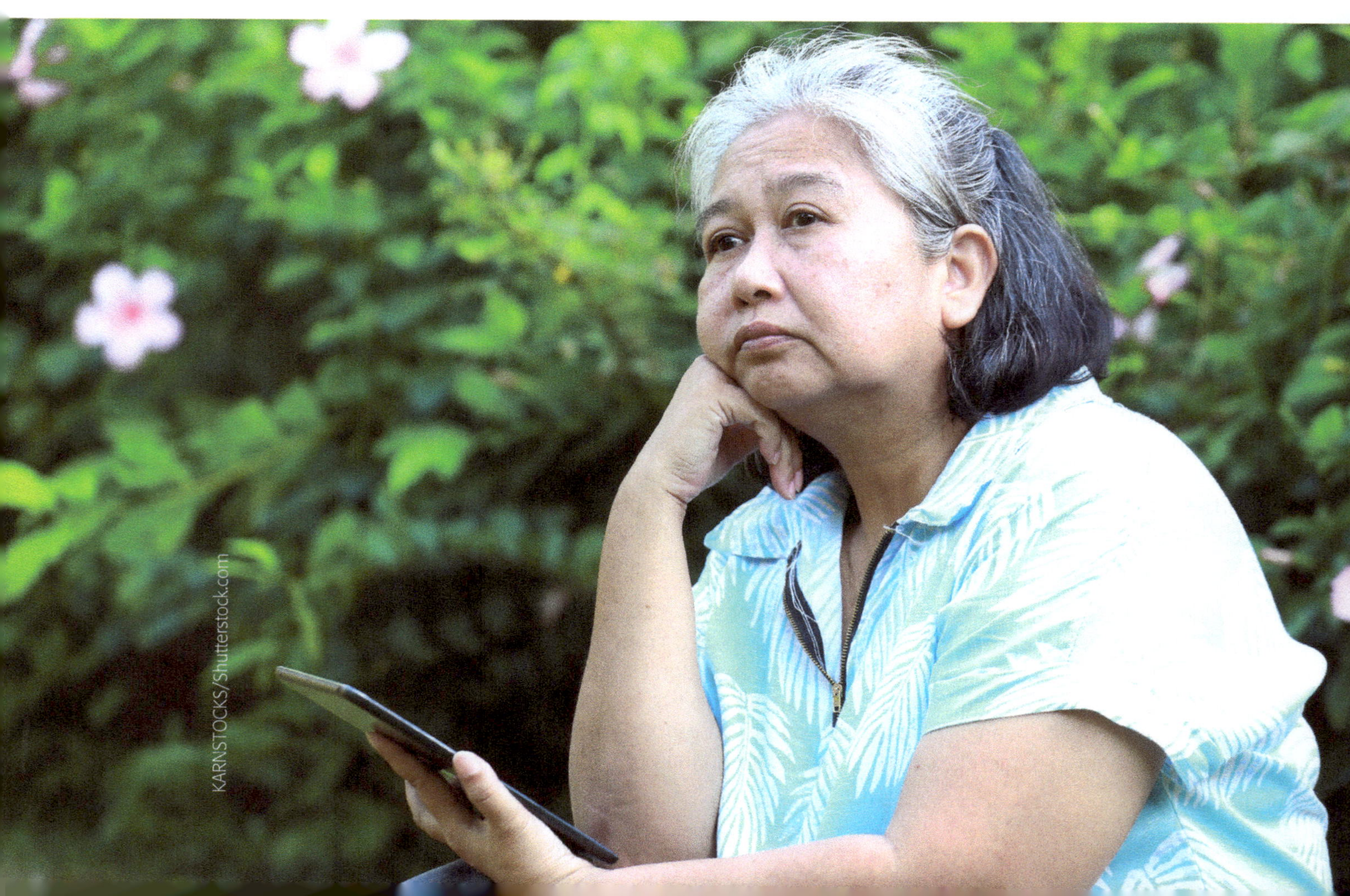

KARNSTOCKS/Shutterstock.com

It's easy to feel like you are alone in experiencing symptoms, such as hot flashes, mood changes, struggles with body image, weight gain, decreased interest in sex, and vaginal dryness, if you aren't talking to others who have had these symptoms. Sharing openly and honestly with other midlife and older women helps to normalize what you are experiencing, helps break the stigma associated with some menopausal symptoms, and can help you gain a sense of perspective during this time. Women who honor you for who you are, who see you as your authentic self, can help you be your best self and live your life to the fullest.

Midlife also allows you to reflect upon how you "show up" to your relationships with others. Earlier in life, you may have felt the need to fit into a certain image to form or maintain relationships. Hopefully, with age has come wisdom and the realization that your authentic self is the gift you give to others in high-quality connections. When you behave in ways that align with your authentic self, you attract friends and possibly a partner that "fit" and have similar goals and mindsets.

As an experienced woman, you can get along with a spectrum of individuals and realize that you can form connections with almost anyone. Even though you won't form high-quality relationships or long-lasting friendships with everyone, you can honor and respect those around you. You don't have to take everything as personally as you may have done years ago. You can celebrate differences, reach out to others, and create connections that help you walk through life's journey as part of a group. These connections take work and effort, but the results are worth the investment you will make.

Reflect

❑ When do you feel most lonely?

____

____

____

❑ Compared with a decade ago, a year ago, or a month ago, do you feel more, or less lonely?

____

____

____

❑ What do you think has contributed to this change (illness, loss of a loved one, kids leaving home, business with your career, retirement, not enough time, etc.)?

____

____

____

- ❑ After you engage with social media, do you feel more, or less connected?

___

___

___

- ❑ How does the feeling that you get from looking at social media pages of friends or acquaintances differ from when you spend time with someone in-person?

___

___

___

- ❑ When do you feel most connected (at work, place of worship, in nature, with family or a group of friends, your pet, etc.)?

___

___

___

- ❑ To whom do you feel most connected? List the individuals:
  - Acquaintances:

___

___

___

  - Friends:

___

___

___

  - Family:

___

___

___

- Spouse or partner (if you have one):

____

____

____

- Places:

____

____

____

- Projects:

____

____

____

- Books:

____

____

____

- Causes, advocacy, and community service initiatives:

____

____

____

- Ideas and beliefs:

____

____

____

❑ Who are women you are connected to in your life, who are going through the same stage as you?

____

____

____

❑ Do you have support from women in this age group, or would you like to foster other relationships? Explain.

____

____

____

❑ Who is a woman who has already gone through menopause or your stage in life, who could serve as a mentor to you?

____

____

____

Acquaintances and Daily Interactions With Others

It's great to have friends and loved ones; however, you can also enhance your well-being by connecting with acquaintances and others who cross your daily path. Smiling at the person who bags your groceries, engaging in small talk with the person sitting next to you on the airplane, or waving at someone walking their dog while you're on a walk can all add a little joy to your day. If you start to smile and try to be friendlier to those you see throughout the day, you will probably notice they return many of your smiles.

With mindfulness, you can look for opportunities to connect with strangers, wave to others, smile at others, and make the world a better place through these short, sweet interactions.

It's also easy to take your many acquaintances for granted. The owner of your favorite neighborhood store, the waitress at your favorite restaurant, and the woman who has delivered your mail for years are within your acquaintance circle. The next time you see them, consider how you could make their day a little brighter with a word of gratitude, inquiring about their day, or even just a smile.

If you feel lonely, get out of your house, and go somewhere else. Consider walking in the park, going to a coffee shop with a good book, or going to the library. It's not about what you do, but about being around other people. You don't need to become best friends of the people you pass on the street but see if you can find ways to acknowledge and uplift those whose paths cross yours every day.

❑ How do you relate to people who are your acquaintances? Do you usually say hello, smile, and ask them about their day, or are you typically silent?

___

___

___

❑ How do you relate to people you don't know but whose paths cross yours throughout the day? For example, do you typically smile at them, look downward, rush by, or pause to say hello?

___

___

___

Just because you've behaved a certain way until now does not mean that you have to continue in this same manner. As a midlife or wiser woman, you can reflect upon your past and decide how to move into your future. This is a great time to investigate, experiment, and try new ways of interacting.

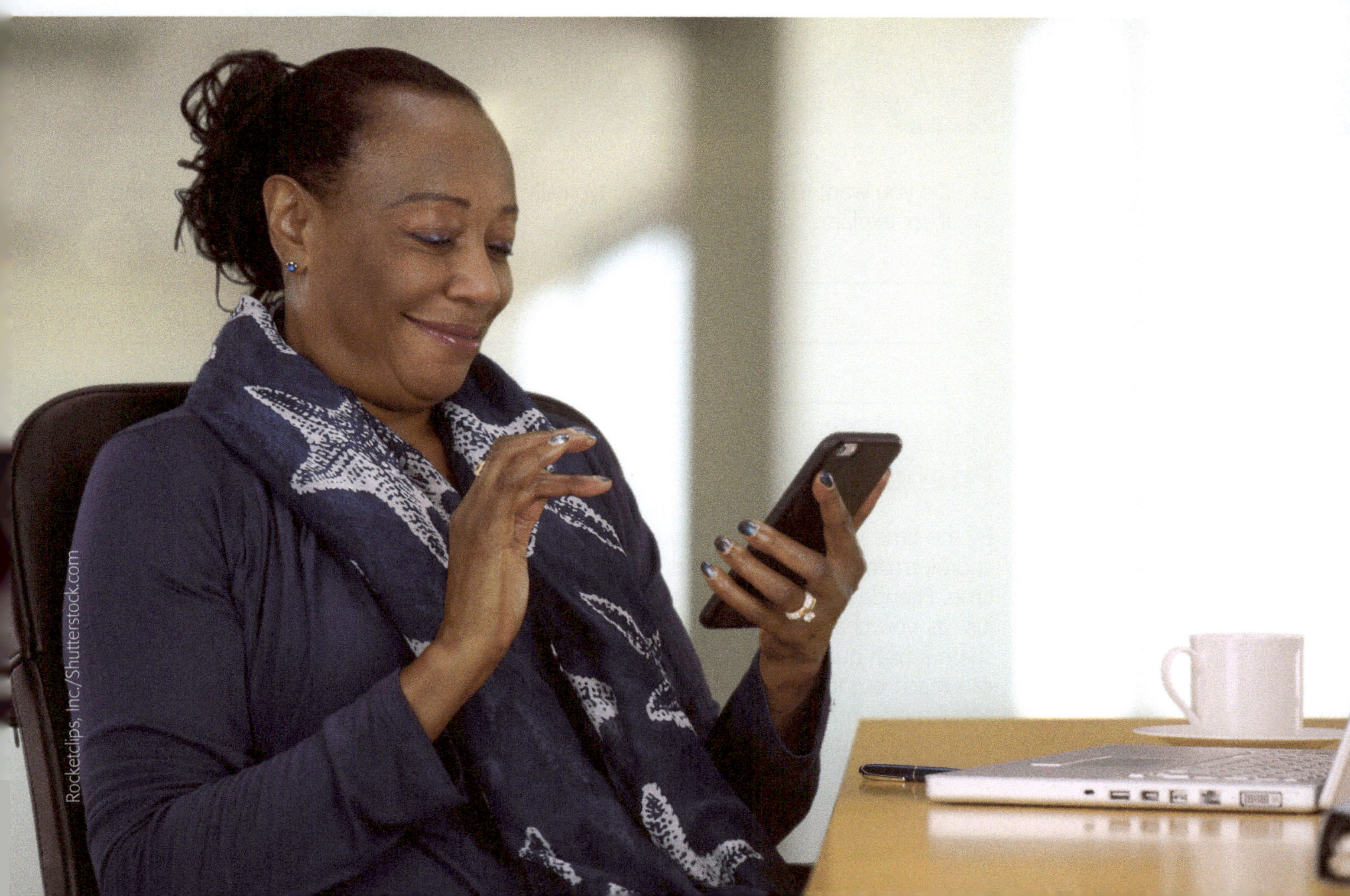

Rocketclips, Inc./Shutterstock.com

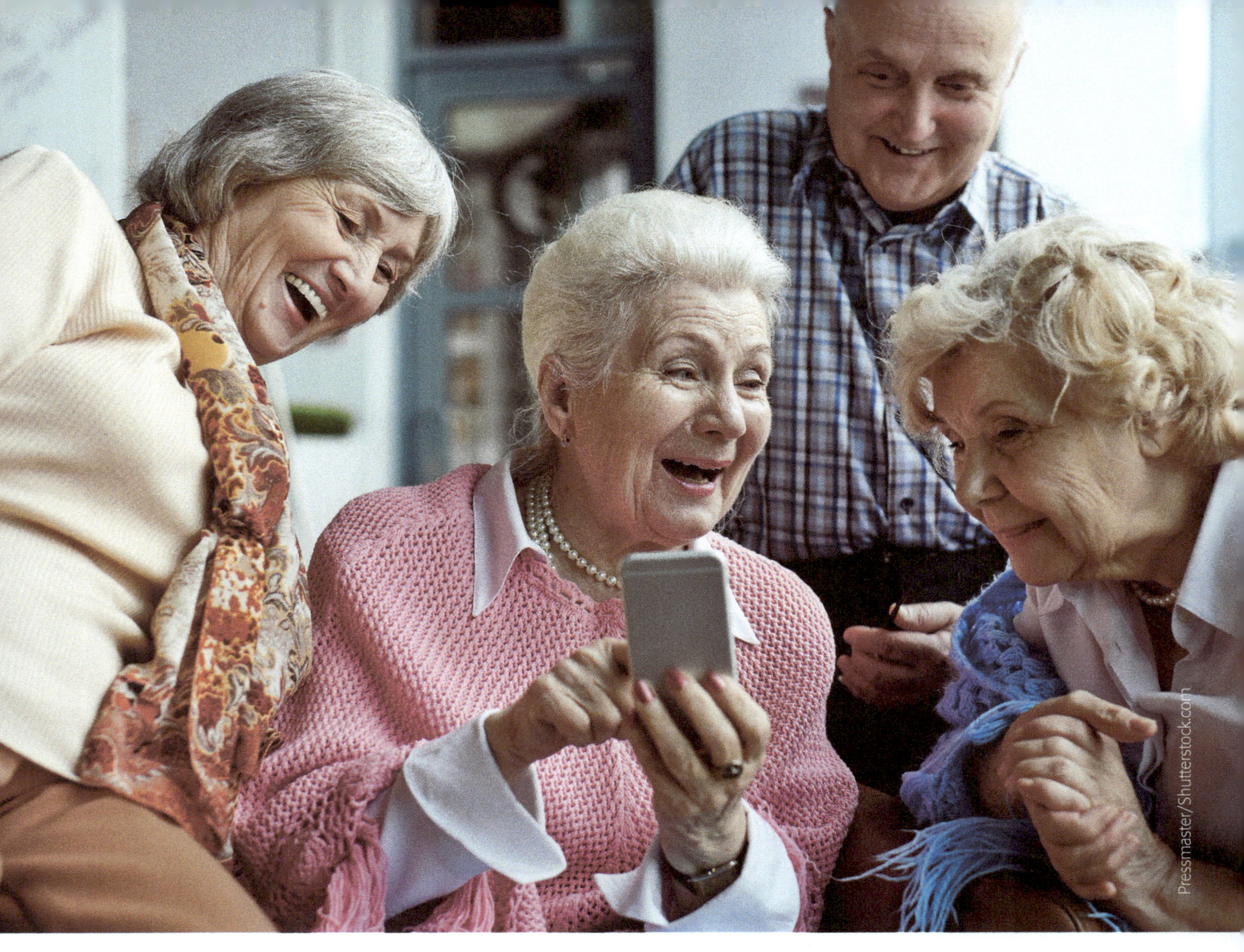
Pressmaster/Shutterstock.com

- ❏ Do you want to change how you typically interact with strangers and acquaintances? If so, explain.

____

____

____

Friendships

By the time you reach menopause, you've probably had friends come and go. You have short-term friends, long-term friends, old friends, and new friends. Relationships change with time. Friends move away, life gets busy, and circumstances cause friendships to change, just as you change with time. Hopefully, you have at least one person with whom you share a high-quality connection. It may be a partner, a family member, or a friend that you can reach out to when things are going well or when life becomes challenging. Although social media may convince you that you need many "likes" or friends to be happy, it's not about the number of relationships you have, but their quality that matters most.

List close friends who you've had during each of the periods in Table 13-1:

Childhood: ______________________
____
____
Adolescence: ______________________
____
____
Early Adulthood: ______________________
____
____
Middle Age: ______________________
____
____
Now: ______________________
____
____

Table 13-1. Close friends you've had over the course of your life

- ❑ What are some commonalities, qualities, or connections you've shared with your friends? Consider what drew you together and kept you together.

____

____

____

____

❑ How have your friends made your life better? Have they helped you through tricky times? Have they been there to celebrate with you? Have they helped you feel good about yourself? Have they listened to you with honesty, care, and concern?

____

____

____

Women often get so busy that they don't pause to consider how fortunate they are to have friends. Remember, it's not about your number of friends, but hopefully having at least one person with whom you feel a strong connection.

❑ Explain why you are grateful for the friends you have had in the past and have now.

____

____

____

❑ If you can still reach these people you just listed, do they know the positive impact they've had on your life? If not, do you want to share this with them? How could you let them know how meaningful their relationship has been in your life?

____

____

____

Sharing your gratitude for friendship with someone is a beautiful gift you can give that person. Plus, it's free and will positively impact both of you.

If you've lost touch with some past friends, this is normal. There is no shame, blame, or guilt. Sometimes, friendships end due to difficult circumstances. In some cases, these old friendships can be worth reestablishing, and sometimes they are better left in the past.

❑ Do you want to try to reestablish contact with any past friends?

____

____

____

- [ ] If so, what will your next steps be to do so?

____

____

____

After considering the traits that you value in your friends, spend a few moments thinking about the type of friend you are to others.

- [ ] Are there things that you want to change to be a better friend? For example, maybe you want to be better about reaching out regularly to see how your friend is doing or try to put your phone on silence and set it down, limiting distraction, when you meet for lunch.

____

____

____

____

During midlife or older age, you may notice that your friendships are decreasing due to life changes such as the death of friends, illnesses (yours or theirs), problems with mobility, living far apart, retirement, or other reasons. However, whether you are struggling with loneliness or feel like you have enough supportive friendships, you can still benefit from putting yourself into situations that invite the formation of acquaintances and, potentially, friendships.

- [ ] What activities you engage in, places you go, or groups you belong to allow you to make new connections with acquaintances and possibly develop friendships? For example, consider places of worship, your job if you are still employed, clubs, organizations, neighborhood, community service activities, classes you take, or local events.

____

____

____

____

Don't feel embarrassed if you don't have as many friendships as you would like. Many, many other women struggle with this too. It's just that women often struggle in silence, thinking that they're the only ones who are lonely. Making new friends takes work. Rarely does someone knock on your door asking if you want to be friends.

- ❑ How do you feel about the number of opportunities you have to interact with others regularly?

- ❑ If you want more opportunities, what are the next steps you can take to create these opportunities? For example, join local organizations and clubs, take your dog on a walk, talk with others at a park, connect in your neighborhood, register for a class, or learn a new hobby.

Don't pressure yourself to become best friends the first time you attend a class or join an organization. Instead, focus on being friendly and open to connecting with others. Often friendships develop from acquaintances and they typically happen over time. Any positive connection with others is beneficial to your overall well-being.

- ❑ Have there been times you've been let down by a dear friend? This may still be a source of great pain and why you're remaining hesitant to develop new relationships. Everyone has suffered betrayal and disappointment by midlife. Men and women included. The question is what can we learn from these experiences? How can we make sure to not experience the same type of pain or create this type of pain for someone else?

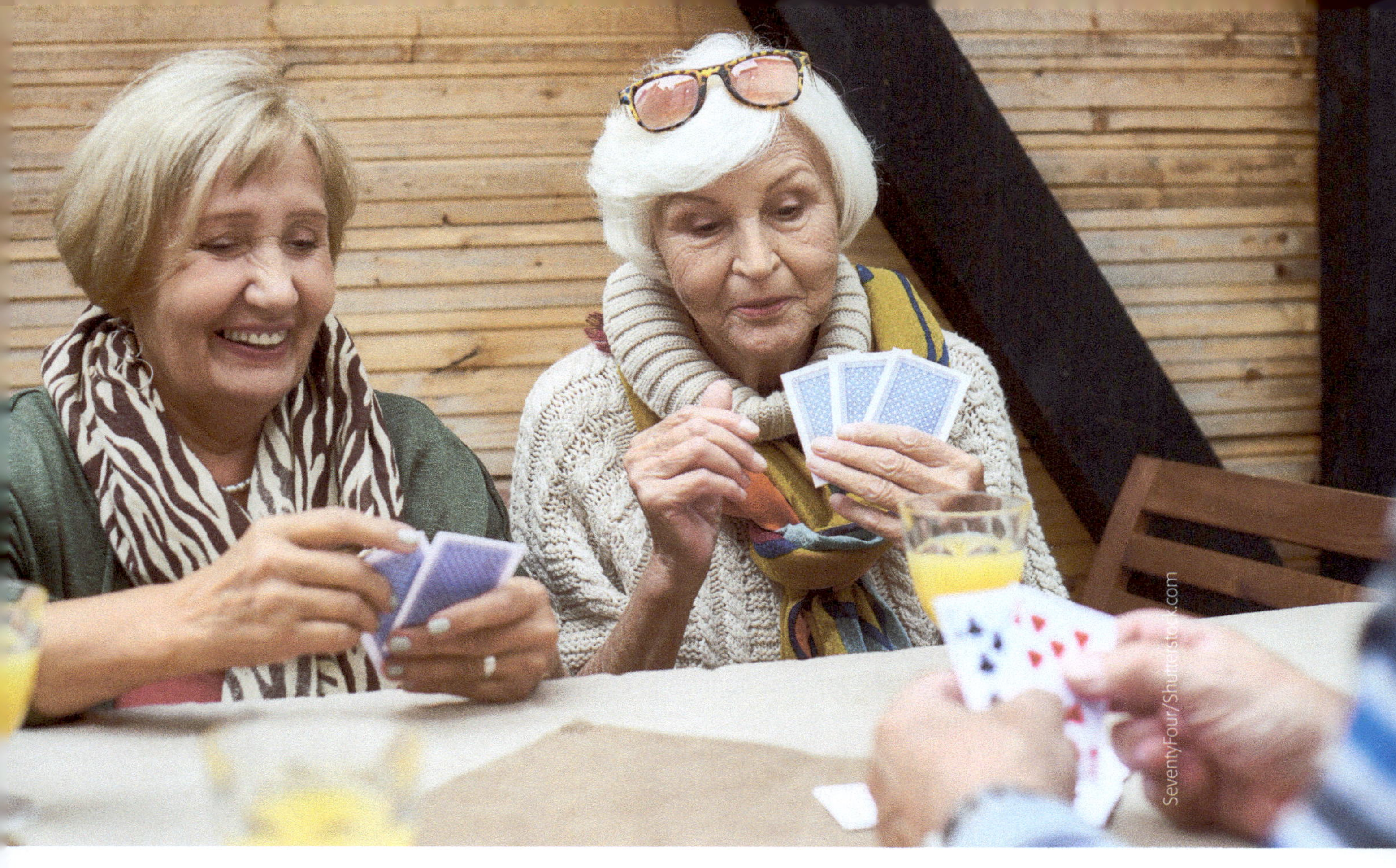
SeventyFour/Shutterstock.com

- ❑ Have there been times when you have acted in a way that may have hurt or disappointed another inadvertently or even purposefully? If so, take the time to understand that your past behavior does not define who you are in this moment. You can always change or apologize. It doesn't necessarily mean that it will resurrect a friendship that you may have sabotaged, but like you learned in the chapter on attitude, you can use mishaps to learn and grow. You can reflect on the behavior that may have put you in this tough spot and consider ways that you can make amends and move forward.

Without reaching out and spending time with others, you risk being misunderstood as being uninterested or not thoughtful. We all get busy. That's why it's important to make sure to allot time for reflection about the people and projects that are important to you.

- ❑ Is there anyone that you want to reach out to and connect with soon? Remember, everyone wants to feel loved and understood.

Among the steps you can take to improve your connections with others are the following:

- Silence and put down your phone while talking.
- Make eye contact with others, especially when you talk with them.
- Ask the other person some questions about themselves.
- Look for commonalities or areas of shared interest.
- Don't limit potential relationships to people who are just like you; branch out.
- Be open to opportunities to connect.
- Approach others with positivity and openness.
- Try to see their point of view, even if it is different than yours.
- Come to interactions with an open mind and heart.
- Schedule time to meet for tea, lunch, or a walk.
- Call, email, or text someone, asking how they are doing.
- Use FaceTime to actually see the person you're talking to.
- Take a few deep breaths before entering a new environment.
- Be grateful for opportunities to connect and express this to others.
- Smile.
- Find a way to share a laugh.
- Tell a joke if you are comfortable with that or share a funny story.
- Let the past go and move on.
- Slow down if you've had a busy, hurried day.
- Put yourself in places where it's easy to connect.
- Engage in positive self-talk.
- Remind yourself of your value, and that others are fortunate to have the opportunity to connect with you.
- Call old friends that you've lost touch with, and invite them to reconnect with you.
- Join a women's group or get more involved at your church, synagogue, mosque, or house of worship.
- Join a community-sponsored agriculture (CSA) group.
- Do a 5-K walk or run with an organization that is donating money to support research for a health condition, such as breast cancer or stroke.
- Take a class at your local university or community college; some even offer free classes for seniors.
- Take a fitness class at your community center or local YMCA.
- Take a cooking class.
- Join an online support group.
- Take lessons to learn a new hobby.
- Join an organization for people who enjoy the same hobbies or interests that you do.
- Look in your newspaper for local gatherings that you might enjoy.
- Join a book club.
- Join a supper club.
- Join a group that meets regularly to play cards or board games.
- Play bridge or scrabble.
- Connect outside of work with your current or past co-workers.

- Attend or host a neighborhood gathering.
- Consider going to a bingo night; it sounds cliché but it could be fun.
- Invite an acquaintance out for coffee.
- Take dancing lessons (ballroom, line dancing, etc.).
- Go to a yoga, barre, Pilates, or Zumba class.
- Remember that by connecting with others, you're giving them the gift of yourself too.
- Consider trying a "dating" app for finding an intimate partner or for connecting with friends (e.g., Bumble, Me3, or Peanut), but remember to be safe if meeting someone new in person (tell another friend or relative where you are, meet the new person in a public place and stay in public places).

Intimate Relationships

If talking about sexual intimacy brings up past trauma, please reach out to your primary care practitioner, gynecologist, or a mental health hotline. You may skip this section and move on to the rest of the chapter.

NOTE: READ THIS SECTION IF YOU ARE NOT IN AN INTIMATE RELATIONSHIP AND YOU HAVE NO DESIRE FOR ONE AT THIS TIME.

If you don't have an intimate relationship and are not interested in having one at this time in your life, know that this is perfectly fine and normal for many midlife and older women. Having an intimate relationship is not a requirement for happiness. Feel free to skip this section and move on.

NOTE: READ THIS SECTION IF YOU ARE NOT IN AN INTIMATE RELATIONSHIP BUT HAVE A DESIRE FOR ONE AT THIS TIME.

If you desire to have an intimate relationship but don't currently have one, know that you are not alone. Many midlife and older women are in this situation due to divorce, death of a loved one, separation of intimate relationships, or never having been in an intimate relationship before now. Finding a romantic partner during midlife and beyond, presents challenges.

Women in this situation may feel awkward when looking for an intimate partner due to stereotypes of close relationships being only for younger people. This assumption is not valid. Your age has nothing to do with your desirability and ability to have a close partner. Women may also struggle with body image due to menopausal body changes, surgical scars, mood changes, sagging body parts, hot flashes, and other symptoms of menopause that can negatively impact their self-esteem.

Uncertainty regarding changes in sexual function or how a woman views herself in a sexual way can affect a woman's mindset as she considers intimate relationships. However, not all intimate partnerships include vaginal intercourse. The vaginal dryness that many post-menopausal women experience can make women uncomfortable, if they desire vaginal intercourse as part of an intimate relationship (or if they think their potential intimate partner wants this).

To address these concerns, first, engage in positive self-talk and remind yourself that what you are feeling is common for women looking for intimate partnerships in midlife and beyond. If you struggle with self-esteem or feelings that make it challenging to connect with potential partners, consider talking to women in your situation, joining groups of single women, or talking to a health professional. When considering vaginal dryness and concerns about intimate sexual encounters, talking with a gynecologist about vaginal health may be helpful.

Gynecologists deal with this issue frequently. They are waiting for you to bring this up. Vaginal moisturizers and lubricants discussed later in this chapter can help. If your vaginal opening has narrowed or you are concerned that your vagina would not be able to have intercourse (if desired), a gynecologist or pelvic floor physical therapist may be able to help you with vaginal dilators. Also, realize that if you are not interested in intercourse or feel that you would be unable to have intercourse comfortably, many intimate partners also are not interested in intercourse (sometimes due to erectile dysfunction). There are many ways to express love to an intimate partner that do not involve the vagina. These will be covered in more depth later in the chapter.

NOTE: READ THIS SECTION IF YOU ARE CURRENTLY IN AN INTIMATE RELATIONSHIP.

If you have or are struggling with your intimate relationship during menopause or beyond, know that you are not alone. Menopause can bring mood changes, decreased self-esteem, body image issues, and changes in vaginal health that can make intimate relationships more challenging. In addition, intimate partners often have their own health challenges (physical, such as erectile dysfunction, and mental health issues, such as depression, and excessive stress in midlife) that make intimacy challenging.

As people age, the likelihood of taking medications that can negatively impact sexual desire (such as some medications used for hypertension or to treat depression) increases, and chronic medical conditions, such as type 2 diabetes, can negatively impact sexual function. Medications and conditions, along with societal sexual scripts, make it more difficult for older women to view themselves as sexual beings and can create challenges with intimacy in relationships. Some women also find that boredom happens in and out of the bedroom, and sexual desire decreases.

Nevertheless, about half of all women in their 50s have vaginal intercourse, and this fraction decreases further as women age. So, if you and your intimate partner are not having vaginal intercourse and you're alright with this, don't worry, as it is typical for many intimate partnerships. Vaginal intercourse does not equal happiness in a relationship. Though you may not desire or be having intercourse, most partners still want intimacy.

The following are some suggestions for sexual intimacy in midlife and beyond.

(Note: As you read through these lists, put a star next to any that you want to ensure that you remember or that you want to consider trying.)

SEXUALITY AS YOU AGE:

- There is no "right" way for these intimate connections.
- Listening to your internal signals is key.
- The way that works for you and your partner is the one to follow and explore.
- If you think you are not happy or satisfied, believe in yourself and seek out opportunities to learn more about your sexual life.

- Society has many "sexual scripts" that women often feel they need to fit. Focus on doing what is best for you and what works for you and your intimate partner.
- Don't compare yourself to others. Most women do not have wild sex every day.
- The frequency of intimate relations and contact varies and even depends on the person's experience that day, that week, or that month.
- Try to embrace your sexuality during midlife and beyond. What sexual well-being looks like for you is different from other women, and it is probably different from what sexual well-being meant for you in your past.
- Define sexual well-being for yourself.
- Realize that there are a variety of cultural and religious norms when it comes to sexual expression. This discussion may be uncomfortable for cultures or religions where these topics are private and not openly discussed.
- Be patient; sexual arousal takes time, especially as you age.
- Understand that for women, sexual desire often happens after sexual arousal, which is alright.
- Know that the female sexual response cycle is different from the male cycle and that women more frequently engage in sexual activity to feel more emotionally connected with their partner.
- Understand that sexual self-stimulation is a common behavior that can be explored and practiced in privacy. It can help decrease sexual inhibition and maximize sexual satisfaction.

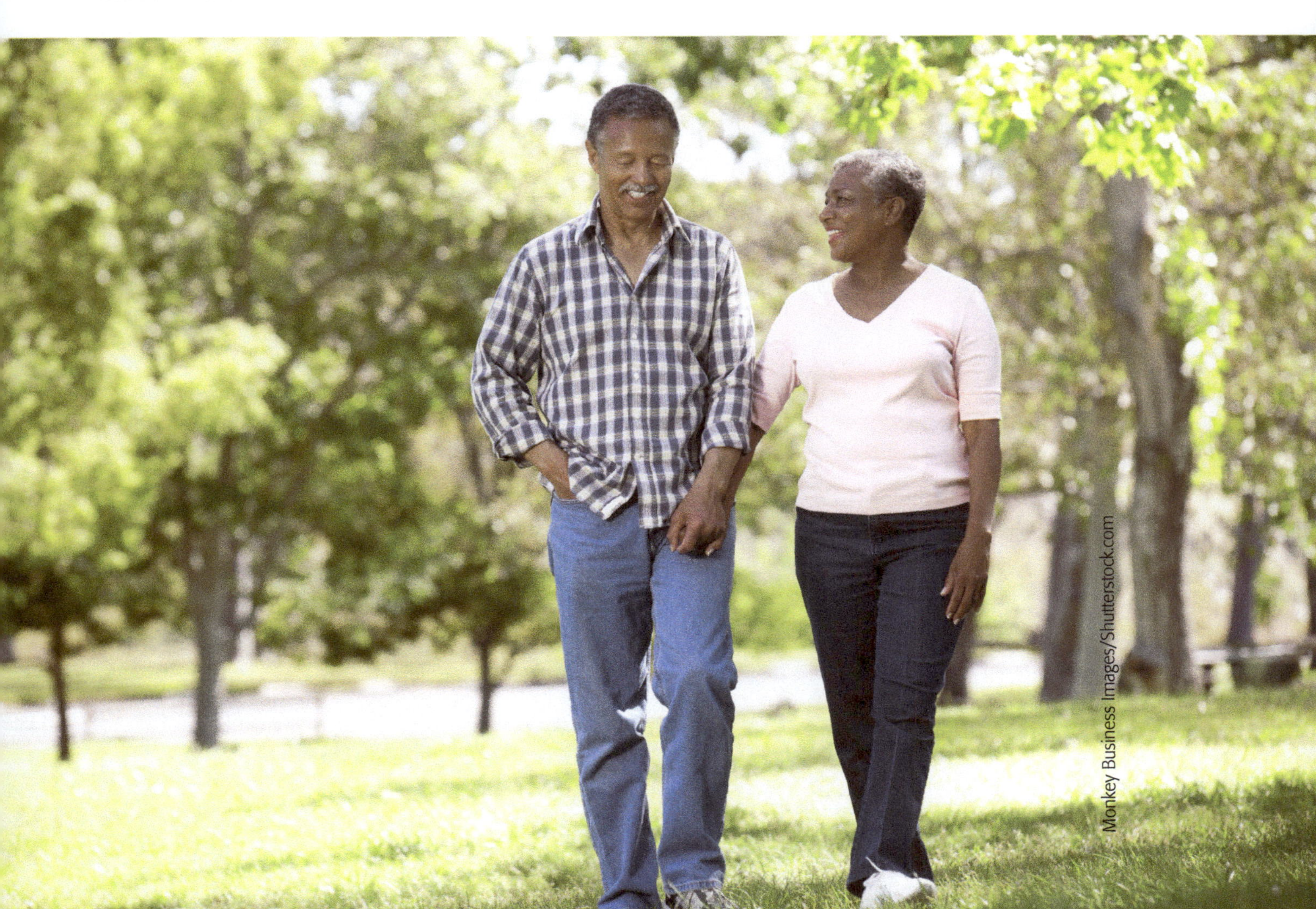
Monkey Business Images/Shutterstock.com

HEALTHY HABITS AND SEXUAL INTIMACY:

- Care for your overall well-being through adequate exercise, nutrition, sleep, and stress management. If you're not sleeping well, work to prioritize sleep as this can positively impact sexual health.
- Eat a nutrient-dense, whole food, and plant-rich diet, such as the Mediterranean diet.
- Avoid "junk" food, drinks, and foods with added sugar.
- Engage in regular physical activity before sexual activity as it may improve sexual desire.
- Decrease excessive sitting and sedentary behavior.
- Try yoga or Pilates, either alone or with your partner.
- Remove distractions and decrease stress as much as is possible, as distraction and anxiety make sexual arousal and enjoyment more difficult.
- Engage in relaxation techniques such as progressive muscle relaxation, guided imagery, diaphragmatic breathing, or mindfulness-based stress reduction for sexuality.

COMMUNICATION AND SEXUAL INTIMACY:

- Communicate, communicate, communicate.
- Prioritize honest and open communication with your partner.
- For some partners, communication is challenging. In the bedroom, it is often even more complicated. Thus, working on expressing yourself to your partner is critical for a satisfying sexual life. Always remember that the brain is a woman's most important sex organ; communicate and work on strengthening your relationship.

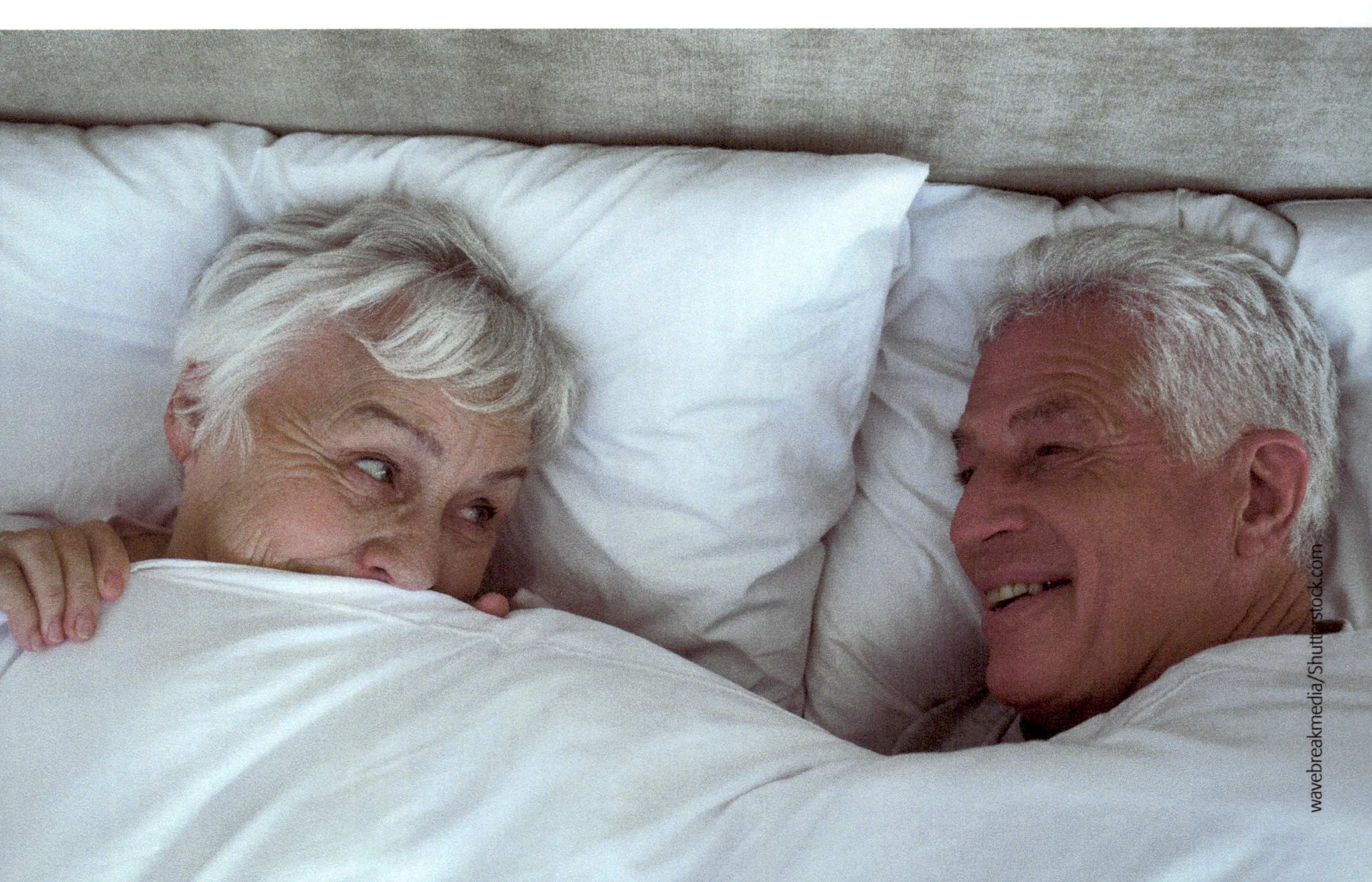

wavebreakmedia/Shutterstock.com

- Use positive and encouraging self-talk around sexual well-being and other aspects of health.
- Work to increase your emotional closeness with your partner, which often leads to increased sexual satisfaction.
- Address any underlying emotional issues that are causing distance between you and your partner.
- Use the element of surprise by leaving love notes, a small present for your partner, or planning an unexpected day of fun that might include a couple's massage.
- Use self-talk to remind yourself that you are valuable, attractive, and deserving of sexual well-being, regardless of your age, body shape, or health status.
- Don't let resentment, frustration, or anger harm your sexual well-being.
- Get professional help from a sex therapist, marriage counselor, or another mental health professional, if appropriate.
- Try mindfulness-based cognitive behavioral sex therapy, if you need support.

PARTNER IDEAS FOR SEXUAL INTIMACY:

- Be open to exploring your changing body and your partner's body too.
- Schedule time for date nights and intimate encounters.
- Have fun with your partner!
- Regular sexual activity helps vaginal tissue to stay more elastic.
- Extend foreplay before engaging in vaginal intercourse, or skip vaginal intercourse altogether and simply enjoy foreplay.
- Don't rush; it takes an average of about 30 minutes for women to be able to reach orgasm after menopause.
- Try to decrease distraction, as it decreases sexual arousal and the ability to have an orgasm.
- Incorporate mindfulness into your sexual encounters.
- Add variety to your sex life by trying a "toy" or another form of erotica from an adult boutique or online, if both you and your partner want to include this in your sexual experiences.
- Try different sexual positions after discussion with your intimate partner about what you would like to experiment with.
- Experiment with sexual intimacy at different times of the day or in other private locations (such as a hotel while on vacation).
- Try different forms of intimacy besides what you are used to doing.
- Consider using all of your senses to enhance your sexual experience (for example, lingerie or sheets with a different texture, essential oils in a diffuser nearby, romantic music, your favorite fruit).
- Express intimacy in ways other than vaginal intercourse, such as hugging, kissing, cuddling, romantic talk, oral sex, manual stimulation, massage, and sensual baths.
- Change positions for vaginal intercourse. Women may benefit from being on top, as this gives them greater control over the depth of penetration and alignment.
- Remember that sexual experimentation is normal and can be beneficial for many relationships, if both partners agree.
- Consider the use of erotica, fantasy, play, sexual devices, and toys, if both you and your partner desire experimentation.

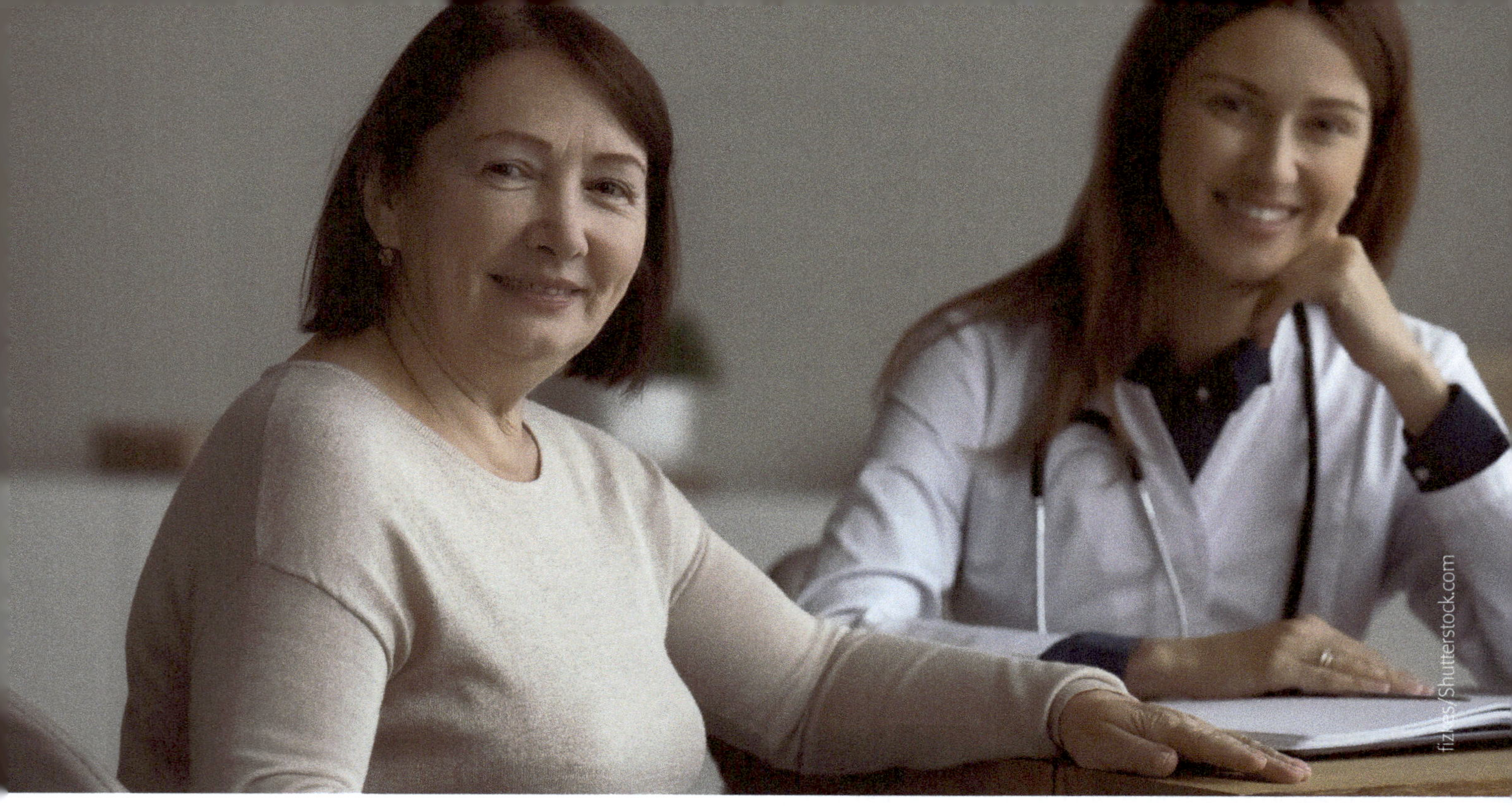
fizkes/Shutterstock.com

GYNECOLOGIC HEALTH AND SEXUAL INTIMACY:

- See your gynecologist or your primary care provider to discuss sexual health.
- See your gynecologist, if you're experiencing vaginal dryness that is not relieved with vaginal moisturizers (used regularly and not just when having vaginal intercourse).
- See your gynecologist or primary care provider, if you are experiencing vaginal discomfort, bleeding, or pain during intercourse. Any vaginal, vulvar, rectal, or urinary bleeding must be investigated.
- For some women, using vaginal estrogen or other prescription medication is beneficial for genitourinary syndrome of menopause (vaginal dryness and sometimes discomfort). Talk to your physician.
- Use a mirror to explore your vulva, clitoris, and opening to the vagina. Many midlife and older women are still unaware of their genital anatomy. Feel free to ask your gynecologist to help you better understand your anatomy, if you want to learn more.
- Regularly do pelvic floor muscle exercises (Kegels), as this strengthens them and makes it easier to contract them, as desired, during sexual activity (see the chapter on physical activity).
- Educate yourself about sexual health and midlife changes. Some of my favorite books are Dr. Jen Gunther's *The Vagina Bible, Come as You Are, Becoming Orgasmic, Getting the Sex You Want,* and *Naked at Our Age.*

❑ Review the items that you placed a star next to on the preceding lists. Is there anything that you want to focus on during the next week? Explain.

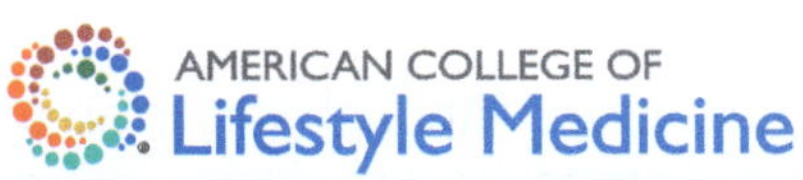

Improve Female Sexual Health

Problems with sexual function are common. Nearly 1/2 of women report issues with desire, arousal, lubrication, orgasm, pain, satisfaction, or intimacy.[1]

DIET

The same whole food, plant-based diet that supports cardiovascular health, also supports sexual health broadly. Eat a diet rich in vegetables, fruits, nuts, whole grains, and legumes, that is high in antioxidants and low in saturated fat and refined carbohydrates.[3]

Choose the type of physical activity you enjoy the most.

PHYSICAL ACTIVITY

Regular physical activity promotes sexual health both in the short and long term. It improves mood and the health of your blood vessels.[4,5]

In addition to aerobic and resistance exercises that are recommended for most women, consider pelvic floor strengthening exercises (kegels).[6] These exercises involve contracting and relaxing the muscles of the pelvic floor several times daily. In addition to supporting urinary continence, these exercises may help you become more mindful of the muscles that support and surround the vagina. Research has shown improvements in sexual arousal and satisfaction in some groups of women who do kegels regularly.

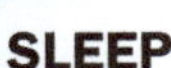

SLEEP

Aim for at least 7 hours of high quality sleep nightly. Women who regularly get enough sleep report higher arousal, less vaginal dryness, more sexual activity, and better satisfaction.[7]

STRESS MANAGEMENT

Daily stressors can distract from interest and enjoyment of sexual activity. Mindfulness-based stress management techniques such as diaphragmatic breathing, progressive muscle relaxation, and yoga help many people.[8,9]

RELATIONSHIPS

The most important relationship you can work to cultivate is with yourself. For those in partnered relationships, intentional communication and regular affection are linked to better female sexual health.[10]

SUBSTANCE USE

Tobacco, cannabis and alcohol can have negative effects on female sexual health and function. Tobacco damages blood vessels, while cannabis and alcohol negatively affect orgasm due to their "depressant" effects.

Lifestyle practices can help by supporting metabolic, cardiovascular and mental health.

DID YOU KNOW?

Vaginal lubrication and orgasm, in part, require healthy blood vessels.[2]

The well-known connection between heart health and sexual function in males appears to hold true for females too!

Sexual problems are even more common in women with chronic diseases like high blood pressure, diabetes, metabolic syndrome, high cholesterol, and problems with mood. Healthy lifestyle practices are a win for your general health AND sexual health.

Talk to your doctor if you have questions or problems related to your sexual health. They may be able to help you or refer you to other experts such as a dietitian, pelvic floor physical therapist, sex therapist, or couples counselor.

Figure 13-1. Improve female sexual health

Emotional Intimacy

Emotional intimacy does not necessarily mean intercourse. Although this is an integral part of sexual expression for many women, some women do not desire intercourse. For some women intercourse is no longer possible for them or their partner, and some prefer different types of intimacy. Regardless of what kind of physical intimacy you engage in with your partner or choose not to, emotional intimacy is a vital component of an intimate relationship.

Emotional intimacy plays a prominent role in maintaining relationship quality while supporting sexual well-being. Emotional closeness is associated with increased sexual desire, arousal, lubrication, and orgasm. Intimacy is also associated with longer telomeres and a longer life expectancy.

It's easy to take emotional intimacy for granted, especially in a long-term partnership. However, couples with high-quality relationships typically prioritize communication and show mutual respect. Communicating about sexual concerns, needs, and desires, as well as awareness of your partner's concerns, needs, and desires, can enhance intimacy and long-term sexual health in a relationship.

If you and your intimate partner are struggling with intimacy, please consider getting help by reaching out for counseling or therapy with someone who is qualified to support you. Some people may choose to see a religious leader or spiritual director for help with their relationship. Although typically it's ideal for both partners to participate in counseling, it can still be beneficial, even if your partner will not attend.

Among the indicators that you may want to consider getting help are the following:

- Feeling uncomfortable expressing yourself emotionally
- Feeling unappreciated in your relationship
- Difficulty or inability to express concerns about your sexual health
- Hiding your feelings from your partner
- Not wanting to spend time with your partner
- Emotionally withdrawing from your intimate partner
- Feeling more intimately connected to people other than your partner
- Not being intimate, if this is something that you desire, and it bothers you
- Fears or seeing signs that your partner has withdrawn from you
- Pretending that you are enjoying your intimate encounters
- Wanting to have deeper conversations but not feeling comfortable
- Feeling controlled or pressured in your relationship
- Feeling anger or bitterness toward your partner for some reason
- Experiencing abuse, physical, emotional, or sexual. In this case, this is an emergency, and you need to seek immediate help through a crisis line: call 1-800-799-7233 (SAFE) or text "START" to 88788.

It's better to reach out for help early and address issues before they fester and become larger than they need to be. Sometimes, one or two sessions with a counselor can be enough to repair or reignite intimacy.

Decreased Sexual Desire

It's common for midlife and more mature women to feel distressed by decreasing sexual desire for their intimate partner. Women are much more likely to have reduced sexual desire than men. It becomes even more common in women who have gone through menopause and are in long-term relationships. However, decreased desire does not mean that something is wrong with you or your relationship with your partner.

Research shows that the sexual response cycle is different for men and women. Suppose you want to be sexually intimate with your partner, though you lack sexual desire. In that case, you may consider being open to being sexually intimate with your partner, knowing that desire often happens only after sexual stimulation. In addition, many women benefit from genital vibratory stimulation, especially after menopause, which may also lead to increased sexual desire.

If you are still experiencing decreased sexual desire, and this is causing personal distress, reach out for professional help. A gynecologist, your primary care provider, a sex therapist, or a marriage counselor can assist you or connect you with someone else who can help. Some medications (such as those often used for treating depression and hypertension), health conditions (such as urinary incontinence and type 2 diabetes), past circumstances (such as trauma or other abuse), or other issues (such as a negative body image) may be the cause of decreased sexual desire too. Many women are looking for help, guidance, and support in this area, postmenopausal women or not.

Words of Wisdom From Dr. Michelle Tollefson

As a gynecologist, I often treat menopausal women referred to me for vaginal dryness and irritation. Many of these women are experiencing painful intercourse due to dryness, while others have stopped having intercourse because of discomfort. After talking to them about their symptoms and doing a pelvic exam, I share with them various treatment options. Many choose to use vaginal estrogen in a cream, vaginal ring, or tablet form, while others prefer not to use prescription medication to treat their symptoms.

It's only through a conversation with a gynecologist or other healthcare provider that you can fully understand your treatment options as they relate to your body and decide what is best for you. Unfortunately, I've seen too many women who have suffered and did not reach out for help with vaginal dryness, painful intercourse, or inability to have vaginal intercourse with their intimate partner due to these symptoms. Women frequently ask questions when they learn that there are treatments for their condition. Why didn't my other healthcare provider tell me about this earlier? Why don't more women talk openly about this? Why did I suffer so long with symptoms when there were treatment options?

Unfortunately, without the use of vaginal estrogen, vaginal use through vaginal intercourse, vibratory devices, or vaginal dilators, some women develop vaginal stenosis (narrowing and partial closure of their vagina), preventing them from having vaginal intercourse, even if desired. However, many women return to a relatively normal level after treatment, especially with vaginal estrogen, and appreciate the improvement of genital tissue elasticity and decreased vaginal dryness. Often, these women can resume vaginal intercourse if desired or have intercourse without discomfort again. There is hope for most women.

If you have vaginal dryness, please see your healthcare provider. Even if you cannot or do not want to use hormones, other treatments are available. Whether or not you decide to use prescription medication to treat vaginal dryness, you may benefit from using a vaginal moisturizer and lubricant. Please reach out to your healthcare provider sooner rather than later.

As a gynecologist, I'm on a mission to educate post-menopausal women about genitourinary syndrome of menopause and evidence-based treatment options, empowering them to decide what is best for their body and overall sexual health. Please feel free to share this information with any of your friends or family members. The more people who know, the better. Although the topic may be a sensitive one, we must work together as women to empower each other so that we can thrive at any age.

Vaginal Dryness (Genitourinary Syndrome of Menopause)

We've previously discussed genitourinary syndrome of menopause (also called atrophic vaginitis or vulvovaginal atrophy), which is a leading cause of vaginal dryness and discomfort in midlife and post-menopausal women. Although it is prevalent, preventable, and treatable, most women do not discuss it with their healthcare providers, and their healthcare providers rarely bring it up without patient initiation. This shouldn't be accepted as the destiny of all women after menopause.

Genitourinary syndrome of menopause impacts more than just the vagina. The decrease in estrogen that happens due to menopause causes the tissue in the vagina, vulva, urethra, and other estrogen-responsive tissue to thin, become less elastic and be more susceptible to trauma. Symptoms, such as vaginal pain, itching, dryness, and discomfort, especially during vaginal intercourse, discomfort when exercising (such as when riding a bicycle or horse) and discomfort with urination, are common with this condition that impacts most women who do not use hormone therapy, at some time after menopause. Even though they are often due to low estrogen, these symptoms can be due to conditions that are not the result of genitourinary syndrome of menopause and deserve evaluation by a gynecologist or primary care provider.

Some women struggle with urinary tract infections after the loss of estrogen. Using prescription estrogen locally can sometimes help this too. It's also important for women to fully empty their bladder, especially before and after having vaginal intercourse. If you experience burning with urination, urgency, or urinary frequency at any time, reach out to your healthcare provider, as bladder infections should be treated with appropriate antibiotics and failure to do so can lead to more serious medical problems. You may need to visit the office and give a urine sample so that the optimal treatment for your specific type of infection can be prescribed.

Women who experience recurrent urinary tract infections are sometimes given prophylactic antibiotics to prevent recurrences. You won't know if this is appropriate for you without talking to your primary care provider or gynecologist. Some women use cranberry juice to decrease the risk of recurrence. While there is no definitive research on if it will help, it won't hurt. On the other hand, it should not be used as a substitute for antibiotics or medical evaluation.

Due to its ability to cause discomfort with vaginal intercourse, genitourinary syndrome of menopause deters many women from wanting to have sex with their partners. It can lead to a vicious cycle as pain during intercourse leads to a woman tensing the muscles surrounding the opening to the vagina to protect herself from the pain. This tightening of muscles surrounding the vagina can make intercourse even more uncomfortable, increasing tension.

Even after genitourinary syndrome of menopause is treated, some women still struggle with relaxing these muscles and benefit from pelvic floor physical therapy, sex therapy, or cognitive behavioral therapy to change their thought patterns. It's common for women to want to try non-prescription remedies for vaginal dryness. Also, even women using hormone therapy may still benefit from vaginal moisturizers and lubricants.

Vaginal moisturizers are used regularly and are not specifically for vaginal intercourse. They increase vaginal moisture, which is beneficial, since menopause makes vaginal tissue dryer due to decreased estrogen. They also help keep the vaginal pH low, which is essential for vaginal health. The following text details several examples of some vaginal moisturizers that are commonly available at local stores.

Women typically use vaginal moisturizers a few times each week and apply them in the vagina and around the opening of the vagina. There are a variety of different vaginal moisturizers. You can even use coconut oil as a vaginal moisturizer, if you want to use something very natural and inexpensive.

Vaginal lubricants are typically applied before vaginal intercourse or manual stimulation to decrease friction and make intimacy more comfortable. Just like vaginal moisturizers, you can buy them without a prescription at local stores, such as Walmart, Walgreens, Target, or CVS.

The North American Menopause Society (NAMS) recommends using water-soluble products, since petroleum jelly and other oil-based lubricants may irritate the vagina. They also recommend using products that are only designed for vaginal use, which means avoiding creams or lotions intended for use on different parts of the body that often contain perfume and alcohol. In addition, they recommend avoiding lubricants that are warming, tingling, or flavored, as these may be irritating too.

If you try a new product, especially if it is flavored or has ingredients that you haven't used before, test it on an area of your body, where the skin isn't as sensitive as the vagina (such as on your thigh or behind your ear) to ensure that it is well tolerated. When you use it for the first time on the vagina or vulva, try it on a tiny area first. After knowing that it is well-tolerated, you can use it liberally before vaginal intercourse, in the vagina and around the vaginal opening, and on your intimate partner, if you have one.

Vulvar care is vital for all women, but this becomes even more essential, if you are experiencing genitourinary syndrome of menopause. Many products are sold to women with promises to help their vagina, vulva, or other "female parts." However, these products are often not beneficial, and in some cases, such as with vaginal douches, they may even be harmful.

The vagina and vulva do not need "cleaning" with special products, "deodorizing," "refreshing," or "scenting." Unfortunately, an entire industry profits from selling women products that are unnecessary and can potentially upset the pH balance of the vagina, which is necessary for vaginal health. In addition, these products can sometimes kill the "good bacteria" that are supposed to live in the vagina and help keep it healthy. Therefore, it can cause an overgrowth of "bad bacteria" and lead to other vaginal symptoms, if this happens.

If desired, consider using vaginal moisturizers and lubricants, but don't use vaginal douches or other products that your healthcare provider hasn't recommended. If you notice that your smell changes, see your healthcare provider rather than trying products to mask it. An odor is often an indicator of infection; thus it's recommended that you have a thorough evaluation.

There's only so much that vaginal moisturizers can do for genitourinary syndrome of menopause. For some women, vaginal moisturizers and lubricants may be sufficient. Vaginal estrogen and other prescription medications, however, are beneficial for many women, especially if vaginal or vulvar symptoms persist despite the use of these products. There are a few conditions where vaginal hormones may be contraindicated, such as hormone-receptor-positive breast cancer, so it's essential to talk to your healthcare provider to get more information, if you are interested in using prescription medication.

Women are often hesitant to use vaginal estrogen and assume it has the same risks as estrogen taken in a pill or patch form. However, this is not true. The potential side effects of using vaginal estrogen are much less than systemic estrogen, since most of the hormones only reach the vagina and surrounding tissues when used locally.

There are various delivery methods for vaginal estrogen including creams, vaginal tablets, and a flexible vaginal ring. For women who are bothered by the feeling of vaginal cream, the tablets or ring may be preferred. There are also non-hormonal prescription medications that your healthcare provider may prescribe for you if you are having painful vaginal intercourse.

Regular sexual stimulation through intercourse, genital vibratory stimulation (a vibrator), or self-stimulation supports vaginal health too. It promotes blood flow to the pelvis and female genitals, which is important for maintaining the health of these tissues, if vaginal sexual intercourse is desired in the future. Without regular vaginal stimulation after menopause, the vagina becomes shorter and narrower over time, increasing the risk of vaginal pain with intercourse. Regular vaginal stimulation helps preserve the vagina's width and length, typically allowing for more comfortable vaginal intercourse.

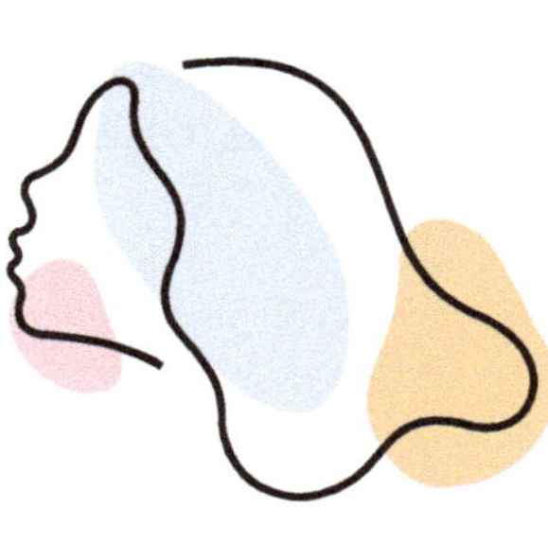

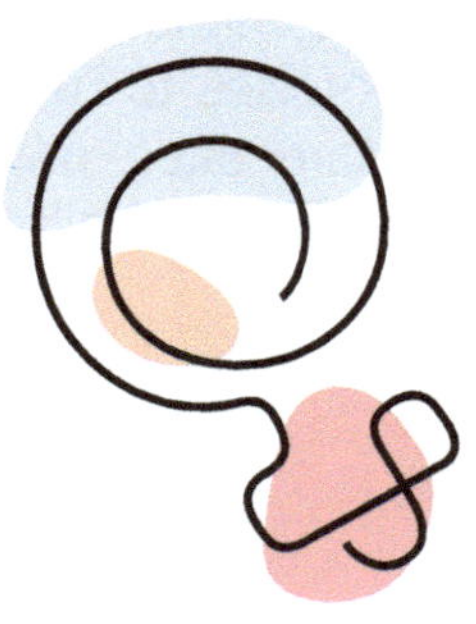

Alexander Ryabintsev/Shutterstock.com

NONHORMONAL OPTIONS FOR GENITOURINARY SYNDROME OF MENOPAUSE

LUBRICANTS*

- Water-based:
  - ✓ KY
  - ✓ Astroglide
  - ✓ Good Clean Love
  - ✓ Sylk
  - ✓ Pjur
  - ✓ YES
- Silicone-based:
  - ✓ Uberlube
  - ✓ Eros
  - ✓ Pink
  - ✓ ID Millennium
  - ✓ Wet Platinum
  - ✓ Pjurmed Premium Glide
- Oil-based:
  - ✓ Elegance Women's Lubricants
  - ✓ Oils (olive, coconut, avocado, vitamin E, Crisco)
- Moisturizers
  - ✓ Replens
  - ✓ RepHresh
  - ✓ Luvena
  - ✓ Lubrigyn
  - ✓ Sylk natural intimate moisturizer
  - ✓ Yes vaginal moisturizer
  - ✓ Canestima
  - ✓ Femallay Moisturizing Suppositories

*Peters KJ. What is genitourinary syndrome of menopause and why should we care? *The Permanente Journal.* 2021;25. Used with permission from The Permanente Federation. http://www.thepermanentejournal.org

The vulvar tissue thins during menopause and beyond due to hormonal changes. This thinning can lead to increased sensitivity and irritation, but practicing vulvar hygiene, as recommended by obstetrician-gynecologist Dr. Kelly Jo Peters, can help protect this area. Scented detergents, soaps, bubble baths and creams often contain chemicals that irritate the vulva. Other products marketed to address odor including feminine hygiene sprays and douches can also harm the tissue and should be avoided. Wearing or using products that rub on the vulvar tissue including tight underwear, pantiliners, washcloths, baby wipes, or cleansing wipes can cause significant inflammation and irritation. Instead, consider cotton underwear during the day and looser fitting clothes. Some women with vulvar sensitivity prefer sleeping without underwear at night. When looking for detergents and soaps, use ones that are fragrance and dye free, and also pH neutral. The vulva can be gently cleaned after urinating or in the shower with water using your fingertips, a peri-bottle, bidet, or sports bottle. Pat the vulva very gently to dry. By practicing these vulvar hygiene recommendations, the vulvar tissue will hopefully stay healthy. If you have any irritation of the vulva or vagina, reach out to a gynecologist or your primary care provider for evaluation and treatment.

VULVAR HYGIENE*

- Things to avoid:
  - ✓ Tight-fitting clothing
  - ✓ Synthetic underwear
  - ✓ Scented soaps, body wash, and bubble bath
  - ✓ Scented detergents
  - ✓ Laundry softener, dryer sheets
  - ✓ Baby wipes, flushable wipes
  - ✓ Feminine hygiene sprays, douches, and wipes
  - ✓ Dyed/colored toilet paper
  - ✓ Constant use of pantiliners
  - ✓ Washcloths, scrubbies, and loofahs
- Try instead:
  - ✓ Loose-fitting clothing
  - ✓ Cotton underwear in daytime
  - ✓ No underwear at night
  - ✓ Fragrance-free pH-neutral soaps/detergents
  - ✓ Tub bath without additives and at a comfortable temperature
  - ✓ Use fingertips for gentle vulvar washing, ideally with water only.
  - ✓ Try a sports water bottle, perineal bottle, or bidet.
  - ✓ Gently pat vulva dry.

RETAIL WEBSITES*

- Intimate rose (www.intimaterose.com)
- MiddlesexMD (www.middlesex.md)
- Good Vibrations (www.goodvibes.com)
- Eve's Garden (www.evesgarden.com)
- Adam and Eve (www.adamandeve.com)
- Babeland (www.babeland.com)
- Target (www.target.com; sexual health)
- Walgreens (www.walgreens.com; sexual lubricants)
- CVS (www.cvs.com; sexual health)
- Sexuality Resource Center (www.sexualityresources.com)

*Peters KJ. What is genitourinary syndrome of menopause and why should we care? *The Permanente Journal.* 2021;25. Used with permission from The Permanente Federation. http://www.thepermanentejournal.org

RESOURCES FOR PROFESSIONAL HELP

- American Association of Sexuality Educators, Counselors, and Therapists
  http://www.aasect.org/
- American College of Obstetricians and Gynecologists
  https://www.acog.org/womens-health/find-an-ob-gyn

Genital Vibratory Stimulation

Typical, age-related changes occur in the sexual responses of both men and women. Women often experience decreased lubrication and increased time needed for genital stimulation before sexual excitement and orgasm. Women may need more than 30 minutes of stimulation and foreplay before orgasm. Also, most women do not have an orgasm with vaginal intercourse alone. Most women need clitoral stimulation, and the amount of stimulation needed to become sexually aroused typically increases as women age.

What type of stimulation is adequate for sexual arousal and orgasm is different for each woman. Men often experience decreased penile rigidity and increased time needed for stimulation as they age too. Therefore, extended foreplay can be beneficial for both men and women as they age.

Although discussing genital vibratory stimulation, often referred to as using a vibrator, might seem taboo, many midlife and more mature women benefit from understanding how such stimulation can benefit their sexual health. If the word vibrator brings up negative connotations, another phrase to describe this is genital vibratory stimulation. With age, especially after menopause, vaginal sensitivity decreases, erectile tissue in the clitoris decreases, clitoral sensitivity decreases (though not as much as vaginal sensitivity), and increased stimulation is often needed to become sexually aroused and to have an orgasm.

For women who experience this, genital vibratory stimulation with a vibrator increases the blood flow to the vagina, clitoris, and pelvic floor. As a result, it can make the sensation more intense and pleasurable. Although typically sold as novelty devices, some vibrators are considered medical devices to treat sexual dysfunction by the Food and Drug Administration (FDA). These devices can also help women better understand their sexual response, allowing women to more effectively communicate this to their intimate partners, if they have one. Genital vibratory stimulation also increases blood flow to the male genitalia, and couples often enjoy using these devices when intimate.

Genital vibratory stimulation can be used in the vagina, on the vulva, and clitoris. There are various sizes, shapes, and speeds of vibrators. When exploring genital vibratory devices, self-stimulation, or manual stimulation by your intimate partner, you may benefit from understanding that the clitoris is much larger than just the area that protrudes above the urethra (opening where urine exits the body). Clitoral tissue extends to both sides in a V shape and surrounds the opening to the vagina, on the side that is closer to the urethra than the rectum.

Stimulating this clitoral tissue can help midlife and more mature women to become sexually aroused and potentially have an orgasm, especially when this becomes more difficult with vaginal stimulation alone. Many women cannot become sexually aroused through vaginal stimulation alone, even before menopause, but this becomes more common after menopause. Also, it's important to note that not all women orgasm nor is it mandatory for sexual health.

For this reason, experimenting with genital vibratory stimulation can allow women to remain sexually active, sexually aroused, and enhance their sexual well-being, if they desire to incorporate this device. Genital vibratory stimulation amplifies arousal, since the amount of erectile tissue in the clitoris decreases with age. Genital vibratory stimulators (vibrators) can also help increase sexual desire and satisfaction, reduce boredom, and add variety to your sexual encounters if you and your sexual partner are interested in incorporating them.

Genital vibratory simulation is not just for women who have intimate partners. Women can also use and enjoy them, regardless of whether or not they are currently in an intimate partnership, to increase pelvic blood flow. They are typically inexpensive, can be purchased without a prescription, and are available online through Amazon or Intimate Rose (a company owned by a physical therapist with expertise in this area), and adult stores. It's important to follow their instructions for cleaning and maintenance.

Kegels or Pelvic Floor Muscle Exercises

Pelvic floor muscle exercises, otherwise known as Kegels, can support sexual health too and were covered in the chapter on physical activity. They can enhance sexual arousal in women and give women increased control over the muscles involved in sexual activity.

Other Areas of Connection

Connections with acquaintances, friends, and intimate partners contribute to the richness of our lives. However, we don't often consider other areas of connection. Dr. Edward Hallowell, the author of the book, *Connect,* reminds readers that there are many areas where they can experience connection beyond their friends and partners. His suggestions are detailed in the following list.

As a mature woman, you have your past experiences to draw upon in each connection domain listed. There may be some areas where you used to feel very connected in the past but where you no longer have a desire to be connected. That is alright. There may be areas where you've always felt deeply connected and others where you've never felt a strong connection. If this disconnection doesn't bother you, that's okay too. As you age, mature, and your life changes, it's normal for connections in all these areas to change.

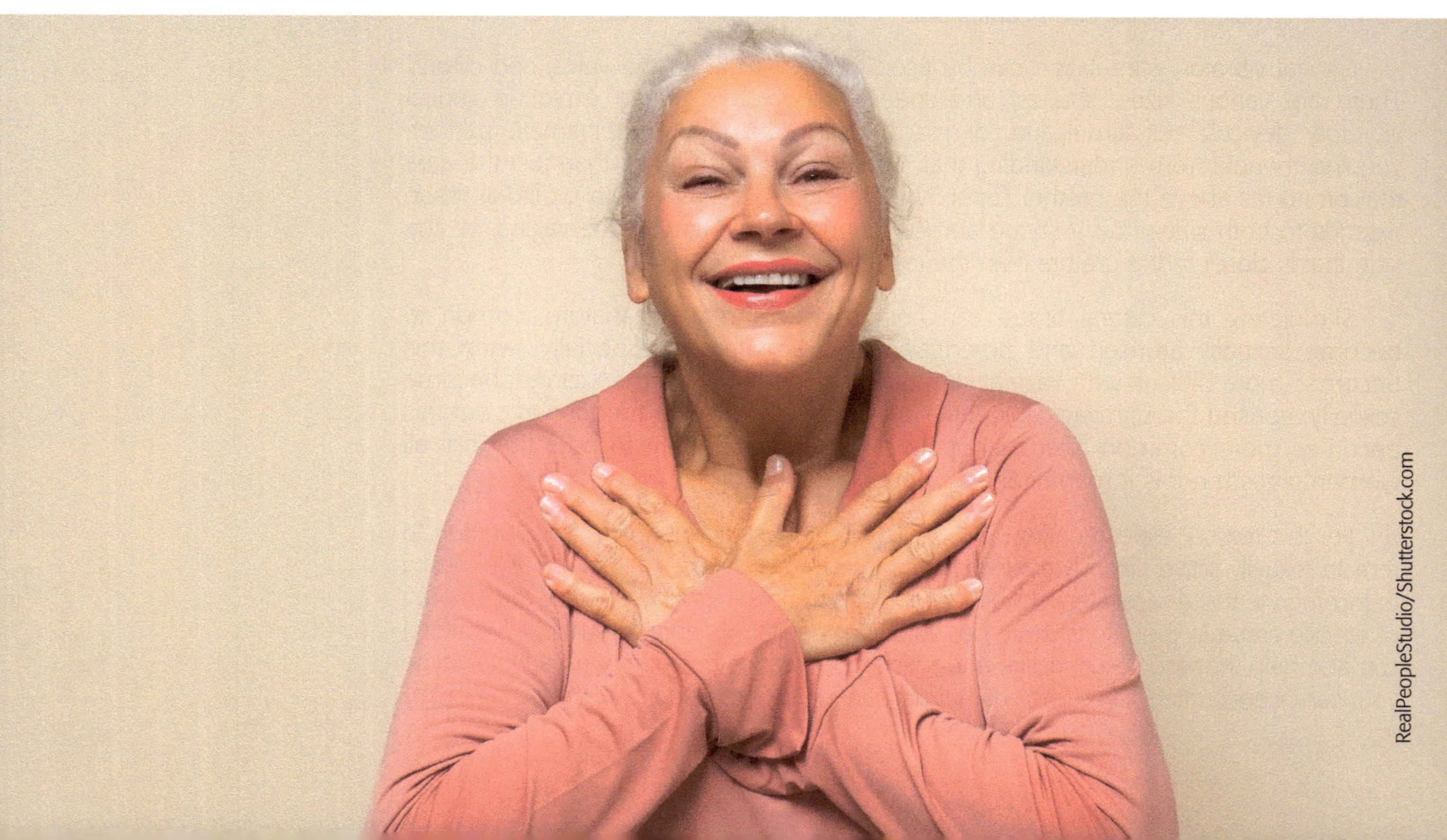

RealPeopleStudio/Shutterstock.com

AREAS OF CONNECTION (2)

- Family
- Neighborhood
- Friends
- Work
- The past
- Nature/outdoors
- Pets/animals
- Art and beauty
- Activities, hobbies, past times
- Information and ideas
- Institutions, clubs, organizations, other groups
- Spiritual connection
- Connection to self
- Connection to life
- Other connections

❑ On a scale from 1-5, 1 feeling extremely disconnected to 5 feeling extremely connected, rate each of the aforementioned areas of connection.

____

____

____

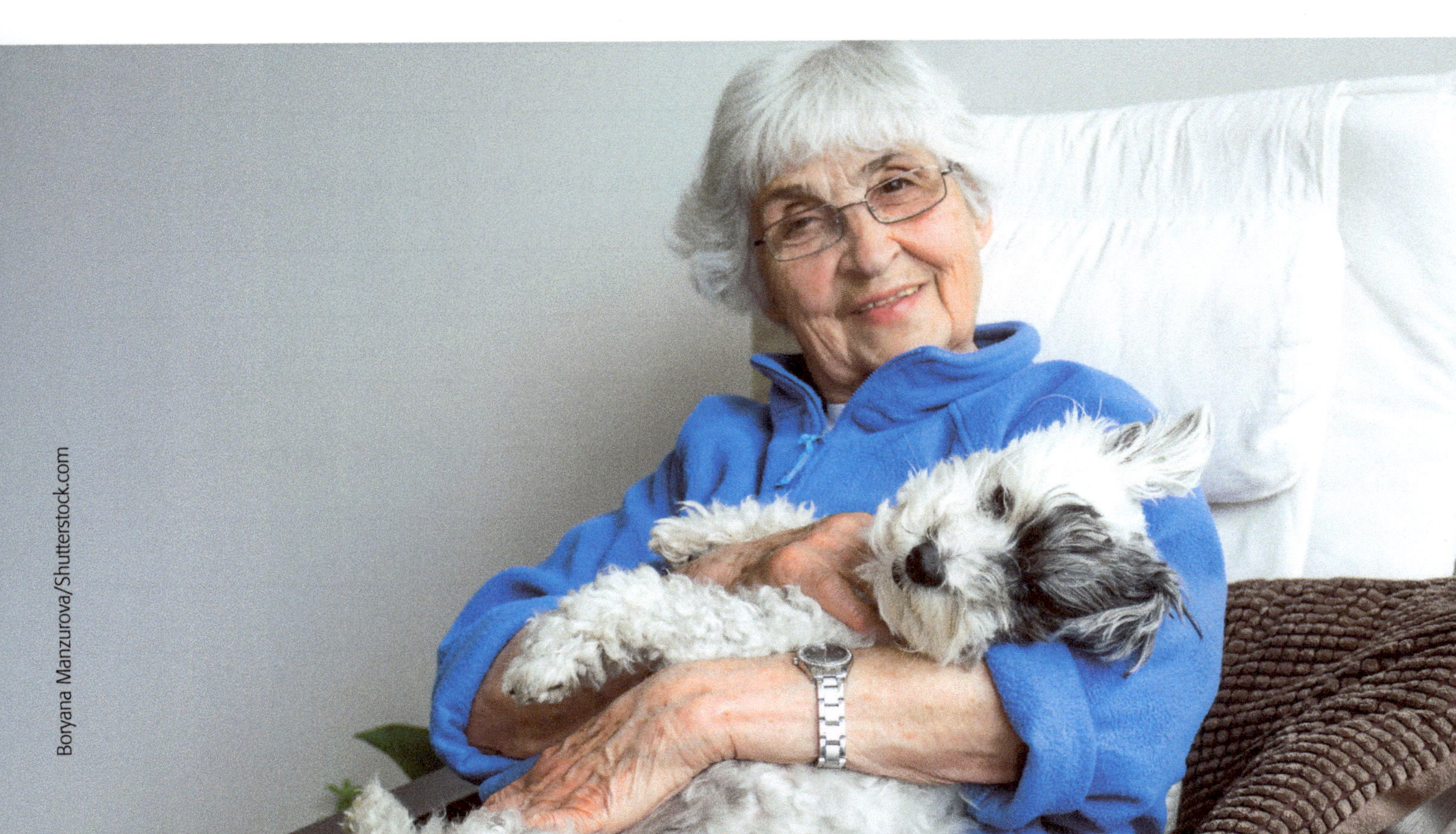

Boryana Manzurova/Shutterstock.com

Next, pick three of the areas to address with the next few prompts. Just because an area of connection received a low number does not mean you need to pick this area. Also, most people do not feel fully connected in all of these areas. Like with the PAVING Wheel, there is no right or wrong way to rate these.

- ❑ What are the three areas of connection that you would like to address? Choose areas that you feel excited about or motivated to work on during the next month.

  ____

  ____

  ____

- ❑ Describe how you feel connected or disconnected within these domains.

  ____

  ____

  ____

- ❑ Create a vision for how you would like to feel connected within these three domains.

  ____

  ____

  ____

  ____

- ❑ Write a SMART goal for each of these three domains to help you achieve your goal.

  ____

  ____

  ____

- ❑ What next step(s) do you want to take this week to work toward your goal(s)?

  ____

  ____

  ____

Coaching Yourself on Social Connection With the COACH Approach

CURIOSITY

You can successfully achieve the PAVING pillars through independent work. However, through working on the pillars with another person with whom you have a meaningful relationship or sometimes with even someone who you just met, you may be able to take your well-being in that area to the next level.

- ❑ Could the PAVING areas of physical activity, nutrition, or stress management benefit from greater attention through social connection? For example, if you've been exercising alone, could you ask a friend to join you or take a group class? Could you invite a friend to join you to take an online or in-person group cooking class? If you've been trying to meditate alone, consider taking a mindfulness-based stress reduction group class.

  ____

  ____

  ____

  ____

- ❑ After reading this chapter, what do you feel curious about regarding your social connections, intimate relationships, sexual health, or your connection to nature?

  ____

  ____

  ____

  ____

- ❑ How will you explore these areas further?

  ____

  ____

  ____

  ____

OPENNESS

Relationships don't magically grow deeper, or new friendships appear without any effort on your part. Sometimes you may not put yourself in a position to be open to connecting with others.

- ❑ You may say that you want deeper intimacy with a spouse or a partner, a closer relationship with a friend, or to meet new people; however, are you open to taking the following steps and putting energy toward making these changes and connections? Explain.

  ____

  ____

  ____

- ❑ If you aren't as open as you want to be, what can you do to address this?

  ____

  ____

  ____

Relationships are personal and often private with regards to emotional and physical intimacy. Your healthcare provider is someone with whom you can be open and honest about all topics related to mental and physical health. Even if they don't have expertise in this area, they can refer you to someone who does.

- ❑ Now is a good time to ask yourself, are you fully open with your primary care provider? Is there something that you've been wanting to discuss but are hesitant to do so? Please list.

  ____

  ____

  ____

- ❑ Would you be open to sharing this chapter with your intimate partner (if you have one)? Yes or no, and why or why not?

  ____

  ____

  ____

Is there anyone you believe would be open to reading this chapter and could benefit from reading it? If so, please make it available to them.

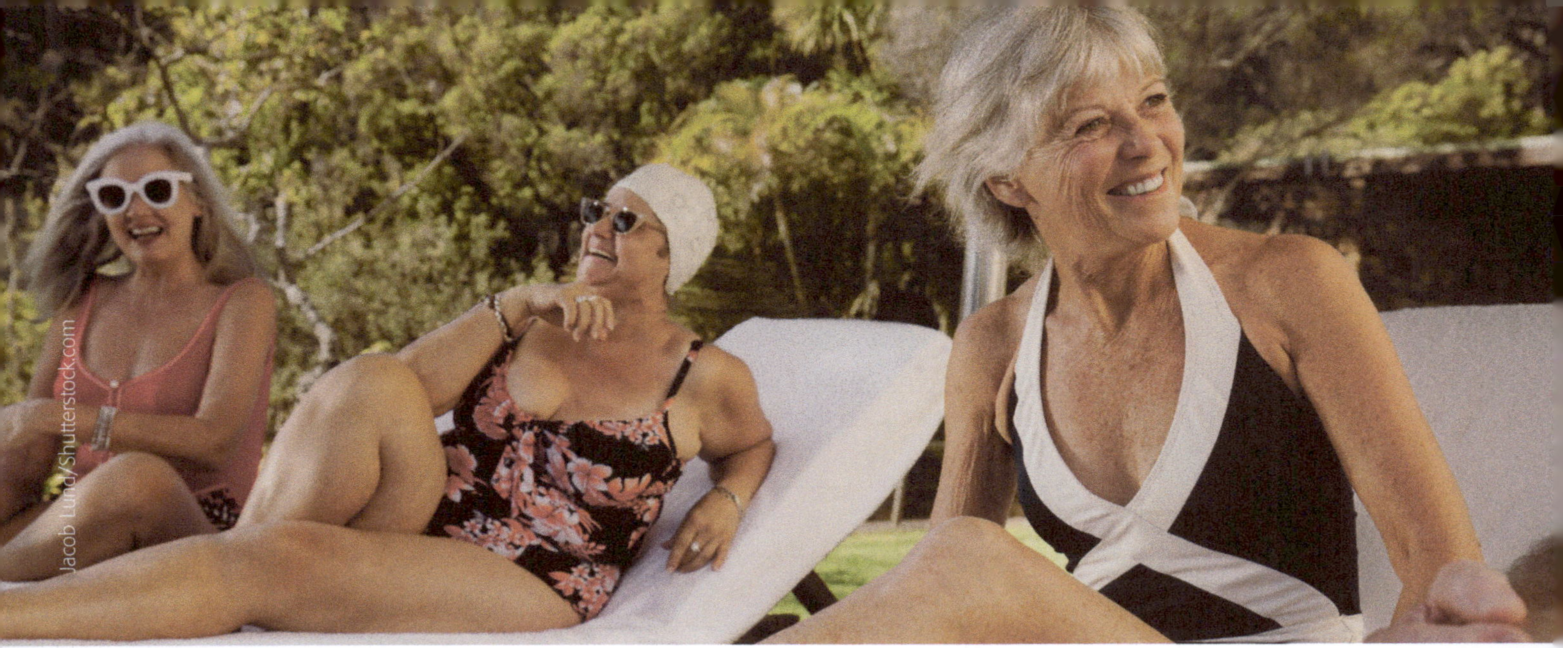

Jacob Lund/Shutterstock.com

APPRECIATION

❑ Please list the most precious connections in your life right now.

❑ What is it about these connections that make them precious?

❑ If you haven't shared this information with your friends or loved ones recently, would you be willing to express this appreciation with them this week or in the near future?

❑ What is it about yourself that allows you to develop high-quality connections? Please list these strengths and take a moment to be grateful for them.

Putting yourself in a position to meet new people or trying to deepen your relationships can be scary. Even if you've had over half of a century of making friends behind you, there is always a risk of hurt, loss, or potential rejection when you put yourself forward to connect with others.

- ❑ To what degree does fear of hurt, loss, or potential rejection prevent you from making connections that you desire?

____

____

____

- ❑ Is there anything that you want to do to address this?

____

____

____

COMPASSION

Embracing loving-kindness for yourself allows you to express it with others. This loving-kindness is often the most important ingredient to initiate and sustain relationships of any kind. It is important to note that thinking about relationships can be challenging, especially if you've had a difficult ending to a relationship, such as with a divorce or the death of a loved one. In addition, it can make it challenging to try to put yourself in a position to meet new people, make friends, and deepen relationships that already exist.

- ❑ Self-compassion is a key component to self-care. Self-care includes cultivating close relationships. How can you use your self-compassion to further deepen your connections?

____

____

____

- ❑ Are there areas where you are experiencing hurt from losing a relationship or changes in a relationship?

____

____

____

- ❑ How can you be compassionate to yourself regarding the change in this relationship?

___

___

___

- ❑ Is there anything that you can do to help yourself heal?

___

___

___

HONESTY

Honesty, compassion, and love are components of high-quality relationships. It can be difficult to consider which of your relationships need your attention and energy, especially if they are suffering from a lack of honesty, compassion, or love on your part. However, reflecting upon this and making changes so that your actions better align with your true self and your authentic purpose can help you achieve deeper meaning in your life and the lives of others.

- ❑ Which relationships need your honest attention?

___

___

___

- ❑ What steps do you want to take to address these issues?

___

___

___

In some situations, people benefit from professional support in their relationships, such as couple's counseling. Relationships can be complicated, they can change, and sometimes they are associated with hurt. If you need help, don't be afraid to reach out and ask. You deserve to be in relationships that support your well-being, are safe, and honor your authentic self.

Be honest, while answering the following questions:

- ❏ Are your relationship needs fully satisfied? Yes or no.
- ❏ Are your intimacy needs fully satisfied? Yes or no.
- ❏ Are your sexual needs fully satisfied? Yes or no.

If you answered no to any of these questions, it's time to find help and solutions. Furthermore, if you are struggling with sexual intimacy, please seek help, if the suggestions given in this chapter do not address your needs. Low sexual desire and difficulty with sexual arousal and orgasm are relatively common in midlife and more mature women, but please reach out to your gynecologist, a sex therapist, or your primary care provider, if the situation is bothersome. They either will have resources to support you or will be able to refer you to someone who can help. Pelvic floor physical therapists have training in assisting women with vaginismus (tight muscles around the opening to the vagina), some types of pain during intercourse, and other sexual problems. If you don't seek the help of a professional, you may suffer in silence for something that is treatable.

NATIONAL DOMESTIC VIOLENCE/INTIMATE PARTNER VIOLENCE HOTLINE:
FREE, CONFIDENTIAL, 24/7

- Call 1-800-799-7233 (SAFE)
- Text "START" to 88788
- Or visit https://www.thehotline.org/ to chat live

Social Connection Wrap-Up

You have gifts that this world needs. You are unique, beautiful, and worthy of love. We're so glad you've connected with us through this book and the PAVING the Path to Wellness program. We hope it has helped you connect with yourself, others in your local community, and potentially others in the PAVING the Path to Wellness community.

Connection with yourself is one of the most important connections you'll have in your lifetime. This book is meant to provide you with time to reflect and time to get to know yourself even better at any age or stage of life. In fact, you could read this book today and read it in five or ten years to get to know yourself better. We are different people from one year to the next. With the 12 steps in the PAVING Program that you've completed, we hope that you'll be able to appreciate yourself and others while cultivating high-quality connections that stand the test of time. Prioritizing the people that are precious to you will provide you and them with moments to cherish and memories that can carry you through the times ahead. Connection is key for a healthy body, peaceful mind, and joyful heart.

References

1. National Academies of Sciences, Engineering, and Medicine. Social isolation and loneliness in older adults: Opportunities for the health care system. *National Academies Press*. 2020 Jun 14.
2. Dr. Hallowell, Inventory of a Connected Life. http://www.drhallowell.com/dr-hallowell-inventory-of-a-connected-life, accessed March, 2022.

CHAPTER 14
IN CONCLUSION

Congratulations on making the PAVING the Path to Wellness journey for midlife and more mature women, who are using their wisdom and experience to thrive. If we were with you in person, we could celebrate together with a high-five or a hug. Since we're not there with you, hug yourself right now. We're serious. Wrap your arms around yourself and give yourself a hug. You deserve it!

The following are a few closing thoughts about each pillar, using the two key acronyms—PAVING and STEPSS—as you wrap up this part of your journey and explore how to move forward beyond the end of this book.

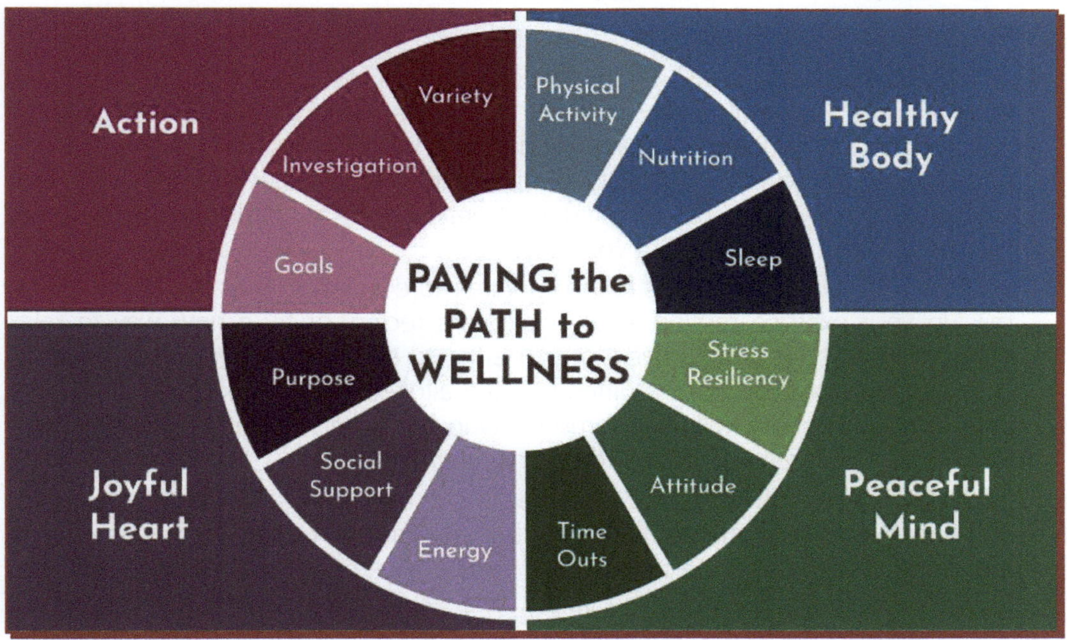

Figure 14-1

PAVING:

- *<u>P</u>HYSICAL ACTIVITY:* Hopefully, you've embraced the joy of movement and are trying to move more each day. Every minute counts. Start where you're at right now and find ways to increase your level of physical activity. Don't sit for too long without standing to stretch or take a walk. Your body is beautifully designed to move. Only you can let it do what it is meant to do. Your body and mind will thank you for moving more.

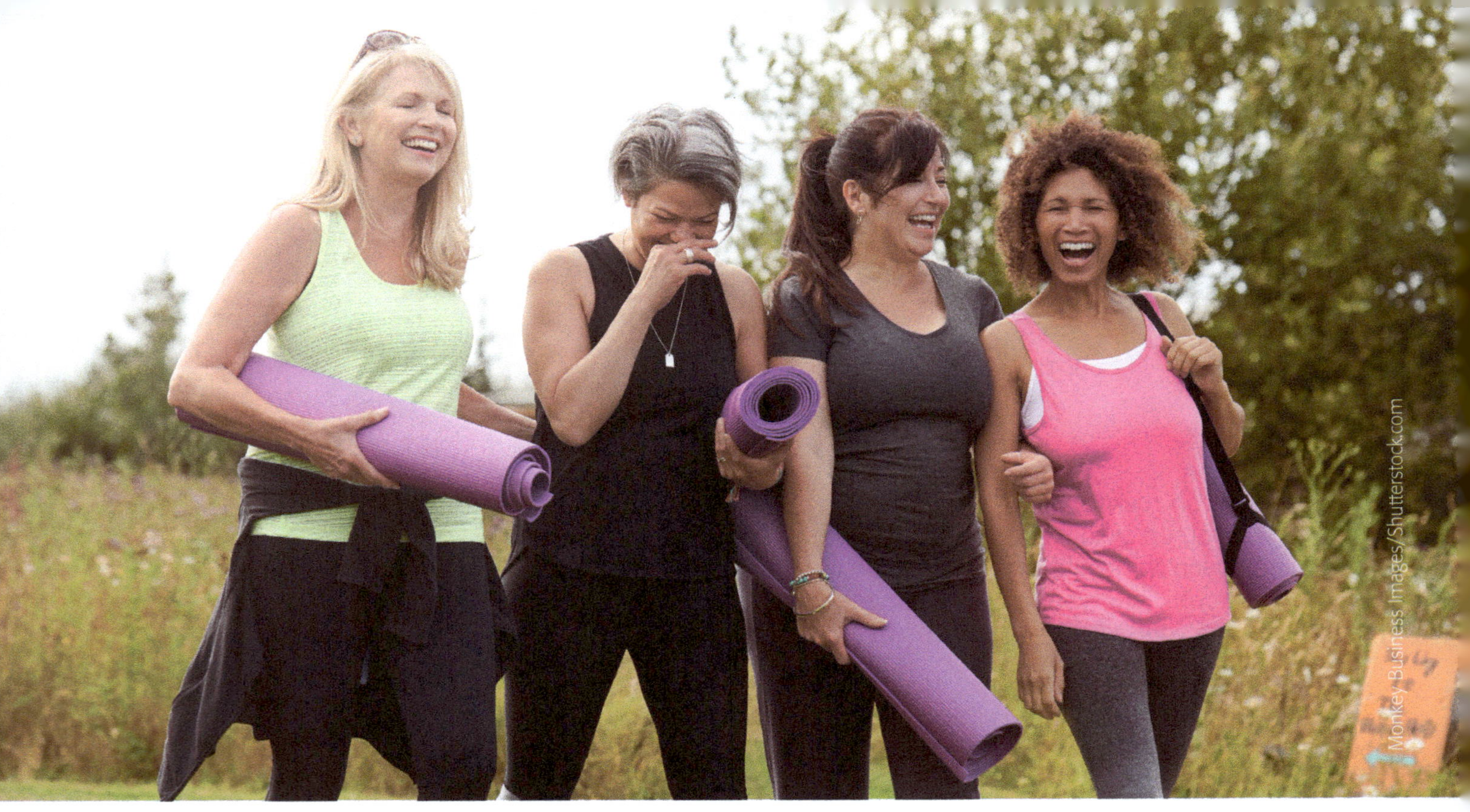

Monkey Business Images/Shutterstock.com

- *ATTITUDE:* You don't always get to choose your circumstances, but you do choose your attitude. Be gentle with yourself. Keep away shame, blame, and guilt by practicing loving-kindness to yourself and others. When things don't go the way you had planned, try to have a growth mindset and look for ways to learn from what happened. Finally, embrace an attitude of gratitude by mindfully looking for what you are thankful for throughout your day.
- *VARIETY:* Actively look for ways to incorporate more variety in your life. For example, mix up your exercise routine, cook a different recipe, or try a new way to relax before bed. Engage in activities that you enjoyed as a child. Drive a new route to your grocery store (or go to a different store altogether) or walk along a different path on your morning walk. Call someone who you haven't talked to in a long time. The possibilities are endless. Just do something different.
- *INVESTIGATION:* You may have over half a century of likes, dislikes, preferences, and habits accumulated over the years, but you can still benefit from investigating and experimenting. Learn a new hobby. Take a class on a topic that interests you. Find a new podcast. Explore the library. The world has treasures just waiting for you to discover. If you don't explore different activities and locations, you will never experience their beauty. So, have fun investigating what truly interests you.
- *NUTRITION:* Nourish your body with high-quality, nutrient-rich foods. Eat a rainbow of fruits and vegetables and make most of your grains whole grains. Eat foods that look like they did when they were grown. Get adequate protein and fiber each day, and experiment with adding beans, nuts, seeds, lentils, and soy foods to your diet. Don't forget to stay hydrated with water. Avoid ultra-processed foods, candy, unhealthy snacks, fast food, fried food, and processed meat.
- *GOALS:* Regularly set goals for yourself. Consider where you want to be in a week, year, and decade, and then work backward. Remember to make your goals SMART: specific, measurable, action-oriented, realistic, and time-sensitive. Tell others about your goals so that they can support you and help hold you accountable. Be gentle with yourself, if you don't succeed at reaching your goal. Use your growth mindset.

STEPSS:

- *STRESS:* Some stress is beneficial and can enhance performance. However, chronic, high levels of stress drain your joy and energy. Engage in activities that help you healthfully manage your stress, such as going for a walk, meditating, praying, spending time in nature, practicing mindfulness, focusing on your breath, reading a calming book, relaxing in the bathtub, or playing with your dog.
- *TIME-OUTS:* Use time-outs to recharge. You deserve time-outs that allow you to return to your regular schedule with a more peaceful mind and joyful heart. If fitting time-outs into your schedule is challenging, block time on your calendar for rest. Ask yourself what type of time-out you need right now. Do you need time alone, spent in silence, or focusing on your spiritual health? Prioritizing self-care through relaxation is essential to long-term well-being.
- *ENERGY:* Remember to use your "spoons" wisely. Energy management is just as important as time management. Avoid energy drainers, such as junk food, a lack of exercise, insufficient sleep, excessive stress, too much sedentary time, toxic relationships, gossip, and excessive screen use. Instead, look for healthy ways to boost your energy, such as spending time in nature, connecting with loved ones, eating nourishing food, prioritizing sleep, volunteering, and moving your body in ways that feel good.
- *PURPOSE:* The entire PAVING the Path to Wellness program will hopefully help you thrive, both now and for decades into the future, to fully live out your purpose. Consider keeping a purpose journal and actively look for ways to live out your purpose. Start each day by setting an intention for the day that is consistent with your values and priorities. Also, remember to care for your spiritual well-being, which can be intricately woven into your purpose.
- *SLEEP:* Prioritize sleep, even though society doesn't prioritize it. Go to bed and wake up at approximately the same time each day. Try to get bright outdoor light in the morning and keep the lights dimmer toward bedtime. Find a relaxing bedtime routine that works well for you. Keep your bedroom like a cave: dark, quiet, and slightly cool. Avoid heavy meals, alcohol, exercise, stressful conversations, bright lights, and using electronic devices close to bedtime.
- *SOCIAL CONNECTION:* Look for ways to create and cultivate high-quality relationships with people who honor your unique gifts. Reach out to people who you've lost touch with over the years. Look for opportunities to join groups, take a community class, or spend time in a location with others around you. Take the initiative to reach out and say hello to someone you don't know. If you don't know what to talk about, tell them about the PAVING program!

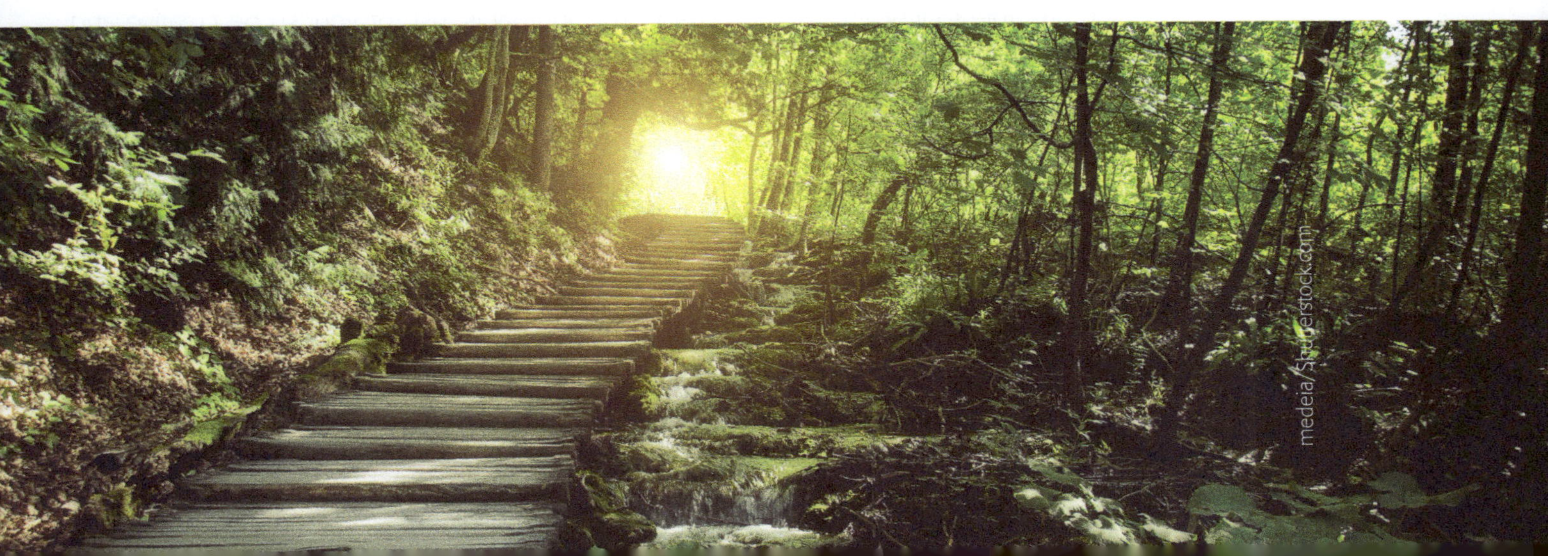
medeia/Shutterstock.com

Thriving With the PAVING Program Now and for Decades to Come

The workbook that you hold in your hands can be a resource for you anytime you need it. You may want to return to it when you're struggling with a particular aspect of the PAVING STEPSS or when you feel called to address a specific area. Taking the PAVING questionnaire at regular intervals, such as monthly, quarterly, or annually, can give you a way to reflect on what areas of your life may benefit from additional attention.

If this sounds like a good plan to you, take out your paper calendar now and put it on your schedule to remember to do this or put a reminder on your phone calendar. When you experience a challenging time, a new health diagnosis, or a time of transition, you may return to this book to reexamine where you are with your well-being and where you want to go now.

It should be noted that there are other books in the *PAVING the Path to Wellness* series planned for publication in the next few years (yet further supplemental texts to the original *PAVING the Path to Wellness Workbook),* including the *PAVING the Path to Wellness for Breast Cancer Survivors Workbook* and the *PAVING the Path to Wellness Cookbook*. Explore these, as well as other books by visiting our website and learning more. Another great resource is the *Lifestyle Medicine Handbook*, 2nd edition, by Beth Frates, Jonathan Bonnet, Richard Joseph, and James Peterson. The proceeds from all of the PAVING books go to the PAVING the Path to Wellness non-profit organization, while royalties for the *Lifestyle Medicine Handbook* are given to the non-profit organization, the American College of Lifestyle Medicine.

You may want to purchase and utilize a special journal to be your PAVING the Path to Wellness Journal, where you can regularly reflect on your PAVING Journey. For example, when changing your diet or exercise routine, it's beneficial to be mindful of your changes and how they've made you feel. You can use it as a sleep diary to record when you go to bed and wake up, if you're working on your sleep.

Writing any questions for your physician or members of your healthcare team in your journal can benefit you at your next healthcare appointment. In addition, writing about the stress management techniques you've learned and others that you want to try could be included in your journal, as can ways to add variety to your life. Your journal can consist of topics that you want to investigate and what you learned when you did the research. It's also an ideal place to write your goals and your progress in achieving them. Consider journaling regularly about what you are grateful for and how you are able to live your purpose daily. This journal is just for you, so be creative and have fun using it on the next part of your journey as a PAVING program graduate.

Now that you've experienced the PAVING the Path to Wellness program through this workbook, you are invited to join the PAVING the Path to Wellness community. You may have used this workbook in conjunction with an online PAVING the Path to Wellness group for women during menopause, midlife, and beyond. If not, consider joining a PAVING the Path to Wellness group that meets online or in person. For more information, visit www.pavingwellness.org and learn about the available PAVING groups. You can also e-mail us at info@pavingwellness.org for additional information.

We encourage you to follow us @pavingwellness on Twitter and paving.wellness on Instagram if you're on social media. In addition, you are invited to stay connected with the PAVING the Path to Wellness community by signing up to receive regular updates from us, by connecting with us on our website.

We have exciting things planned for the future, and we would love to have you join us on this adventure of spreading the PAVING program to those in need of receiving it. If you feel moved to do so, you can tell others about your wellness journey and the PAVING program, write a review about this book on Amazon (all proceeds from the book go to the non-profit organization and we appreciate your input about the book), or give a copy to a friend. We believe everyone can benefit from this program. Furthermore, if you are interested in donating to the PAVING the Path to Wellness non-profit organization so that others who cannot afford to purchase this book or join the groups can receive assistance, consider donating to our non-profit 501c3 organization PAVING the Path to Wellness (www.pavingwellness.org).

Congratulations on your commitment to PAVING your path to wellness, both now and for future decades. We, the authors, are here to support you along the journey, cheering you on every step of the way on your path. One step at a time, you're PAVING the way to a healthier body, a more peaceful mind, and a more joyful heart, through menopause, midlife, and beyond.

ABOUT THE AUTHORS

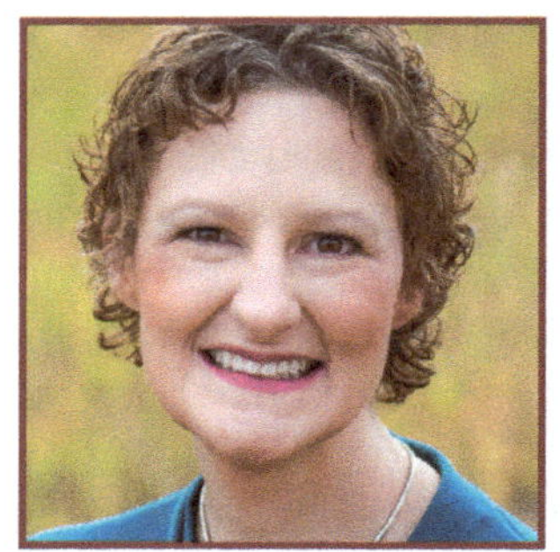

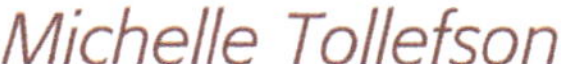

Michelle Tollefson

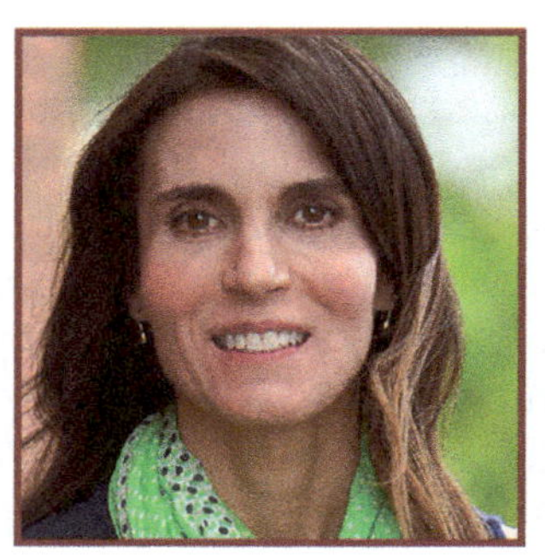

Beth Frates

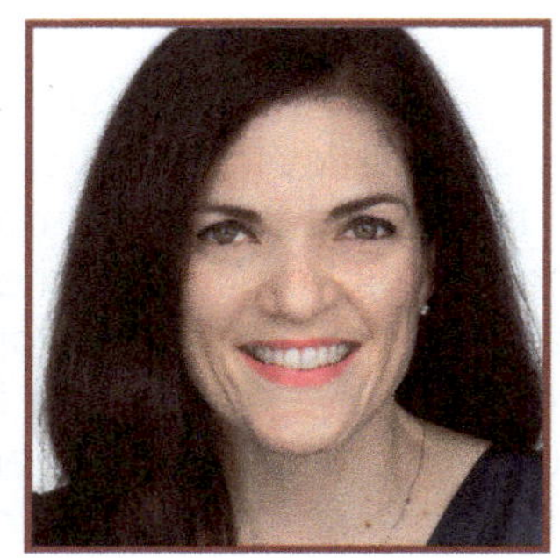

Amy Comander

Michelle Tollefson, MD, FACOG, DipABLM, FACLM, is an obstetrician-gynecologist in Denver, Colorado, and a professor in the Health Professions Department at Metropolitan State University of Denver, where she created and oversees the Lifestyle Medicine Program and the Wellness Coaching and Lifestyle Medicine Pathway.

Dr. Tollefson is a graduate of Creighton University, where she received both her Bachelor of Science and Doctor of Medicine degrees. She is board certified in obstetrics and gynecology and completed her residency at the University of Missouri in Kansas City. She is also board certified in lifestyle medicine and is a fellow of the American College of Lifestyle Medicine (ACLM).

As an ACLM member for over a decade, she founded and co-chaired the Women's Health Member Interest Group, as well as the Pre-Professional Lifestyle Medicine Education Member Interest Group. She currently serves as the ACLM Executive Board Secretary and is on the Education and Membership Committees.

Along with Drs. Frates and Comander, Dr. Tollefson co-authored the *PAVING the Path to Wellness Workbook*. She is on the board of directors of the non-profit organization, PAVING the Path to Wellness.

Dr. Tollefson co-edited *Improving Women's Health Across the Lifespan*, which is part of Dr. James Rippe's Lifestyle Medicine book series. In addition, Dr. Tollefson leads workshops, speaks at national and international conferences, and is a consultant on Lifestyle Medicine and women's health topics.

Dr. Tollefson is also a breast cancer survivor and thriver. She facilitates PAVING the Path to Wellness online lifestyle medicine groups for breast cancer survivors (thrivers) and women who want to optimize their health during and beyond menopause.

Beth Frates, MD, FACLM, DipABLM, is a trained physiatrist and a health and wellness coach, with expertise in lifestyle medicine. She is an award-winning teacher at Harvard Medical School, where she is an assistant clinical professor. A pioneer in lifestyle medicine, Dr. Frates developed and first taught a college Lifestyle Medicine course at the Harvard Extension School in 2014, which is still one of the most popular courses offered at the school.

Dr. Frates is the President of the American College of Lifestyle Medicine. She is on the board of directors of the non-profit organization, PAVING the Path to Wellness, and is the lead author of the original PAVING the Path to Wellness Workbook. Dr. Frates also authored a syllabus on lifestyle medicine, which instructors and professors can download through the ACLM website as a template for their curriculum. In addition, Dr. Frates co-authored the *Lifestyle Medicine Handbook: An Introduction to the Power of Healthy Habits*, which Book Authority ranked in the top 20 medical books released in 2018. To accompany the syllabus and handbook, she also co-created Lifestyle Medicine 101, a full college curriculum, with 12 weeks of PowerPoints and a teacher's manual, both of which are free and accessible through the ACLM website. Most recently, Dr. Frates co-authored *The Teen Lifestyle Medicine Handbook*, published in October 2020, with corresponding slide-decks for faculty use.

As Director of Wellness Programming at the Stroke Institute for Research and Recovery at Spaulding Rehabilitation Hospital, a Harvard Medical School affiliate, Dr. Frates has created and implemented a 12-step wellness program, PAVING the Path to Wellness for patients and health care practitioners. At the present time, she serves as the Director of Lifestyle Medicine and Wellness for the Department of Surgery at Massachusetts General Hospital. In addition, Dr. Frates has her own consulting/coaching practice in lifestyle medicine, where she sees patients 1:1 and in groups.

Amy Comander, MD, DipABLM, is a breast oncologist and the Director of Lifestyle Medicine at the Massachusetts General Hospital (MGH) Cancer Center in Waltham and at Newton Wellesley Hospital. She is the medical director of the MGH Cancer Center in Waltham, and an instructor in medicine at Harvard Medical School. Along with Drs. Frates and Tollefson, Dr. Comander co-authored the *PAVING the Path to Wellness Workbook.* She is on the board of directors of the non-profit organization, PAVING the Path to Wellness.

Dr. Comander is a graduate of Harvard University, where, as an undergraduate, she developed a passion for understanding the biological basis of behavior. Subsequently, she studied neurobiology and psychology as part of the multidisciplinary Mind, Brain, and Behavior Initiative. She then received her Doctor of Medicine at Yale University School of Medicine. She completed her internal medicine residency training and hematology-oncology fellowship training at Beth Israel Deaconess Medical Center and Harvard Medical School. She is board certified in hematology, medical oncology, and Lifestyle Medicine.

As a breast oncologist, Dr. Comander has witnessed the struggles her patients face during and following completion of primary cancer treatment, and she is passionate about improving the overall health and well-being of breast cancer survivors through lifestyle interventions. She is the founding co-chair of the American College of Lifestyle Medicine Breast Cancer Committee. In collaboration with Dr. Frates, she launched the PAVING the Path to Wellness Program lifestyle medicine group for breast cancer survivors. She trains other colleagues at the MGH Cancer Center to run PAVING groups, so that this transformational experience can be offered to a larger group of breast cancer survivors. Dr. Comander practices what she preaches, having run marathons, including seven consecutive Boston Marathons to date. She views running marathons as a metaphor for life, and her favorite running mantra is "Every mile out there is a gift and every finish line is a gift" (Amby Burfoot, winner of the 1968 Boston Marathon).

MW01620782

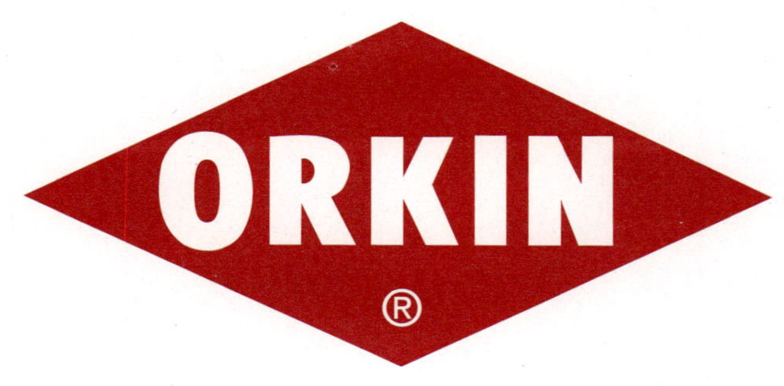
ORKIN
®

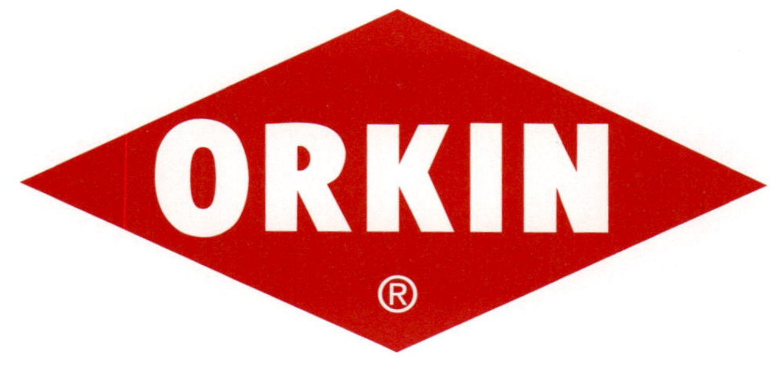

The Making of THE WORLD'S BEST PEST CONTROL COMPANY

Margaret O. Kirk

Note to the reader: This book contains the opinions, recollections, and memories of individuals associated with Orkin, Inc. While an effort has been made by Rollins, Inc. to verify the accuracy of the facts, the opinions and personal statements are those of the subjects quoted.

Published by Rollins, Inc.
Atlanta, Georgia
www.Orkin.com

ISBN: 0-9764862-0-2

Printed in the United States of America by Corporate Printers

Book design by Jill Dible

To the memory of Otto Orkin and O. Wayne Rollins, and to all the Orkin Men and Women who have made Orkin, Inc. the world's best pest control company

Over more than one hundred years, countless Orkin Men and Women have had an important role in creating the company, its culture, and its numerous achievements. It would be impossible to mention all of them by name and locale; however, it is important that they be thanked and recognized. This book is a tribute to all the individuals who have made Orkin great.

CONTENTS

ACKNOWLEDGMENTS

The idea to publish the history of Orkin, Inc. has always belonged to Gary W. Rollins, an Orkin Man who advanced through the company to be its president and chairman. Over the years, Mr. Rollins worked with various writers to bring this history to life, encouraging not only their historical research but also their efforts to interview a wide range of Orkin executives, employees, and customers in order to record their stories. Early manuscripts and interviews by Loyce Sandifer and Robert Snetsinger provided the foundation for writer Margaret O. Kirk to ultimately research and write this final book. Editor Carol Molnar ushered the book into print, working closely with copy editor Alexa Selph and designer Jill Dible. Appropriately, Mr. Rollins provided the name for this history — *Orkin: The Making of the World's Best Pest Control Company.*

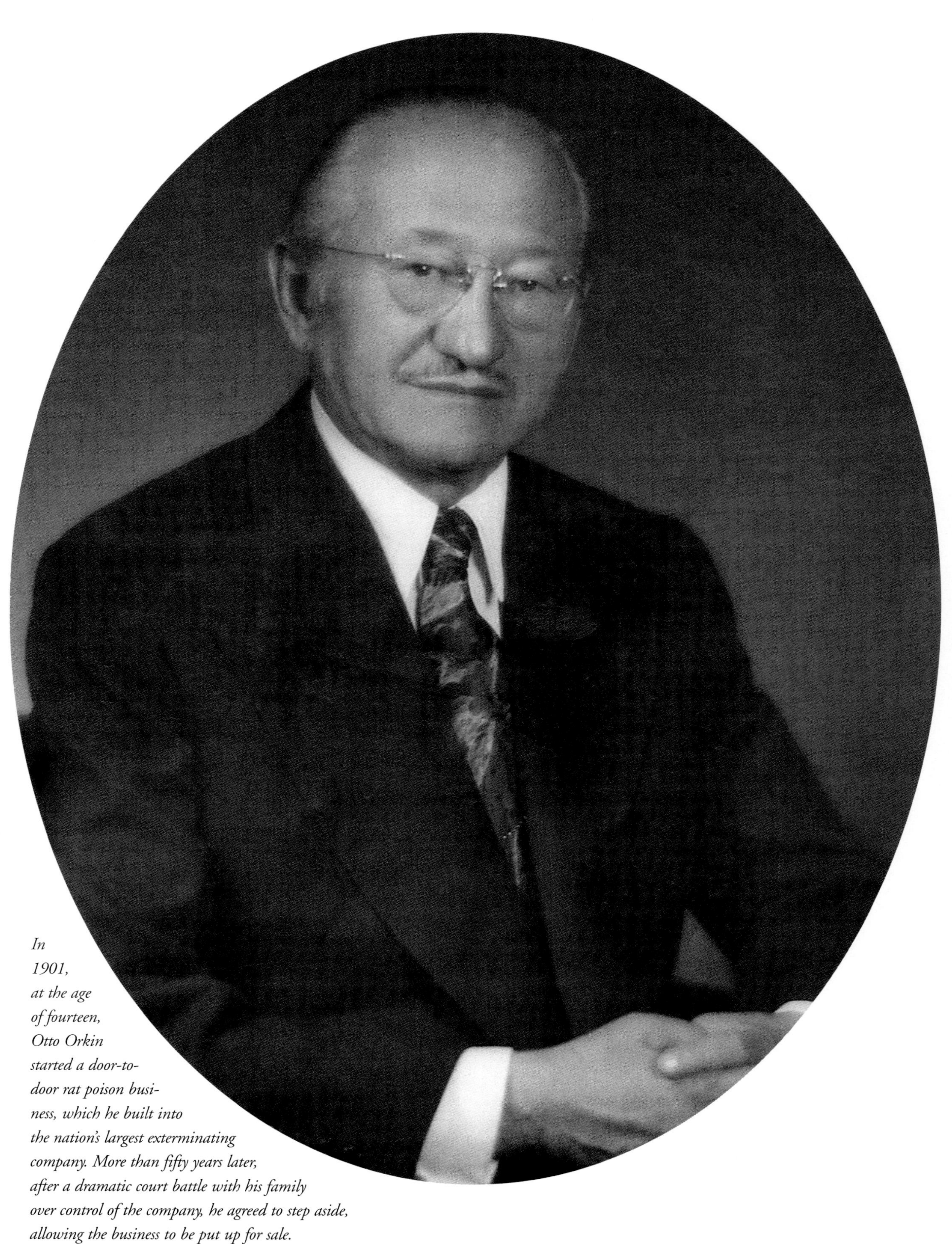

In 1901, at the age of fourteen, Otto Orkin started a door-to-door rat poison business, which he built into the nation's largest exterminating company. More than fifty years later, after a dramatic court battle with his family over control of the company, he agreed to step aside, allowing the business to be put up for sale.

Introduction: "Jonah Swallows the Whale"

In the spring of 1964—during the season when subterranean termites begin to swarm, around the time little black ants venture outside their colonies to forage for protein, when the female carpenter bees start to drill into wood to lay their eggs, and just before the smoky brown cockroaches decide to come indoors—the rumors began.

The Orkin family, the owners of the world's largest pest control company and the purveyors of an American service icon named Otto the Orkin Man, had decided to sell the company founded by their father, Otto Orkin.

No matter where they turned, the employees of the Atlanta-based pest control company had to confront the rumors, which surfaced regularly in newspapers and magazines around the country and in the whispers that floated up and down the long, quiet hallways of the company's Piedmont Road headquarters. Company president Sanford H. Orkin developed a standard, practiced reply, and it played out over and over in the press: "Sanford H. Orkin declined to confirm or deny the report at that time," reported the *Atlanta Constitution* on May 6, 1964. *The fifty-three-year-old company was in fact up for sale. The Orkin family—sons Sanford and William, daughter Bernice, and son-in-law Perry Kaye, who collectively controlled 85 percent of the company's stock—had found a buyer.*

To all but the most unobservant Orkin employee, however, the evidence to support the rumors was overwhelming. Allen Post, the Orkins' Atlanta-based Rhodes scholar lawyer, who had a flair for dramatic presentations, was in constant contact with the Orkin family members, outlining the pros and cons of what close associates were calling a "major transaction." For nearly a year, it had been rumored that a wealthy New York investor named Lewis B. Cullman had offered to put together a deal to buy the entire company for $26 a share—for a total purchase price of $62.4 million. The Orkin family had supposedly accepted his offer, and Cullman was reportedly working to develop potential buyers not only to finance the deal but also to manage and run the company. Cullman's business connections had apparently led him to a businessman from Delaware who might be interested in buying and managing Orkin. The rumor seemed all the more substantial on Memorial Day, when what could only be described as a very important meeting took place inside the Orkin Atlanta headquarters, around Perry Kaye's rectangular, highly polished desk in the center office of the east side of the second floor. Here, Kaye, vice president of operations, William Orkin, executive vice president, and Sanford Orkin, president, met for several hours with John and O. Wayne Rollins, cofounders of Rollins Broadcasting, a successful radio, television, and outdoor advertising company based in Wilmington, Delaware. The rumors concerning a Delaware investor, it seemed, were true.

O. Wayne Rollins, as everyone would confirm, was a country gentleman with a brain for business and a sophistication that transcended his humble beginnings. Born in the north Georgia mountains near the town of Ringgold, Wayne and his younger brother, John W. Rollins, had grown up on the family farm. As young men, they worked as farmers, laborers, and eventually entrepreneurs, and in 1948 they formed the business partnership that was the beginning of Rollins, Inc. John operated automobile dealerships in Virginia, Delaware, and Maryland, while Wayne opened their first radio station in Virginia. As he acquired more radio stations in other markets, Wayne became one of the first in radio broadcasting history to tailor programming to specific community segments—a practice known today as niche marketing. From their success in radio broadcasting, the Rollins brothers entered the television industry in 1956. Rollins Broadcasting of Wilmington, Delaware, went public in 1960 and was listed on the NASDAQ Exchange. The next year, Rollins stock began trading on the American Stock Exchange.

Wayne Rollins's introduction to Orkin was actually triggered by a media business deal that had gone sour.

In April 1964 Wayne Rollins's introduction to Orkin was actually triggered by a media business deal that had gone sour; at the last minute, Wayne's $29 million proposal to buy three Dallas-based businesses—a radio, television, and newspaper property—had unexpectedly fallen apart. On the airplane home from Dallas to Wilmington, a business associate named George Weymouth looked at Wayne and said, "I'd like to show you another deal, for Orkin Exterminating Company. Are you familiar with it?"

Wayne dismissed the idea without much consideration until a few weeks later, when Weymouth urged him to take another look. He encouraged Wayne to go down to Atlanta on Memorial Day, when no Orkin employees would be around to speculate about the visitor and when he could tour the entire facility without any restrictions. Weymouth assured him he could arrange a meeting with the Orkin family.

By all accounts, the first meeting between the Orkin family and Wayne Rollins began somewhat dubiously. To begin with, Wayne Rollins had always been skeptical of the $62.4 million price tag that had been established for the deal, more than double the cost of his unfulfilled Dallas proposition. Wayne Rollins had doubts as to whether he could finance such an enormous transaction, and he wasn't even sure that he wanted to. By the end of the Memorial Day meeting, the rumor mill was abuzz with stories that Kaye had inadvertently offended Rollins with his blunt manner and somewhat colorful language. After a perfunctory handshake, he asked Wayne, "What kind of business are you in?"

"We're in the radio and television business," Wayne replied.

"That's a helluva business to be in," retorted Kaye. Momentarily taken aback by this rather unprofessional outburst, Wayne Rollins maintained his composure and continued the business discussions until the meeting was interrupted by the unexpected appearance of the company founder, Otto Orkin. The seventy-six-year-old small and wiry man with graying hair and rimless glasses was no longer directly involved with the company. He was widely thought to be estranged from his family, following a dramatic court battle for control of the company that ended in 1960 when Otto Orkin agreed to be bought out of the company. Wayne was shocked to see Otto Orkin, and thought that the son-in-law treated the company founder with disrespect, something that made Wayne very uncomfortable.

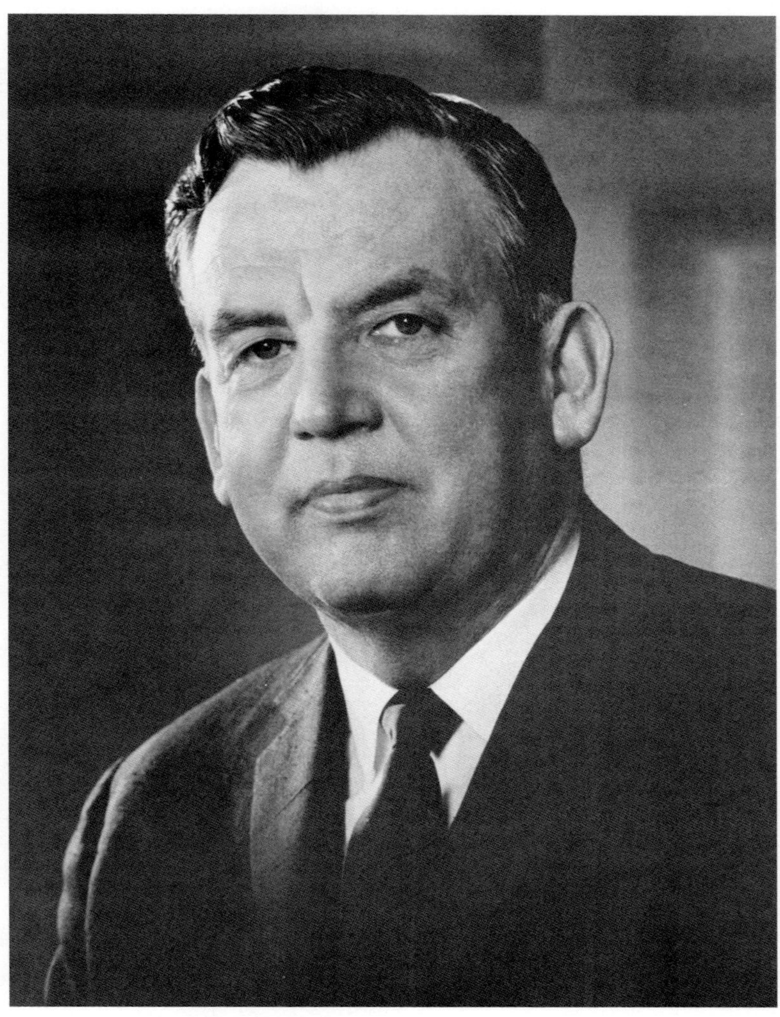

In 1964 O. Wayne Rollins, in the first recorded leveraged buyout, orchestrated the purchase of Orkin Exterminating Company for $62.4 million. Up to that time, his company, Rollins Broadcasting, had operated in a totally different industry—radio and television.

But despite some shaky introductions, Kaye's manner, and Otto Orkin's sudden unexplained appearance, Wayne Rollins was genuinely impressed with Orkin by the time he left the meeting. Compared with Rollins Broadcasting, Orkin was a giant: Orkin's sales of $37.3 million for the previous fiscal year were four times Rollins's $9.1 million, and the exterminating company's profits of $3 million were more than three times the Rollins earnings. What specifically appealed to Wayne Rollins was the rapid and consistent climb of Orkin sales and earnings; the company, for instance, was reporting a 14 percent gain in revenue over the same period in the previous year. The company had a

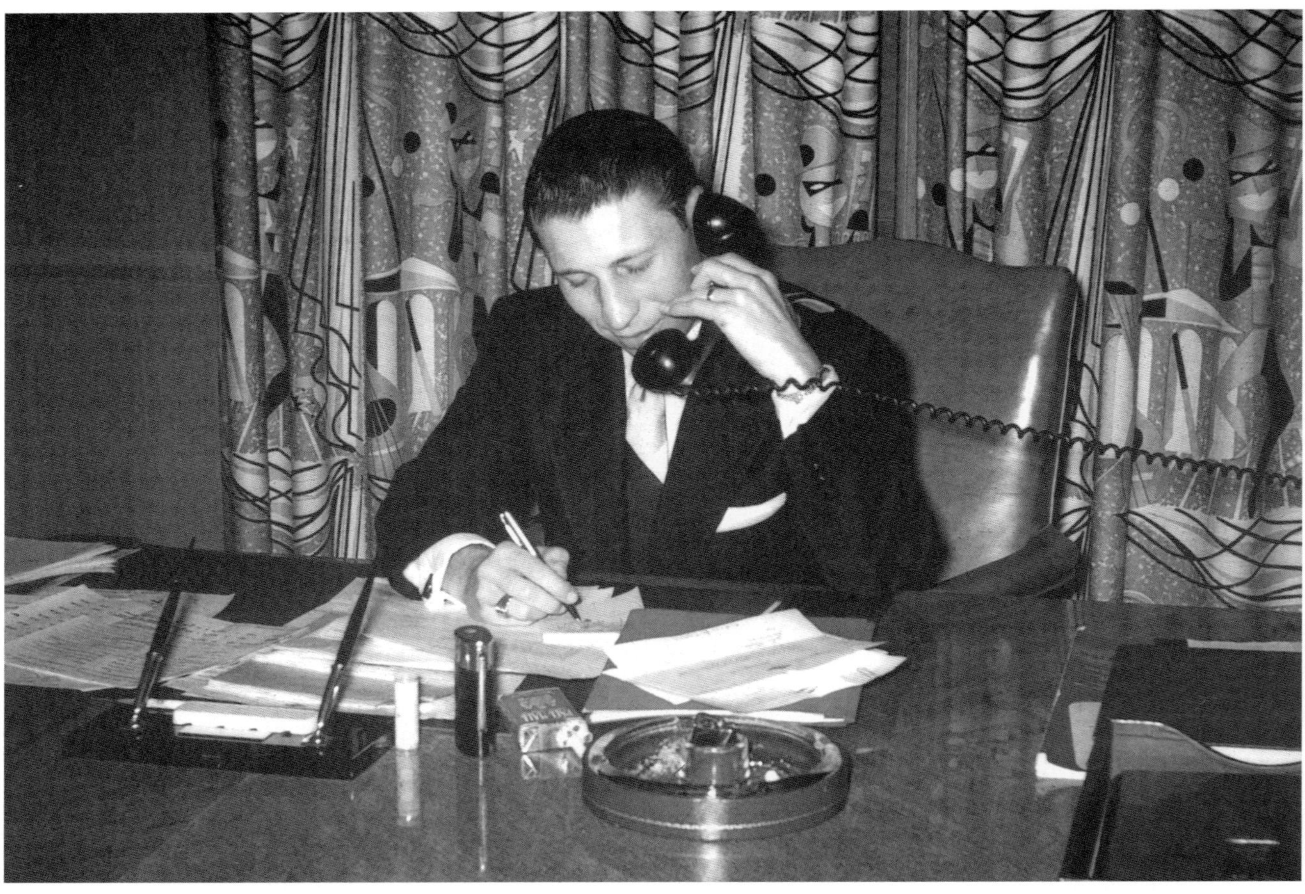

Perry Kaye, who was married to Otto Orkin's daughter Bernice, headed up the day-to-day operations of the company in the early 1960s, eventually negotiating its sale in 1964.

consistently strong pretax profit margin, it billed for services in advance, and it had an amazing list of seven hundred thousand customers.

What especially attracted Wayne Rollins to Orkin, however, was something that *didn't* appear in the books. From his days in radio and television, Wayne had developed an uncanny ability to pick companies that were underperforming and poised for growth. When he analyzed Orkin's records, he recognized the traits of a business that could achieve remarkable growth at an accelerated pace if it were managed aggressively. What exactly then did Wayne Rollins see that wasn't in the company records?

First, when he analyzed the competition, Wayne Rollins simply wasn't worried. While the Orkin family had been intimidated when Sears, the department store giant, had recently entered the pest control business, Wayne concluded that there was no possibility that the product-oriented company could operate a service business effectively. The two businesses were just too different, he reasoned. And Orkin was larger than its next ten competitors combined. Orkin's number-one status in the industry was extremely important to Wayne, because it suggested that the company could demand top dollar for its pest control services. "People will pay more for quality," Wayne explained in talking over the Orkin deal with his associates. "And they'll pay more for good service."

Second, despite Orkin's size, Rollins executives concluded that the market for pest and termite control had barely been tapped; 53 percent of Orkin's accounts were concentrated in only five states, which meant that a potentially greater market existed for new customers. When he looked at the numbers, Wayne saw only room for growth. "If we just did as much business in the other states as we're already doing in Georgia and Florida," Wayne realized, "then we would double our business."

And the third point, ironically, reflects how Wayne Rollins saw his own expertise as it could be applied to Orkin. Wayne had concluded, somewhat arrogantly perhaps, that Sears couldn't succeed in the service-oriented pest control business because the mission was so unlike its product-oriented business. But this media executive had decided that the same logic didn't apply to his own very similar situation. Any service industry, he rationalized, was all about pleasing the customer. "If you have a customer and that customer has a complaint and you take care of it, you have a more loyal customer than one who never had a complaint," Wayne said. "So you turn that into an asset." Wayne then argued that like Orkin, Rollins Broadcasting was "essentially a service company. With Orkin, we can apply advertising and merchandising knowledge to ensure specialized future growth."

From his days in radio and television, Wayne had developed an uncanny ability to pick companies that were underperforming and poised for growth.

In American business circles, research was now beginning to focus on the South and its growth since World War II. Wayne Rollins was no doubt aware of some of the historians' scholarly conclusions. In widely publicized articles during the 1960s, the development of the South had been attributed to three modern conveniences: screen doors and windows, air conditioning, and managed pest control. Without being scholarly at all, Wayne Rollins had come to the same conclusion. In fact, he eventually took the entire pest control industry and the South's dependence on it and reduced it to one simple, economic conclusion: "A housewife just isn't going to put up with bugs. It's way down on the list of things she'll cut to save money. People want to protect their investment in a house from termites. They won't cancel that. Pest control is recession-proof."

By the middle of June, a letter of intent was signed for Rollins to pursue buying Orkin, a move that gave Rollins complete access to Orkin's business records. And there was no more denying the rumors when, on June 19, 1964, an "Immediate Action Memorandum" was sent from the Orkin executives to "All Offices." From first glance, the memo was most unusual. Perry Kaye, who ran the day-to-day operations of the pest control company, usually sent out the company's Immediate Action Memos under his signature alone, incorporating a series of exclamation points and lots of capitalized words to emphasize his typically curt executive orders. But this memo carried three signatures—those of Sanford Orkin, William Orkin, and Perry Kaye. Its tone was formal and surprisingly cold, hardly what one would expect when saying good-bye to the employees of a company that not only carried the family name but had created the family's wealth. The memo's message was clear: the Orkins were selling Orkin.

> *Gentlemen: Attached is publicity which is being released immediately to the news services. You may be sure that only after long considered thought and deliberation for the best interests of all members of the Orkin Company was this decision agreed upon. We wish to emphasize most strongly that the company policies and programs of progress, growth and personal security of all employees will be continued and expanded by the new owners. We will, of course, expect your continued loyalties and cooperation in fulfilling and achieving company goals and objectives and maintaining leadership within the industry.*
>
> *Sincerely,*
>
> *Sanford H. Orkin   William B. Orkin   Perry Kaye*

The "attached publicity" was a press release that gave a few key details that weren't included in the Action Memo: the Orkin family had agreed in principle to sell Orkin Exterminating Company to a wholly owned subsidiary of Rollins Broadcasting, Inc., a Wilmington, Delaware, corporation, for $62.4 million.

Business analysts around the country labeled the acquisition the "deal that captured the imagination of Wall Street."

"We essentially are a service company," O. Wayne Rollins, president of Rollins, announced in the press release, "and we have acquired a service company to which we can apply our advertising and merchandising operations towards specialized future growth."

The announcement stressed that the Orkin company's "policies and personnel," as well as its products and services, would be continued under the new owners. Beyond that, Wayne Rollins tried to keep the announcement focused on the two companies' similarities. "Both companies have had outstanding growth," said Wayne. "In the past ten years, Orkin's revenue has increased by an average of 14 percent annually, and this year's first-quarter profits exceed those of last year by 15 percent. Rollins's earnings were up 41 percent from 1962 to 1963, and according to a company spokesman, preliminary figures which are now under audit indicated that earnings will be up 50 percent for the fiscal year ending April 30, 1964, over 1963."

The press release was all the more interesting, however, for what it *didn't* say. Neither the Rollins nor the Orkin company president mentioned what was so obvious about this unusual sale, a feature that would lead business analysts around the country to label it the "deal that captured the imagination of Wall Street." At the time of the announcement, Orkin was the world's largest pest control business, providing residential, commercial, and industrial services in twenty-nine states and the District of Columbia, with revenues of $37.3 million. Rollins, on the other hand, reported revenues of $9.1 million through its television, radio, and outdoor advertising ventures in ten states.

When Wall Street analysts started looking at these figures, they couldn't believe what they were seeing. Here was a small, albeit successful, communications company buying a business more than four times its size. The press held a field day with the image of this $5 million company with revenues of $9 million acquiring a company worth $62.4 million with revenues of $37.3 million.

"Mighty Gulp for Rollins," reported one national newspaper.

"Jonah Swallows the Whale," said *BusinessWeek* magazine.

"Can a small radio-TV chain buy a giant exterminating company and find financial happiness?" asked yet another headline.

And that wasn't all. The revenue-size discrepancy was just one element that made this business deal one for the history books. Throughout the summer the challenge of financing the $62.4 million purchase loomed over the transaction. In 1964 financial institutions were primarily willing to lend money based on hard assets, which were not abundant in a service business. To counter this notion, Wayne Rollins consistently argued that the fixed assets associated with this business deal were not as important as the stream of earnings from Orkin. The debt in this transaction, Rollins proposed, should be financed based on the company's earning stream and not on its fixed assets.

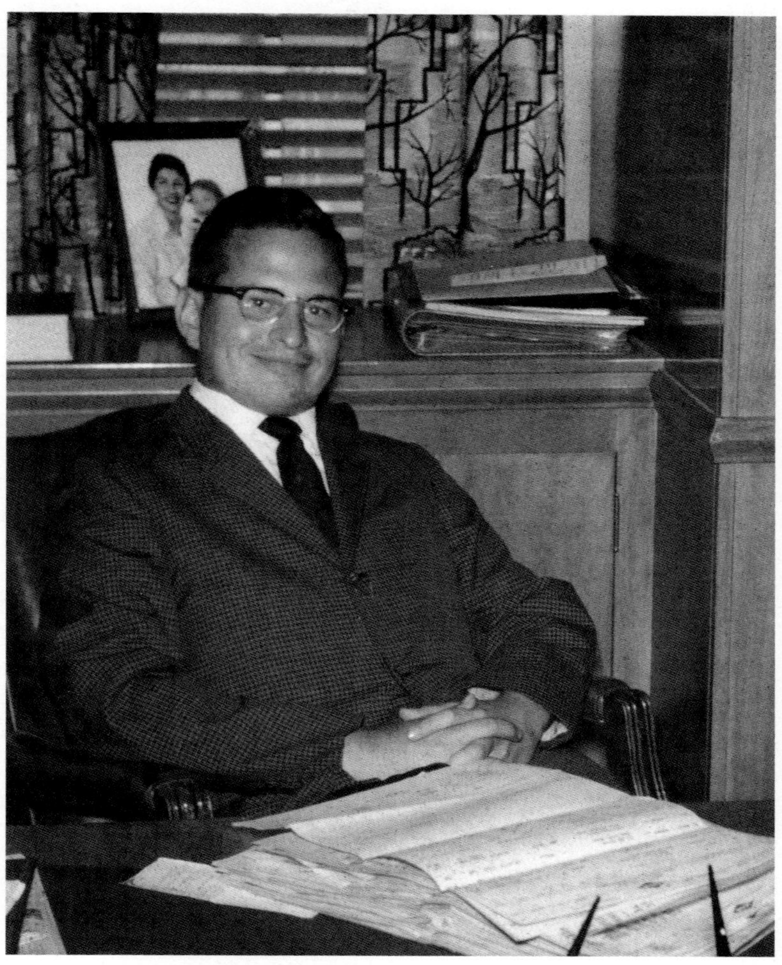

Sanford Orkin, Otto's older son, was named president of Orkin in 1961, when the company went public, and served in that capacity until its sale in 1964.

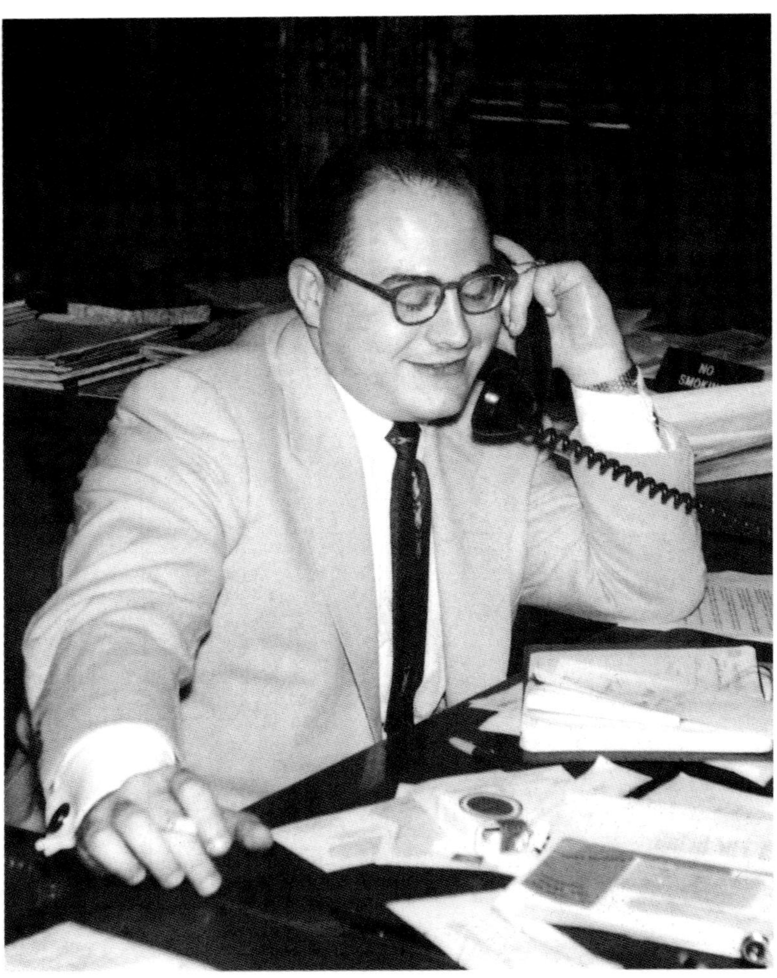

William Orkin, Otto's younger son, was vice president of the company from 1952 to 1964. Collectively, William, his brother Sanford, and his sister Bernice and her husband Perry Kaye owned 85 percent of the company stock at the time of the Rollins buyout.

As the numbers were crunched, the true impact of this deal began to emerge. This transaction, as one magazine reported, "seemed to violate all the canons of the business world." Rollins had structured the transaction such that most of the purchase price for Orkin would be paid for by borrowing money from others. Even the $10 million that Rollins would put into the deal was borrowed. In financial terms this deal represented "the high use of leverage to finance a purchase." This particular type of transaction would become known as a "leveraged buyout." And the Rollins purchase of Orkin was considered the first documented leveraged buyout in the country—a history-making business transaction that would later be a case study at the Harvard Business School.

The deal clearly marked a turning point for Orkin. Just as Wayne Rollins had predicted, the company he purchased was capable of remarkable growth. Orkin's rapid expansion of customers and services would propel the company into the twenty-first century, still managing to honor the efforts of a company founder who called himself "Otto the Orkin Man." Its success would far surpass his dreams for the company he started from a black satchel stuffed with paper bags of rat poison. The very name "Orkin" would one day represent a true American icon, a name as familiar to American consumers as Ford Motor Company, Oscar Mayer, and Motorola. And when all was said and done, the development and success of this pest control enterprise named Orkin mirrored the remarkable contributions of two families—and the thousands of capable, talented individuals who worked by their sides.

The hundred-year-plus history and success of Orkin is "much broader than somebody being at the right place at the right time who had a lot of luck," explained Gary W. Rollins, the younger son of O. Wayne Rollins, who worked his way up from positions as an "Orkin Man" in service, sales, and branch management to be named president, chief operating officer, and chairman of the company. "I think Mr. Orkin made his own luck. He strikes me as the kind of person who, if it hadn't been pest control, would have likely been extremely successful in anything he chose. I don't believe you can have that many skills and that much energy and not be successful."

When his father orchestrated the purchase of Orkin, Gary Rollins instantly saw his father in a new light. "I knew that Dad was a successful businessperson," he recalled years later. "But I think the Orkin acquisition signaled to me that Dad was willing to bet it all on something that was major in the form of size, and major in the form of locations and number of employees. And also that he had the wherewithal to raise the money to be able to execute a transaction like that. He was willing to go outside of the media industry and get into something totally different. It was really a bold move.

Gary Rollins was always aware of the importance of Otto Orkin's legacy to the company and would one day choose to honor the company's founder by helping to establish the O. Orkin Insect Zoo at the Smithsonian Institution in Washington, D.C. (Photo from the 1983 Rollins Annual Report)

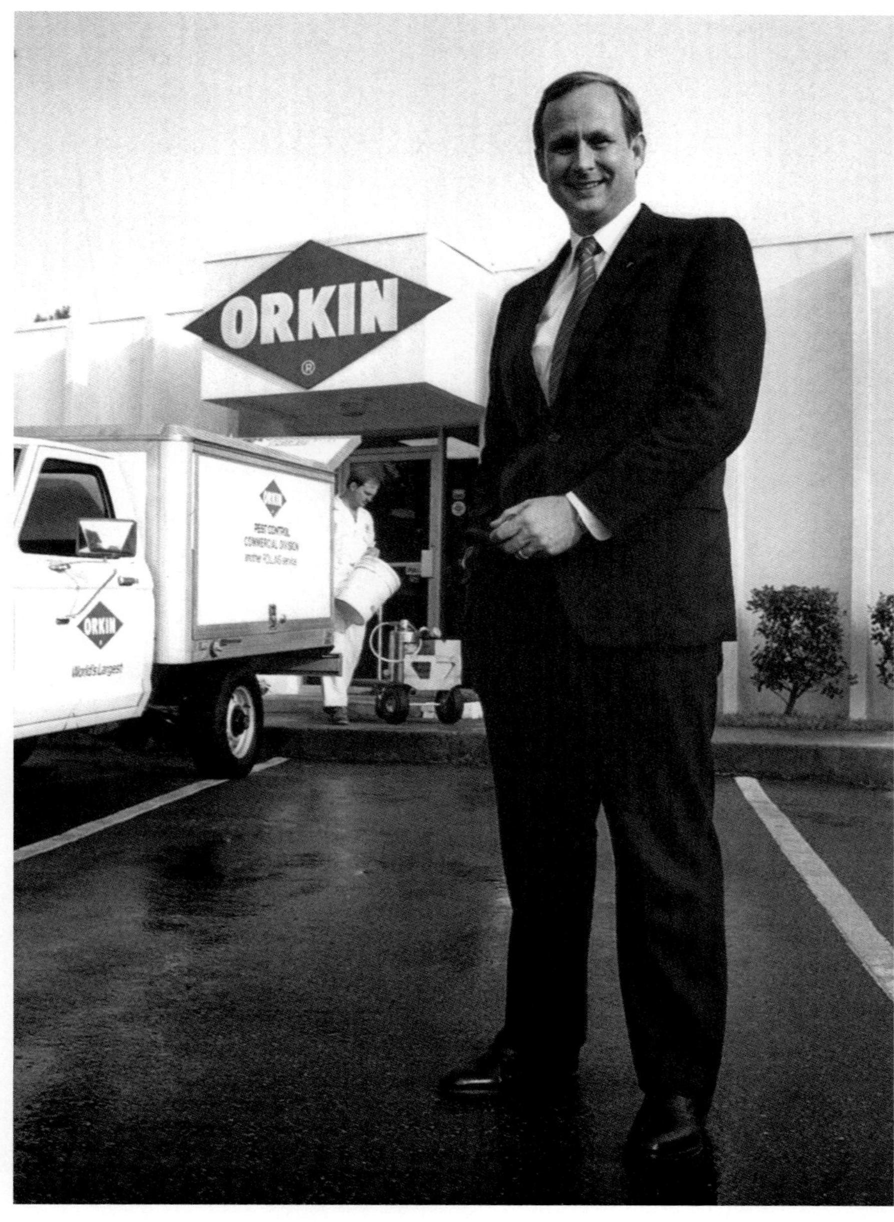

"I realized that this was really a unique individual. I think the Orkin deal really made me realize how unique his business skills were, and how he had the courage and the willingness to continue to extend himself. And even with all this boldness, Dad pretty well understood what had to be done, and he had the capabilities to do it and didn't need to rely on somebody else. I think that's really when it sunk in to me that my father was more than a successful businessperson. I realized that he was extraordinary."

To truly understand and appreciate why the Rollins purchase of Orkin represents a historical business achievement, it's important to go back over one hundred years, to look at the very beginning of a company that would one day grow to be the largest and best pest control company in the world.

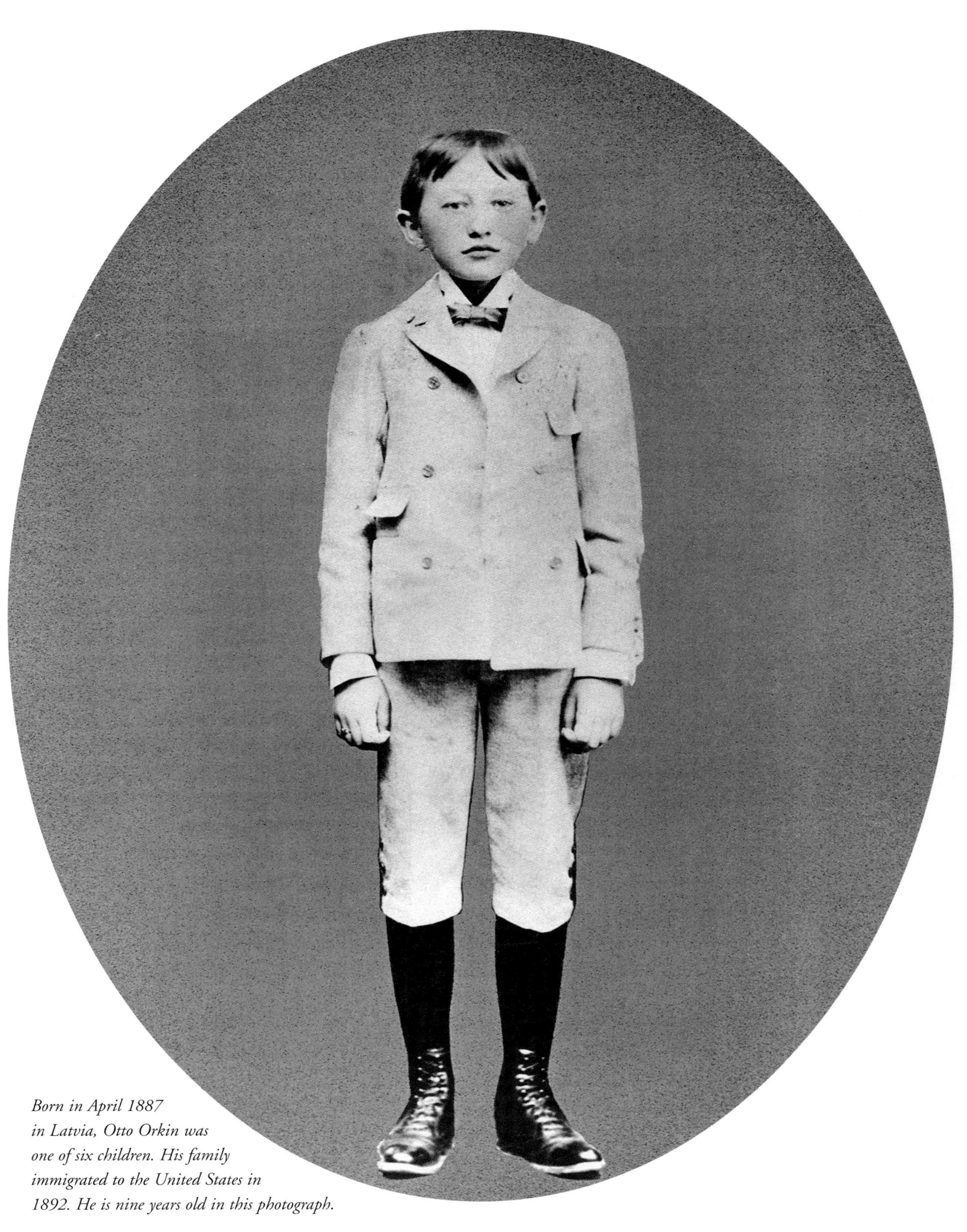

Born in April 1887 in Latvia, Otto Orkin was one of six children. His family immigrated to the United States in 1892. He is nine years old in this photograph.

Chapter 1

1901 to 1912:
A Pest Control Empire Begins

The story of Orkin and the man who developed the company into a multimillion-dollar business begins on a farm in the foothills of Pennsylvania, in a small rural community where a lot of pests lived alongside a boy named Otto. Designated the family rat catcher, Otto Orkin soon discovered that nearby farmers and neighbors were willing to pay him for his special blend of rat poison. From 1901 to 1912, Otto's unique sense of entrepreneurship and business savvy helped him expand his business into parts of the Northeast and as far south as Richmond, Virginia, where the young businessman soon became the rat exterminator of choice. In just twelve short years, Otto Orkin had become "Orkin The Rat Man."

In the mid-1890s, the Orkin family lived on a small, six-acre farmstead in rural Pennsylvania. The farm was basically a clump of land on the side of a hill in a community known as Lockport, about twenty miles northeast of Allentown. Some cherry, apple, and plum trees, along with many kinds of berries, grew on the property, and a vegetable garden was planted to one side of the two-story unpainted farmhouse that was separated from the barn by an underground spring that ran through the property. No crops grew in the fields around the house, and the land was used primarily as pasture for dairy cows and livestock. Piles of scrap metal and odds and ends were scattered across the landscape, junk piles that the Orkin family regularly peddled to make money.

Ironically, the unkempt pastures, crowded barnyards, and piles of junk invited the unwelcome intruders that would prove to be the key to success for the Orkin family.

In a word? Rats.

In Lockport rats flourished in the family's junk piles and barnyards, where too many animals were kept in too small a space. Here, Otto Orkin, one of six children in the Orkin family, first learned to shoot and poison rats in order to keep them away from the farm animals and their feed supplies, and out of the family's winter supply of flour stored in the attic. With his keen eyes that were once described as "always taking things in," Otto's designation as the family rat catcher seemed a perfect fit for the small and wiry youngster with the ruddy complexion. He quickly learned to shoot a gun and kill the rats, one by one, outside in the yards and fields. He was a good marksman, no doubt crouching just inside the barn door, waiting for the rodents as they made their final sprint from the one-story shed the Orkins built for horses and a wagon along the barn's east side. Or he may have aimed for the doomed rats as he sat amid the tools and farm equipment in the workshop, a small, forgotten building nestled in the hillside between the barn and house.

When he was about twelve years old, Otto began experimenting with poison to kill the pesky rodents that got inside the family home, into the attic where the family often stored as much as a hundred pounds of flour for winter baking. "My parents put the flour in the attic, where they thought it could be stored safely away from the rats," Otto once said. "But the rodents found it and ate their way into all four bags." Otto was particularly miffed by rats in his house, and he was determined to get rid of them. First, he tried traps, but they "wouldn't work," he said. "The old rats would keep their young back, crawl underneath—and snap the trap harmlessly." Otto knew that the family used sugarcoated arsenic, a substance called Paris Green, to kill potato bugs. Why wouldn't the same concoction work on rats?

Otto first learned to poison rats to keep them away from the Orkins' farm animals and their feed and away from the family's winter supply of flour stored in the attic.

Otto tried different mixtures of the poison, spreading it between slices of bread and setting out the sandwich bait on the attic floor. Otto thought it would look tempting to a rat, but the rats refused to bite. Otto knew all of this because he used to hide for hours behind the supplies, patiently watching the rats and learning their habits from his secret attic refuge. He quickly realized that the rats were amazingly cunning. "They didn't want anything that was out in the open," Otto figured out. "If you make them think you don't want them to have something, they want it worse." So Otto decided to put the sandwiches in paper sacks, tempting the rats to sneak up, chew through the bags, and taste the seemingly forbidden treat. The method worked. The rats ate the poison and died, and Otto soon eliminated the rats from the family home.

In 1901 Otto began to sell his rat poison to neighboring farmers in the Lehigh Valley, carrying the bags of carefully measured poison inside a signature black satchel that became his personal trademark. A fourteen-year-old entrepreneur, Otto unwittingly took the first steps along a business path that would eventually make "Orkin" synonymous with pest control throughout the country.[1] It was a turn of events that no one could have predicted nearly ten years

1. For information about the origins of pest control, see Appendix A.

earlier, when the Orkin family immigrated to the United States from the small Eastern European country called Latvia. From the very beginning, no one in the Orkin family ever imagined that this young man's quest to be a modern-day pied piper would one day make Orkin a household word.

THE EARLY YEARS

Otto Orkin was born in April 1887 in the flat countryside of Latvia, a slip of land near the Lithuania border that was part of Russia from 1795 to 1917. His parents, Hessel and Annie Levine Orkin, were farmers and lived with their growing family in a Jewish community thought to be about a day's journey by horse and wagon from Riga, Latvia. Unlike the Russian farmers, who lived close together in rural villages, Latvian farmers resided in isolated farmhouses, generally two-story houses with slate or red tile roofs. Their main crops were rye, wheat, barley, oats, flax, clover, sugar beets, and potatoes, with fruit trees and flowers planted around the houses. Latvian farmers like Hessel Orkin were known as fine herdsmen who tended horses, sheep, poultry, pigs, and milk cows. During the 1870s and 1880s more than 70 percent of Latvians were farmers and lived in the country, away from cities and towns. Nearly 5 percent of the population was Jewish. The Courland Jews, as the Jews around Riga were often called, were strongly influenced by their German neighbors and spoke a combination of German and Yiddish in their homes. The Orkin family spoke Yiddish and German, and so strong was their German association that they actually identified themselves as coming from Germany in the 1890 U.S. Census.

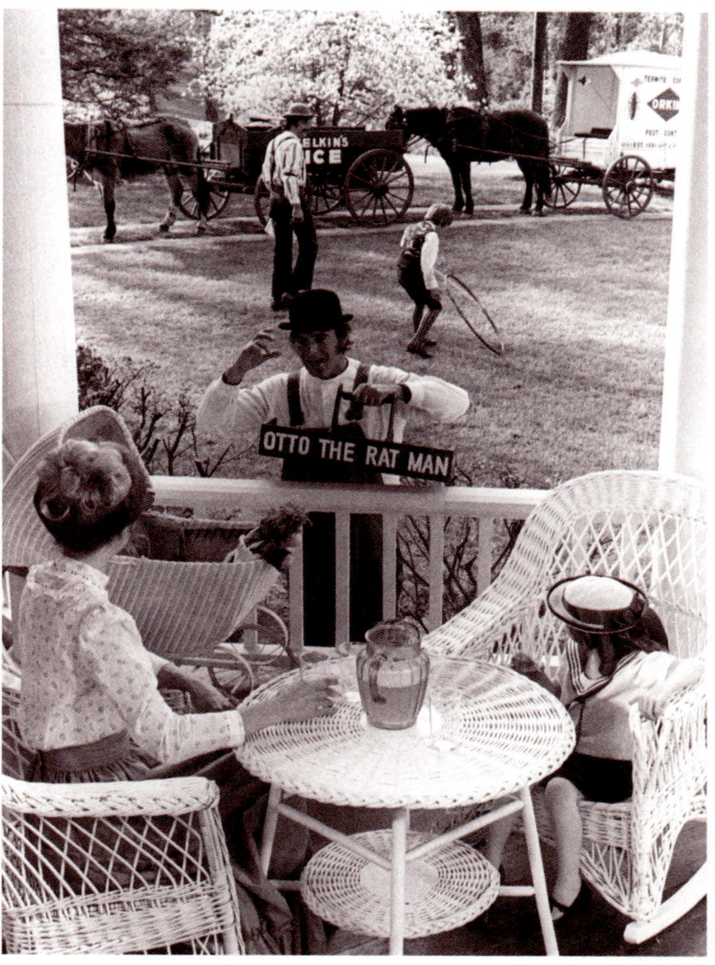

Otto traveled from farmhouse to farmhouse trying to convince neighbors to use his product. Bits of the Orkin company history were later reenacted for television.

From 1880 to 1898 over a half million Jews made their way to the United States, and in 1892, when Otto was five years old, the Orkin family was among them. By then, there were six children in the family: Jacob, Celia, Bertha, Otto, Harry, and an infant named Florence (also known as Fannie or Florsene). Exactly why this family decided to immigrate is not known, but the hostile, anti-Semitic conditions in and around Latvia at the time offer some clues. During the 1880s, for instance, the Russian authorities tried various means to eliminate the Germanic influence in Courland, and insisted that all citizens speak either Russian or Latvian; Jews were penalized for speaking Yiddish, their native language, which was written in Hebrew but borrowed from German and other languages. In 1881 the head of the Russian Orthodox Church began a series of campaigns of persecution and massacre to "solve the Jewish problem." Official Russian policy at the time did not allow anyone to depart from a country without a special government permit, and disobedience was considered a criminal offense. However, in January 1882 a notice was published that the Jews could immigrate to the western front of Russia and the government would not interfere. Within months, in an effort that all but forced Jews to consider leaving their homes, the Russian government began to expel Jews from rural villages, driving them into cities where jobs were scarce and they were usually unwelcome. Many small towns were reclassified as villages and closed to Jews; in fact, Jews who left their village for any reason were often unable to return. The threat of military conscription for their three sons must have worried Hessel and Annie Orkin. According to government law, males between the ages of twelve and twenty-five were required to serve in the Russian army for twenty-five years, and the law particularly discriminated against Jewish males. In 1890, the year the Orkins left Latvia, their oldest son, Jacob, turned thirteen.

Any one of these hostile conditions was reason enough for Hessel Orkin and his family to sell everything they had, leave Latvia, and make the long, often dangerous, two-year journey to America, first through Germany and then to New York City. The fact that the entire family immigrated at the same time is a tribute to Hessel's success as a farmer, because he obviously had saved enough money to pay for everyone to travel together. According to some estimates, the trip may have cost the Orkin family nearly four hundred dollars, a remarkable sum at the time for a family that likely considered itself poor. Many families could only afford to send the father or an oldest son to America, where he would work and send money back to the remaining family members to pay for their own journeys. It could take years, even decades, for families to be reunited. Hessel and Annie Orkin were apparently determined to keep their family together, and they succeeded.

When they arrived in the United States in 1892, the Orkin family probably stayed with relatives named Oser, Orkin, or Kramer in New York or New Jersey until Hessel could buy some land and resume farming. He quickly settled on six acres in a rural community called Lockport in the Lehigh Valley of eastern Pennsylvania, not too far from some of Annie's relatives in Allentown. The hilly, wooded homestead was nothing like the flat countryside of Latvia, but the surrounding Pennsylvania Dutch neighbors spoke German-English, which may have reminded the Orkins of home. The farm was only a short distance from the Lehigh Valley Railroad, which ran along the south side of the Lehigh River canal. There was a lock on the north shore of the canal, which gave Lockport its name and also made barge traffic and transportation possible. And while Otto was growing up, the railroad maintained a stop-on-demand passenger station in Lockport, an ideal situation for a young man who would one day travel frequently from home to make his fortune.

The Orkin farm was located on the north side of the road that ran in front of the property. The modest, two-story frame house faced south. As they had done in Latvia, the Orkins planted fruit trees around their farm, something not usually noted in the Lehigh Valley. In addition to the horse shed and workshop, the property also included a goat shed, a poultry house, and an outhouse. Across the road were two neighboring farmsteads and a blacksmith's shop. Further north up the road stood a one-room schoolhouse. Records show that Otto and his siblings attended this school, where one teacher often taught students of many ages and grade levels. As an adult, Otto sometimes claimed that he only had a third- or fourth-grade education, but the 1890 census shows that Otto was "at school" when he was at least thirteen years old. The census also states that he could read, write, and speak English, even though everyone who knew Otto would agree that he always spoke with a very heavy accent.

As an adult, Otto sometimes claimed that he only had a third- or fourth-grade education. . . . He always spoke with a very heavy accent.

By 1900, only eight years after coming to the area, Hessel Orkin owned his farmstead mortgage-free. Though he was known as a quarrelsome man who often disputed property lines with his neighbors, everyone acknowledged that Orkin earned money through a most novel way of dairy farming: Hessel would breed heifers, and when they were ready to freshen, he would "lend" them to a farmer to feed in exchange for the farmer getting the milk. This arrangement worked particularly well for small farmers who only had an acre or two of land. The heifer would be bred three months after giving birth, and Hessel would get the calf. A heifer, which cost forty to forty-five dollars, would eventually produce seven to nine calves, worth about seven or eight dollars each. This meant a 15 to 20 percent annual return to Hessel as long as he got a calf. Eventually, he sold the cow, too. Hessel's grandchildren once declared that their grandfather "mated cows" for a living. And when he died, sometime around 1920, it was rumored that he had 140 cows "rented" out.

"Grandpa Hessel was a fine upstanding man," remembered a granddaughter, Ruth Orkin Miller, the oldest daughter of Harry and Ethel. "He would sit me on his knee and try to teach me the Hebrew alphabet. We would sit under the cherry trees on the side of the house and enjoy the beautiful flowers in the garden, such as peonies and bleeding heart. On the fence dividing the property from the street was sweet-smelling honeysuckle."

In addition to his unconventional cow business, Hessel turned to scrap metal to earn money, selling the contents of his junk piles for additional family income. Indeed, the 1890 census for Lehigh Township, Northampton County, lists Hessel's occupation not as "Farmer" but as "Junk Dealer." And after taking care of the children and the house, Annie Orkin also worked to bolster the family's coffers. It wasn't unusual to see Annie going door-to-door, peddling household items, piece goods, needles, pins, and anything else she could sell to help support her large family, which numbered anywhere from eight to fifteen family members including several in-laws and a handful of grandchildren, all living under one roof. Some days Annie would walk so far away from home that she would have to spend the night along the road, or perhaps in someone's barn or home before returning to her family the next day. Family stories about the feisty, determined matriarch often include the fact that Annie developed terrible bunions on her feet, and she always pointed to her long days of walking as the cause of her foot problems.

Whether or not Otto expressed an interest in exterminating wasn't important; killing rats was his designated family job.

The family's penchant for junk dealing and scrap metals was eventually passed on to the sons. Otto's older brother Jacob identified himself as a "Peddler" in 1890, and as a "Junk Dealer—Iron, Rubber and Rags" in 1910. And Otto's younger brother, Harry, started his own scrap business in nearby Slatington.

The way the Orkin family worked, it's pretty clear that the appearance of chaos—junk piles, crowded barns, pastures worn thin—masked a fairly orderly system that allowed the family to thrive. Each sibling had responsibilities and, from an early age, was expected to contribute to the family's well-being by taking care of younger children, picking up scrap metals, cooking and washing, gardening, helping with the cows, or keeping rats off the farm. It wasn't much fun, and it was never easy; health care was poor, and a few children inevitably died of childhood diseases. Annie lost a child who was born in America, and her daughters Bertha and Fannie each lost several children.

Whether or not Otto expressed a natural interest in exterminating wasn't important; killing rats was his designated family job. In the summer and fall of 1900, Otto accepted a welcome break from his routine and went to work in Allentown at the Globe Department Store for three dollars a week. He probably lived with nearby Oser family relatives.

But in 1901, when he was only fourteen years old, Otto saw a chance to leave the department store job and develop his rat poison business for good. Arsenic, now a prime ingredient in his poison mixture, was produced commercially for the first time in the United States in 1901. Otto borrowed fifty cents from his parents to buy a bulk amount of this poison powder. He experimented with the right proportions and mixing ingredients, and was known to consult with local apothecaries (now known as pharmacists) about formulas, since these early druggists were important sources not only of medicines but of recipes for poisons and pest control substances. Moreover, Otto could have obtained some rodenticide products from the Rose Exterminating Company out of Cincinnati, the extermination and poison mail-order company established by Solomon Rose around 1865, and considered one of the oldest pest control companies in the country. During Otto's youth the company was well known for developing a phosphorus rat paste used to kill rats, roaches, and mice, as well as a pyrethrum powder that was used to kill bedbugs, roaches, and body lice. With Otto's limited financial resources, however, it appears unlikely that Otto invested in other products in a crude attempt to do market research. Rather, his knowledge of pest control, it appears, came from his parents and his own experiments on the family farm.

And he ran with it. Gradually, the young Otto began to introduce his bags of poison to his Pennsylvania Dutch neighbors. Luckily, he understood their German.

"I offered to get rid of their rats," Otto once recalled in a newspaper interview.

"*Du bist verruckt* (you're crazy)," they told Otto. "*Was fuer die Ratzen? Wir haben die Katzen* (Who cares about rats? We have cats)."

"*Es kostet nicht* (for free)," he replied.

"*Komm' sie herein* (come on in)," they replied.

If the rat poison worked and the customer wanted another application, Otto would charge them a small amount the next time he dropped by.

From the moment Otto took his business on the road, he measured his poison into paper bags labeled "POISON" and bearing a sketch of a skull and crossbones. With his bags safely tucked away inside his black satchel, Otto traveled from farmhouse to farmhouse, trying to convince his neighbors to use his product. "I was timid, nervous," he remembered. Giving away his bags of poison for free was an introductory marketing ploy that Otto continued to use for many years and one that foreshadowed his future customer service approach ("I guarantee to rid your home, office or store of rats or mice BEFORE I get one cent"). And within six months after he started selling poison door-to-door, Orkin had regular customers. A one-pound bag, which contained enough poison to kill about seventy-five rats, sold for one dollar. There were so many rats, however, and so many customers who wanted the poison, that Otto soon raised his price to three dollars a bag.

"I wasn't very good at speaking the English language," he once said. "But when my customers saw what my product could do, it did my speaking for me."

There is some debate over how Otto developed his highly successful rat poison formula. Otto claimed to be "the sole manufacturer of the 'Orkin Method'—a powder guaranteed to rid any premises of rats and mice." His first rodenticides were arsenic and phosphorus paste, which he mixed with fresh baits such as fish, cheese, bread, sweet potatoes, cantaloupe, and meat. Some arsenic was coarse and grainy and easily detected by rats, so he also mixed it with flour, sugar, and a red coloring, so it could not be mistaken for flour in kitchens or pantries. The sharp particles of arsenic were irritating to the rats' paws; the rats would often ingest the poison while licking and cleaning themselves, and die. Otto's first label for the "Orkin Method" rat poison cans was printed in black and red on orange, and contained this message: "Orkin Method will do the work. It has never failed in any case. Beware of Imitations."

But according to *The Ratcatcher's Child—The History of the Pest Control Industry* by Dr. Robert Snetsinger, Otto wasn't the family's only or first rat exterminator.

"The Orkin family was related by marriage to David 'Red' Kramer (a brother-in-law to Otto's mother), who also had emigrated from Europe and settled in Slatington (Lehigh County) Pennsylvania, across the Lehigh River from Lockport," Snetsinger wrote.

"The Kramer family had been involved in formulating rat poisons in the 'Old World,' and according to one family member, one of Red Kramer's brothers formulated rodenticides in Germany. Shortly after 1890 Kramer began formulating and packaging a rat tracking powder and a phosphorus paste for rodent and cockroach control; Jacob Orkin, son of Hessel, soon joined him. Brother Otto was invited to join the twosome as a salesman in 1901. . . . The tracking powder that was peddled door-to-door, first in eastern Pennsylvania and later across much of the United States, was packaged by the Kramer/Orkin families. This enterprise at different times involved about a dozen nephews, nieces, sons-in-law, uncles, aunts, etc., some of whom later worked for the Orkin Company and established their own pest control firms.

"I wasn't very good at speaking the English language. But when my customers saw what my product could do, it did my speaking for me." —Otto Orkin

"The rodenticide was a formulation of arsenite, flour, sugar and vermilion coloring, costing about fifty cents to make six pounds. This quantity was packaged in a 'lard can' with a pink 'Kramer' label and sold for fifteen dollars. The phosphorus paste was marketed as 'Roach Doom' and purchased from a Detroit formulator."

There are several interesting points to be made here.

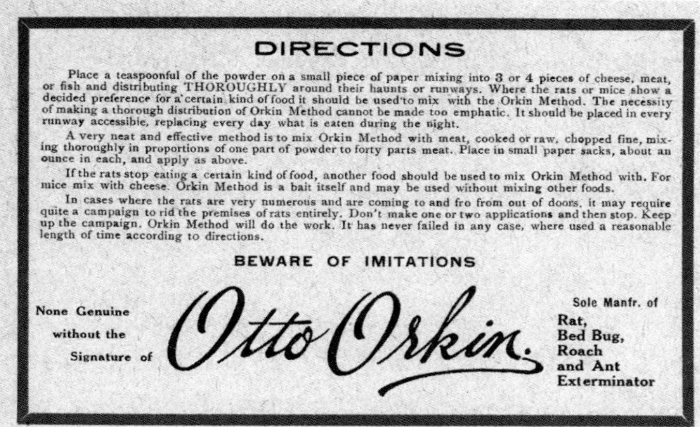

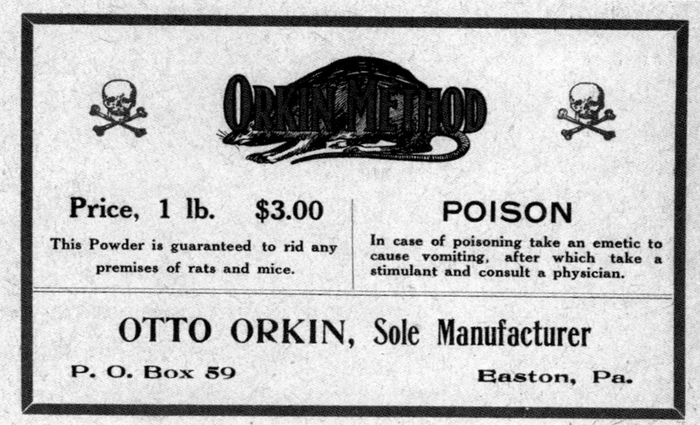

A label from the first commercial rat poison developed by Otto Orkin.

First, Otto always claimed that he was the "sole manufacturer of the Orkin Method"; he never gave a nod to any other family member as being a joint partner in his business and/or a coproducer of his poison formula.

Second, Otto's brother Jacob identified himself as a "Peddler" and a "Junk Dealer"—but never as an exterminator. Harry's daughter, Ruth Orkin Miller, remembers clearly why her father didn't go into the business: "In the beginning," she said, "Otto peddled the rat poison all over the country. Dad would accompany him, not knowing how the weather would be. Once he and Otto were in one of the northern states, and he didn't even have earmuffs. Harry was walking around in the tiny town with his ears uncovered, and a farmer in the general store said to him, 'Say, young fellow, you better cover your ears or they will freeze stiff and fall off.' He took the farmer's advice; however, when he got home, he decided to stay there. But that is why we didn't go into the pest control business. Harry came home and started to help his father in the junk business and Otto went on selling the rat poison. He was a very dandified person and wouldn't have liked the junk business. It was beneath him."

And third, census records show that the Kramer family did not immigrate to the United States until 1905, four years after Otto started peddling his rat poison door-to-door and about the time Otto was handing out business cards that read "Otto Orkin—Creators of Sanitation. Exterminators for Rats, Mice, Roaches and Vermin." Even if Otto had met Red Kramer before leaving Latvia, he was only five years old at the time; it's hard to imagine that he would have been interested enough to steal the family's rat poison recipe.

No one doubts that Red Kramer formulated rodenticides in Germany before he came to the United States. Pest control was a traditional Jewish profession in Eastern European countries, and knowledge of exterminating passed from generation to generation and eventually traveled to the New World. At one time over fifty members of the Kramer, Orkin, and Oser families were involved in the field of pest control, with at least twenty relatives working directly for Otto Orkin. But none of this suggests that Otto ever worked for Kramer, or that he stole the Kramer formula and used it as his own. It does help explain, however, some of the animosity that eventually developed between the family members when Otto became remarkably successful, and why some surviving members of the Kramer family continue to begrudge the Orkin legacy.

When Otto started out, however, the main factor in his success wasn't family connections. It was hard work, pure and simple. By living in Lockport just above the Lehigh Railway, which ran from New York City to Buffalo, Otto was able to hop on a train and travel to just about anywhere in the United States—north to Chicago and beyond and south to Philadelphia, Washington, D.C., and eventually Richmond, Virginia. "I chose Richmond to move to because it was the first city I came to on my way South," he said

Rat Catchers: *Pied Pipers*

In the seventeenth century an important element was added to the fight against vermin: the professional rat catcher. In Italy the rat catcher distinguished himself by carrying a pole topped with a square flag, decorated with rats and mice. Several dead rats hung from a sword that he carried at his side, and he often carried a box of poisoned lozenges. The Royal Rat Catcher in Great Britain wore a special costume of scarlet, embroidered with yellow figures of rats destroying wheat sheaves. In Shakespeare's time it wasn't unheard of for the seemingly lowly rat catcher to be an honored citizen of his town. Such an honor was given to the rat catcher who carried the most rat pelts—particularly the soft black rat fur used in the Middle Ages to make inexpensive coats and trim for garments. There were so many rat catchers during the Middle Ages that they were organized into guilds. However, their "secret" formulas and carefully guarded methods were often passed from father to son, or kept within the family circle.

The rat catcher, or Pied Piper as he came to be known, was depicted in drawings, paintings, and writings from the sixteenth through the eighteenth century by such notable artists as Shakespeare, Goethe, and Rembrandt. The medieval Pied Pipers were shown as almost carnival-like characters—with their colorful costumes, tall hats, and poles carrying both flags and rat carcasses. The Pied Piper was often seen playing a reed or flute, with a stream of rats following both the man and his music. It's more likely, however, that this romanticized version of the rat catcher had less to do with his music skills and more to do with the poisons he carried in his pockets or in the box by his side.

In 1803 Goethe wrote a poem called *Der Rattenfanger* (The Rat Catcher), which was put to music by everyone from Schubert to Berlioz:

I am the bard known far and wide,
The travell'd rat-catcher beside;
A man most needful to his town,
So glorious through its own renown.
However many rats I see,
How many weasels there may be,
I cleanse the place from ev'ry one,
All needs must helter-skelter run.

simply. But Otto was no fool. His research and travels had shown him that rat catchers and exterminators were already well established in many cities. There was Solomon Rose in Cincinnati, Cleveland, New York, Boston, Philadelphia, and Baltimore; Adolph Isaacsen and Son in New York; and Getz Exterminators in St. Louis and west of the Mississippi. Otto no doubt chose Richmond because it was a city without an established extermination business—and one where Otto could make his mark.

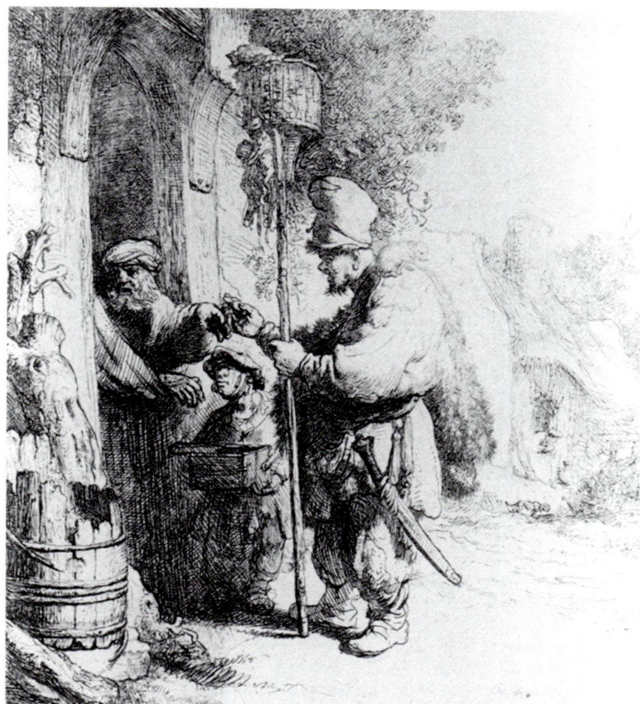

Rembrandt's etching Le Marchand de Mort aux Rats *(The Merchant of Death to Rats) shows a professional rat catcher of the seventeenth century. His tools were the sword hanging from his belt and the ferret on his shoulder. The dead rats hanging from the basket on top of the pole served as testimony to his skill. (Etching from Connecticut College's Wetmore Print Collection)*

As Otto traveled, he was never without his little black satchel, ready to knock on doors and convince customers to try his product. "Behind every door is a prospect," he always said. In cities Otto focused not on residential customers but on commercial clients—warehouses, grain stores, hotels, schools, and government buildings. He continued to pledge to guarantee customer satisfaction or he wouldn't charge them a dime, a pledge that became as important a trademark as his black satchel. If customers were still reluctant, he offered his service on a free-trial basis of thirty to sixty days. Within five years, Otto once boasted, he had accumulated an amazing list of satisfied customers, and he was making nearly five hundred dollars a week. With such receipts, it's no wonder that he had soon saved the remarkable sum of twenty-five thousand dollars—money that he would eventually use to expand his business and open his first office.

Before 1910 it's likely that Otto had already hired additional salesmen to peddle the Orkin Method and grow his customer base. And it was during a sales trip to Richmond that Otto began the second phase of his business: not just sales, but service, too.

A GROWING BUSINESS

In 1909 Otto knocked on the door of E. A. Saunders Jr., a food wholesaler in Richmond, Virginia. Saunders immediately challenged Otto to demonstrate his product by getting rid of the rats in his warehouse. "No one can get rid of my rats!" Saunders reportedly cried. Years later, Otto admitted that Saunders was "dubious. They said they'd tried everything, as had everyone else in those days. But they gave me the chance when I said I wouldn't charge anything. All I wanted was a recommendation."

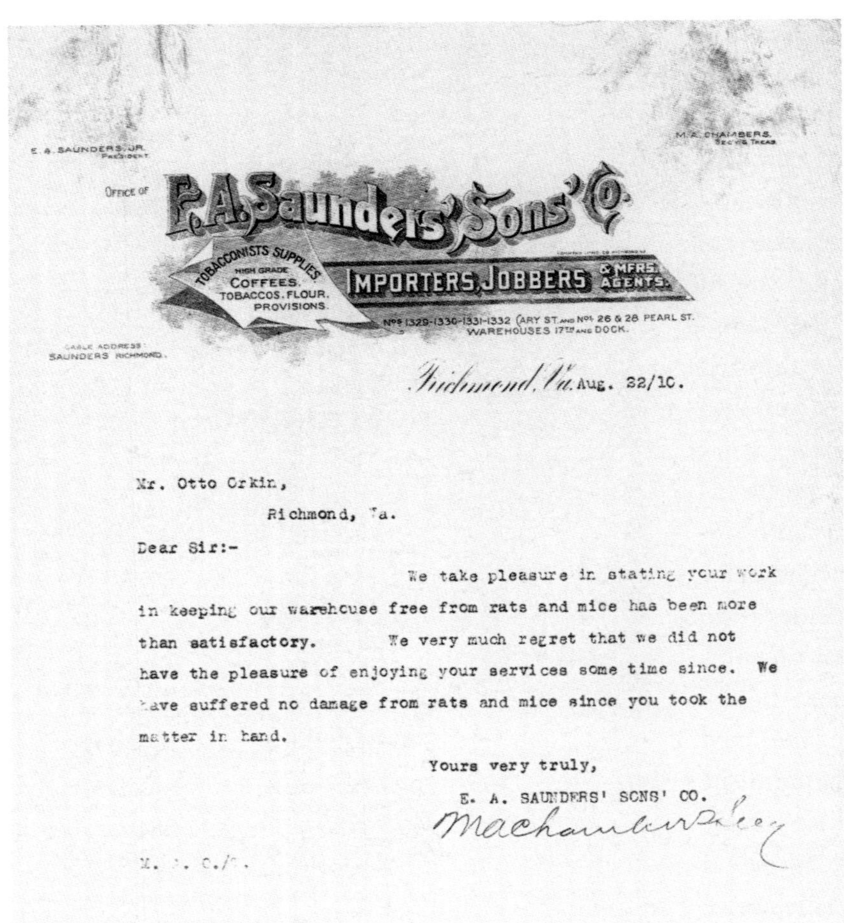

E. A. SAUNDERS, JR.
PRESIDENT

M. A. CHAMBERS.
SEC'Y & TREAS.

OFFICE OF
E. A. Saunders' Sons' Co.

TOBACCONISTS SUPPLIES
HIGH GRADE
COFFEES.
TOBACCOS. FLOUR.
PROVISIONS.

IMPORTERS, JOBBERS & MFRS. AGENTS.

NOS. 1329-1330-1331-1332 CARY ST. AND NOS. 26 & 28 PEARL ST.
WAREHOUSES 17TH AND DOCK.

CABLE ADDRESS:
SAUNDERS RICHMOND.

Richmond, Va. Aug. 22/10.

Mr. Otto Orkin,
Richmond, Va.

Dear Sir:-

We take pleasure in stating your work in keeping our warehouse free from rats and mice has been more than satisfactory. We very much regret that we did not have the pleasure of enjoying your services some time since. We have suffered no damage from rats and mice since you took the matter in hand.

Yours very truly,
E. A. SAUNDERS' SONS' CO.

E. A. Saunders' Sons' Company of Richmond, Virginia, was a very special customer in the history of Orkin Exterminating. They were the first customers for whom Orkin performed exterminating services as opposed to simply supplying rat poison. This letter dated August 22, 1910, shows their satisfaction with that service.

Otto quickly discovered that the rat problem was not confined to the Saunders warehouse but extended to the barn across the street, which housed the mules that pulled Saunders's food delivery wagons. Not only were the rats destroying the stored foods, but they were harassing the mules. The infestation was so heavy that Otto had to set traps every night and come back the next morning to remove the traps and dead rodents.

Within months, Otto had cleared every rat out of Saunders's warehouse and barns. Saunders was so thrilled, he gave Otto more than a recommendation. He hired Otto to regularly service the Saunders company and keep it pest-free, an agreement that lasted for the next twenty-five years.

Otto's pest control service business had begun. Instead of just selling rat poison, Otto began selling pest control as a service—the same way a utility company might sell gas or electricity. Over time, Otto's greatest commodity became his service to his customers, and weekly or monthly pest control service became his trademark. And as he developed his business, Otto's unique emphasis on regular service would distinguish Otto The Rat Man from other pest control businesses. He would be recognized as the one who initiated this business concept.

Otto no doubt saw dollar signs in the South. The weather was warmer, and the pests were everywhere. Until 1912 Otto serviced his accounts in Richmond as a "road agent"—a name then adopted by traveling pest control servicemen. Rats were his stock in trade, but Otto also guaranteed to get rid of roaches, mice, bedbugs, and many other objectionable pests by providing service on a regular basis to his customers. To control rats, he used three main methods: he shot them, trapped them, or poisoned them. For insect control, he used roach-powder bellows and a garden sprayer for bedbug treatments.

Monthly pest control, Otto once said, "costs but a few cents a day. It would be far more expensive to have us come out for what we call a 'clean-out' once or twice a year. Without regular service, pests are given a chance to get a real foothold."

If pests—particularly rats—did secure a foothold in any building serviced by Orkin, Otto would go to almost any lengths to find out why, including staying up nights in warehouses in order to observe the habits of rats and to study their "rat runs." Rats, Otto knew, marked their "runs" with urine and returned to similar tracks each night; by watching the rats and mice, he could figure out how to trap them. The practice came naturally to the young man who once hid behind flour sacks in his family attic, just to figure out why rats

Exterminators and Entomology

The Pied Piper image of the rat catcher made its way across the Atlantic Ocean to America, but the mystery of rodents was quickly displaced by new knowledge and science. An early group of farmers, ministers, physicians, and teachers in the Colonial Period began to study insects and pests, along with their economic impact. One of the most prominent individuals to study insects was William D. Peck, a Massachusetts naturalist who was born in Boston in 1763. In 1805 he became the first professor of natural history at Harvard University and continued to pursue his study of bugs. As a result, he became known as America's first native entomologist.

Entomology is the branch of zoology concerned with the study of insects and related animals such as spiders, mites, fleas, etc. Economic entomology includes rodents and other animals that are destructive or dangerous to the welfare of human beings. Entomology as a profession in the United States actually began in 1854 when two important events happened: Townsend Glover became the first entomologist to work in the new federal Bureau of Agriculture, and Asa Fitch went to work as an entomologist for the state of New York.

As knowledge in the field increased, rat catchers, or pest management professionals, as they now preferred to be called, had more information about the poisons and formulas that they used. And as the business grew, it attracted regulations and professional organizations. The oldest known group of exterminators and fumigators was the New York Vermin Exterminators Association, organized in 1910 by Nathan N. Sameth, one of the most highly respected pioneers of the pest control industry. (Like Otto Orkin, Sameth got his start in Richmond, Virginia, but there are no records to show that he was still operating in the southern city when Otto arrived in 1909.)

And just when Otto Orkin began to hand out his business cards, Congress enacted the first federal legislation affecting the pest control industry. The Federal Pure Food and Drug Act, effective in 1907, and the National Insecticide Act, approved in 1910, sought to control the overuse and unauthorized branding of commercial preparations for insecticides and fungicides. Before long, the entire industry would be subject to licensing requirements and governing regulations.

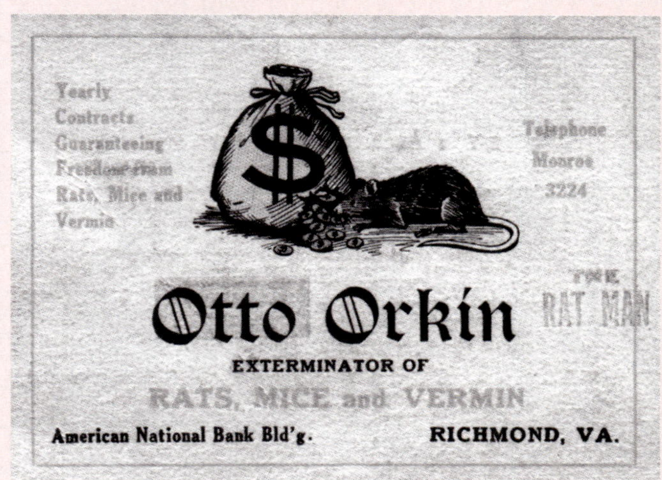

Otto's business card from his first office, which he established in Richmond around 1912.

kept avoiding his poisoned sandwich bait. "Thinking like a rat is indeed the only way to beat the wily rodents, experienced ratcatchers say," wrote Robert Hendrickson in a history of rats and men called *More Cunning Than Man.* Alone at night in the warehouses, Otto no longer hid behind flour sacks; instead, he often hid in a big box cut with peepholes big enough for him to peer out and observe the rats, but small enough to keep the rats from spotting him. Based on what he witnessed, Otto developed specific theories about where to place baits and traps; unlike other exterminators, he never indiscriminately tossed bait around. He continued to put rat poison in paper bags—eventually called "throw packs"—which was the perfect tease for rodents. The bags gave the mice something to gnaw and the sensation of finding something, which Otto knew they preferred. And the paper bags enticed the rats, which liked to investigate anything new in their surroundings.

If all else failed, Otto kept a double-barreled shotgun beside him, perhaps reminiscent of his rat-shooting days on the Lockport farm. Though Otto often resorted to shooting rats that eluded his traps, the practice came to a halt in Richmond one night when Otto got angry and fired both barrels at the stubborn rodents. Suddenly, there was a loud hissing noise, and the room filled with gas. Otto had killed the rats all right, but he had also zeroed in on a gas pipe. The damage was quickly contained by the Richmond Fire Department, and from then on Otto left the shotgun at home.

These long hours and late nights left Otto with some battle wounds—rodents twice bit him on the nose and the palm of his hand, and he had the scars to prove it. But these "shotgun watches" reinforced many things that Otto knew to be true about rats. They could climb walls, jump as high as three feet in the air, and swim half a mile with ease. They had an uncanny ability to recognize poison, unless it was disguised within an appetizing food like rolled oats, cornmeal, or peanuts. Since the baits were perishable, Otto had to service the traps as often as three to six times a week during the warm weather. To help trap rats in warehouses, Otto used wooden rat traps or steel rabbit traps baited with salmon, meats, and other cooked foods. For mice, he used snap traps with toasted bacon that he often cooked over a candle. Usually, Otto would set the traps in the evening after the employees had gone home, and he would pick up the traps and fresh kill the next morning, before his customer's employees returned to work. Otto knew that the sight of dead rats, and the smell of rat kill, could be really unpleasant. It went without saying that part of his customer satisfaction efforts included keeping the results of his work out of sight.

This unsavory aspect of his profession probably bothered Otto. How could he put a better spin on catching rats, on being a rat catcher? What if he appealed to a customer's desire for a cleaner, healthier environment—a public relations ploy that would instantly elevate what Otto did for a living, and also put the man behind the rat business in a more favorable light? Late one night in a Richmond department store, Otto laid the groundwork for what would become his "sanitation" campaign. Here, he observed rats literally bypassing his baited traps in favor of the poison-free morsels of food left by employees in their desk drawers! From then on, Otto told anyone who would listen that simple, sanitation practices—storing food in containers, keeping trash and food scraps out of buildings—would ease rat and vermin problems and help eliminate health problems. To bolster his claims, he obtained a one-paragraph letter from Dr. Ennion G. Williams, the health commissioner for the Commonwealth of Virginia in the early 1900s, and this is what he said: "Rats and mice not only destroy about ten million dollars of property a year in the United States, but it is also possible for them to carry contagion from the sick room to the kitchen and store room." Before long, Otto changed his business cards. He was still an exterminator, but now his company was described in red letters as "Creators of Sanitation."

How could Otto put a better spin on catching rats? By appealing to a customer's desire for a cleaner, healthier environment—a public relations ploy that would instantly elevate what he did for a living.

Business down south was so good, apparently, that in 1909 Otto opened his first unofficial office in Richmond. He lived in a five-dollar-a-month room in a boardinghouse at 501 North Fourth Street, where he mixed his pesticides and stored his service equipment. He kept his records in heavy paper files, alphabetically arranged in three dresser drawers: one drawer held "Paid Bills," another held "Current Bills," and the third held "Letters." His only business expenses were rent, telephone, chemicals, and traps.

When he wasn't in Richmond, Otto continued to live at home in Lockport, a single, twenty-two-year-old businessman who in the 1910 Census described himself as a self-employed "Traveling Salesman, Disinfectants." In 1911 Otto was listed as an exterminator and "Creator of Sanitation" with a post office address in Easton, Pennsylvania, a small town not far from Lockport. But no matter where he traveled, Otto began to collect proof of his customers' satisfaction by asking for letters of recommendation on their letterhead. He would then take the letters, have them photographed, and print them on linen-backed paper that was sturdy enough to show to potential customers. No doubt, these were the "Letters" that Otto kept filed away in the third drawer of his dresser in his Richmond boardinghouse. For example:

Virginia Bonded Warehouse Corporation—August 25, 1911

We take pleasure in advising that your work in our warehouse exterminating rats and mice has proven satisfactory in every respect. We contracted with you reluctantly, as we had very little faith in your proposition at the time you presented it to us.

We believe you have done everything and more than you claimed to do, and heartily recommend your system of ridding any building of rats and mice.

Smith, Moncure & Gordon, Attorneys At Law—May 2, 1911
I take pleasure in stating that you have complied fully with your promise to rid my premises of rats and mice, and I can recommend you to the citizens of Richmond generally along this line. It is a consolation to know we have somebody in the community who can protect us from this pest.

E. W. Gates & Son Co. Wholesale Grocers—May 10, 1911
When you took hold of our building three months ago, we were fairly overrun with rats and mice, and I must confess that I had no great confidence in your ability to do away with this pest. Within less than ten days' time, you had them exterminated, and now, after three months, I can safely say that you have lived up to your contract in every detail.

Your price, I must say, is very fair, and but a very small fraction of the expense to which we were put by the depredations of the rats and mice. I can recommend your services as a splendid investment to any business house which is bothered the way we were before employing you.

As this ad from the Richmond Times-Dispatch *(March 16, 1924) shows, Otto relished being called "the rat man." His wife, Dora, however, was embarrassed by it.*

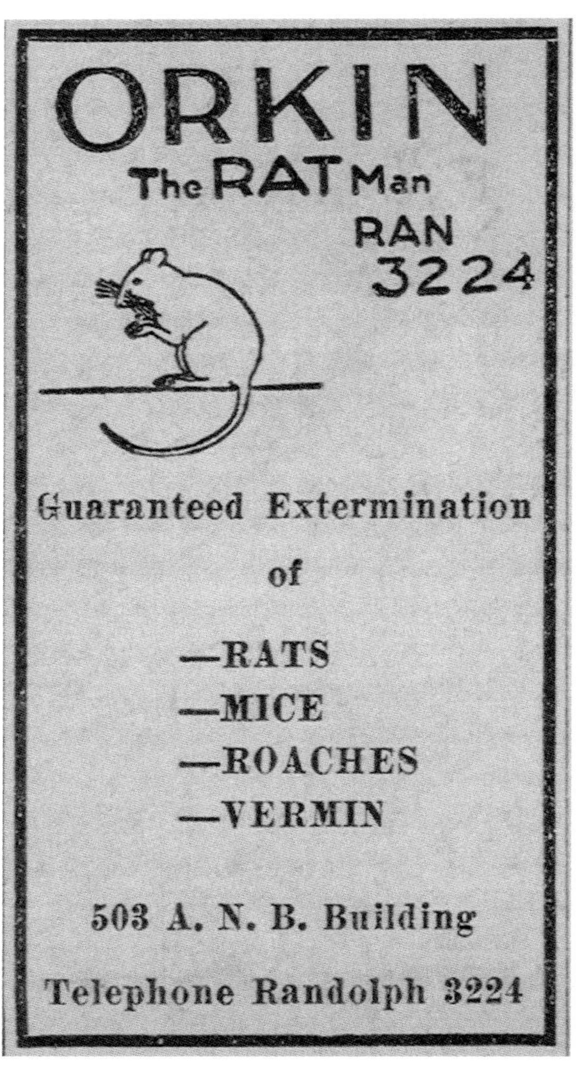

Otto wasn't content to merely copy the letters and use them as testimonials for his service. He often copied checks, too, to show that he had actually been *paid* for his services. "I continue to provide good service," he told prospective clients. "Otherwise, these customers would not continue to pay me."

Orkin's reputation as the professional rat exterminator of choice soon spread throughout Richmond. He was so popular that an unusual catch might lead to some publicity. On April 6, 1911, the local newspaper and one of Otto's customers, the *News Leader,* ran a story and a picture of a "saber-toothed rodent with tusks over an inch long" that Otto caught in the Chesapeake and Ohio warehouse building. "Otto Orkin, the professional rat exterminator, captured this curiosity and says it was the only rat of uncounted thousands he has killed that had such a remarkable dental formation." The rat's two front teeth had literally grown out of its mouth and curled around its head until the teeth looked like elephant tusks; in the newspaper article, a naturalist explained that the rat's teeth probably grew this way because the bottom and upper teeth didn't meet and the upper teeth couldn't be ground down by use. Otto preserved the rat's head in alcohol, and the newspaper ran a picture of it with the article, which cast Otto as something of a mysterious character who "keeps his methods to himself."

Otto clearly recognized the value of advertising, because the *News Leader* was one of his first customers. "We made a bargain," Otto explained. "The rats were eating the glue and paste, so the newspaper agreed to run my advertising in return for my extermination service."

By 1912 Otto had established an official office in the American National Bank Building at 1001 East Main, the heart of downtown Richmond. The location helped Otto make contacts with attorneys, bankers, businessmen, and members of the Richmond Chamber of Commerce, and gave his business a certain professional cachet that was hard to ignore. Otto had cultivated a reputation as a shrewd, if somewhat eccentric, businessman, one who dressed in expensive, handsome suits and fine leather shoes. Even his advertisements —this one from page 37 of the Richmond, Virginia, telephone directory— began to reflect his growing self-confidence, based no doubt on both his expertise and his growing list of satisfied customers:

OTTO ORKIN, Rat Exterminator AMERICAN NATIONAL BANK BUILDING

TELEPHONE 3224 MONROE RICHMOND, VA.

"Let me Rid Your Place of Rats and Mice. I can do it quickly and effectively and in a thoroughly sanitary way. **I GUARANTEE** *to rid your home, office or store of rats or mice* **BEFORE I** *get one cent."*

With his business thriving, Otto took some time to put his personal life in order. In 1912 he married Dora Levine, who was from the same Jewish community outside Allentown that the Orkin family belonged to. For most of their first year of marriage, Dora remained in Allentown with her family while Otto traveled back and forth to Richmond. It wasn't long, however, before Otto and Dora moved to Richmond and lived at 305 East Clay Street, in a boardinghouse that was operated by Dora's widowed sister, Bessie Baker. And though the family connection must have made Dora feel more comfortable about the move, it's fairly clear that Otto Orkin's bride wasn't prepared for the reception they received.

Otto, after all, absolutely relished being called "The Rat Man," a moniker that more and more Richmond citizens were beginning to attach to this energetic, determined young businessman. But on Friday nights, when Otto parked his truck in front of a movie theater with the sign—*Orkin The Rat Man*—prominently displayed to get everyone's attention, Dora was totally embarrassed. She was happy to be identified as Mrs. Otto Orkin, but being greeted as "The Rat Lady" was a bit too much for Dora.

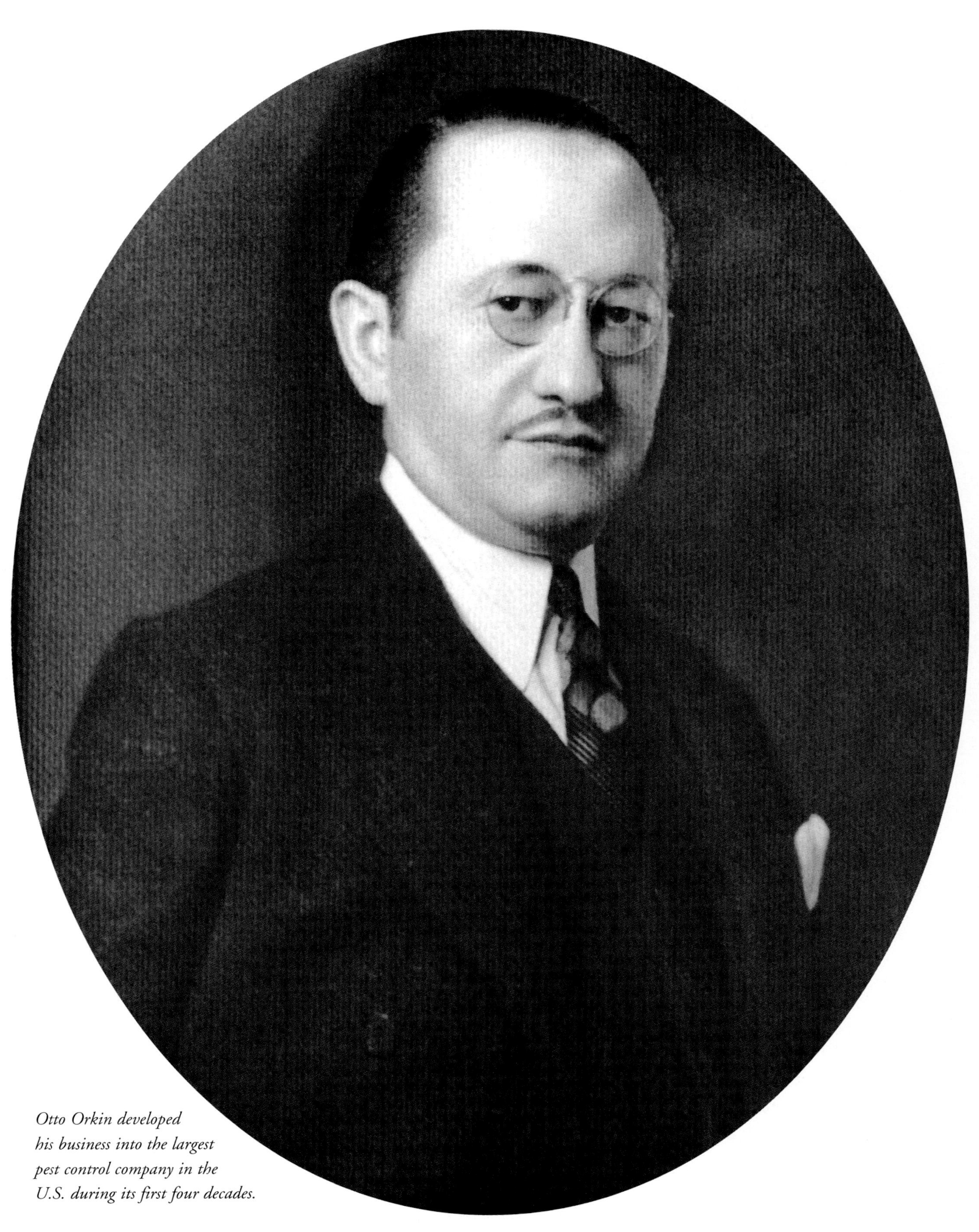

Otto Orkin developed his business into the largest pest control company in the U.S. during its first four decades.

Chapter 2

1913 to 1940:
Building the World's Largest Pest Control Company

From city halls to executive mansions, from family homes to thriving businesses, Otto Orkin began to expand his pest control business. Long known as "The Rat Man," Otto gradually expanded into general pest and termite control for both residential and commercial customers, increased his staff of service technicians, and secured his first government contract. Forever trusting his instincts, Otto headed further south, expanding his branch system and establishing exterminating services in state after state. "Bugs go south," Otto reasoned. In Atlanta, Georgia, Otto established the new headquarters for his Orkin Exterminating Company, developed the Orkin diamond logo, and cemented his reputation for "satisfaction guaranteed" service. His push for sales and advertising advancements reflected business patterns and maxims that he followed his entire business life. By 1940, Otto Orkin's quest to make Orkin the world's largest pest control company was firmly in place.

From his office at the American National Bank Building in Richmond, Otto began to build what would become the world's largest pest control company. The cornerstones of his growing enterprise were based on what Otto often described as "hard thinking, persistent salesmanship and advertisement"—not to mention complete customer satisfaction. And as he sought to develop every aspect of his business, these principles became apparent to all who knew Otto Orkin.

His company letterhead, for instance, carried the "Orkin The Rat Man" trademark at the top of the page, with the names of prominent customers printed along the side. Otto used the letterhead for his contracts, like the one he presented on May 11, 1914, to executives at the First National Bank Building:

> I will agree to exterminate the rats, mice, roaches and waterbugs from the First National Bank Building, also the Whitlock Building Annex, for one year for the sum of Four Hundred and Twenty Dollars ($420), payable at the rate of Thirty-Five Dollars ($35) per month, provided the work is satisfactory. This Agreement is entered into "conditionally" that the work is entirely satisfactory to the First National Building Corporation, otherwise this agreement becomes null and void.

As Otto worked to secure the business of hotels, banks, and warehouses throughout Richmond, his efforts caught the attention of City Hall. In 1915 the Richmond Administrative Board hired The Rat Man to fight the rats that infested City Hall, an administrative maze of a building with Gothic architecture. Not only did Otto rid City Hall of its rat problem, but his work so impressed city officials that they signed a contract with him for monthly service. The local newspaper, the *Richmond Times-Dispatch*, announced the transaction with these headlines:

"Professional Rat Killer Gets Contract From City"
"Otto Orkin Agrees To Rid City Home of Rodents and Insects"
"Will Receive $25 A Month"
"City Hall Clerks Praise His Workmanlike Job in Ridding That Building of Pests, Which Were Said To Be as Large as Kittens"

The verbose but unusually descriptive and highly amusing story that followed illustrated the extent of the rodent infestation. And in a day when little was known about extermination, it points out the public's near-reverent appreciation of Otto's talents:

> Otto Orkin has the most peculiar avocation in Richmond. His business is contracting for the extermination of rodents and insects that infest private and public buildings, mostly the latter.
>
> Yesterday the Administrative Board awarded to Mr. Orkin a contract for exterminating the rats, mice, roaches and water bugs that are colonized in several buildings that comprise the City Home. For this work he will receive during the year the sum of $300, payable in $25 monthly installments.
>
> Chief Clerk W. W. Dunford, of the Administrative Board, paid an eloquent tribute yesterday to Mr. Orkin's efficiency, as evidenced by the thoroughgoing manner in which he rid the City Hall of the rodents that one time infested that spacious Gothic pile.
>
> "I don't know how he did it, but he did," said Mr. Dunford. "It used to be so bad in this office that it was impossible to leave anything on the tables or desks overnight without coming back in the morning to find it gnawed to pieces. The rats would eat the glue out of the backs of books and gnaw away the mucilage brushes. They had a particular fondness for postage stamps, and would invariably gnaw them to pieces if we failed to lock them up. Now, as far as I know, there isn't a rat in the building."
>
> Assistant Clerk J. B. Puller corroborated Mr. Dunford in the statement that the City Hall rats often attained the size of full-grown kittens.

> A. C. Brown, statistical clerk of the board, suspected that some of the rats that frequented the board's office were addicted to ink-drinking, having frequently found the ink wells half empty, surrounded by the desk wreckage that bore evidence to another stamp orgy.
>
> Whatever their special tastes, it was well known that the City Hall rats, in point of stature and rapaciousness, were the Huns of the city's rodent colony. The Hustings Court was afraid to store its records in a basement room because of their anticipated depredations. They stalked through the silent corridors, devouring everything except departmental reports.
>
> Those who have seen Mr. Orkin work say that he sprinkles a certain green powder where the rodents are accustomed to roam. After that, they don't roam.

With the success of his City Hall contract well publicized, Otto next received a call from Virginia Governor Henry Carter Stuart to get rid of all rodents in the Executive Mansion. His contract included one of Otto's favorite bargaining and public relations chips—payment *after* satisfied service. "In consideration of a cash payment to be paid within six months *after* the premises becomes ratless, Otto, The Rat Swatter, contracted to exterminate every rodent that infests the Executive Mansion," read one newspaper report. "For many years, robust and vandal rodents have held high carnival within the actual precincts of the state home of Virginia's executives. It would appear now, however, that a period is about to be placed upon their further activities. Professor Otto, the rat killer, has taken a vow that no rat shall remain within the mansion building following cock-crow time today."

The green powder that Otto used in both City Hall and the Executive Mansion—a certain sugarcoated arsenic called Paris Green—was one of the many ways in which Otto would get rid of rats. His original tracking powder formula was "one-half pound arsenic to one pound powdered sugar and the rest flour to fill a one-gallon paint can"; he added "coloring" to ensure that the mixture was not confused with flour. The poison mixture was combined with ground cheese or food scraps. But not just any food scraps. Otto had a theory that rats were attracted to food that had been handled by human hands. Instead of just using scraps and wastes from grocery stores, he preferred to furnish galvanized pails to restaurants. The kitchen staff members were asked to scrape leftover food into the pails, which meant the scraps carried the scent of a human touch. Orkin paid the restaurants for each pail of waste food and supplied them with another pail. The Orkin servicemen would pick through the scraps to get their bait and mix it with the rat poison. Smelly, slimy, and unappealing, picking through food scraps was one of the servicemen's least favorite assignments.

During his first twenty years in business, Otto clearly focused on rat control. And something about those down and dirty, try-anything-once early days of his business often made Otto nostalgic. "I used to go into a cellar armed with a baseball bat to clean out the rats," he once said in a newspaper interview, a look of sheer wonder crossing his face. "When it comes to exterminating household pests—that's just business to me. But when we deal with rats—that's a personal affair. I wasn't the first to fight the rats, but I was the first to declare war on a large scale."

In time Otto moved into general pest control—services to exterminate not just rats and mice but roaches, fleas, ants, moths, bedbugs, silverfish, earwigs, and something called the confused flour beetle. To get rid of insects and roaches, Otto combined pyrethrum, sodium fluoride, and borax or ground pumice stone. For ants, he boiled together sodium fluoride, arsenic, sugar, or glucose. Sometimes he recommended spraying the ants and fleas with a mixture of carbolic acid, mineral spirits or kerosene, and perfume to kill the odor. Kerosene, Otto knew, was a successful larvicide used to control flies and mosquitoes.

"When it comes to exterminating household pests—that's just business to me. But when we deal with rats—that's a personal affair." —Otto Orkin

It's important to remember that the extermination business was still an unregulated industry. There were not yet any state licensing requirements or health department permits for exterminators, though federal legislation had been developed to try to govern the use of hazardous chemicals around food. But in truth, anyone could produce a poison and call himself a rat catcher. "It was possible for any man with a smattering of exterminating knowledge, a few tools, and a little bait to open up for business," wrote Dr. John J. Davis, of the Department of Entomology at Purdue University, in his 1961 essay "A Contribution to the History of Commercial Pest Control." And according to Davis, the exterminators' techniques and applications were just as varied:

> In the early days, there was no such thing as flashlights; only candles were used for light when getting into dark places to do exterminating work. Equipment and materials used were somewhat crude. We used the old formula of roach powder, which was known as pyrethrum powder instead of Persian insect powder. Other products included phosphorous paste . . . used as a control for the large American Roach and the Black Oriental Roach . . . also as a poison for rat and mice bait, in addition to a mixture of finely ground white arsenic. We also packaged a bedbug powder, which was a pure pyrethrum power. In addition to this, we had a bedbug poison liquid, which contained corrosive sublimate, wood alcohol and turpentine. It was a very poisonous substance and could not be

> sprayed or come in contact with metals; it had to be applied with a brush and it was painstaking work.
>
> Fumigation was practiced with sulphur dioxide commonly used, particularly for bedbug work. Hydrocyanic acid gas was introduced for indoor structural fumigation. On smaller jobs, spraying was done with a solution of corrosive sublimate, ether and wood alcohol. This liquid was placed into a one-quart bottle which had a rubber atomizer inserted (later described as a turkey baster) and sprayed into baseboards, moldings, joints of beds, etc.

From the beginning Otto had a conservative streak when it came to poisons. He apparently believed, and instructed his assistants, that all baits and liquids should be applied with care and positioned according to information Otto knew to be true about the rodents' or insects' behavior. Though many of his pest control contemporaries dabbled in the practice, Otto apparently never relied on the use of ferrets to flush out rats from their nesting places or to bring out rat carcasses. Otto and his servicemen obviously preferred chemicals, which were cheaper to obtain than ferrets and worked faster. As a rule, Otto appears to have avoided pest control chemicals when they were first introduced, preferring to wait until more was known about their success rate, danger, and proper application. He often avoided some chemicals completely—for instance, he was one of the last exterminators to use strychnine, because he thought it was unsafe. But in addition to his hand dusters and fireplace bellows, it appears that Otto did use a competitor's applicator—the Getz insect powder blower. Offered to the public in a marketing campaign after the 1904 St. Louis World's Fair, the Getz duster was no bigger than a soup can. But it was recognized as one of the most convenient and economical distributors of powered materials in the extermination field.

When Otto Orkin started his business, exterminating was still an unregulated industry. No state licensing or health department permits were required for exterminators.

With the use of such techniques, Otto continued to add clients to his growing business in the Richmond area. In December 1916 the Miller & Rhodes Department Store signed a contract for six hundred dollars per year. The Jefferson, one of Richmond's largest and more prestigious hotels, signed a contract in October 1918 for three hundred dollars per year. The Rat Man serviced the Confederate Soldiers Home in Richmond, and provided free service to the Jewish synagogues and some Christian churches. In the 1920 census Otto identified himself as a "Vermin Exterminator," and his success in getting rid of vermin from rats to bugs had won him the business of most of the hotels, hospitals, feed mills, baking companies, and warehouses in Richmond.

A NEPHEW ARRIVES

By now Otto was working eleven to twelve hours a day, and every weekend. His Orkin accounts were scattered from Pennsylvania to Washington, D.C., and on to Richmond, and he employed a team of service employees to keep his business running: Horace Byrd, Paul Mende, Walter Moore, and G. J. Walpert. But when a twelve-year-old nephew named Theodore Oser came from Pennsylvania to live with Otto and Dora in Richmond in 1916, Otto began a personal and business relationship that would play a unique role in the development of the Orkin company. Ted, or Theo as he was called, became Otto's shadow—a young boy who would become not only Otto's confidant but also his highly trusted business partner, someone constantly by his side as Otto developed and grew the company.

Ted was the second son of Otto's sister Bertha and her husband, Barnet Oser, who apparently moved with their four children to live with Otto's parents in

Ted Oser: *An Early Orkin Man*

Ted Oser was only twelve years old when he came to live with his aunt and uncle in Richmond, and only fourteen years old when he started working for his family's pest control company. Once a week Ted was excused early from school to treat for bedbugs at the Confederate Soldiers Home. Years later, Ted still remembered the old-fashioned bellows that he used to spray roach powder and the garden-variety sprayer he used to treat for bedbugs with a special concoction of kerosene, carbolic acid, oil of mirbane, and oils of eucalyptus or citronella to cover the odor. On Tuesday nights during the summer months, Ted, Otto, and the other servicemen would often go to Richmond's city dump and practice shooting rats with .22-caliber rifles to improve their aim. Otto's infamous shot at a gas line in a Richmond warehouse had slowed his use of guns to kill rats, but he still resorted to the practice when he had to, going so far as to get special permission from the city to use a silencer on the rifles.

Clearly a surrogate son to Otto, Ted Oser was hiring and making management decisions for the company before he turned eighteen. From then on, his contribution to the company and the industry was almost as great as Otto's, but he never ran the company, and he was never given the title of president. Though he performed every conceivable job at Orkin—from serviceman to branch manager to executive—Ted Oser was eventually displaced by Otto's biological sons.

Years later, when Ted Oser was asked to revisit the history of Orkin's expansion, he judged it shrewdly, if not harshly. Otto's contract with the U.S. government for the Wilson Dam project, he once wrote in a letter, changed everything for his uncle. "It was this contract for Rat Control on Wilson Dam in Alabama that caused Mr. Orkin to stop off in Atlanta and when he found no one in the exterminating business, he decided that we would open up a branch. If not for this contract, I doubt if Mr. Orkin would have done anything other than staying in Virginia to run his little 'Rat Factory.' As far as I am concerned, this is the (contract) that made Pest Control History."

Lockport around 1910. It wasn't an easy time. The house was crowded, and eventually the Oser sons were sent to live with relatives: Maurice, the oldest son, went to Philadelphia to live with his paternal grandparents, and Ted moved in with Otto and Dora in Richmond. By now Hessel Orkin was openly feuding with his neighbors over a strip of land between the Orkin family farm and a new road that ran south of Hessel's property line. When the road that previously ran in front of the Orkin property was replaced, Hessel's property became landlocked, and Hessel was never able to reach a settlement with his neighbors. The house burned down in 1918, and Hessel and Annie moved in with their son Harry, who had started a successful hauling and junk business in nearby Slatington. The Orkin farm was abandoned and stood empty until Hessel died and it was sold in 1926. Ironically, Peter and Grace Hnath bought the property, the son-in-law and daughter of the family involved in the feud with Hessel over egress to the new road.

Ted was barely settled in Richmond and enrolled in school before Otto put him to work. And why not, his uncle must have reasoned. After all, Otto was Ted's age when he started peddling his bags of rat poison door-to-door in the hills surrounding Lockport, and barely fourteen when he started his own business. He immediately set his nephew on a similar path, teaching him to observe rats and how to use chemicals effectively. By 1921 the Richmond Directory listed Otto Orkin as manager of Orkin The Rat Man, with Theo Oser listed as assistant manager. Ted was only seventeen years old, and already he was helping manage and run the business, and even making some personnel decisions. While on a service run to Washington, D.C., in 1921, Ted hired Cliff Green to work in service and sales out of Richmond. Ted's hire was a good decision; Green would have a long and distinguished career with Orkin, and he helped the company improve its sales. According to sketchy records, Orkin's gross annual sales were more than sixty thousand dollars when Green came to work for the company.

As Otto's business grew, he had less and less time for Dora and the traditional home life she had always wanted. Increasingly, Dora was bored, restless, and unhappy. In 1921, after nine years of marriage and no children, Otto and Dora divorced. When he was younger, Ted would occasionally remark that his aunt left Otto because she hated being called "The Rat Lady" by the women in Richmond. The situation was no doubt more complicated than that. Dora, for instance, was an Orthodox Jew and wanted a home that reflected her Jewish traditions; Otto put business ahead of Jewish observance and was rarely home with Dora to start the Sabbath observance on Friday nights. After the divorce Dora returned to Allentown; she never remarried and continued to attend the same temple as many of Otto's relatives.

Ted continued to live and work with Otto. For several years after the divorce, Otto lost some interest in his work, and business was slow. In 1922 and 1923 city directories list G. J. Walpert as manager of Orkin The Rat Man, with Ted as assistant manager. Family rumors from this time period describe how Otto even tried to sell the business to a lawyer, but the deal fell through when it was suggested that the lawyer had embezzled money from a client to finance the deal. At one point, Ted grew bored just working with his uncle, and started his own company in Richmond called "Sanitary Mop & Specialty Co." while he continued to work for Otto. But by 1924 Otto's enthusiasm had returned, he was again listed as the manager of his company, and he was looking to expand the company even further.

As a mentor to Ted, Otto presented himself as a successful, ambitious businessman, but one who obviously had some eccentric tendencies. When it came to advertising, Otto insisted on having his ads placed at the top of the page—in telephone directories or newspapers. He insisted on easy-to-remember phone numbers for all of his offices. When it came to telephone calls, he expected all business to be completed in three minutes—no longer. He was a shrewd businessman who could calculate figures in his head, but he had little understanding of the basic principles of accounting. Soft-spoken and polite in public, Otto was not above using some harsh words in the privacy of his own office. And it's been said that no one was more customer-conscious than Otto Orkin. He was not a fast talker or a slick showman, nor did he make expansive promises. But he wanted customers to be satisfied and retained, arguing that a satisfied customer was Orkin The Rat Man's best advertisement.

But above all, Otto was a salesman—someone who inspired confidence and trust from customers and employees alike. He believed in cutting the price, if necessary, to get a prestigious account, knowing that an important and satisfied client would attract more customers. He encouraged reciprocity—in other words, Orkin did business with companies who did business with Orkin. Otto never hid the fact that he would often eat in restaurants in order to get to know the staff and eventually the owner or manager. And once he secured them as Orkin customers, Otto would start eating at another restaurant, looking for that next satisfied customer.

Toward that goal, Otto gave these instructions to the service and salespeople:

Smile!
Keep your shoes shined.
Thank the customer.
Be sure the customer knows your name, and you know theirs.
If the customer likes you, they will like the company.
Talk when the customer is listening. If he is not listening, "shut up."
Keep your customers happy and you will have no collection problems or bad debts.
Behind every door there is a customer.

OTTO'S FIRST GOVERNMENT CONTRACT

One particular satisfied customer would prove invaluable to Otto in 1925, when he got a call from the Army Corps of Engineers about a serious rat problem at the Wilson Dam in the Muscle Shoals area of northwest Alabama. Named for President Woodrow Wilson and started in 1918 by the U.S. Army Corps of Engineers, it was the first dam constructed on the Tennessee River. At the time, the $46.6 million dam was needed to provide electricity for two plants that provided nitrate for ammunition during World War I. At the beginning of the project, construction was rapid, and the dam project employed more than five thousand people in various shifts, with work continuing around the clock.

By 1925 the entire area had a tremendous rat infestation problem. Thousands of laborers brought their lunches or dinners to work, which

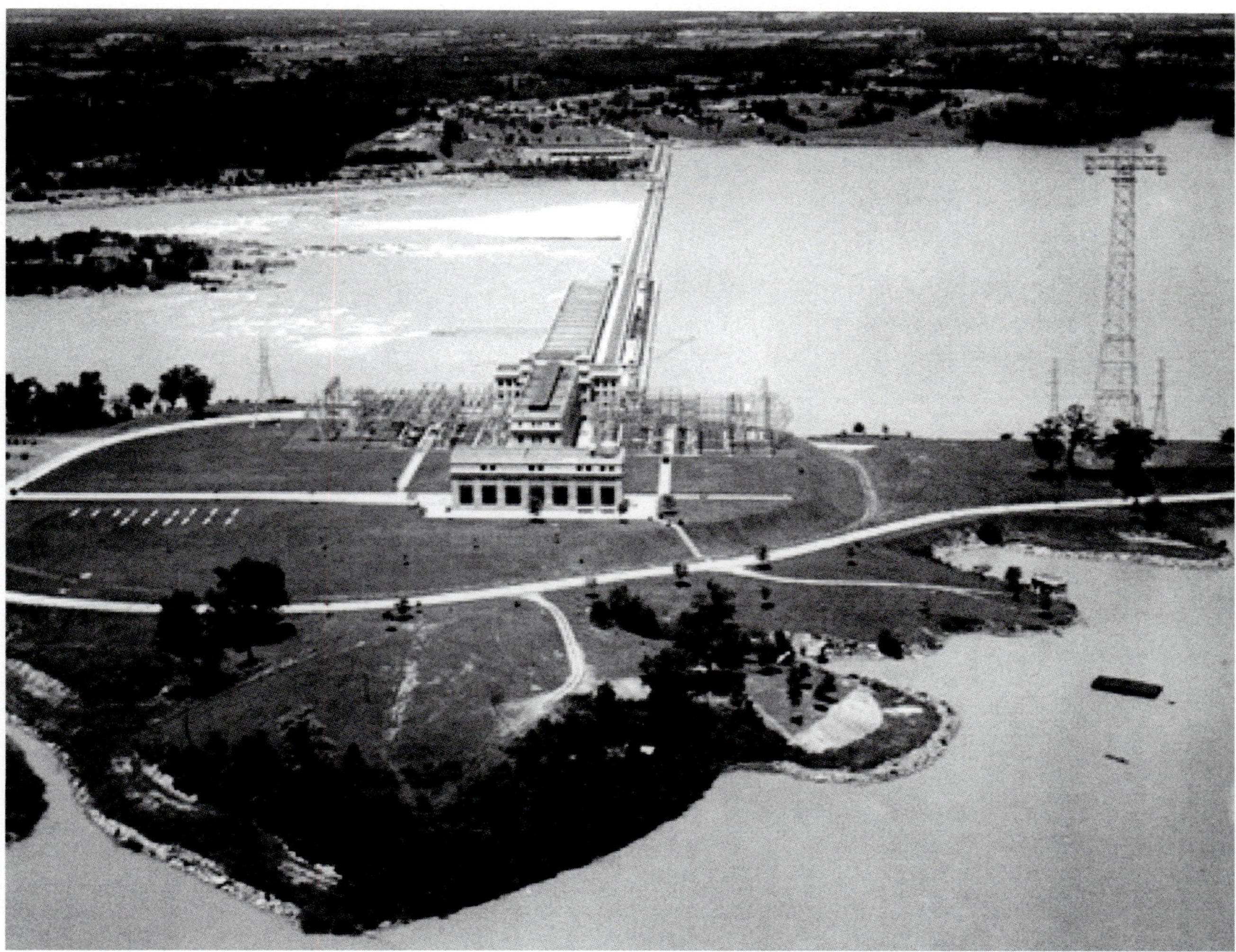

Wilson Dam. Otto stopped off in Atlanta on his way to Muscles Shoals to carry out his contract for rat control on the Wilson Dam. When he found no one in the exterminating business in Atlanta, he decided to open up a branch there. Ted Oser, once Otto's right-hand man, said, "If not for this contract, I doubt if Mr. Orkin would have done anything other than staying in Virginia to run his little 'rat factory.'"

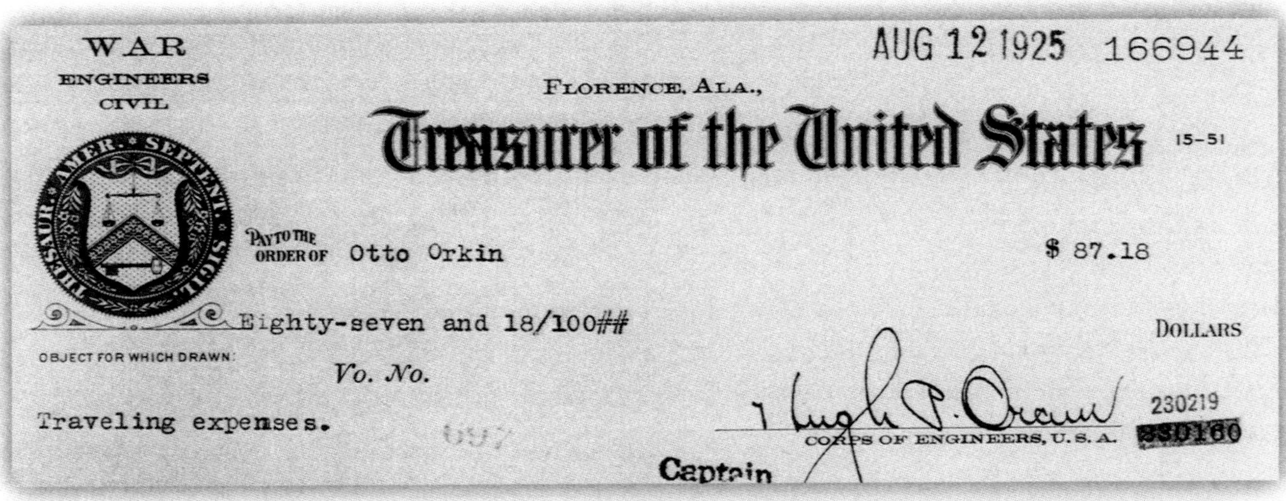

WAR
ENGINEERS
CIVIL

AUG 12 1925 166944

FLORENCE, ALA.,

Treasurer of the United States 15-51

PAY TO THE ORDER OF Otto Orkin $ 87.18

Eighty-seven and 18/100## DOLLARS

OBJECT FOR WHICH DRAWN:

Vo. No.

Traveling expenses. 697

230219

CORPS OF ENGINEERS, U.S.A. 330160

Captain

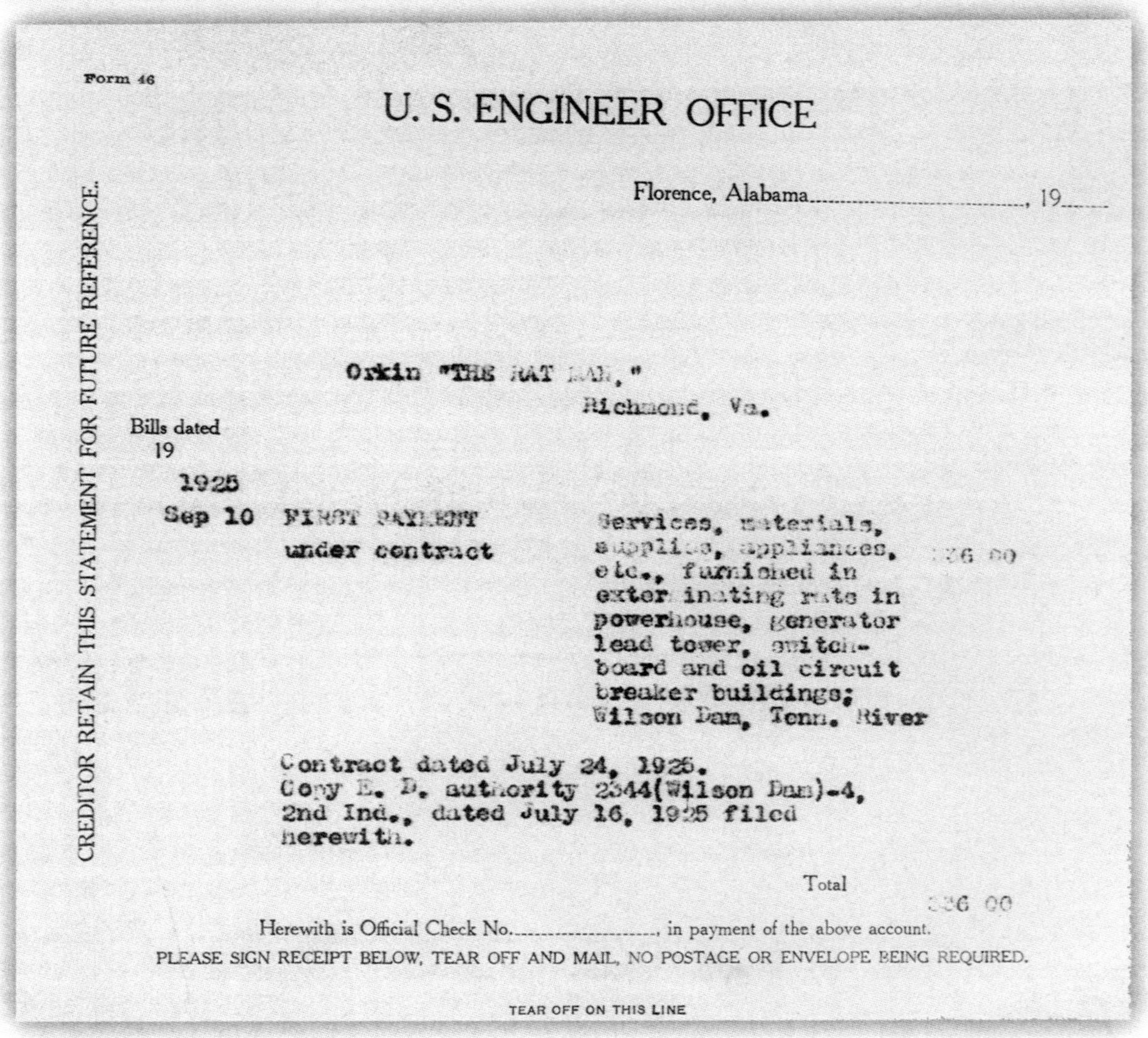

Form 46

U. S. ENGINEER OFFICE

Florence, Alabama............................., 19......

Orkin "THE RAT MAN,"
Richmond, Va.

Bills dated
19

1925
Sep 10 FIRST PAYMENT under contract

Services, materials, supplies, appliances, etc., furnished in exterminating rats in powerhouse, generator lead tower, switchboard and oil circuit breaker buildings; Wilson Dam, Tenn. River 336 00

Contract dated July 24, 1925.
Copy E. D. authority 2344(Wilson Dam)-4,
2nd Ind., dated July 16, 1925 filed
herewith.

Total 336 00

Herewith is Official Check No....................., in payment of the above account.

PLEASE SIGN RECEIPT BELOW, TEAR OFF AND MAIL, NO POSTAGE OR ENVELOPE BEING REQUIRED.

CREDITOR RETAIN THIS STATEMENT FOR FUTURE REFERENCE.

TEAR OFF ON THIS LINE

The contract for the Wilson Dam project in 1925 was worth $1,986. Otto's expense check for his trip from Richmond to inspect the dam was for $87.18. The first payment on the contract was for $336.

meant that they were leaving food scraps and trash anywhere and everywhere within the construction site. True to Otto's theory that rats can't resist food touched by human hands, rats from the nearby woods and farmland virtually invaded the site—from the power house and lead tower to the circuit breaker buildings. The pests made nests out of the paper construction wrappings in the wooden frames used during construction and, worst of all, in the open ends of the electric motors that operated the oil and water pumps for the huge generators.

The rats created an absolute nightmare on a day in 1925 when a group of high-ranking army and government officials were invited to witness a test run of sections of the dam's generating equipment. After the appropriate ceremonies were held for the assembled dignitaries, it was time to throw the switch and start the machines. But nothing happened—or rather, nothing happened that was supposed to happen. Not only did the machines never start, but the inner workings of the machines caught on fire. Flames burst out from the electric motors, where the rats had built their nests. The electric current, set in motion by throwing the switch, had set the countless rat nests on fire and electrocuted the rats. Apparently no one had inspected the generators for the nests. Before they left for Washington, the officials had one order: solve the rat problem.

The Orkin Exterminating Company, Inc. became a Georgia corporation in January 1926, opening an office in the heart of downtown Atlanta.

As the story goes, a captain in the Corps of Engineers told his commanding officer about a certain exterminator in Richmond, Virginia, who rid his father's house of rats. On August 12, 1925, the Corps of Engineers paid $87.18 for Otto Orkin to travel round-trip by train from Virginia to Alabama to inspect the Muscle Shoals dilemma and suggest a solution. As a result of Otto's inspection, the Office of the Corps of Engineers in Florence, Alabama, awarded Orkin The Rat Man a six-month contract for "services, materials, supplies, appliances, etc. furnished in exterminating rats in power house, generator, lead tower, switchboard and oil circuit breaker buildings." The contract, dated August 21, 1925, was worth $1,986, and the first payment of $336 was issued to Orkin by the treasurer of the United States on September 10, 1925.

To complete the job, Otto immediately recruited more family members to go with him to Alabama. Ted convinced his older brother Maurice to join him, along with Louis Kotler, who was the son-in-law of Celia, one of Otto's sisters. Otto was courting a young woman from Richmond named Miriam Berz (whom he soon married), and so he hired his future brother-in-law Ted Berz to join him in Alabama as well. Within six weeks, the men had the rat problem at Wilson Dam under control. So impressed were the officials that they rewarded Otto with a nine-month contract extension to provide maintenance to the site and keep the dam free of rats.

The Muscle Shoals project was beneficial to Otto in several ways. First, it gave him an important government connection and was one of the biggest-name contracts he had acquired to date. And second, the job in Alabama gave Otto the chance to explore the South, something he had been thinking about for quite a while. Without benefit of focus groups or surveys or business consultants, Otto knew intuitively that his expanding southern business and his southern strategies would prove to be the backbone of his business.

Why south? someone once asked Otto.

"Bugs go south," he said.

ATLANTA

In the mid-1920s, Atlanta was known as the railroad hub of the South, a city on the move. Candler Air Field was being developed, Southern Bell was expanding, and automobiles were crowding the streets. The Atlanta Planning Commission was trying to develop a master plan for road construction, and a bond issue had been passed for the construction of bridges and viaducts. The Pullman Company had just put the finishing touches on a new million-dollar plant for the maintenance of its equipment; the Pullman train made its first run between New York and Atlanta on April 26, 1925. The new Forward Atlanta Commission was luring new businesses to town. The commission's nationwide advertising campaign proclaimed that "if the world knows of Atlanta's advantages, more of the world's businesses will come here."

While traveling back and forth by train to Alabama, Otto and Ted had a perfect opportunity to visit Atlanta and other parts of Georgia and analyze its business climate. Out of habit, Otto looked in the telephone directories and was probably surprised to find no exterminating company listed in Atlanta. One of Orkin's main extermination competitors, the Getz Company, retained a traveling representative in the city to service some of Atlanta's hospitals, food establishments, and other institutions, but Getz did not have an office in Atlanta. And Otto could clearly see that the Forward Atlanta Commission was working to draw businesses to its city limits. In 1925 R. H. Macy affiliated with the Davison-Paxon department store and started construction on a new building on Peachtree Street in the downtown area. Sears, Roebuck & Co. was new in town, and Rhodes-Haverty had a twenty-one-story building at Peach and Willow Streets. Between 1926 and 1929, approximately 760 new enterprises opened in Atlanta, and Otto Orkin's company was one of them.

The Orkin Exterminating Company, Inc., became a Georgia corporation in January 1926, with Otto Orkin as president and Theodore Oser as vice president in charge of sales. On January 2 Orkin opened an office in the 609 Candler building in the heart of downtown Atlanta, where, true to his strategy in Richmond, Otto could mingle with the city's elite businesses. In addition to Otto and Ted, the office staff included Barnet Oser (Ted's father and Otto's brother-in-law), who was responsible for service, and an office secretary. In the early months of 1926 Otto hired two additional servicemen, Charles Loudermilk and Henry Grady Bennett, to deliver handbills and solicit business door-to-door. Repeating his Richmond business tactics, Otto produced letters of introduction from Richmond customers and business associates who vouched for his expertise. When he began servicing accounts, Otto's pest control service was delivered door-to-door by the "walking exterminators." If customers were located beyond a reasonable walking distance, the servicemen rode bicycles or the company's sidecar motorcycle, or they drove the 1926 company Chevrolet. Otto added a truck two years later.

In August 1926 the red and white Orkin diamond first appeared in Orkin advertisements, and the symbol has been used continuously ever since.

There's no doubt that Otto, who had been contemplating his expansion for some time, came to Atlanta well prepared with both cash and strategies. After years of living frugally and spending little, one of his first moves was to deposit fairly large sums of money in several Atlanta banks, a step that showed he was serious about investing in Atlanta and that he wanted the bankers to help him get established. Company employees later said that Otto entered Atlanta with one hundred thousand dollars, and split the money into twenty-thousand-dollar deposits in five banks. An early believer in advertising, Otto advertised aggressively—running regular ads in the Atlanta newspapers and various business-oriented publications. For his full-page ad in the 1926 Atlanta City Directory, Orkin tapped into his recent association with the Wilson Dam project to describe Orkin as "Creators of Sanitation" and "Endorsed by the United States Government." His eye-catching advertisement started like this: "War on Pests! . . . The Menace to Health . . . The Destroyer of Dollars." And by April 1926, he used a listing of twenty-four major Atlanta clients as part of his advertising copy in the *City Builder,* the prestigious magazine for the Atlanta Chamber of Commerce:

> **"These Atlanta Firms Are Among the Many Clients We Serve!"**
> J. P. Allen & Co. | Howard Theater | Forsyth Theater | Rialto Theater | Lowe's Theater | Constitution Pub Co. | Atlanta Georgian | Hotel Winecoff | Kimball House | Norris, Inc. | Atlanta Baking Co. | A & P Tea Co. | Gate City Dairy | Cudahy Packing Co. | White Provision Co. | Ivan Allen-Marshall | and others.

In Atlanta Otto continued his Richmond tradition of using his company letterhead to list many well-known names. But it wasn't long before Otto discontinued a business approach that had worked well in Richmond. Granted, the Orkin logo—"The Rat Man"— had put the company on the map in Richmond, but Otto wanted another image in Atlanta. In August 1926 the red and white Orkin diamond first appeared in Orkin advertisements in and around Atlanta, and the symbol has been used continuously ever since.

Atlanta welcomed Orkin's decision to move its headquarters to the city, as this Atlanta Journal *article from January 17, 1926, shows.*

JANUARY 17, 1926.
THE ATLANTA JOURNAL

WAR ON RODENTS BUSINESS OF NEW ATLANTA CONCERN

Killing rats has really attained the proportions of a business in Atlanta, and a full-fledged company, having a corporation charter and everything, is now in the field, it was announced from the chamber of commerce Thursday by Frederick T. Newell, secretary of the industrial bureau.

Otto Orkin is president of the company and Theodore Oser is vice president. Offices have been opened at 609 Candler building, and the systematic business of ridding Atlanta buildings and homes of rats, roaches and other pests is under way. The company is known as the Orkin Exterminating Company, Inc.

Officers of the company this week began directing the spreading of a mysterious, secret formula chemical in certain part of Atlanta, and it was stated that one contract was for ridding a nationally-known Atlanta company's place of rats.

Efforts of cats, and even the mythical prowess of the famous Piper of Hamlin, do not compare with the accomplishments mentioned in scores of indorsements which Messrs. Orkin and Oser brought with them to Atlanta.

The Atlanta office is to be permanent headquarters of the organization, thus affording at all times this unusual service to Atlanta industrial and public buildings, it was stated.

An indorsement which is being displayed by the company is that of Governor Stuart, of Virginia, who contracted with Mr. Orkin to rid the official mansion of rats in 1915.

A number of indorsements from department stores, the United States Engineering corps and numerous other public and private concerns make up a folio which is treasured.

Their service, Mr. Newell mentioned, really should be of great value to Atlanta, as the property damage from rats runs into hundreds of thousands of dollars every few years, and diseases are often spread by rats and insect pests which are exterminated by their secret process.

Orkin Exterminating Company was the only exterminating company listed or advertising in the Atlanta City Directory from 1926 through 1928. The company was obviously growing because Otto kept hiring new staff. Fred McColl, an accountant, joined Orkin in 1927. Years later, when asked what made the company grow so successfully, McColl didn't hesitate: "It is my opinion that one of the major factors was the old maxim that 'the customer is always right,' which Otto Orkin adhered to and so thoroughly instilled in the minds of everyone connected with the company. I remember several incidents regarding the length to which Mr. Orkin would go to satisfy and retain a customer." For instance, when Orkin once lost Atlanta's Rialto Theater to a competitor, Otto regained the account by accepting payment in theater tickets.

In 1928 Otto purchased a new Ford truck for the Atlanta servicemen to use on their routes (complete with an Orkin diamond painted on the door panels), and he hired another serviceman, Eugene Cunnard. A new and larger business office was needed, and in 1929, apparently showing no adverse effects from the stock market crash and the Depression of 1929 and the 1930s, Otto moved a few blocks south to 82 Courtland Street. From here Otto managed his growing pest control business, which by 1930 included thirteen branches in eight states: Virginia, Georgia, Alabama, Tennessee, Florida, North Carolina, Mississippi, and Louisiana.

Just who ran these offices? Since the Wilson Dam project, Otto had retained the many relatives who worked for him and employed them to open the new branches. Otto and Ted Berz opened the Chattanooga office in early 1926. Otto actually lived in Chattanooga for a few years while he and Berz also opened offices in Nashville, Memphis, Knoxville, and Charlotte. Maurice Oser opened an office in Birmingham, followed by offices in Mobile, Alabama; Jackson, Mississippi; and Louisville,

Kentucky. Oser spent six months with Louis Kotler, developing a branch in Memphis. Kotler began managing the Memphis office in 1928 and opened other offices in Tennessee (Nashville, Knoxville, and Jackson); New Orleans, Louisiana; Jackson, Mississippi; and Charlotte, North Carolina. Time and again, Kotler proved to be one of Orkin's strongest and most successful early managers, appreciated for his fiscal management skills and ability to keep expenses under control. Very quickly, he expanded his territory into Mississippi, Arkansas, and parts of Kentucky and Alabama. Barnet Oser, Ted's father, was named the Atlanta office's service superintendent in 1929 and would become general manager in 1932. Elwood Orkin, Otto's nephew and the son of his older brother Jacob, ran the "Orkin The Rat Man" exterminating branch in Richmond.

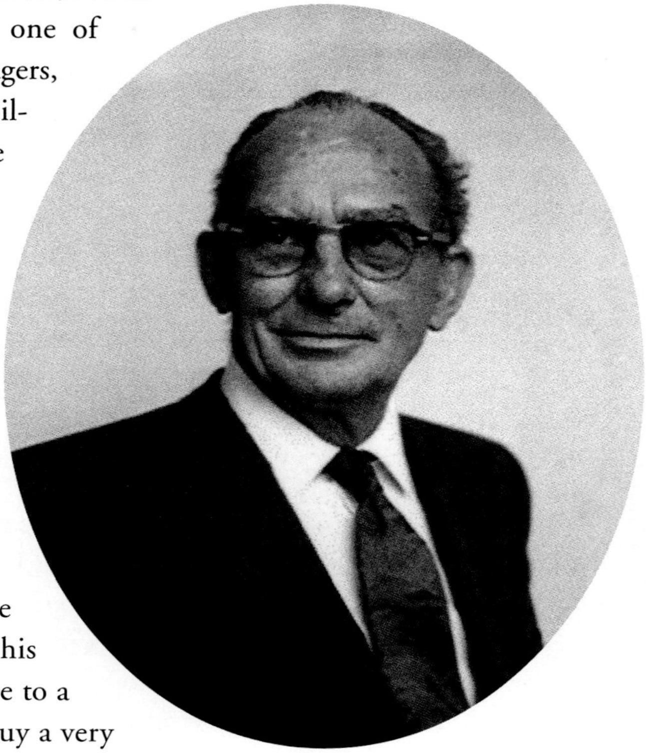

From early records and office manuscripts, Otto's method for opening each individual branch office emerges. He allowed an initial investment of five thousand dollars to start each branch. Otto and his branch partner—usually a relative—would each agree to a salary of fifty dollars per week. Otto preferred to buy a very modest building in a suitable location for the branch office, but would agree to rent office space if a purchase wasn't practical. The branch manager had to buy a service truck, hire an office manager and possibly a service technician, purchase service tools and supplies, and pay for advertising. On average, the ledger balance would have been reduced to about two thousand dollars, which was used to keep the branch afloat until it had enough customers to become self-sufficient. Routinely, Otto (or one of the more experienced managers) would spend the first six months or so with the new branch managers, helping them learn the various service techniques and how to attract customers. Building a customer base took time; as the funds dipped lower, Otto often couldn't afford to take his fifty-dollar-a-week salary, so he customarily accepted an "IOU" from the company, which allowed him to continue to grow his equity in the business. When the office did make money, Otto would take interest on his investment and use the money to start another branch.

Fred McColl joined Orkin in 1927 as an accountant and in later years served as the company's first historian.

It's been said that one of Otto and Ted's greatest talents was their ability to recognize exceptionally bright, ambitious people who could make the company successful. Indeed, Otto was very persuasive if he wanted someone to work for him, going after the individual with the same tenacity that he often used to secure clients. To further convince talented people to work for

Advertising through the Ages:
From Rats to Diamonds

From the very beginning, Otto Orkin believed in advertising. He even developed his own methods for what would years later be called product branding: he religiously carried around his trademark black satchel, filled with paper bags of rat poison with a skull and crossbones printed on the outside. His first telephone directory advertisements and his original calling cards proudly included the picture of a rodent. And Otto's signature company name, "Otto The Rat Man," was proudly displayed on stationery, business cards, advertisements, and on every service vehicle he owned.

With his company poised for growth, however, Otto Orkin wanted a new image when he opened offices in Atlanta in 1926. Specifically, Otto wanted to be rid of his company's "rat killer" label and his own identification as "The Rat Man."

It's unclear why Otto had soured on the image that had made him so successful, though a newspaper interview once quoted Otto as saying, "People don't like to see pictures of rats or other pests in telephone directory advertisements or elsewhere." But it was probably more complicated than that. His business had grown beyond rats to include roaches, termites, and other insects. The "Rat Man" advertising scheme was the idea of a very young Otto as an inexperienced entrepreneur, one more concerned about catchy phrases than lasting professional images. Otto was well aware that his first marriage had failed in part because his wife had loathed the "Rat Man" reference and the image. When he expanded into Atlanta, Otto probably no longer saw himself as the "Rat Man" who once hid in dark places to observe rats; he was a thirty-nine-year-old businessman with nearly fifteen years of successful business experience, a rapidly growing family, and a desire to be accepted within his community. For a time Otto used the "Modern Pied Piper" logo, but the public didn't respond to rats following a piper. And the Pied Piper metaphor implied that rat control was the only service that the Orkin Company provided, even though the company was now dedicated to total pest control and had launched a service to rid homes and businesses of termites.

To help produce a new image for his company, Otto made yet one more deal: in return for regular pest control service at the *Atlanta Georgian-American* newspaper, Merle A. "Tommy" Thompson, the paper's advertising and promotion manager, agreed to create a new advertising campaign for Orkin. And it appears that Tommy created the symbol that would forever be associated with Orkin: the red and white Orkin diamond. The first known Orkin ad with the diamond logo was used in the August 1926 issue of the *City Builder*, establishing what would become a long association between Tommy and Orkin and the launch of a new corporate logo. Tommy included the word "RATS!" in the advertisement—but no picture of a rat. The new visual symbol for Orkin was not a rodent but a red diamond with white lettering.

After 1926 Orkin Exterminating Company never produced advertising, printed material, or signs from Atlanta without the Orkin diamond. Why a diamond? As Otto reportedly once said, "We are the diamond of the industry." Within a year, the Orkin diamond appeared on signs, advertising, printed materials, and vehicles throughout most of Orkin's territory. Even "Antipest Control Company," owned by Otto in Norfolk, Virginia, had the name "Antipest" inside a blue—though not red—diamond. Otto's nephew, Elwood Orkin, had a company registered as "Orkin Exterminating Company" in Norfolk until the mid-1950s, which meant that Otto could not use the company's national name in that territory. Similar problems occasionally cropped up throughout Orkin, due to different incorporation names and different relatives' business spin-offs. It was confusing, to employees and customers alike. "You can imagine the problems we had explaining that we were not Orkin in Norfolk, but that we *were* Orkin from Atlanta, and then provide Antipest guarantees," said Don Holt, who first joined Orkin through the Norfolk branch.

After 1927 the images of rats, roaches, and vermin would occasionally show up in newspaper advertisements and city directory listings for Orkin. But the Orkin diamond was there, too. Sometimes, the words "Creators of Sanitation" and "Exterminating Company Inc." were printed on the edges of the diamond, but often the red diamond stood alone with the white letters of ORKIN stamped inside.

The Orkin diamond was the first step in an advertising campaign that would one day achieve truly amazing results. In fact, the Orkin diamond logo would become one of the most readily recognized icons of American business.

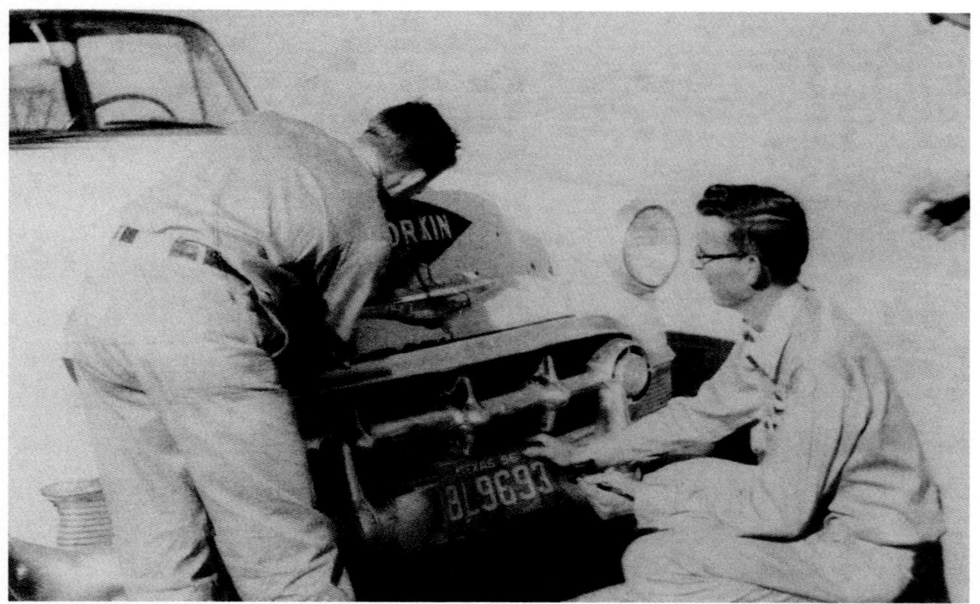

Orkin vehicles, uniforms, and branches all eventually sported diamond logos. Gene Imington, left, and S. E. Hill attach decals to a truck at the Lubbock, Texas, branch in 1956.

Orkin, Otto established company benefits such as medical insurance and pension plans long before the days of obligatory employee benefit plans. And well before the era of affirmative action, Otto hired black and white employees alike.

Once hired, each manager was personally trained by Otto or Ted, but then the manager was encouraged to develop his territory in a somewhat autonomous manner—hiring and training his own staff, making deposits, paying bills, printing his own stationery and statements, and handling his own advertising. Most districts were a collection of various branches formed under separate corporations, and each manager had his own unique compensation arrangements; in some cases, a manager would negotiate for a generous percentage of gross deposits, while some even had stock options.

While many exceptional people worked for Otto during the late 1920s and 1930s, four other individuals on his management team proved invaluable to Otto: Owen Kelly, Gertrude N. Walker, Abraham S. Krawcheck, and J. L. "Jake" Pressman.

Kelly joined the management team in 1928 and opened branches in Macon, Georgia, and Jacksonville, Florida. Otto trusted him completely, and Kelly became a close, personal associate of Otto's and expanded the company into south Georgia and all of Florida. He traveled extensively—acquiring businesses, hiring and training staff, and managing territories not covered by other managers. Like Otto, he was competitive by nature and was probably the person who convinced one of Orkin's main Georgia competitors—William H. "Uncle Billy" Crawford—to sell his Columbus, Georgia, pest control company to Orkin in 1935. Crawford remained with the company as a branch manager in Columbus and, for a number of years, produced one of the best service-sales records in the company.

Gertrude N. Walker joined Orkin The Rat Man (which remained the name of the company in Virginia until 1956) and was named office manager of the Richmond office in 1930. She was highly regarded by the people she supervised at Orkin, and by the people she worked with throughout the pest control industry. She represented Orkin during the formation of the National Association of Exterminators and Fumigators (later known as the National Pest Control Association) in 1932–33, and was on its board of directors through 1935. She managed the Richmond branch until 1944, when she reluctantly resigned to devote more time to her husband, who was ill. Mrs. Walker will always be remembered as the one who hired three of the five renowned Hall brothers to work for Orkin, the most members from a single family ever to be employed with Orkin at one time (outside of the Orkin family, of course): Berkley Hall (1937 to 1971); Dorsey Hall (who never missed a day of work in thirty-two years with Orkin from 1941 to 1973); James Wesley Hall (1942 to 1983); and Floyd Hall (1943 to 1973). Mrs. Walker actually hired Dorsey, Wesley, and Floyd Hall, along with their brother-in-law, Nathaniel Mills (1943 to 1978). A fifth Hall brother, Alfred, and a grandson, James Wesley Hall, would one day work for Orkin, too.

Abe Krawcheck had a promising newspaper career until he met Otto Orkin in Charlotte, North Carolina, in 1931. Otto quickly convinced him to come to work for him, and Krawcheck was soon training in the New Orleans

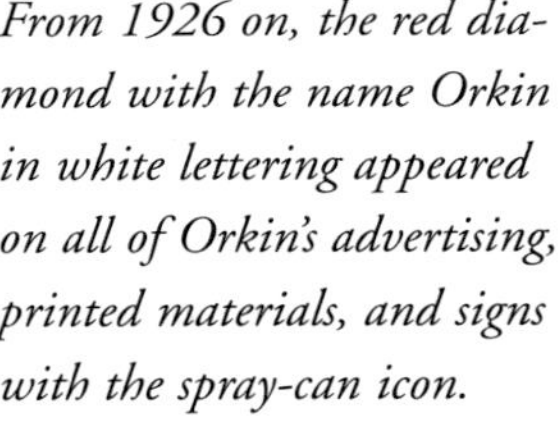

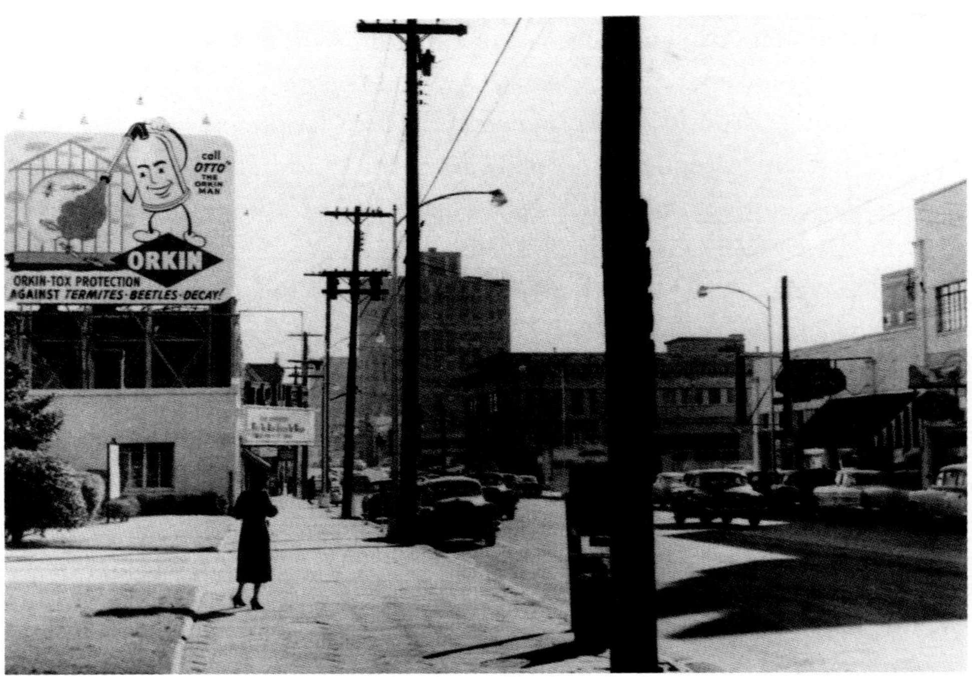

From 1926 on, the red diamond with the name Orkin in white lettering appeared on all of Orkin's advertising, printed materials, and signs with the spray-can icon.

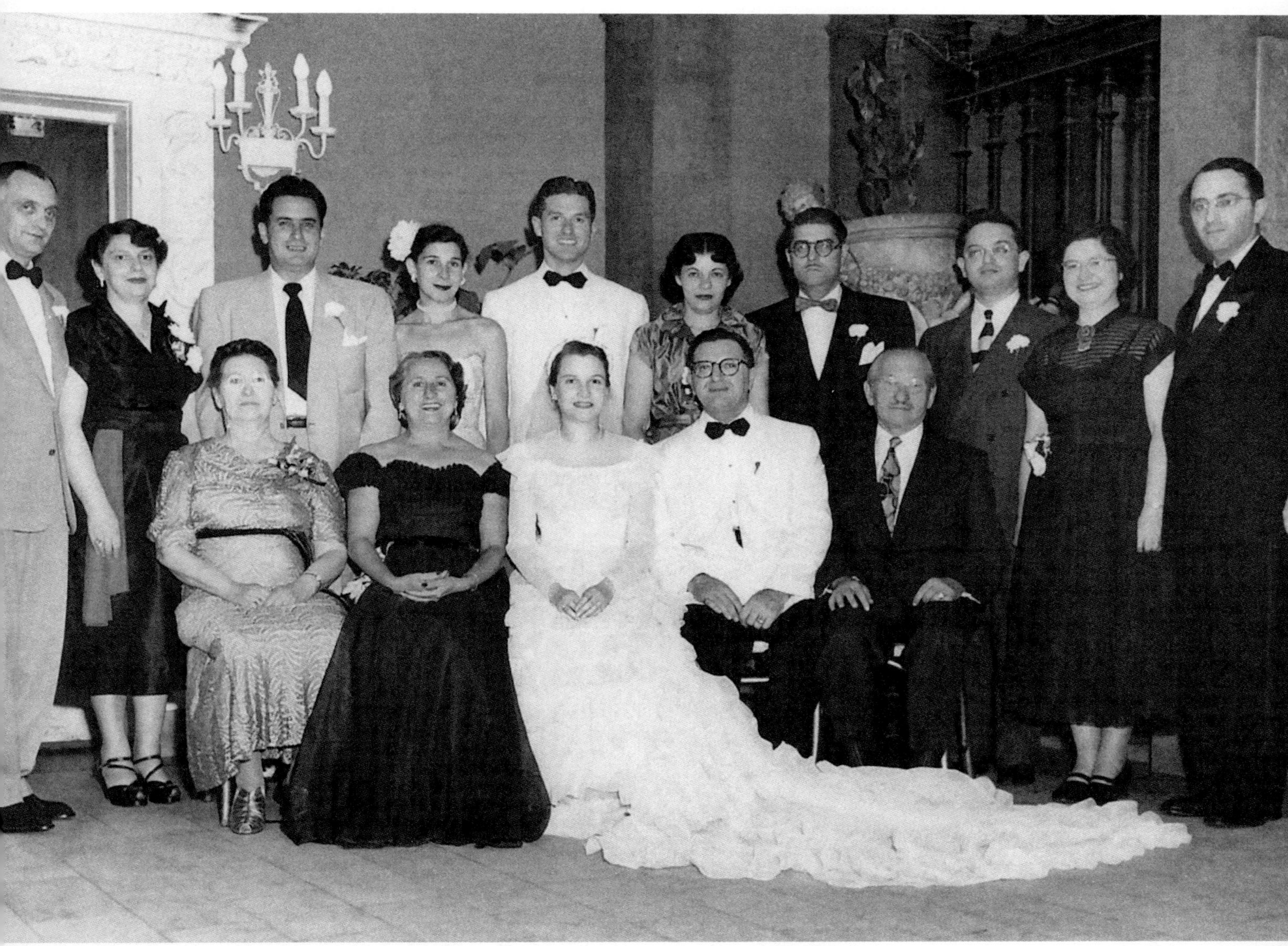

Otto Orkin (seated front row right) combined business and personal life by having many of his relatives work for him. Here he is shown at the wedding of Dave Kotler (standing, in the white dinner jacket), son of Louis Kotler (seated next to Otto). Louis was the son-in-law of one of Otto's sisters and opened offices in Memphis, Nashville, Knoxville, Jackson, New Orleans, and Charlotte.

branch before being tapped as branch manager in Birmingham. Krawcheck became one of Otto's most trusted advisors; it wasn't unusual for Otto to summon Krawcheck to Atlanta to handle a touchy personnel situation that likely involved a employee confrontation. It was widely known that Otto didn't like conflict or unpleasant personnel encounters; Krawcheck became one of his favorite "hatchet men." Krawcheck's compensation reflected both his considerable business skills and his value to Otto: his employment agreement gave him a percentage of the gross revenue, which in some years amounted to more income than Otto earned. During his twenty-five years with the company, Krawcheck expanded his territory to include all of Alabama and the Florida Panhandle.

By 1932 nearly a hundred pest control companies were established around the country. Otto's was still growing. And while expanding his company, Otto continued to personally service accounts, too. A. M. Martin of Rosemary Drug Company, in Roanoke Rapids, North Carolina, remembered that in 1932 Otto would ride a train from Richmond to Roanoke Rapids every month to service his drugstore. On these trips Otto scouted out new business and new talent for his company. One was Jake Pressman, hired in 1932 to manage the Charlotte office, and this aggressive yet generous manager developed the Carolinas into one of the largest districts in the company. He openly courted businesses in districts that were under the jurisdiction of other Orkin managers—but he didn't care. If he thought other managers

Ted Oser, front row, second seat from the left, shown here at an Orkin meeting in 1946 in Memphis, personally trained many of the early managers recruited into the company.

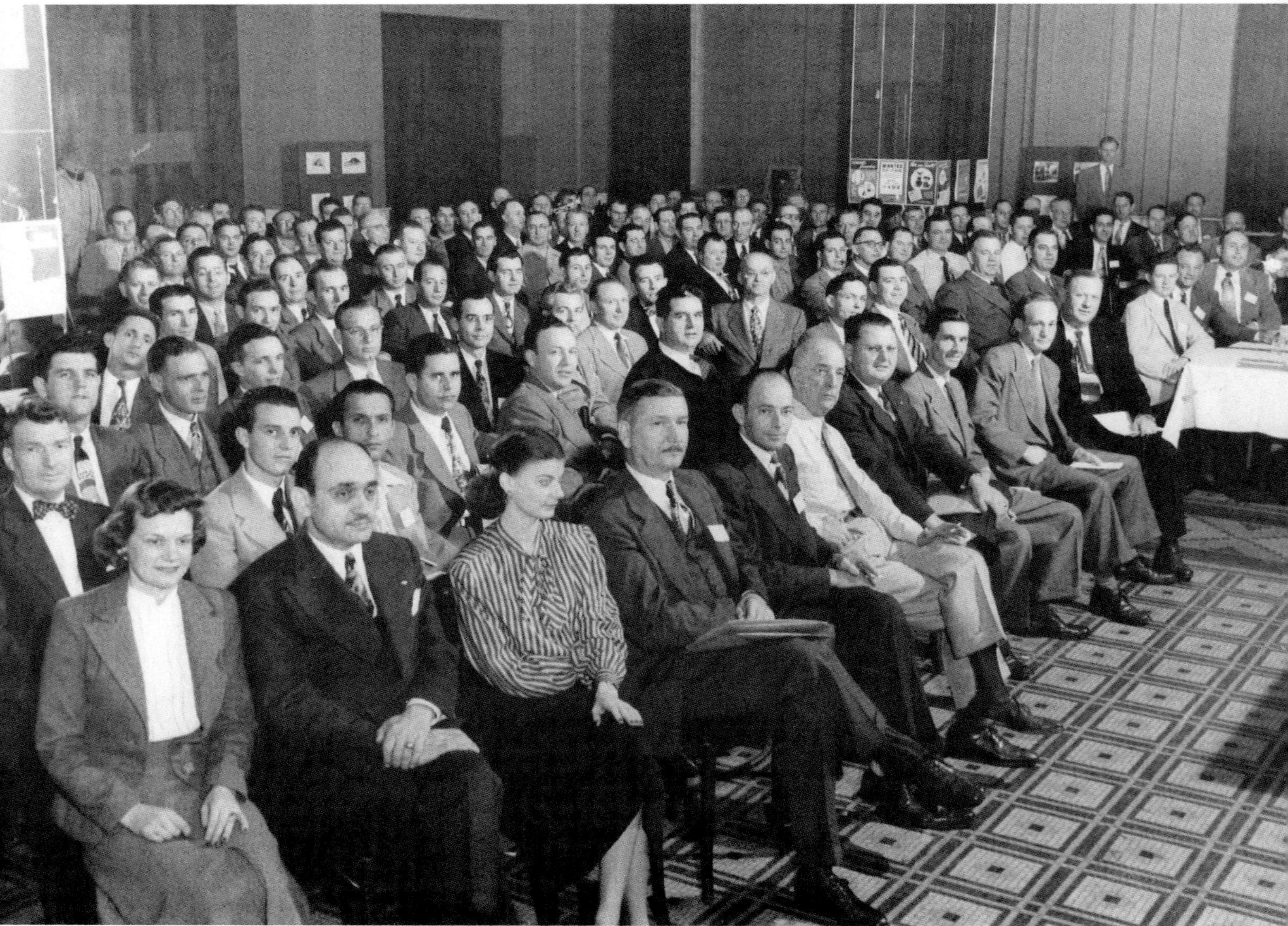

weren't doing their jobs, then their area was open territory (a practice that actually continued within Orkin into the 1970s). Otto and Ted were often called in to settle disputes between Pressman and other managers, but it was difficult to argue against Pressman's methods. He kept detailed maps of his territory on his wall, and he knew every route and income. His staff claimed that he could "sew up a contract in no time." And Pressman had a talent for hiring good people. His assistant, Louis E. Killough, was general manager of the two Carolinas for many years and made sure the Orkin service was handled professionally and that the customers were satisfied. He frequently rode the three-wheeled Orkin motorcycle from Charleston to Charlotte and back, servicing customers.

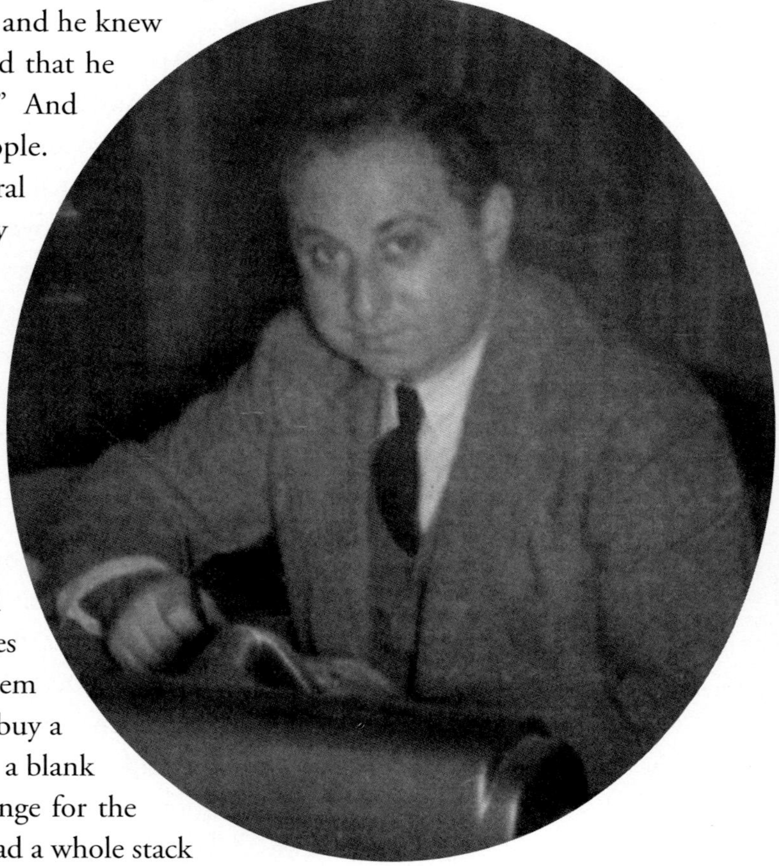

Not only did Orkin's business expand rapidly and profitably under Pressman's leadership, but his staff adored him. Pressman's close bond to his employees often included making personal loans to them or arranging loans for them so they could buy a car or a house. He would literally draw up a blank note for the employee to sign—then arrange for the necessary funds. At one point, Pressman had a whole stack of signed notes from people he had loaned money to. Otto was extremely impressed by this practice, and recommended that his other managers provide financial assistance to their employees. If they didn't, he didn't hesitate to let them know that he was disappointed in them. His nephew and Orkin employee, Ted Berz, once felt Otto's wrath on this very subject. Through the grapevine, Otto heard that Berz was reluctant to cosign a loan for a new employee named Stone, even though Berz had already loaned him seventy-five dollars and provided him with a furnished house. Otto wrote:

Hired in 1932 to manage the Charlotte office, Jake Pressman developed the Carolinas into one of the largest districts in the company.

> *I don't appreciate the attitude that you have towards the loans of your men. All the other managers in every branch are always perfectly willing to cosign their men's notes and always do sign them. You are no different. Have you ever realized that the men who work in your office earn your living, so to speak? Were it not for them we would have no need of a manager, and that holds true in every territory. So you should be willing, and glad, to do anything that you can. The note for Mr. Stone's loan is enclosed and I will thank you to cosign it for him.*

No matter who Otto hired, however, his nephew Ted Oser remained his closest associate and confidant during the years they were developing Orkin The Rat Man and The Orkin Exterminating Company. Since he was twelve years old, Ted had absorbed his uncle's knowledge and techniques for selling. He was totally dedicated to helping his uncle achieve success. From 1932 to 1937 Ted lived in Richmond and was general manager of Orkin The Rat Man, continuing to expand the Virginia territory and develop national commercial customers. An early advocate of safety measures for the industry, he worked to develop both national and regional pest control associations—professional contacts that would prove beneficial to Orkin in the years ahead. The Atlanta Exterminators and Fumigators Association was founded in 1935, with Glenn H. Burnett as the first president. Ted maintained close ties with Burnett and William O. Buettner, who led the national association for many years and is considered by some to be the father of commercial pest control.

In many ways Ted and Otto were amazingly similar. Both were driven businessmen—each possessing boundless energy, strong business skills, unwavering devotion to the company, and a competitive drive that would take them to the top of their profession. But Ted and Otto also complemented each other, allowing the strengths of one to cover for the weaknesses of the other. Ted, for instance, wasn't very good with details; Otto never forgot anything. Otto was not well educated and was very uncomfortable speaking in public; Ted was well read and dabbled in philosophy and religion. And he was an inspiring speaker who expressed his ideas well in both public settings and in private conversations with just a few people.

But it was clearly Otto who set the tone for the company, and his business mantra was reinforced by his steadfast devotion to the thousands of people who stood under the red diamond: the Orkin Customers.

OTTO'S CUSTOMER POLICIES, SERVICEMEN, AND PEST CONTROL TECHNIQUES

To Otto, it wasn't a cliché: he truly believed that the customer was always right. From the very early days of his business, he offered customers an unqualified "satisfaction guaranteed" and would go to great lengths to keep his customers—through discounts, extra services, or extended contracts. He often boasted that his very first Richmond customer—food wholesaler E. A. Saunders—retained Orkin's services for twenty-five years until Saunders was sold, a benchmark that seemed to set the standard for Otto's expectations. Keeping a customer happy and on the books was paramount to Otto. When he talked to a manager, he was always more concerned about lost customers than new sales, and nothing would make him madder than losing an account. One manager reported how upset Otto got about a district report showing seven lost accounts, even though the same report also showed sales of about seventy-five new accounts. Another manager dared to brag that he had just sold a hotel service contract for $50. Otto reportedly replied, "That was very nice; you have $50, but rather we have ten $5 accounts than one $50. If we lose an account of $5, we still have $45, but if we lose $50, we have nothing."

According to Orkin legend, Otto once caught a manager cheating on his financial reports, and he forgave him. Later the same manager gave a careless reason to explain why a certain account was canceled. Otto fired him, with this explanation: "You can get back money, but a customer you may not get back."

Otto would not tolerate cancellations. He would call his managers between 1 A.M. and 3 A.M. to find out why a specific account had been canceled and what the manager was going to do about it.

Otto kept up with the customers and sales records the old-fashioned way: he pored over the books. When he went to work every day, the first thing he did was to get the daily cash balances in every bank account; he kept the information on a white piece of paper tucked inside the breast pocket of his suit, and he never hesitated to let someone know that he always knew his bank balances. The second thing Otto did every day was review the daily reports—reports from every branch that documented sales, service, and cancellations. Any cancellation—big or small—bothered him enormously, and Otto developed a rather eccentric method to let everyone know that cancellations would not be tolerated: he would call his managers in the middle of the night, usually between 1 A.M. and 3 A.M., and demand to know why a specific account had been canceled and what the manager was doing to get the customer back.

Though he started this infamous early-morning cancellation inquisition in the 1930s, managers well into the late 1950s remembered Otto doing exactly the same thing. Many learned to keep their reports of canceled accounts by their bedsides, so they could have answers for Otto when he called and demanded to know why someone had canceled. For many years the staff thought that their boss just never slept—and often questioned themselves to see if they should be working harder. But the truth eventually came out: Otto went to bed at 9 P.M., and set his alarm clock for 2 A.M., just so he could place the call in the middle of the night and make an impression on his staff. It worked.

Otto apparently tried to intimidate his competition as well. In the 1930s the Atlanta Getz manager recalled that their office was across the street from the post office where Otto picked up his mail. Otto would stand at a table in the post office, in view of the Getz office, while going over his mail. This made the Getz receptionist extremely nervous, and she began picking up her telephone repeatedly, as if she were talking to a lot of customers. Why? She was sure Otto was trying to see how busy they were!

The Other Orkin Family

Otto Orkin may have been the original 24/7 workaholic. To the public, building a company seemed to be his only interest, particularly after his first marriage ended in divorce. But that didn't mean that Otto didn't want a family and a home. Ted Oser, who had always been like a son to Otto, was by now grown and would soon be married. In the mid-1920s Otto was alone, and his only interest other than working seemed to be eating out in restaurants. And it was his longing for home-cooked Jewish food that actually gave him the opportunity to meet his second wife, Miriam.

A beautiful, dark-haired teenager, Miriam was the daughter of Bella Rosen Berz, a widow who ran a rooming house at 524 North Eleventh Street in Richmond. Mrs. Berz served delicious Jewish food to help make ends meet for herself, Miriam, and Miriam's two brothers, Ted and Phillip. Otto returned again and again to the Berz home for his favorite dishes, and it was soon fairly obvious that Otto was falling in love with young Miriam. Otto, who was thirty-nine or older, and Miriam, aged seventeen, married around 1926.

There were soon four young children in the Otto Orkin family: Bernice, born in 1927; Gloria in 1929; Sanford in 1931; and William in 1932. Eventually, Miriam's mother, Bella, came to live with her daughter in Atlanta. Everyone loved Miriam—she was known as a gracious hostess to family, friends, and Orkin employees, who were always welcome in the Orkins' home. Occasionally, in the early days, Miriam would assist in the home office and often accompanied Otto to conventions and meetings. But Miriam's priorities were her home and family. When she had time, Miriam was an active member of Atlanta society, and in the Ahavath Achim Synagogue. She loved to play cards—particularly bridge and canasta.

A black-and-white photograph of the Orkin family, taken when the girls were probably just teenagers and the boys nearly ten and eight, shows a very handsome and relaxed family. But it's not clear how precisely the picture mirrors the reality of the Orkin family life. Otto was a complex person—shy and usually reticent, strict and sometimes hard to get along with, but generous and kind-hearted when he chose to be. And he was demanding: he didn't allow drinking, playing cards, or smoking, rules that caused repeated disagreements between Otto and his wife.

Granted, work often kept Otto away from his family. But even when he did manage to be at home he was constantly on the telephone and conducting business, his son Sanford later recalled. "He wasn't exactly the kind of father who went out and threw a baseball around with you. My father just lived, breathed, and slept the business," said Sanford, who always felt that the age gap between his mother and father (Otto was over twenty years older than Miriam) and the age differences with his children (Otto was in his forties when his children were born) kept the family from being close and sharing interests. "He did not like to read, and he did not like music. He had what he said was a third-grade education, and he knew very little about accounting procedures or how to set budgets and goals. But he had instincts, and he knew in his own mind what he was attempting to accomplish. His determination was just unbelievable. He was always thinking of the business, always working at it, wondering what he could do to make it bigger and better."

Whenever he was in Atlanta, Otto often took his children into work with him. Gloria remembered "playing office" at the Orkin headquarters. From the age of ten or so, Sanford remembers going on Saturdays to work with his father, and being introduced to technicians and salesmen. When Sanford was about fifteen, he traveled with Otto to visit his former home in Lockport, Pennsylvania, and remembers that his dad pointed out the one-room schoolhouse and several other childhood landmarks. Gloria recalled that her father liked to take them to see the trains. "The railroad is what brought me to Atlanta," he told them. "All trains stopped in Atlanta."

As teenagers, each of Otto's children was given a job to do in the company, reminiscent of Otto's own father's insistence that each child should have a chore. The girls remembered filing and bookkeeping. Sanford and William did a little bit of everything until they joined the administrative offices in the 1950s. "I just knew that that's what my father wanted me to do, without him having to say it," said Sanford. "He expected me to do that. It was just there, and in his own way, yes, he encouraged me."

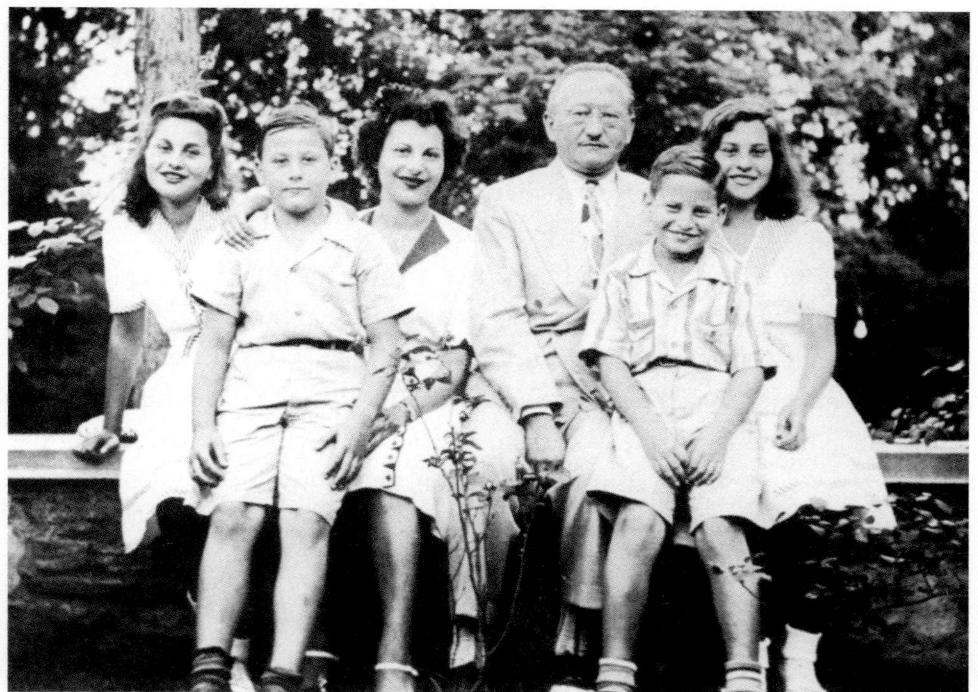

Otto Orkin's family. Left to right: daughter Bernice (born 1927), son Sanford (born 1931), wife Miriam Berz Orkin, Otto Orkin, son William ("Billy," born 1932), and daughter Gloria (born 1929).

The pencil-posted logs for the Orkin Atlanta office in 1937 and 1938 provide some interesting insights into the customers' needs and the daily calls, service, and collection records. For instance, during the spring, summer, and fall of 1937 and the winter of 1938, new services or service problems reflected these categories: 28 percent rat problems; 18.5 percent bedbugs; 17 percent roaches; 9.6 percent mice; 9 percent ants; 6.2 percent fleas; 5.1 percent termites; and 1.8 percent moths. The biggest callback complaint from customers was "dead rat odor." On about 15 percent of the rat jobs, the customer wanted the serviceman to return and remove the dead rats. A few problems concerned excessive residues on walls or claims that the pesticides were not working. The only damage claims during 1937 and 1938 seem to have been to repaint furniture for a customer and a report of two stray dogs being killed, perhaps due to rat poison.

With Otto's insistence on customer satisfaction, the early Orkin servicemen worked long hours. And because the insect and pest control industry was relatively new, people were not always clamoring for the service or even able to grasp that they needed pest control on a month-to-month basis. Eugene Loyd, who was hired in Atlanta in 1929 and remained a valued Orkin employee for over forty-one years, either walked or rode a motorcycle to service his accounts. He worked from 7 A.M. to 7 P.M. on both residential and commercial accounts. After a quick supper at home, he would go back to work for several hours, servicing restaurants after they closed for the night. When Marcus Kaplan started in 1936, he remembered walking "door to door, trying to sell contracts. I'd have to explain to people just what pest control entailed. Restaurants that definitely needed pest control, but weren't *required* to have it, would wait until the roaches got so bad that they would *have* to call us."

Records show that a serviceman during the 1930s in Richmond or Atlanta earned about ten to twelve dollars a week; a branch manager was usually paid about fifty dollars; and a district manager had various pay arrangements set up with Otto, ranging from a percent of gross deposits to a salary plus a percent of revenue. A typical workweek was six days from 7 A.M. to 5 P.M., with an additional three to four hours after dinner during busy seasons. (Loyd once noted that if he worked to help his fellow servicemen during the evening hours, they paid him an additional twenty-five cents an hour.) On Sundays, as many as four hundred to one thousand traps—particularly those

Otto's Challenges: *Health and Extended Family*

An early proponent of exercise and healthy eating, Otto recognized exercise as the key to good health. Clearly ahead of his time, Otto was considered something of a quack in the early 1930s for his memberships in health clubs and his exercise program, which included walking, lifting weights, and jogging. He was so devoted to exercise that he religiously left the office for the gym every day around 11 A.M., and didn't return until around 2 P.M. He worked out not only to control his weight but also to be physically fit. On the weekends, his personal secretary, Clyde Young, would often drive Otto to a health club—first the Bill Daily Club and, after that closed, the Progressive Club.

Otto's home life reflected his penchant for physical fitness and meals that included lean meats, fish, and lots of fruits and vegetables. Gloria, Otto's daughter, once noted that her father gave his children a medicine ball because he wanted them to exercise and stay healthy. And son Sanford remembered that his father was an adamant antismoker long before such a stance was considered politically correct. He even kept a sign in his office that read, "NO SMOKING." The fact that Miriam smoked against Otto's wishes caused considerable friction in the Orkin home.

That Otto was loyal to his family is, however, without doubt. At one time or another nearly fifty relatives from the Orkin, Oser, and Berz extended families worked for the company, and Otto's two sons-in-law and two sons would eventually be employed at Orkin as well. But the family connections did not necessarily make for a blissful existence. As with any family, there were difficulties—no matter which side was telling the story.

Paul Berz, Ted's son and nephew to Otto and Miriam, recalled that Otto was "domineering, persuasive, aggressive, and overbearing." The family believed that Otto treated Ted Berz, Miriam's brother, unfairly. Otto first offered Ted a job when Orkin signed the contract for Wilson Dam, and Ted later opened Orkin's Chattanooga

set in large warehouses—had to be checked and removed before 7 A.M. on Monday mornings, so the customer would not have to see dead rodents.

The starting salary for the first branch managers was thirty-five dollars a month plus a percentage of sales. The monthly salary rose to fifty dollars by the 1930s, but the branch managers were concentrating on their percentages instead of on monthly wages. As long as they could collect their charges and expand their customer base, the branch managers made increasingly more money.

The rates for Orkin services in the late 1930s ranged from three dollars for treating a small apartment to seven dollars to fifteen dollars for service to a home, restaurant, or other small business. If a customer wanted to discontinue service, the logbook would typically give as reasons "moving," "poor service," "no further trouble." If the explanation made no sense to Otto, his

office. Apparently, Ted did not have the same lucrative contract agreement with Orkin that other district managers had, nor did he make the kind of income other managers did. This particularly rankled the Berz family because Ted had actually trained many of these better-paid managers—like Krawcheck and Kotler—from Chattanooga. According to former employees, Otto was constantly worried when his managers got together, knowing full well that their different contractual arrangements would surface and that someone would be unhappy. Another of Ted's sons, Robert, once referred mockingly to his "beloved" Uncle Otto and noted that his father had some "rather unpleasant dealings with Otto."

To Otto, family members were as different as night and day, and so were their results with the company. He hired three of his sister Celia's sons—Karl, Sidney, and Charles Rosenthal. Karl and Charles worked out fine, but family members recalled that Otto eventually fired Sidney. Otto's experience with Celia's son-in-law, Louis Kotler, who was married to her daughter Lillian, turned out much more positively, and Kotler became a valued member of the Orkin team in Memphis and later went into business for himself. But Otto had to fire another sister's son-in-law, Jack Besbris, who was married to Helen, Otto's youngest sister's daughter. Otto, however, reportedly continued to provide financial support for Helen and her one son, and even paid for him to go to military school and law school.

Throughout his life Otto gave without fanfare to charities, family members, and many of his employees. He was particularly sensitive to employees and their families with expensive medical needs and to those who experienced family tragedies, and he had a genuine soft spot for children, often handing them quarters or fifty-cent pieces, just because he happened to see them. But there was never any doubt, really, that Otto's first love—his true passion—was for his business and making Orkin the most successful pest control company in the world.

determination to keep that customer would quickly be reflected in his notes in the logbook margins: "See to this problem immediately!"

Though the extermination industry was beginning to see the first traces of regulation, the chemical treatments used by servicemen in the 1940s were carried out primarily on a trial-and-error basis. Mixing techniques and methods used by many competitors were surprisingly casual and notoriously dangerous, considering the hazards of the chemicals. For instance, Orkin's servicemen knew that effective pest control service depended on a good "powder man"—one who was able to squeeze and direct poison dust effectively with equipment like the Hudson sprayer and the Getz Duster. The Atlanta office bought chemicals in quantity; as service manager, Barnet Oser was no doubt in charge of mixing the chemicals and shipping them to other branches. Eugene Loyd, who worked for Oser, remembers mixing the chemicals, a job that Otto secured for him once his debilitating arthritis kicked in and he could no longer service his route. "The ingredients would arrive by truck in large barrels," he once said. "There was a finely ground powdered arsenic called Red Cross Rat Embalmer, obtained from a company in Detroit, Michigan. A second rodenticide was a phosphorus paste called Murray's Doom. Mr. Orkin never used strychnine because he considered it too dangerous."

The typical week for an Orkin technician during the 1930s was six days from 7 A.M. to 5 P.M. with an additional three to four hours after dinner during busy seasons.

Barnet Oser trained Loyd to mix the Orkin materials, using what he called a "mixer-sifter" that Barnet Oser designed to formulate the final products. But other servicemen, like George Huffman and E. P. Bragg, recalled other mixing methods and some rather unorthodox techniques.

George Huffman, who was hired in Knoxville, Tennessee, in 1936, said an old milk churn was used to mix borax, sodium fluoride, and pyrethrum for roach powder. The servicemen also thinned phosphorus paste with light corn syrup to make a solution which could be painted onto a surface. "A-dust" (calcium cyanide fumigant) was used for rat burrow treatments, and barium carbonate was used as a mild rodenticide. In Knoxville they made their own glue boards by painting pieces of roofing, approximately eight by twelve inches in size, with rat glue, which they purchased in gallon cans.

E. P. Bragg could tell some fairly exciting tales of trying to control rats by using razor blades, fish hooks, and broom handles, as well as arsenic. Bragg, who joined Orkin in Jacksonville, Florida, in 1936, claimed to have success with two additional methods. First, he soaked flower seeds in poison, wrapped them in tissue paper, and hid the small packages in a shoebox. Following in Otto's footsteps, Bragg had learned that rats would eat bait if they thought they were stealing it. If this method didn't work, his next most unconventional method for catching rats was, well, barbaric, but inspired. Bragg would cut notches into a board and insert fish hooks into them. Then he'd take the board and tie it to an overhead pipe or in the path of a designated rat run. When the rats ran over the board, the fishhooks would snag their tiny little feet or sagging stomach pouches, and Bragg would stop the tricky rodents, quite literally, dead in their tracks.

Given the nature of some of these unorthodox methods—and the industry's lack of regulation—imagine the slight irony of an article in the *Atlanta Georgian* on October 10, 1938:

> Orkin Exterminating Company Protects Atlanta Homes. . . . This war on pests, roaches, ticks, spiders, bedbugs, mice and rats and all the revolting annoyances of this kind is constantly being waged by the Orkin Company, with their staff of experienced men *and the expert technique perfected only after years of trial and experiment.*

EXPANDING SERVICES: FUMIGATION AND TERMITES

With his business growing steadily, Otto was slow to enter the field of fumigation. As dangerous as the direct-application chemicals could be, the compounds used in gas fumigation techniques were even more lethal, particularly when used or stored inappropriately. Fumigation involved sealing vacant buildings, releasing the fumigants, and keeping the building sealed for eight hours or more before opening windows and doors to air out the building. For smaller jobs, there were special fumigation vaults where mattresses, stuffed chairs, or even pianos could be placed for fumigation. As protection, servicemen involved with either method were required to wear gas masks when performing fumigation or clearing out buildings after a treatment.

After World War I, for whatever reason, Otto began using several different fumigation techniques that involved chloropicrin and hydrogen cyanide gas. Used primarily to control bedbugs, chloropicrin had a very disagreeable odor, and it was highly irritating, not to mention dangerous. In fact, following one chloropicrin fumigation, an Orkin assistant was driving back to the office with the application pans and other materials in the back of the truck. The jarring of the truck activated some of the fumigant residue, and fumes quickly filled the truck. The frightened driver jumped from the moving vehicle, which then crashed into a tree.

Around 1930 Orkin started using hydrogen cyanide (HCN) gas—a chemical widely used by exterminators since 1898 for household pests—to fumigate for moths, bedbugs, and beetles. But even this method proved tricky. To begin, buildings were vacated, tightly sealed, all pilot lights extinguished. Then, starting at the area farthest from the exit, the servicemen would drop the hydrogen cyanide blocks in a pan that contained muriatic acid or water and sulfuric acid that would activate the HCN gas. Moving quickly, and often not wearing protective gas masks, the servicemen would continue dropping blocks in solution pans throughout the building until every square inch of space was in the process of being fumigated. They immediately left the building. After eight or more hours, the servicemen would enter to air the building.

After two particularly close calls, Gene Loyd never forgot the dangers of fumigation jobs. He tells about one job where he was waiting in the Orkin truck while Barnet Oser opened up a building that had just been fumigated. Oser's only mistake? He entered the building—no doubt thinking it was safe—without his Acme full-vision gas mask. This equipment was approved by the State Bureau of Mines and was required equipment for all Orkin servicemen when working around hydrocyanic acid gas. Soon a janitor came running out of the building, shouting, "There's a man in there. He's unconscious!" To his credit, Loyd remembered to grab a gas mask before running in, found Oser, and pulled him out of the building. Though he had no training in artificial respiration, Loyd managed to massage Oser's chest while someone ran to a nearby drugstore for ammonia to try to revive Oser, who was starting to foam at the mouth. The ammonia revived him, however, and Oser was fine in a few hours.

In another incident, Loyd was alone, fumigating a piano in one of Orkin's many fumigation vaults where the servicemen placed mattresses and pieces of furniture to get them pest-free. Carpet beetles, for instance, often attacked the felt pads in pianos, and it was all but impossible to get them out without fumigation. It wasn't long before Loyd was experiencing some classic HCN poisoning symptoms—nausea, headache, and nearly blinded by eye irritations. He managed to crawl out of the vault, and the fresh air revived him. Eventually, he was fine.

When the National Association of Exterminators and Fumigators was founded in 1932–33, Otto urged the association to focus on safety practices as absolutely essential within the industry.

No doubt the public rarely heard of these early fumigation nightmares. Fumigation was simply not big business until tarps were introduced in the 1950s. Rather, the newspapers frequently carried photographs of Orkin termite servicemen—always wearing ties—as they held up the proof of their fumigation, trapping, and baiting: a pole, held horizontally, with hundreds of dead rats dangling by their tails. "Expert Orkin Exterminators Clean Out Warehouse," began one photo caption from the late 1930s. But the realization that the pest control industry sometimes puts workers in close contact with dangerous chemicals—and that customers could be adversely affected by their service materials if used incorrectly—was something that Otto, and especially Ted, thought about constantly.

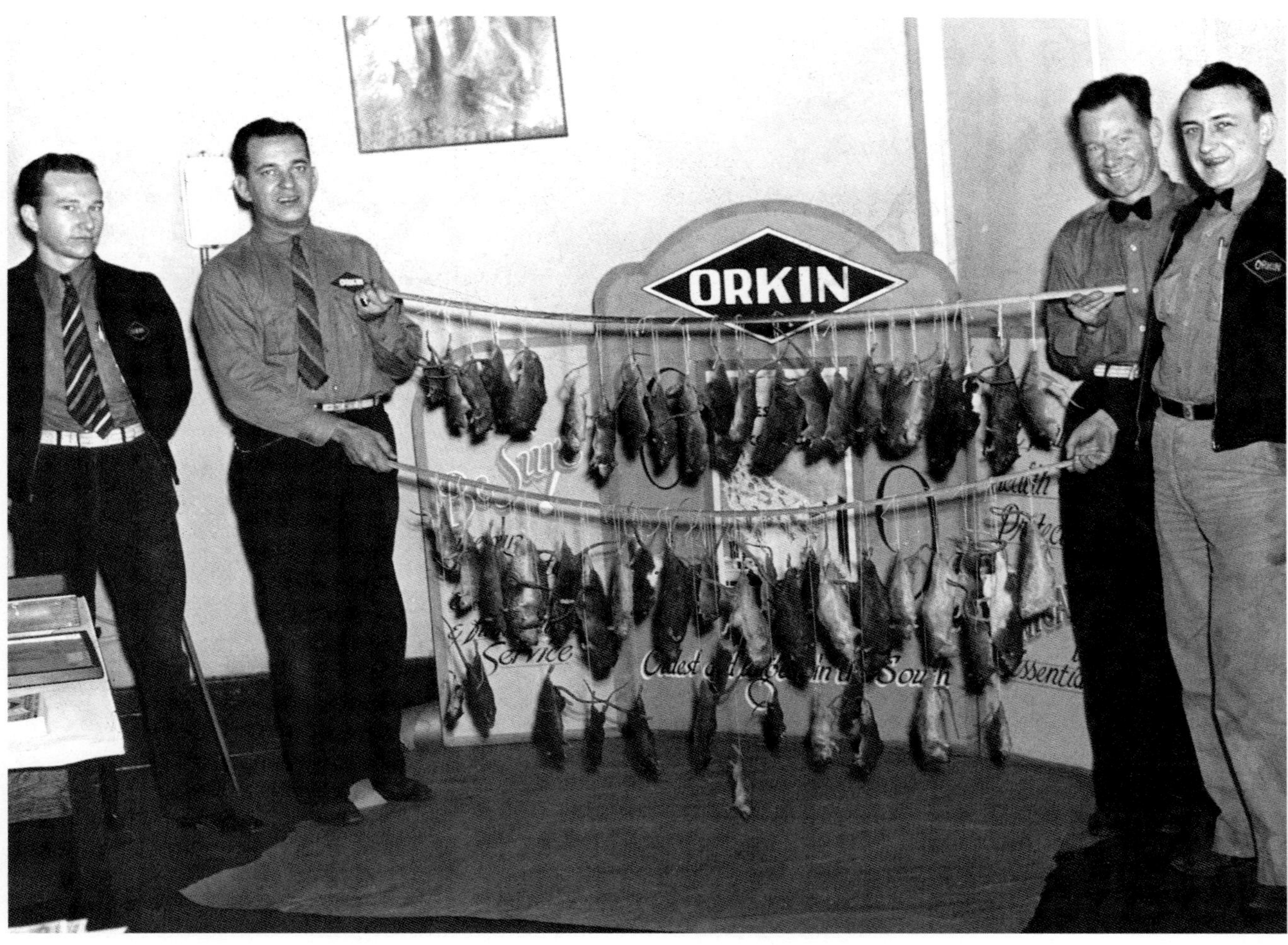

Newspaper stories about Orkin in earlier days were often accompanied by pictures of technicians displaying dead rats dangling by their tails.

When the National Association of Exterminators and Fumigators was founded in 1932–33, both Otto and Ted joined others in urging the association to focus on safety practices as absolutely essential within the industry. From the very beginning, Orkin was well represented in the national association—Mrs. Walker was the only woman elected to the board of directors in 1933, a position she held until 1935; Otto was elected a regional vice president that same year, and served in that position until 1941. When the association met for a convention in Memphis in 1937—the year it changed its name to the National Pest Control Association (NPCA)—Orkin's Louis Kotler was chairman of convention arrangements and Mrs. Louis Kotler was chairwoman for the women's program. Otto always encouraged spouses to participate in the conventions, and his message really hit home: at the Memphis convention, his second wife, Miriam, was on the organizing committee.

Orkin's efforts to adhere to industry safety standards did not go unnoticed by the press. In December 1938 the *Charlotte Observer* ran a story on Orkin's fumigation process, and noted the following:

> Orkin Exterminating Company fumigated entire homes for insects such as moths, roaches, bed bugs, etc., using Hydro-cyanic Acid Gas. . . . This is one of the deadliest known gases and is the only gas that will penetrate into over-stuffed furniture and walls, to get to the hidden eggs laid by these destructive pests; however, it does not kill bacteria. The gas does not affect household furnishings or foodstuffs and airs out rapidly, leaving no after effect. The men using this gas wear gas masks. These Acme full-precision gas masks are approved by the United States Bureau of Mines. The fumigation methods adopted and practiced by the Orkin Exterminating Company are those laid down by the National Pest Control Association and manufacturers of this gas.

For nearly three decades the name "Orkin" had been synonymous with exterminating rats, mice, and all kinds of pernicious insects. And while its pest control and fumigation services continued to grow through the 1930s, Orkin quietly added some additional services to tackle a relatively newly recognized pest: termites.

TERMITES—A NEW BUSINESS

While the pesky rat had been labeled a pest for centuries, the termite (or "flying ant" or "white ant") wasn't even recognized as a menace until the 1920s. After all, termites were considered natural recycling elements, living primarily in forests and woodlands, where they devoured old stumps and fallen trees and helped convert the remains back to soil. But when development and builders moved in on the forests, the termites continued to pursue their new next-best source of food: buildings and houses made of wood. At first, even the exterminators weren't aware that termites—which resemble ants with wings that typically appear every year in early spring—were causing any damage. By the 1930s, however, no less an authority than the U.S. Department of Agriculture's Bureau of Entomology had declared that termites wrought "enormous destruction" to properties—to the tune of $45 million a year.

And termites represented what those in the exterminating businesses called "seasonal business," particularly in the spring and fall after a rainstorm, when they can be seen swarming as "white flying ants." Said one report: "They swarm in silence—there's no sound equipment that can detect their approach. Soon they dig in, barricade themselves in the timbers of the foundations of your homes. Slowly . . . the termites wreak destruction."

Otto actually approached the termite business much later than some exterminators—it's been said that he was leery of the chemicals involved, not to mention the predominantly trial-and-error approach of the smaller termite industry. When Otto finally entered the termite business, he did so through the proverbial back door, a competitor's back door, to be precise. In the process of developing a preservative for its lumber, the E. L. Bruce Lumber Company in Memphis, Tennessee, had developed a system of termite control, which the Bruce Company patented as Terminix. Bruce then proceeded to sell the rights to this patented system through franchises, and in 1931 and 1932 Orkin *Terminix* Company, Inc., operated in a number of locations. The "Terminix News" on October 15, 1931, printed a list of the top Terminix companies, and several Orkin locations were among the leaders: Orkin Terminix Company in Richmond ranked number three in sales; the Norfolk office ranked number four; the Atlanta office number eight; and the Birmingham office was listed as number fifteen.

Though clearly successful, Otto discontinued the Terminix franchises after a year or two. Why? There are two schools of thought, and both seem plausible. First, the franchise agreement required that a Terminix company must be completely separate from general pest control service, which meant that Orkin could not offer all of its other services to its customers—a business situation that Otto simply couldn't go along with. And second, industry rumors persisted that Otto

Orkin approached the termite business much later than some companies, but in 1938 Otto made the bold move of offering a five-year bonded guarantee on his termite service. This scene from Industry on Parade, *the 1953 television film about Orkin and its services, features Atlanta termite supervisor Jack Wheeler, left, and termite serviceman Oscar Roberts uncovering termite-damaged timbers.*

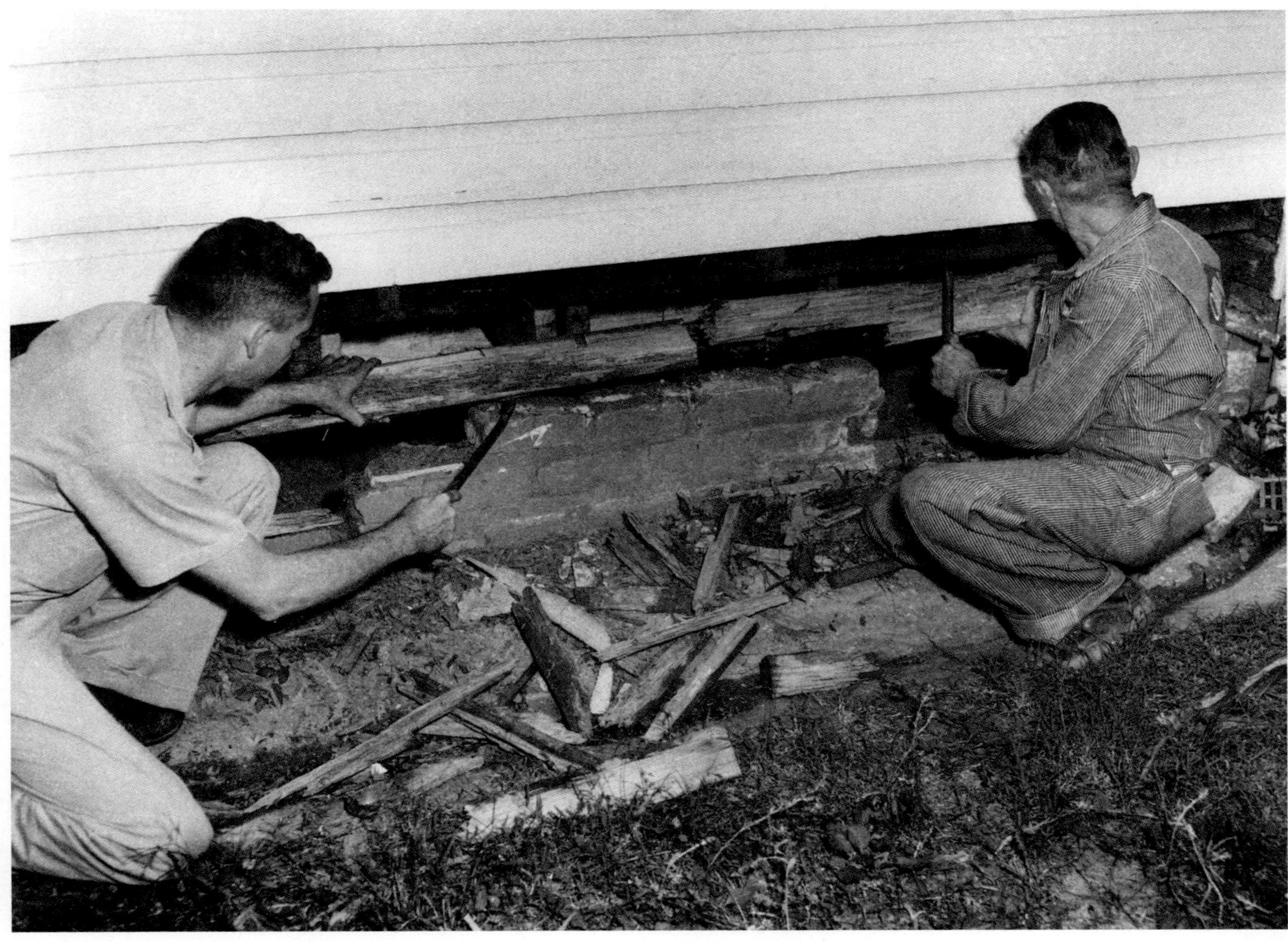

intentionally bought the franchises in order to learn all there was to know about termites from Terminix. When this was accomplished, he sold the franchises and focused on growing the termite business within his own company.

Orkin began advertising for termite business in the Atlanta City Directory in 1930 and was the only company listed in the directory as a termite service provider until 1936. The first chemicals used for termite control had limited effectiveness, and the odors were offensive. One early termite treatment consisted of one part creosote mixed with three parts kerosene, which was then mixed into the soil or poured around the foundation walls. Another common chemical for termite control was sodium arsenite, mixed into the soil to create a barrier between the termites and the structure. (It didn't take long to realize, however, that seepage through the soil could also kill adjacent vegetation.) By 1932 Orkin's service trucks were outfitted with large chemical storage tanks, and the message "Specialists in Termite (White or Flying Ant) Eradication" was written on each side of the flatbed trucks. The Orkin diamond, of course, was painted on each door panel. When the *Chattanooga News* ran a story about

Advertising through the Ages: *1950–1965*

One of Otto Orkin's initial advertising schemes was to personally hand out copies of complimentary letters from satisfied customers. This simple act of self-promotion to prospective clients was one of the first steps the company took to establish one of the most successful brands in advertising history. And though the company eventually advertised widely in newspapers and telephone yellow pages and on billboards, its advertising legacy would be grounded in a medium that offered the greatest advertising reach—television. In time, Orkin would be recognized as the first pest control company to produce television ads that effectively promoted its services. And there's no doubt that Orkin's early television experiments distinguished it from its competitors, and helped create a brand that would establish Orkin as the world's best pest control service.

Television advertising was in its infancy in the 1950s when Orkin launched its first animated commercials. Anita Ritchie, assistant director of advertising, created such characters as Rags the Ruinous Rat and Toothy the Terrible Termite for "Otto the Orkin Man" to exterminate to a jingle based on the "Popeye the Sailor Man" song. "It was determined that the audience would be squeamish about seeing live rats and bugs and that cartoon pests would be less offensive," she wrote in a history of her Orkin years. "We could deal discreetly with the touchy subject of extermination by portraying the pests as tough, criminal types. Otto would mow down the repulsive thugs with a blast of smoke."

By the early 1960s, television comedian Arnold Stang began appearing in a series of humorous "sit-com" commercials that ended with the near infamous phrase, "Stop Squawkin.' Call Orkin." Next came a series of commercials that featured hand puppets. But after Rollins purchased Orkin, the company revived its earlier successful animation commercials, adding color to update the "Otto" character.

Orkin's termite business, it also ran a picture of the new termite service truck and proclaimed it the "Weapon Used Against Termites."

Compared to its pest control service, however, Orkin had few termite jobs in the 1930s (the Richmond office only reported $78.82 for termite work in 1933), and callbacks were common. But as the chemicals became more effective and Orkin could offer a reliable service (one promoted through advertising), Orkin's termite business began to grow; in 1936 Otto tapped Owen Kelly to manage the company's termite business and to fight "enemy No. 1." Two years later, around the same time that the Orkin Atlanta home office moved to its new location at 315–317 Peachtree Street, Otto made a bold move: he began offering a five-year bonded guarantee on his termite service. The surety bond was issued from the Massachusetts Bonding Company, and Orkin leveraged the guarantee in its advertisements: *Free inspection and estimate and Bonded Termite Control.* The move dramatically increased Orkin's termite business, and by 1938 Orkin handled a large portion of the market.

As Otto neared the end of his fourth decade in business, sales were growing rapidly, fast approaching $1 million a year. Otto began to boldly advertise his company as "The South's Oldest and Largest Pest Exterminators." For Otto, however, that wasn't enough. He wanted to be the largest pest control company in the country—not just the South. To reach his goal, he realized that he had to make an important change in the Orkin organization. Since he first began developing branch offices, the branch managers had been given autonomy to determine their own policies and methods of doing business. This loosely organized corporate structure gave many customers, in fact, the impression that Orkin was a franchise operation or a collection of independently owned local offices. For years Otto was hesitant to interfere with the branches' or the managers' success, particularly if the district was earning money and making profits. But by 1937 Otto realized that in order to grow, his company needed to be more organized and centralized.

Naturally, Otto turned first to Ted Oser and asked that he and his wife Rose move back to Atlanta from Richmond, where they had been living since 1932. Otto wanted Ted to be in charge of all efforts to consolidate the general operations of the company. Next, Otto called for a convention of all Orkin managers on December 17–18, 1937, at the Atlanta Biltmore Hotel. Never fond of public speaking, Otto nonetheless stood before his managers and in a soft but clear voice explained to them what the convention was all about.

"The philosophy of business operations is to provide a system or a skeleton," he began. "It is the same as a bridge between cliffs, or high points of business prosperity, and must carry us over the stream of business disaster. Heretofore, our company representatives have followed their own system. Most of these are alike in nearly every respect, but we have not as yet definitely

Nº 1
SPECIALISTS IN
TERMITE (WHITE OR FLYING ANT) ERADICATION
ORKIN

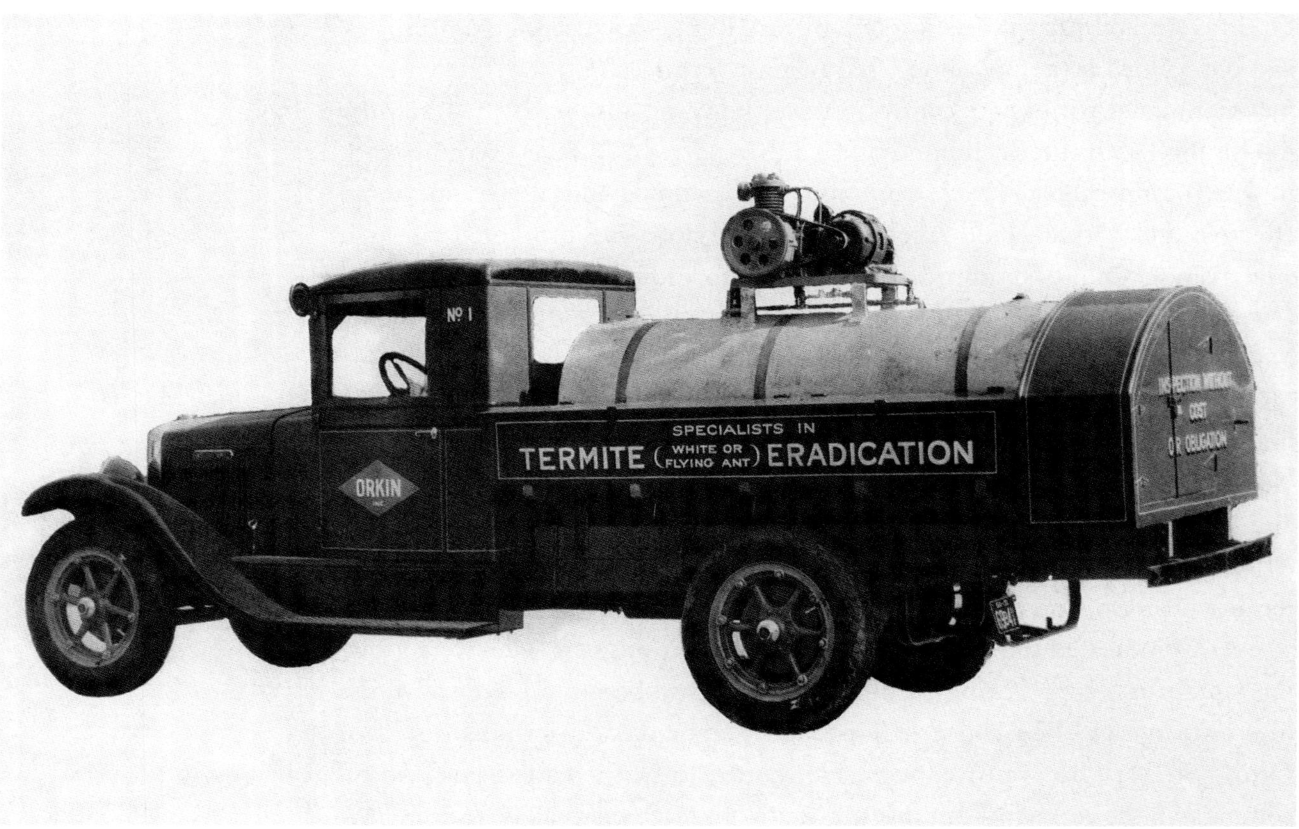

After termites were recognized as a menace in the 1920s, Orkin bought franchises for the patented Terminix system of termite control. And although Orkin discontinued the franchises after a year or two, the company remained in the termite control business.

set down on paper and committed to our minds the main picture of what we must and must not do to succeed in our business. This, I hope, will be accomplished at this meeting and will hereafter be known as the 'Orkin System.'"

For two days, between thirty and thirty-five managers met regularly to work toward standardizing company operations and establishing long-range plans for expansion and reorganization. Though many of these plans would be delayed until after World War II, a code of ethics called the Orkin Creed came out of the meeting and became the cornerstone of the Orkin System:

> I believe in the job I'm doing, in the firm I am working for, and in my ability to get results. I believe that honest goods can be passed out by honest men by honest methods. I believe in working, not weeping; in boosting, not knocking; and in the pleasure of my job. I believe that a man gets what he goes after; that one deed done today is worth two deeds tomorrow; and that no man is down and out until he has lost faith in himself. I believe in today and the work I am doing; in tomorrow and the work I hope to do; and in the sure rewards which the future holds. I believe in courtesy, in kindness, in generosity, in good cheer, in friendship and honest competition. I believe there is a more important job ahead for every man ready to do it. I believe in preparing for that job—right now!

The convention concluded with an elaborate banquet in the hotel, hosted by Otto and Ted for the managers and their wives. The banquet room was festooned with colorful ribbons and decorative holiday bells, with the men in suits and ties and the women in cocktail dresses, proudly wearing corsages from Otto, a gesture that would become something of a company tradition.

After the convention, the managers returned to their branches with the new company vision and the Orkin creed clearly outlined. For the next several years, Ted visited all of Orkin's field offices, working steadily to establish uniform procedures for operations and services. Gradually, the company changed from a loose confederation of district offices to a more unified company. In 1938 Otto called together the first meeting of an informal Council of Managers: Ted Berz (Chattanooga), Louis Kotler (Memphis), Abe Krawcheck (Birmingham), Gertrude Walker (Richmond), Marc Kaplan (Macon), Jake Pressman (Charlotte), Charles Rosenthal (Nashville), and Maurice Oser (Jackson). Expansion continued, based on Otto's philosophy to move from state to neighboring state, never skipping a state. "Like playing checkers," is how he described it. By 1940 Orkin operated fifty branches in fourteen states, with branch offices in most of the major cities in the South. Within the year, billing for all national accounts was centralized in Atlanta, and gross sales were pushing $1.5 million. And most important, perhaps, the Orkin Exterminating Company was recognized as one company.

In 1937, Otto realized that branches had been given too much autonomy. Orkin needed to standardize operations and establish long-range plans for expansion and reorganization.

As Otto celebrated forty years of continuous business in the pest control industry, newspaper articles now referred to Orkin as the "biggest and oldest exterminating company in the United States." Stories and headlines about the business were no longer punctuated by near hysterical "Rats as Big as Kittens" stories or any mention of "Otto the Rat Killer." By 1940 newspaper feature stories about Otto and Orkin Exterminating Company were, in effect, free advertisements—touching on all of the important arguments that Otto now made in his role as advocate and proponent for extermination in general—and for Orkin in particular. After twelve years of operation in Chattanooga, Tennessee, for instance, a newspaper article about the local Orkin Exterminating Company—with a picture of servicemen Raymond Barrett, Thomas Rogers, and Howard McCalla, service manager Leroy Shook, salesman Harry Torch, office manager Irene Buchanan, and general manager Theodore Berz—read like an Orkin company press release, extolling all of Otto's talking points for superior and safe pest and termite control:

> The Advantages of Pest Control: 1) "Instrumental in saving property owners worry, damage and considerable sums of money by ending the activities of destructive insects and rodents." 2) "Insects and rodents are also known to be carriers of many diseases, thus endangering human life. The control of these harmful and annoying insects and rodents should be considered foremost. . . ."
>
> Orkin's Superior Service: 1) "Dependable and efficient service department . . ." 2) "This company is one of the best qualified and equipped concerns specializing in termite control, and the extermination and fumigation of rats, roaches, bedbugs, etc., in this part of the country. . . ." 3) "Highly complimented by many property owners ranging in size from the smallest home owner to the largest mercantile and industrial establishment." 4) "Methods used by Orkin are those which have been approved by the United States Department of Agriculture, Bureau of Entomology and indorsed [*sic*] by the Tennessee State Health Department." 5) "Orkin extends free inspections and estimating service without cost or obligation. The wise property owner will have these inspections made at regular intervals. . . ."

In the Atlanta office, manager Owen Kelly was regularly quoted in the newspapers, singing the praises of monthly exterminating services as a "profitable investment that pays dividends," he said. "Our patrons do get regular returns in savings on their homes, their furniture and fabrics after these have been treated by Orkin. It has been estimated and proven by statistics that this service, rendered with materials which are known to do the work properly, has protected customers from losses amounting to thousands of dollars annually. All types of homes in Atlanta, from the most inexpensive to the most palatial residences, have been serviced."

The public, however, was still struggling with the image of the Orkin serviceman and what to think of him—as well as wondering what their neighbors might have to say about the Orkin service truck appearing in their driveways. Granted, Otto insisted that the servicemen wear short jackets and ties, and that they keep their Orkin trucks spotless. And the notion that pest control service was about clean and healthy environments—and not about the embarrassment of having a house or restaurant filled with bugs—was beginning to catch on. But it was going to take a while before it was enthusiastically embraced.

In Evansville, Indiana, for instance, local newspaper columnist Ernie Pyle reported in 1940 that the Orkin "exterminator boys have to take a lot of ribbing from their friends. People call them 'Pie-eyed Piper' and 'Brother Rat' and 'Joe Rat' and 'Mickey Mouse.' . . . Most merchants wouldn't want to display a sign saying that they were regular clients of an exterminating company, yet the truth is you're much better off trading in a place that is checked by an exterminator every week. . . . Several times a week, the Orkin company gets a frantic call from some housewife (this is a minority 10 percent of the business) saying to come quick, she's got bugs. Nine times out of ten, she says not to park that truck with 'Exterminator' written all over it in front of her house either. So what do the boys do? They either park up an alley, or leave the truck sitting in front of the house next door!"

In Orkin's early days, when the pest control industry was young, many people were not quite sure what pest control service was. And they worried about their neighbors seeing the Orkin service truck in their drive.

But in Chattanooga the Orkin termite servicemen weren't hiding from anyone. Quite the opposite, in fact—they seemed to have developed a bona fide following. The termite servicemen had become known as Orkin's "T-Men," and they were described in near heroic terms as "dealing death to criminals." Consider this story from the *Chattanooga Times* in 1940:

> Lauded for their bravery and courage, their deeds of daring and valor, are our agents of the Federal Bureau of Investigation, or more familiarly known as the "G-Men." Also doing deeds of valor and safeguarding the property of Americans from millions of dollars in damage yearly are the "T-Men" of Orkin Exterminating Company, Inc., 924 Market Street.
>
> These T-men specialize in a particular brand of criminal, a criminal of the underworld surely, that bores from underneath—never letting the thousands upon thousands of homeowners know of its presence until the damage is so completely wrought. That criminal is the termite, and it is mercilessly hounded and destroyed by Orkin's termite eradicating agents, or T-men. . . . Orkin's T-Men, with their modern, sanitary methods of termite control, give the homeowner every protection desired from the hidden foe.

When Otto Orkin read this story in 1940, his agenda was already full. The pest control industry was about to be dramatically affected by the impact of World War II, encompassing everything from changing government regulations to the introduction of new chemicals and applications. But no matter how much Otto had on his mind, it's fairly certain that the idea of the Orkin "T-Men" caught his fancy. It wouldn't be long before Otto elaborated on this newspaper description and embarked on one of the most successful marketing and advertising campaigns in business history.

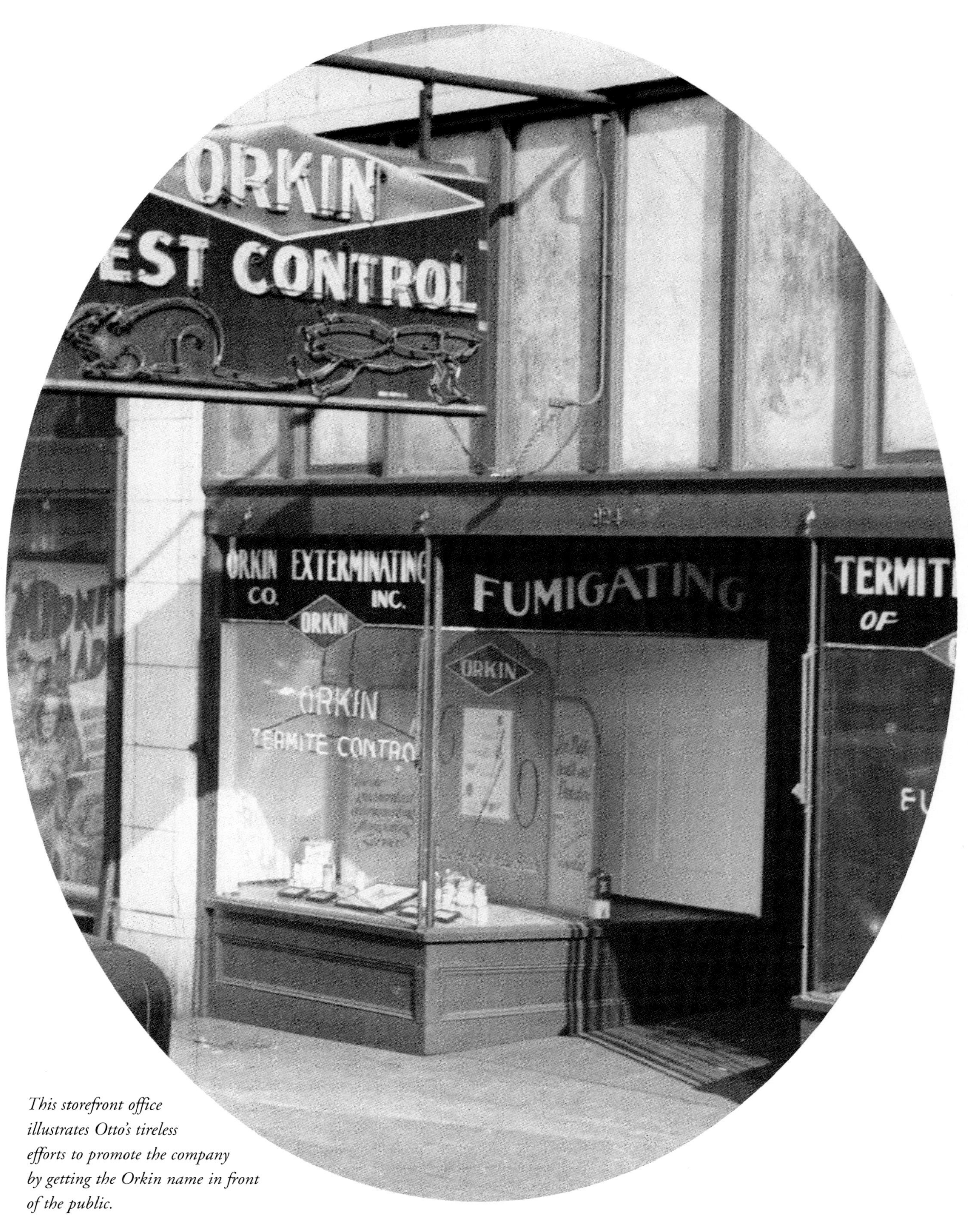

This storefront office illustrates Otto's tireless efforts to promote the company by getting the Orkin name in front of the public.

Chapter 3

1941 to 1963: War and Peace, Highs and Lows

As his company celebrated forty years in business, the emergence of World War II reduced Otto Orkin's resources and employees to a minimum and frustrated his dream of initiating an "Orkin System" of management and control throughout the country. But the war efforts and Orkin's response to it would in time create a golden opportunity for the company to grow when pest control was declared a necessary service. In the 1940s and early '50s, the Orkin company continued to capitalize on postwar chemical applications, cutting-edge technology that changed the pest control industry, and groundbreaking advertising techniques and public relations efforts that put Orkin far ahead of its competitors in both sales and revenue. At a rapid pace, the company continued its continuous postwar expansion into residential and commercial markets nationwide. No less an authority than Fortune *magazine pronounced Orkin the "General Motors of Exterminating" in 1952, as the company grew from coast to coast and grossed over $7 million in sales. But by 1960 the man who built this company from a tiny rat poison business in the hills of Pennsylvania would be forced out by his own family in an ending worthy of a Verdi opera.*

As these remarkable twenty-two years unfolded, an amazing transformation took place at Orkin. Otto Orkin continued to be the hardworking and somewhat eccentric company leader that he had always been. But the company he founded and nurtured to such heights would gradually leave him behind. Otto—who loved nothing more than focusing on the details of lost accounts, office supplies, and branch numbers—was no match for the industry changes, regulations, and scientific advancements that his industry was poised to make. And yet the company he started accomplished some truly significant achievements in the pest control industry. Because this much can be said of Otto Orkin: he may not have been a strategic planner by today's standards, but he never stood in the way of company advancements; he was never afraid to hire people who could move his company forward; and he was in many ways the epitome of a successful chief executive officer, content to create the broad outline of his company and confident enough to step back and allow talented individuals to fill in the canvas.

ORKIN DURING THE WAR YEARS

Otto Orkin recognized his own limitations. After forty years as the head of his own company, Otto had not developed public speaking skills, he didn't easily trust people, and he wasn't always interested in understanding the latest industry advances. At the annual pest control conventions, he enjoyed mingling and observing, but he rarely attended any of the seminars about industry developments or new processes. When he was nominated to lead the NPCA in the 1940s, Otto deferred the role to Ted Oser, who went on to lead the organization for two terms as president. As events unfolded at Orkin, the roles of Otto and Ted became more intertwined than before, with Ted assuming more responsibility and making more decisions at Orkin.

The NPCA convention was held in San Francisco in 1941, just a few weeks before the attack on Pearl Harbor and the start of our nation's involvement in World War II. It wasn't long before there was a shortage of service technicians in the company, and some managers met with draft boards to try to obtain military deferments for their key personnel. The war effort also meant shortages of chemicals and supplies—including gasoline, tires, and repair parts for vehicles and equipment. The shortages were so severe that many Orkin competitors just closed up shop until the war was over. Why? At first, it was a matter of numbers. Like many industries, a service industry like pest control relied on people to run the organization; as more men were drafted into the war effort, there were fewer workers at home. And the need for pest control was not immediately understood by the military or governmental agents. It was necessary to convince military officials that food supplies and the public were endangered by the proliferation of pests, and to convince them that pest control services were necessary to protect water, food supplies, and the public's health.

Ted Oser's industry connections paid off handsomely during the war years. He and William O. "Bill" Buettner, the founder of the national industry association who had always been supported by Orkin's top officials, traveled extensively to meet with legislative representatives, rationing boards, and other important agencies. Their message? Please classify pest control as an "essential service"—ensuring that the industry qualified for draft deferments and was placed on a preference list for chemicals, gasoline, tires, and food ration points for rodent bait. Out of forty-three service industries operating during the war, only two were classified as "essential"—pest control and mortuary service. A lot of the credit for this important classification was tied directly to Oser's and Buettner's efforts.

The war years certainly created special pest control needs. Bedbugs were a constant problem at military training camps, where barracks often had to be fumigated every six weeks as new recruits arrived for training; southern

The Orkin Man during World War II:
Joe Jones

World War II created shortages for everyone, and the Orkin pest control man was no exception. Joe Jones, a serviceman who first started working for Orkin in Columbus, Georgia, in February 1942, recalled how he continued to service his routes around Fort Benning during the war. He had to improvise and, in the process, came up with an entirely new service vehicle:

> *It was during the war, and business picked up rather rapidly at Fort Benning. Gasoline was rationed, and we didn't have enough to go around. Ed Fulford and I were the only PC (pest control) servicemen. Ed's route consisted mainly of Fort Benning and the surrounding area, so "Uncle Billy" Crawford asked me if I'd use a delivery bicycle to service the Columbus customers.*
>
> *My new "service bicycle" was bright red and had a little front wheel with a basket over it. In the basket I put my service grip, which had all my equipment and supplies—a bucket or can of dry rat bait, Argentine ant syrup, a can of sodium fluoride mixed with pyrethrum powder, bellows gun, several sizes of rat traps, and sometimes a small can of cyanide gas and dust gun.*

In Jones's case, the pest control industry's deferment efforts didn't work: he was drafted into the service in January 1943. But when he returned to the Columbus Orkin office in February 1946, he had a surprise waiting for him. Said Jones: "I found the bicycle stored in the basement, right under the office."

Jones retired from Orkin in September 1988, after forty-three years of service.

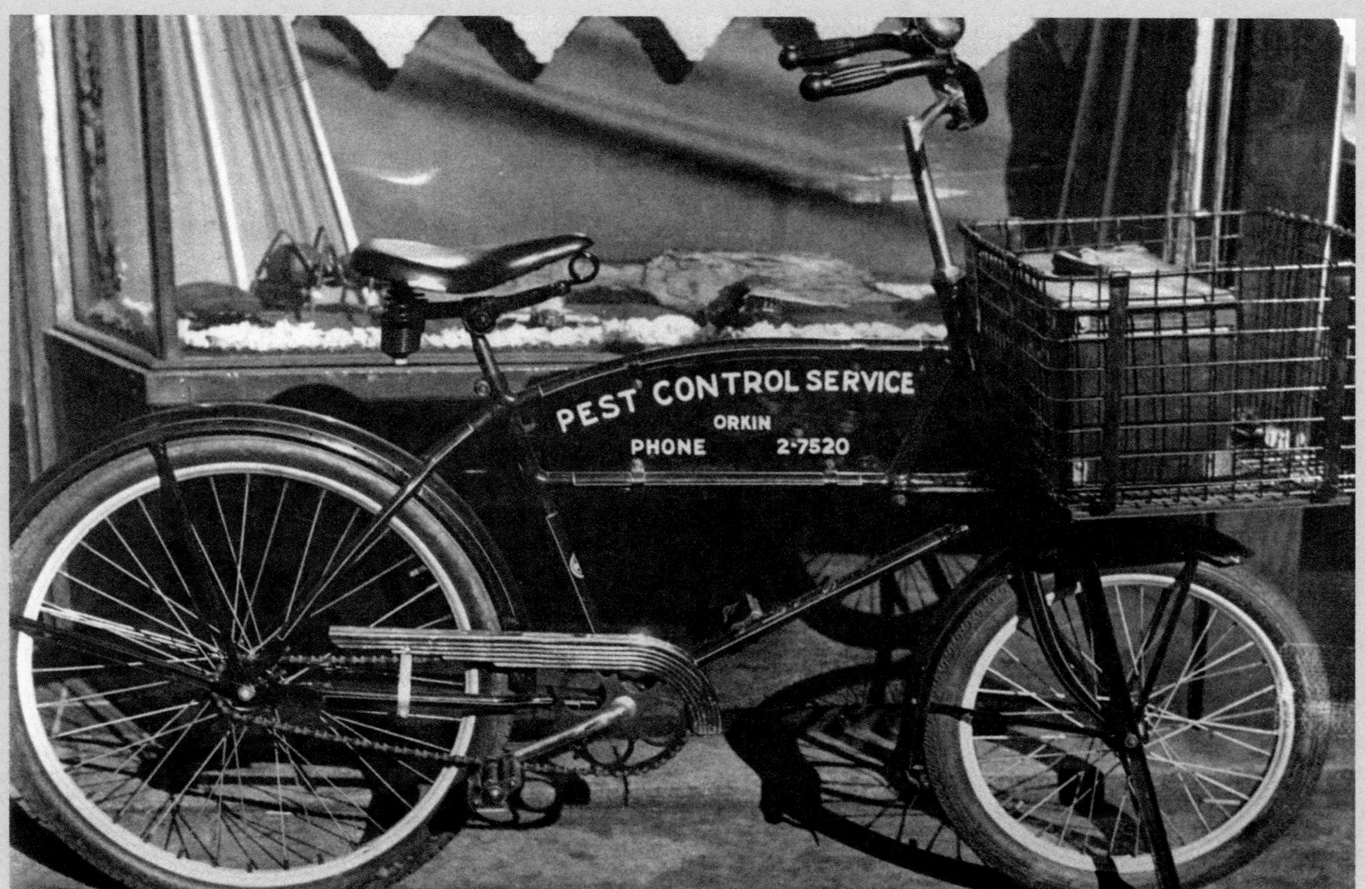

The Columbus, Georgia, Orkin branch relied on a service bicycle when gasoline was rationed during World War II.

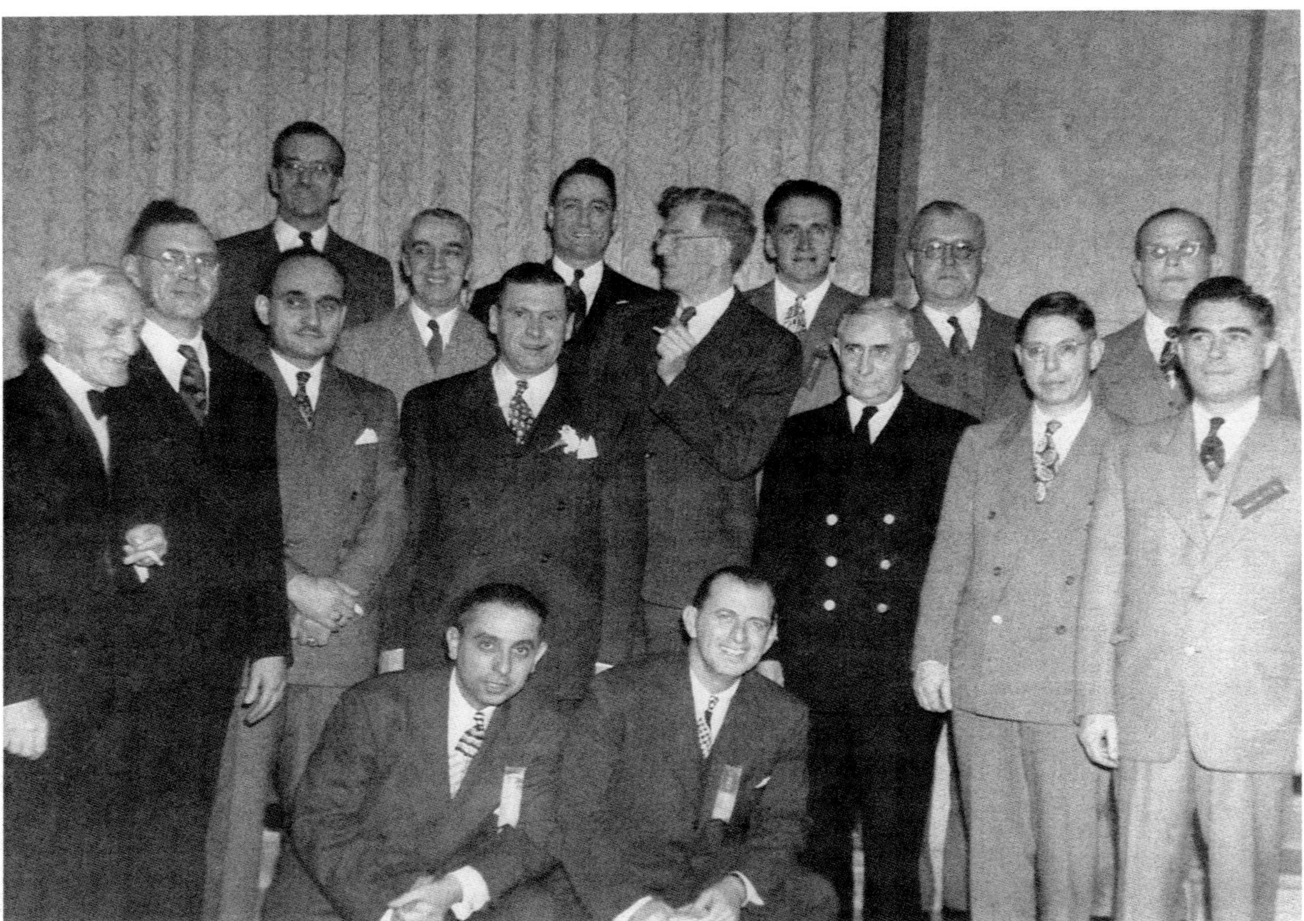

Ted Oser served as president of the National Pest Control Association and was successful in getting the government to classify pest control an "essential service" during World War II. Here he is shown, second row, third from left, at a meeting of the New York Pest Control Association in 1942. Others present included Jacques Hess, Herbert Meyer, Bill Buettner, S. A. Rohwer, Ned Goldy, Harold Shepherd, A. M. W. Carter, Bud Jennings, R. C. Roarkes, and Sidney Wimmer.

military bases reported particularly serious problems with mosquitoes, which required constant monitoring in the humid, rain-prone climate. There were heavy demands to fumigate ships and trains for the War Shipping Administration and the War Food Administration as food and supplies were shipped coast-to-coast. Many railroads needed around-the-clock service in order to maintain their schedules. To keep up with demand, teams of pest control operators would have cots at the railroad yards, rotating shifts between sleep and service for their crews.

At one time, Orkin had nearly 150 military establishments under contract for pest control and fumigation. The company was also called to service related warehouse and shipping companies, and Ted negotiated many contracts for Orkin's pest control services with the army, the navy, and the merchant marine, as well as with manufacturers and food-processing plants. And on the home front, movie theaters, restaurants, hotels, motels, transportation facilities, and residences all needed regular pest control service—war or no war.

The demand for more pest control services created havoc in the industry. Not only were there shortages of chemicals and important supplies, but the sodium fluoride, powdered arsenic, and pyrethrum chemicals that were available were often not very effective. This created the need for more frequent servicing, taxing an already limited workforce. And the political tensions of war had another particular impact on the pest control industry: one of its major insecticides—pyrethrum—was supplied predominantly by Japan. After 1941, as one might imagine, this "natural" pesticide that was derived from a flower was in critically short supply, and the United States turned to Kenya as its new major pyrethrum supplier.

Even with its "essential" service classification, Orkin and other pest control operators felt the pressure. Ted Oser traveled extensively, representing both Orkin and the NPCA to assure that pest control operators secured their needed allocations of supplies and equipment and, when possible, draft deferments for essential personnel. With Ted networking on a national level, Otto stayed closer to the corporate base, visiting field offices, recruiting, training, and overseeing the general operations of the company. Regular meetings with Kotler, Krawcheck, and Pressman helped Orkin map out strategies for handling shortages of material and manpower. Many branches had to be consolidated, and customers were serviced less frequently than before. Even so, just keeping branches supplied with pesticides and rodenticides was quite a challenge.

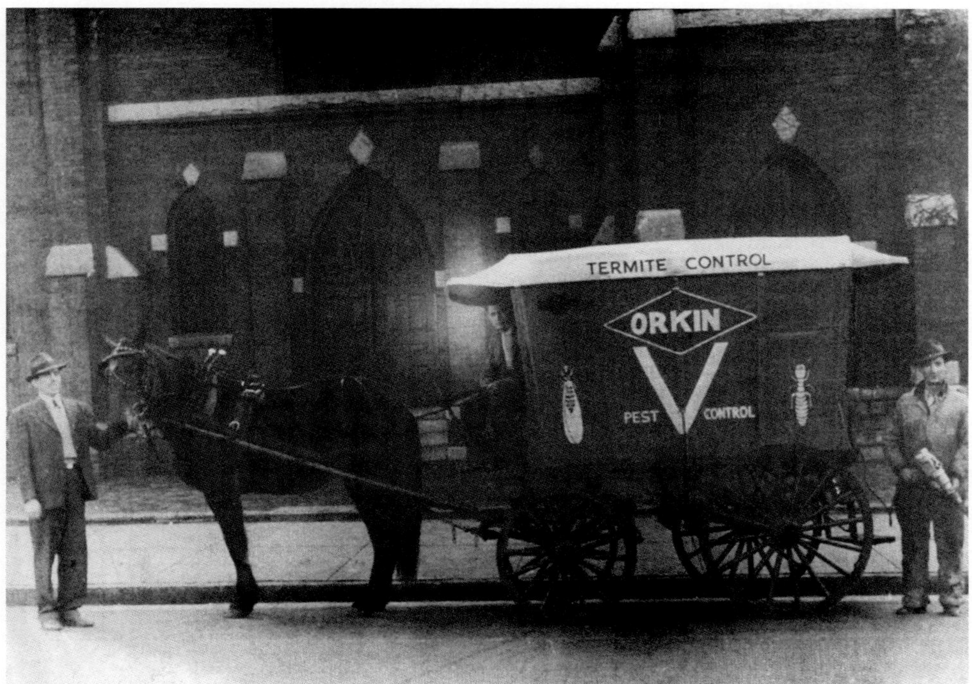

During the gasoline rationing of World War II, this wagon was used to make service calls. The V painted on the side of the wagon stood for victory.

Gertrude Walker ran the Richmond branch by herself during the war, with seven servicemen and one salesman. When Dorsey Hall, one of these servicemen, couldn't get pyrethrum during the war, he reported using phosphorus paste in his work to treat boxcars, warehouses, and grocery stores around the Richmond area. Marc Kaplan, who had established a long-running and successful record for the Macon, Georgia, branch, recalled "being on the road all the time" in order to service accounts and maximize the company's limited man power. When his branch had no car or gasoline, Orkin serviceman Joe Jones rode a bicycle in 1942 to continue to service his Columbus, Georgia, customers. Even the advertisements reflected the war's grip on our country, when an Orkin ad during the early 1940s displayed an army tank with this headline: "Rats are more dangerous than Tanks." It continued, "Cold weather drives rats and other pests inside your home and business establishment. Guard against this destructive and unsanitary condition. We exterminate rats, roaches, termites, fleas, bedbugs, ants."

And even Otto was hard-pressed to try to come up with new methods of pest control during the company's chemically deprived war years. After the 1943 NPCA convention, Otto sent a letter to Levenson Chemical Company in Omaha, Nebraska:

> *While at the convention, you were good enough to tell me of a electric light that you are using in bedbug contracts, and you also gave me the formula of a mixture that contains alfalfa. I made notes of both of these items, but unfortunately misplaced them. I would very much appreciate if you would send me this information in the enclosed stamped envelope. I would very much appreciate this kind favor. Otto Orkin*

In spite of the shortages and hardships, Orkin definitely managed to survive during the war: the military contracts actually helped the company expand. Gross sales of $2.098 million in 1945 were the highest in the company's history and included just over $250,000 in termite work. At the end of the war, Orkin announced that it was "the oldest and largest exterminating company in the South," with eighty-two branches in seventeen states. But the war years had also taken a toll on the Orkin company, and it now faced some major challenges. The company's lack of enough experienced and adequately trained staff was being blamed for some unfortunate fatalities that had occurred during a recent fumigation job, and Orkin's liability insurance was at risk of being canceled. The end of the war would bring the introduction of some powerful new chemicals for use in agriculture and pest control—accompanied by new federal and state regulations designed to control their use. To stay current with the demands of the changing exterminating profession, and perhaps to protect the company from future insurance lapses, Otto and Ted both realized that something entirely new was needed at Orkin after World War II. The company, managed for four decades by uncle and nephews and cousins and hardworking good ol' southern boys, was looking to acquire something it never realized was missing—outside, intellectual prowess. And so the word went out. One of the leading pest control companies in the country was looking to hire academically trained, experienced professionals from the fields of public health, entomology, chemistry, and sanitation engineering.

In 1946 Orkin moved into a building at 590 Courtland Street. Shortly thereafter the adjacent building at 591 Peachtree Street was purchased as well.

ORKIN'S EXPANSION

In 1946, Otto, Ted, and Max Cuba, Orkin's business advisor and attorney, began to change the look of the Orkin company—both figuratively and literally. The company moved to its new Atlanta home office at 590 Courtland Street, which had room for offices and ample storage space for equipment and supplies. Before long the company purchased the adjacent building at 591 Peachtree Street. The two buildings, connected by a freight elevator, allowed Orkin to create a

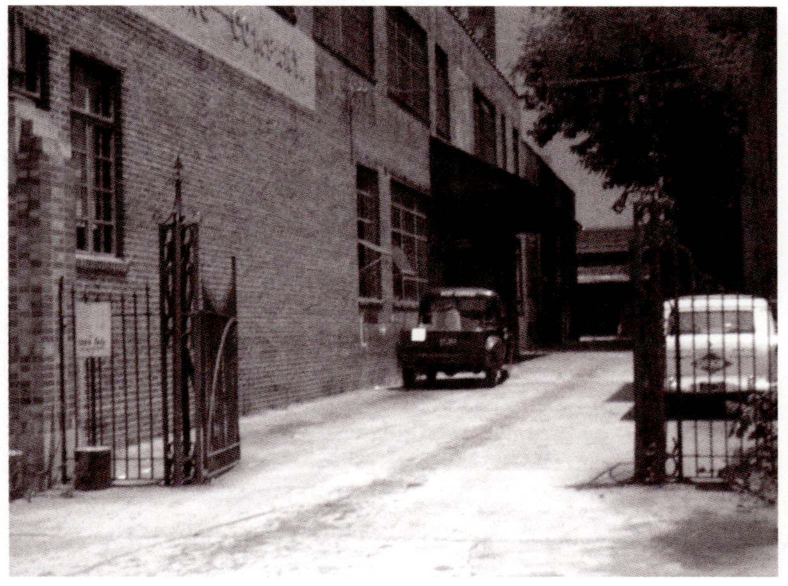

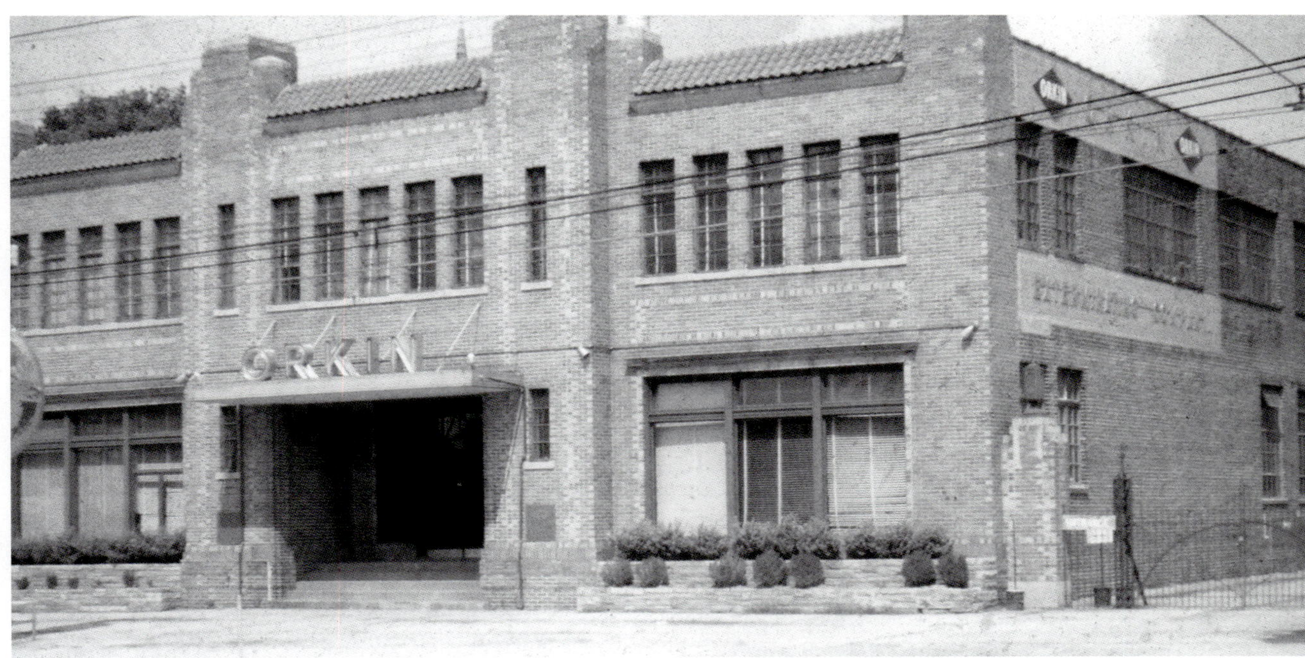

more professional appearance: the executive offices were in the Peachtree building and the service department and storage areas were in the Courtland Street facility. The home office distributed the first issue of a new company newsletter called *Orkin Talkin* in September 1946, following a company-wide "name the paper" contest that was won by Hope Newman in San Antonio.

Following World War II, a new wave of experienced, college-educated professionals was interested in working for Orkin.

But the people coming in and out of the new Orkin headquarters after World War II would do far more to alter the professional appearance of Orkin than a new company newsletter or the orchid-colored paint on the exterior of the Peachtree building. From the resumes that flowed steadily into the company, it was apparent that a new wave of experienced, college-educated professionals was interested in working for Orkin. And Ted, Otto, and Max wasted no time in hiring them. Consider:

- **Robert Couhig** was among the first professionally trained entomologists hired by Orkin after the war. A graduate of the University of Massachusetts in 1937, Couhig had worked for a pest control company in the North before serving in the army. His friend Bill Buettner told Couhig that Orkin was interested in expanding and wanted trained, experienced people. Couhig contacted Ted Oser and was hired in March 1946. He was trained by Abe Krawcheck, then took over one of the company's most profitable territories, the New Orleans branch. Couhig's district expanded to include all of Louisiana and Mississippi and into east Texas and south Arkansas.
- **Bernard Kolkana** graduated in 1939 with a degree in entomology from Purdue University, where he studied with famed entomologist Dr. John J. Davis. He worked with the Jacksonville, Florida, Public Health Department, heading up typhus control and managing that city's campaign against rats. Since Jacksonville was a strategic port city during the war, Kolkana's job had a defense priority. Cliff Green, the Tampa manager, induced Kolkana to come work for Orkin, and Ted Oser hired him in May 1946. After being trained, Kolkana took over the Miami branch, which became one of the foremost income producers in the company. Kolkana helped write the Florida legislation regulating the pest control industry, and he served on the Florida Pest Control Board. In 1956 he became manager of the Tampa branch, which he enlarged from seven routes to forty-six routes, and he was eventually named a regional vice president.
- **Max Isbill** was considered Orkin's "self-made entomologist." He was widely known for insect collections, and his personal collection of

Coleoptera (sheath-winged insects, including beetles) was among the most complete in the United States. First hired in Tennessee in 1939, Isbill served Orkin as a technical advisor from the 1940s through the 1960s, and was on the staff of the Orkin Institute of Industrial Sanitation. His primary areas of expertise were food-infesting insects and rodents in industrial facilities. Isbill developed a number of fumigation techniques that became standards for the industry. He became known throughout the world for his work in economic entomology, and he was

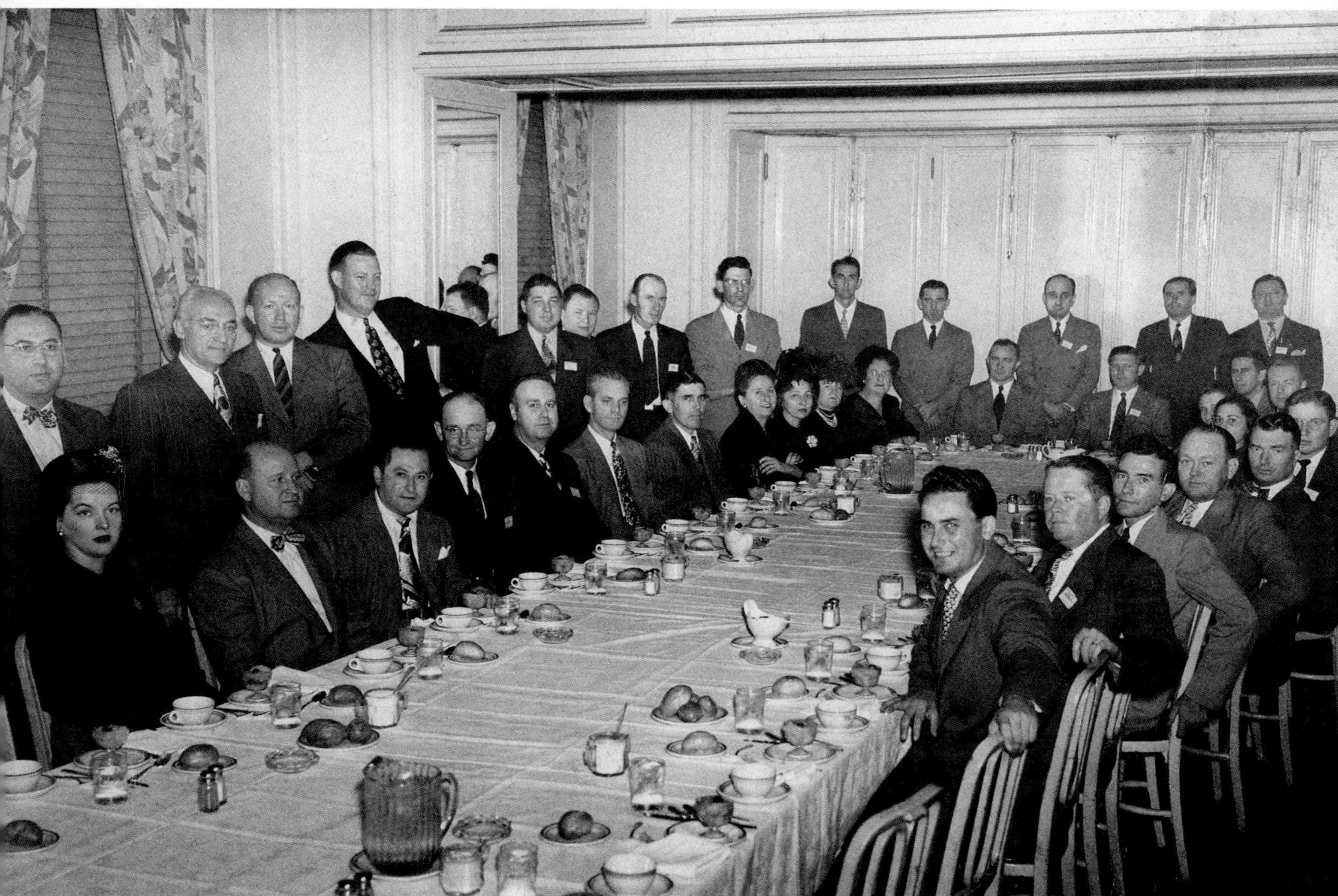

Many of the most-valued early managers attended this meeting in Philadelphia in 1948. Bob Couhig and Herman Fellton are sitting at the head of the table, with Ted Oser standing between and behind them. To their right, next to Ted, stand Jack Dorris and Lou Kotler. Seated on the left side of the table are (left to right) Mrs. Abe Krawcheck, Abe Krawcheck, Jake Pressman, next three not identified, Louis E. Killough, Mrs. Lou Kotler, Mrs. Ted Oser, and the next two not identified. Standing behind them are Ted Berz, Max Cuba, Red Tindol, Ike O'Hanlon, Mike Benton, Mr. Scales, next three not identified, and Jimmy Algood. Seated on the right side of the table are Charles Rosenthal, next person not identified, O. P. Brink, Mr. Hite, Eli Cole, J. D. Adams, Bernice Kaye, Perry Kaye, and next person not identified.

Orkin Talkin

In the fall of 1946 a new company newsletter called *Orkin Talkin* began to circulate throughout the company, pledging to be "Of, By, and For Orkin employees."

In seven quick issues, editor Jean Rooney established such standard features as "The President's Message," where Otto briefly addressed the employees with a pep talk of sorts or a holiday greeting; a "Nibblings" column that dutifully reported new hires, new babies, wedding announcements, and a smattering of company gossip; a humor column called "Orkin Laffin" that reprinted the corniest jokes; and regular features that showcased the writing talents of various employees. Who could ever forget Selethal Finklestein's clever twist on "'Twas the Night Before Christmas" (Do You Have Regular Pest Control Service) in the December 1946 edition?

And just as suddenly as it appeared, *Orkin Talkin* was gone. In March 1947 the newsletter disappeared and didn't resurface again until October 1949. "*ORKIN TALKIN* SAVED FROM UNTIMELY DEATH!" read the headline. Just as before, the same iconic paper scroll rolled out over the top of the page, with a cartoon character holding a megaphone as if to shout, "*Orkin Talkin*!" Otto's "President's Message" corner was back, but "Nibblings" had been changed to "Orkinites Niblets." And there was a new editor—Otto's son-in-law, Petty Bregman, who began his first issue with this promise:

"HERE IT IS!!! Proudly its pages are being seen throughout many branch offices by you and some 800 of your fellow Orkinites. We have waited a long time to see it. At times we thought it had died. But *Orkin Talkin* has survived. It has been born anew with all the vim, vigor, vitality of a newborn babe. . . . We are Orkin. When Orkin is talking, we are talking. This issue is our first in many years."

For nearly ten years, *Orkin Talkin* not only survived but became an important chronicle of company news and announcements, ranging from the mundane to truly significant corporate news.

For instance, "Otto the Orkin Man" was first introduced in the October 1950 issue of *Orkin Talkin*. From then on, the spray-can character was incorporated into the newsletter logo.

And when Otto Orkin celebrated fifty years of pest control service on January 9, 1951, the subsequent edition of *Orkin Talkin* provided complete coverage of Otto's achievement and the celebration it inspired—including the testimonial dinner and banquet held in his honor, with tributes from such distinguished guests as Atlanta Mayor William B. Hartsfield and Assistant U.S. Surgeon General Mark D. Hollis.

But the heart of *Orkin Talkin* was rarely focused on Otto. Instead, this simple company newsletter remained true to its mission to be "Of, By, and For Orkin employees." When Petty Bregman resigned as editor in 1951, associate editor Virginia Cook took over until Frances J. Black was named editor in June 1952. And under Black and her far-flung collection of office correspondents, *Orkin Talkin* covered employee news and corporate events throughout Orkin's growing territory.

When Black decided in 1958 to go back to school and leave Orkin, advertising manager Leon Robbins wrote to John E. Drewry, dean of the journalism school at the University of Georgia: "We would appreciate your letting us know of any young ladies who might be interested in following Miss Black which, to our way of thinking, would be roughly equivalent to speaking at Gettysburg after Mr. Lincoln. . . ."

The post was never filled. After a cost analysis, *Orkin Talkin*, the company's first newsletter, folded after the September 1958 edition.

one of the few Americans ever elected to the Fellowship in the Royal Entomological Society of London. Many of his displays of mounted insects were purchased by educational institutions for exhibits in entomology and natural history.

- **Orvis Griggs**, another experienced entomologist, joined Orkin as manager of the Richmond office in 1946. A graduate of the University of Florida in entomology, Griggs spent twelve years with the Federal Bureau of Entomology and Plant Quarantine. During the war years he was on part-time loan to the U.S. Public Health Service, conducting pest control projects in training camps along the Gulf Coast. After the war, he wanted to work in the private industry, and he chose Orkin.
- **Rufus L. "Red" Tindol Jr.** was an engineer with the Georgia Department of Public Health when he was called into service with the Corps of Engineers in the South Pacific. Because of Tindol's work during the war with classified pesticides, he was able to get supplies of restricted chemicals after the war, and he started his own exterminating company in Atlanta in affiliation with his brother-in-law, Jimmy Allgood, in Dublin and Robert Russell in Augusta. Rapidly, their affiliated companies took over many prime accounts in the Georgia area; after all, they had the new chemicals, which were far more effective than the old materials. Otto resented the competition on his home turf, and he started watching Tindol's operation from the hall outside his office door. Ted Oser finally approached Tindol about selling his company to Orkin, and Orkin's offer was one Tindol said he could not resist. Tindol joined Orkin as Georgia district manager in late 1947. At the closing of the sale of his business, Tindol remembered that Otto was quite agitated when he saw the list of Tindol's customers who had switched from Orkin.
- **Robert M. "Bob" Russell** joined Orkin in May 1947 after serving in the Sanitary Corps of the U.S. Army Engineers, working in the areas of insect and rodent control and in environmental sanitation. After the war he had started his own pest control company in Augusta in conjunction with Tindol, whom Russell had known while in the service. When Tindol sold his business to Orkin, Russell, likewise, sold his company and joined Orkin, first as a salesman in Augusta and Savannah, then as manager of the Atlanta Pest Control branch. He resigned as manager to complete his degree in sanitary engineering at the Georgia Institute of Technology. While going to Tech, he worked part-time as Orkin's purchasing agent; when he graduated in 1949, Russell became a member of Orkin's technical staff and was eventually named vice president of government relations for the company.

One of the company's most progressive hires occurred in May 1946, when Major Herman L. Fellton of the U.S. Public Health Service joined Orkin as the company's new technical director. A registered professional sanitary engineer, Fellton had been prominent in public health work and environmental sanitation for the previous eighteen years, including a stint as the deputy chief of the Health Department at the New York World's Fair in 1939 and 1940. His previous educational training and prior public health service made him a natural to expand the technical scope of Orkin. He would work to centralize purchasing, warehousing, and shipping of chemicals and supplies in order to standardize the use of chemicals in all field locations. But two special contributions made Fellton a unique individual at Orkin: first, he brought some much-needed training and professional expertise to the Orkin servicemen and branch managers, which led to the development of the Orkin Institute of Industrial Sanitation; and second, Herman Fellton is credited as the professional who introduced the use of a new chemical named 1068, later called chlordane.

Headline Highlights from Orkin Talkin

- **December 1952:** Orkin announces pension plan for employees.
- **July 1953:** New uniform introduced.
- **October 1953:** A loaf of bread containing rat poison is stolen from an exterminator's truck in Washington, prompting a story about locking your truck "to prevent something like this from happening to you."
- **December 1953:** Orkin-Tox introduced to the public. "Built-in triple protection."
- **January 1954:** At the managers' conference, advertising manager L. R. Robbins announced that Orkin will soon have four new television commercials, with the two on pest control to be in color. "We now advertise in more than 700 telephone directories and 90 newspapers."
- **April 1954:** "The Orkin Legend" history series begins.
- **May 1954:** "I've always been deathly afraid of even the smallest bugs," wrote Mrs. Ashby McGehee of San Antonio, Texas, to her uncle Marshall Lane, an Orkin salesman in Orlando, Florida. "You can imagine my fright when my little daughter Mimi found a 'crab' which turned out to be a granddaddy scorpion in the house. That did it! I frantically called Otto, the Orkin Man."
- **June 1955:** "King Bee" contest between district managers in full swing.
- **September 1955:** Orkin tackles the largest drywood termite fumigation job on record when it fumigates the fifteen-story Fleetwood Hotel in Miami. The entire operation—sealing, fumigating, and airing out—took three weeks. Horace Reese, technical representative out of Orlando, helped supervise the job. Whitey Hays and Irby Dunwoody of the Orkin termite department in the Miami branch served as foremen.
- **December 1955:** Orkin now coast-to-coast as Otto opens an office in California. Plus, the largest tarp fumigation ever done is described—9.3 acres of tarps

Soon after being hired at Orkin, Fellton began a series of four-day, concentrated training courses for branch managers and supervisors. For the first time in the company's history, he and his staff developed printed instructions for handling and administering chemicals in all branch locations. He visited branch offices to assist managers on technical matters and train service technicians. During his visits he would often contact governmental officials, offering assistance on pest control problems. He frequently met with public health representatives in an effort to alleviate misconceptions about the pest control operators' responsibilities and skills. Fellton was a frequent guest speaker, presenting information about all phases of pest control and taking advantage of every opportunity to elevate the recognition of pest control service from a trade to a science and profession.

"Herman Fellton was a real leader, very positive, very precise," remembered Glenn Burnett, at the time the head of the National Pest Control Association. He credited Fellton with developing some innovative techniques in order to teach extermination procedures. In fact, Fellton could have been

used to wipe out the Kharpa Beetle at the J. B. Hill Company in Fresno, California.

- **January 1956:** Miss Frances Jarrett, who has faithfully ridden a bus every day to work as a secretary since the Tampa Orkin office opened in 1936, wins the office collection contest. Her prize? A 1956 Nash Metropolitan hardtop, with radio and heater. "No more riding the bus for her!"
- **May 1956:** Fiftieth anniversary of the Food and Drug Act, signed into law by President Theodore Roosevelt.
- **June 1956:** New pest control service kits save time from trucks to home. "With my kit in one hand and my spray gun in the other, I can carry all the supplies I need for several stops," said Wilbert Marchand of Baton Rouge, Louisiana.
- **October 1956:** Ed Fulford back at work in his electric wheelchair!
- **February 1957:** Earl Geiger, former sales manager of Bliss Exterminator Company of New York City, profiled as new Orkin manager of the Atlanta exterminating branch.
- **May 1957:** Tommy Thompson, who created the early Orkin ads in the 1920s, dies.
- **August 1957:** Tenth Annual Series of Orkin Service Schools begins. "More than 2,400 Orkinites will go back to school during the next three months," according to Robert Russell, technical director.
- **January–February 1958:** King Bee contest commences, and managers hold their annual meeting.
- **September 1958:** Last publication of *Orkin Talkin*, featuring news of recent branch changes in Charlotte, North Carolina; an Army H-37 helicopter filled with bees and rescued by the Orkin Man in Monroe, Louisiana; and editor Frances J. Black's resignation.

the original "show 'em how, don't just tell 'em how" advocate and a forerunner of an important training technique at Orkin. Under Fellton's leadership Orkin acquired a building on the parking lot of Crawford Long Hospital and used the building to simulate situations that servicemen could expect to encounter on the job—residential and commercial kitchens, an area with upholstered furniture, and different surfaces where servicemen encountered pest control issues. The house served as a testing and training ground for hundreds of managers and supervisors, who traveled to Atlanta for instructions on new chemicals, equipment, application procedures, and safety practices.

In 1948 Fellton's technical department began a series of one-day service schools, conveniently located around the country so employees from six to eight neighboring Orkin offices could attend. The first series of schools were held in Knoxville, Roanoke, Louisville, Raleigh, Charlotte, Greenville, Charleston, Orlando, Birmingham, Memphis, Dallas, New Orleans, and Atlanta. The training included information on new chemicals and instructions for their application and safety. Two or three members of the technical staff would load a station wagon with equipment and models of houses with various types of construction to use in demonstrating treating procedures. By the time the series of schools was completed, all service employees throughout the company had participated. These service schools allowed the technical staff to interact with personnel throughout the company. But more important, it allowed the company to standardize Orkin's methodology and elevate the employees' expertise.

Constantly improving and tracking technological changes in the industry proved to have a financial benefit for Orkin.

The Orkin technical staff also stressed the importance of staying current with reading material and technology. In 1950 Orkin's technical department initiated its *Technical Bulletins* to keep every office informed about the latest service developments and to help technicians better perform their services. Beginning in 1952, the technical department began placing representatives in each region to oversee training, particularly for those taking licensing examinations, and to assist with specialized service and sales situations.

Fellton's "How To Train A Serviceman" publication was widely circulated in the industry. Wrote Fellton: "Pest control is a rather hazardous business, and the best and only way to minimize accidents, with resultant expensive claims, is by the thorough training of our servicemen. . . . The successful pest control firms of the future will be those which incorporate a serviceman training program as an integral part of their operations." Fellton stressed simplicity of information and maximum participation in the training program, which he said should include reading material, periodic meetings, and on-the-job training. "Accident prevention cannot be over-emphasized," he stressed. "A new employee should receive good basic training in all aspects of his job before he is sent out on a route by himself. This training should include a period of apprenticeship working a route with an experienced serviceman. It should also include training in identification of the common rodent, insect and related pests, the proper formulation and use of insecticides and rodenticides, correct use of applicator equipment, safety principles and customer relationship. The pest control industry, operationally, is no better than the servicemen we utilize. Let's advance the industry by ensuring that our service personnel are adequately trained and competent."

James Hutto started his career as a serviceman with Orkin in January 1946 in eastern North Carolina, and he never forgot the difference that Herman Fellton and his training techniques made in the company's service training. "At first there was no written training material," he said. "I just went with a previous service sales representative for two weeks, then I was on my own. Soon after Fellton started we got this typed, recipe-like instruction about how much chemical to mix and how to use it."

Constantly improving and tracking technological changes in the industry proved to have a financial benefit for Orkin. Don Holt, who joined Orkin in 1949 after serving in the merchant marine and public health department, claimed that critical assistance from the technical staff helped him better handle fumigating ships that had been quarantined by the U.S. Department of Agriculture. "A ship's downtime was usually eight days—two days to seal a ship, three days to hold the fumigant, and three days to aerate," said Holt. "With support from Atlanta's technical team, we were able to reduce the sealing time to less than one day and cut the aeration time by using huge blowers to clear the fumigants, thus cutting nearly three days from the ship's downtime, saving thousands of dollars."

CHEMICALS, CHANGES, AND CHOICES

Orkin's emphasis on safety and training had everything to do with the changes in the industry after World War II—changes that Orkin followed closely. As head of the NPCA during the last two years of the war, Ted Oser knew exactly what new technologies and new pesticides had been developed during the conflict. And he knew that the discovery, research, and development of chemicals during these years had produced a slate of new pesticides that would usher in a new era for the pest control industry. This postwar chemical warfare against pests included some of the most famous—if not infamous—chemicals in pest control history in the twentieth century:

- **DDT: Dichlorodiphenyl-trichloroethane** was first identified and tested in 1939. Used during World War II to fight body lice and other pests, it was manufactured in 1943 and soon became the most widely used single insecticide in the world. The first military use of DDT—other than fighting typhus-carrying lice—was to control malaria-carrying mosquitoes. Through its connections with Bill Buettner, Orkin obtained use of DDT after the war and was one of the first pest control operators (PCOs) to do so.

- **Compound 1080: Sodium fluoroacetate** is derived from plants found in South Africa, where its poisonous effects on cattle and rodents were widely known. Subsequent research revealed that it was a very effective rodenticide—highly toxic but accepted by rats and mice because it has no objectionable odor or taste and does not irritate the skin.
- **ANTU: Alpha-naphthythiourea** is a synthetic poison, manufactured by DuPont in 1946. A very effective rodenticide generally, it didn't work on all rodents and sometimes killed pets. Orkin used it, but later discontinued it.
- **1068, or chlordane:** A very effective household insecticide with wide usage in the control of roaches, ants, carpet beetles, termites, and other pests. First given the code identification of 1068, Orkin's own Herman Fellton introduced the use of 1068 and wrote the instruction page for its application; however, a patent dispute kept the chemical from being identified as "chlordane" by the United States Department of Agriculture until the early 1950s.

These new chemicals equaled better, faster pest control—and the result was an incredible boom in sales and services by Orkin. For instance, in 1945, the company sales volume was $2.1 million, including $250,000 in termite work; in 1951, the total sales volume was $7.03 million, including $3.25 million in termite contracts—a figure that represented more than the combined sales for pest control and termites just six years earlier.

Better chemicals available after the war equaled better, faster pest control—and the result was an incredible boom in sales and services by Orkin.

And while pest control continued to be the heart of Orkin's services, the company was expanding in some critical areas. Otto was very proud of the growth of his separate termite company. In 1945 J. Stark "Starkey" Thomas was named manager of the company—a popular, energetic manager who commanded not only Otto's trust but also the respect of his colleagues. During 1949 the much-anticipated *Termite Sales Manual* was completed by Thomas and Bob Russell, with some fifty pages of pictures, facts, and figures about termites and the incredible havoc they bring to homes and buildings. It was a valuable sales tool, and Orkin did approximately ten thousand termite jobs during 1949, ranging from large government projects to small private homes. In December 1949

Ted Oser, who was then vice president of sales, urged that salesmen generate termite sales by knocking on doors, one house after another, and asking permission to make a termite inspection. Until then, most termite sales resulted from advertising, primarily in newspapers and telephone directories and the ensuing phone inquiries. But, said Ted, "The aggressive manager and salesman goes out and looks for business. Don't wait in the office for the phone to ring." Apparently, one sales representative went so far as to lease a house in order to sell the owner a termite contract!

Early methods of termite control included drilling holes in the sills and forcing a preservative (pentachlorophenol) into the wood, then scattering a mothball-like substance around the perimeter of a house. But after World War II, the chemicals and methods used for termite control changed significantly. At first chlordane was mixed with oil-based kerosene (which was a fire hazard) and applied with a hand-pump applicator. Later, chlordane became water-soluble, making it much safer and less smelly, but some old-timers felt it was not as effective. Chlordane and other chlorinated hydrocarbons eventually placed on the market were much more effective in controlling infestations, and they gave longer-lasting protection against future infestations.

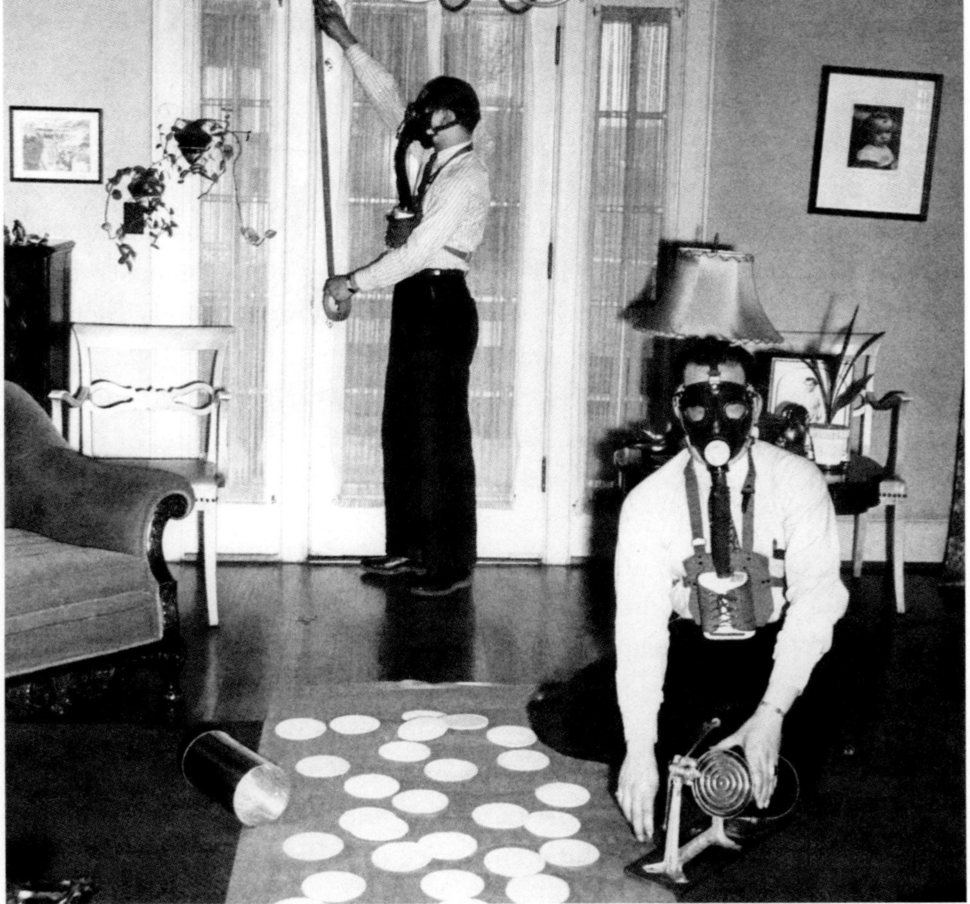

Otto Orkin was originally reluctant to get into the fumigation business because it required the use of lethal gas.

Another area of expansion for Orkin was fumigation. Otto began doing fumigation work in Virginia after World War I—but it was arguably crude, based on sealing windows and doors and dropping hydrogen cyanide blocks throughout the buildings. During World War II, Orkin was known for its fumigation work to eliminate bedbugs, lice, and fleas, particularly at military bases. And in the latter part of the 1940s, when drywood termites were discovered in Florida, Orkin technicians realized that an entire structure had to be tented, sealed, and injected with toxic fumigant in order to destroy the infestation. Bernard Kolkana, Miami manager at the time, met frequently with Dr. Thomas E. Snyder, entomology consultant to the Smithsonian Science Museum in Washington, D.C., to understand the characteristics of drywood termites and how to control them. With additional help from the entomologists at the University of Miami and Bob Russell at Orkin (who specialized in large termite jobs and industrial fumigations), Kolkana devised a fumigation wrap of heavy craft paper, sealed with four-inch tape and fastened on one-by-four-inch stakes at the ground—which proved to be the forerunner of the tarp fumigation system perfected by Orkin in the 1950s. The first wrap-up fumigation job using this system was a house owned by an automobile dealership on Biscayne Boulevard in Miami: the house was wrapped, sealed, and filled with cyanide fumigant to kill the drywood termite infestation. "Sounds impossible, doesn't it?" Orkin advertised in its fumigation literature. "But we are doing it all the time, and have been since we pioneered the tent method of destroying drywood termites, beetles, weevils, wood borers, roaches, rodents and scores of other pests. The tent method makes possible the ultimate in fumigation for home or business."

In addition to buildings, Orkin was frequently called on to fumigate agricultural products and interstate commerce items. Several branches had a mobile fumigation unit; the one in Orlando was called the Drywood Fire Department. It was on call for wrap-up fumigations of any nature, and the truck was equipped with ladders, tarps, and all other necessary equipment, including experienced operators. Max Isbill, with Clyde Sylvester of the Fort Worth, Texas, office and John Veal of the El Paso branch, eventually established a border fumigation station near El Paso, Texas, to take care of quarantined goods for that part of the country.

Back in Atlanta additional services were being developed. Borrowing from Otto's early "Creator of Sanitation" days, the Orkin Technical Department in 1947 began a sanitation inspection and training service for companies that handled food items—such as flour mills and candy manufacturers. A member of the technical staff would assist in making an inspection and work out a program for the particular food infestation. In 1948 the Atlanta office expanded its sanitation service to include janitorial service in addition to its regular pest control work. One of Orkin's custodial customers was the Ansley Hotel, where such tasks as mopping, waxing, and other cleaning duties were handled by Orkin's staff. Ted Oser set up the new service, and coined its motto: "Watch the Corners."

In 1951 Orkin officially established the Institute of Industrial Sanitation as an adjunct to the Pest Control Division. Headed by Herman Fellton and executive director Keith Fitch, the institute offered consulting services to any industry or organization, but particularly to those companies dealing with food or food handling. The institute's staff—composed of experienced professionals in the fields of sanitation engineering, public health, plant pathology, chemistry, entomology, and related disciplines—would inspect a client's premises, provide a detailed written report, and offer to consult with, and give advice to, the client's managers while providing training for the client's employees. The institute staff did not perform corrective services nor did they sell any products—even though the clients were always aware of the consultant's affiliation with Orkin's pest control services.

The industry—killing pests with increasingly toxic chemicals—now required something Otto Orkin never experienced in his days of ground arsenic, phosphorus paste, and rat traps. It now required greater monitoring, more attention to safety, and constant evaluation to determine whether regulations and controls were adequate.

To their credit neither Otto nor Ted ever shied away from this side of the industry. For any number of reasons—from trying to create favorable public relations for Orkin to influencing consumers and regulatory authorities—Ted wrote many letters and editorials during his two terms as NPCA president

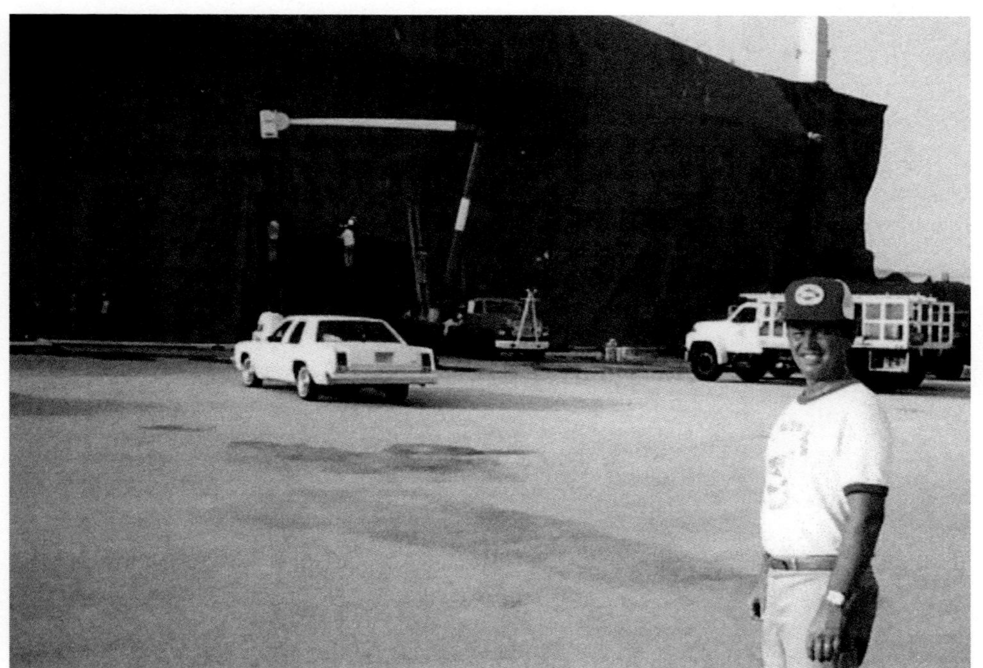

Fumigations were never a big business until Orkin started using tarpaulins to cover the entire building being treated. Here Gordon Crenshaw, manager of the South Florida district at the time, oversees the fumigation of the Pan Am world headquarters in Miami in July 1983. At 6.7 million cubic feet, it was the largest fumigation Orkin ever did.

emphasizing "safety practices" as absolutely essential for the industry. Shortly after being named president of the NPCA at the annual banquet in Chicago in 1944, Oser wrote an editorial in *Pests* magazine that nearly pleaded with his peers to recognize their past mistakes and put safety first:

> There is no other word possibly that means quite so much to us PCOs (pest control operators) as the word *safety.* Unless we can show our customer and the public generally that their health and property are not endangered when they deal with us, and unless we can see to it that our employees and we as owner-operators render services with self-safety, it will not be long before we shall have lost the confidence of the public and, indeed, shall have legislation that will cause us serious technical burdens. And yet, in this completely vital matter of safety, we can look to no one but ourselves. We know our business best. It is definitely up to us to improve our methods, our technique, our standards, and our personnel and thus avail ourselves of new discoveries and developments in the use of rodenticides and insecticides. To "just get by" must be frowned upon by every self-respecting PCO in the nation. The uninformed PCO will unfortunately join the ranks of the "forgotten man."
>
> The members of this association were not content with their lot, and programs were made. This progress has manifested itself in . . . two instruments of progress: "The Good Domestic Fumigation Practices" and "Standards for the Use of Calcium Cyanide in Structures as an Extermination Procedure in Rodent Control," recently adopted at the Chicago convention. These instruments of progress are the result of much hard work, study and unfortunate accidents, and are given to us not to put away in a file drawer, to be forgotten, but to be applied in our everyday work. Our goal for professional recognition means more than just knowing how to do a good job. It means, above all else, that the Professional Pest Control Operator, employed to do a job, is going to do it safely. . . . IN ALL FAIRNESS, I THINK WE ALL KNOW WHEN WE TAKE CHANCES. Let's simply stop taking chances with ourselves, our employees, or with our customers and the public. Remember, IN SAFETY THERE IS HAPPINESS.

By the end of his two terms as association president, Ted was still pressing for implementation of better safety programs. He continually urged that contributions be made to promote industry-wide safety. During the 1946 NPCA convention in New Orleans, Otto Orkin heeded his own executive's advice and announced that he was giving the association a gift of $2,525 to launch a safety campaign.

But safety was not Ted's only platform. He constantly encouraged his fellow PCOs to think highly of their industry, to recognize their contributions to the health and safety of society, and to stop "apologizing" for the industry by using unmarked vehicles. In words that echoed the stance of Otto Orkin, Ted insisted that PCOs should not wait for legislation to force them to mark their vehicles; homeowners, he once said, "should let their neighbors know that the health and welfare of their family and property were protected by regular pest control service." The Orkin Diamond on every Orkin service truck reflected both Ted's and Otto's insistence that pest control be recognized as a valuable public service—not something to be ashamed of.

Ted admitted, however, that the "earlier hit-or-miss methods that once characterized the work of Pest Control Operators had, without doubt, not yet been overcome," he wrote in 1946. "Much remains to be done to establish the industry on a more secure foundation. Nevertheless, so much progress has been and is being made, that the way ahead is clear, and the goal that we have set for the industry is within our grasp. Scientific research and the application of exact and scientific methods have lifted the operations of the industry out of the realm of the economic outcast and we are at last coming into our own as an indispensable part in the modern scheme of things."

In 1947 the enactment of the Federal Insecticide, Fungicide and Rodenticide Act (FIFRA) placed the pest control industry under the regulatory control of the U.S. Department of Agriculture.

As enthusiastic as Ted and many PCOs no doubt were, the industry was given a strong nudge in that direction in 1947 with the enactment of the Federal Insecticide, Fungicide and Rodenticide Act (FIFRA). This act placed the pest control industry under the scrutiny and regulatory control of the U.S. Department of Agriculture; one of the many areas it highlighted was the need for pest control operators to be better trained, more knowledgeable, and more safety-conscious. With federal and state legislation becoming the norm, more and more state pest control associations were being formed to help the industry adapt to the growing regulations and licensing requirements for pest control operators. Many Orkin employees were instrumental in establishing state organizations. To name but a few: Cliff Green, Walter Helms, and Bernard Kolkana were among the organizers of the Florida Pest Control Association; Bob Couhig started an organization in Louisiana; Louis Kotler helped start the Memphis Pest Control Association, while Abe Krawcheck assisted with the association in Alabama; Orkin home office staff started an Atlanta pest control association; Ted Oser and George Huffman started the statewide Virginia State Pest Control Association, while Richard Rottler (Orkin's Norfolk Antipest Company manager) was elected as the first president of the Virginia Tidewater Pest Control Association.

Through these various associations, Ted Oser continued to stress that one of the factors that "contributed to the emancipation of the industry"

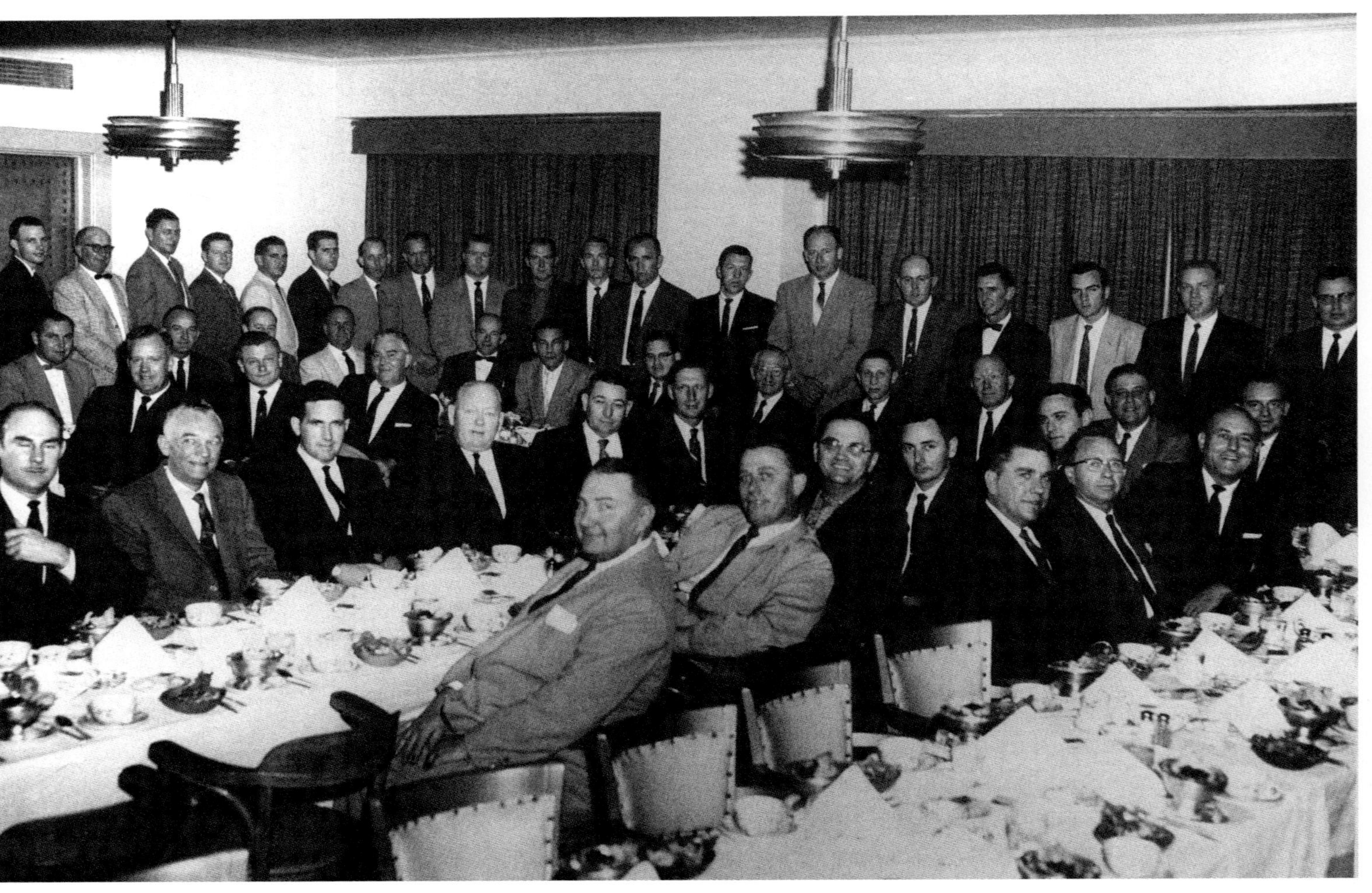

At a meeting in the early 1960s. Left to right, seated at frontmost table: first two not identified, Gerald Ellerbee, and Grady Rogers. Table in center, front side: Starkey Thomas, Jim Jernigan, Horace Anthony, not identified, Carl Prescott, and Marcus Kaplan; back side: Earl Geiger, John Hatcher, Jack Dorris, next three not identified, Otto Orkin, Perry Kaye, and R. L. (Red) Tindol. Back table, front side: Jack Watkins, Ray Chandler, Joe Vining, not identified, and Sanford Orkin. Standing behind Otto Orkin, Butsy Wright. Standing behind Perry Kaye, Duke White. Others not identified.

was the industry's newfound emphasis on technical training. When Orkin hired Fellton—and initiated Orkin's widely recognized technical training programs—Oser showed the company he wasn't afraid to live by Fellton's principles and lead by example. Fellton always gave credit to Ted—and not to Otto—as the visionary behind the push for technical training and for his "good housekeeping" angle of pest control. True, Otto had always emphasized the housekeeping side of pest control, as judged by his early pleas for sanitation reform in warehouses and restaurants and his early advertisements as the "Creators of Sanitation." But to Fellton, Ted was the more farsighted of the two. "He wanted to make the industry a profession to be proud of," said Fellton. "Otto was persistent, shrewd, and determined, but not really a visionary."

GROWTH AND INNOVATION

Through the 1940s and into the early 1950s, Otto's ability to surround himself with excellent people continued to carry the company forward toward a decade that would be known for growth, groundbreaking advertising, and technological advances. And though the entomologists, technical experts, and sanitation-health professionals at the home office would help advance Orkin's prominence in the industry, the district managers, branch managers, and service technicians throughout the country proved to be the backbone of the company, responsible for the company's $6 million in sales in 1950 as Orkin expanded to include over a thousand employees in 141 locations in twenty states.

There were many great Orkin men leading the way. There was George Huffman in Tennessee, who started as an Orkin serviceman and worked his way up to supervisor and then branch manager, the only Orkin manager who could ever claim that he trained two of Orkin's future presidents; Marcus Kaplan of Macon, Georgia, branch manager, who believed strongly in educating the consumer on the value of pest control, and who for years drove his trademark black 1937 Chevrolet coupe with an Orkin diamond on the side; A. B. Hollingsworth of Alabama, who started out as Orkin's one-man manager, salesman, and service operator in Montgomery and eventually became manager of the entire Alabama district; Dan Cauble of the Louisiana, Tennessee, and Texas districts, highly regarded for his ability to stimulate growth through new accounts and for his attention to detail; Walter Helms of Florida, who later opened the Kansas-Missouri-Nebraska districts and served as vice president of the western and the northeast region; James Hutto of North Carolina, who implemented the division of North Carolina into two districts, which allowed managers to better sell and service their customers and allowed Orkin to increase its revenue faster; John W. Hatcher, a salesman in Georgia, branch manager in Savannah and Roanoke, and assistant sales manager to Ted Oser in Atlanta; and Ed Elkins, who answered an Orkin ad for a pest control serviceman in 1946, a move that would begin his incredible career path through a company that would one day name him president of the entire operation.

Their instructions and game plan were fairly uniform and simple. From Helms's days in the Midwest, he recalled these Orkin strategies:

- **Developing territories:** Referrals from existing customers; home shows; word-of-mouth; technicians also sold accounts; accounts serviced on a grid system.
- **Advertising:** Local advertising in periodicals; when Otto visited, [he] wanted to meet editors of the local *Jewish Chronicle.* However, Atlanta headquarters coordinated advertising, which was a relief to local branches.
- **Business operations:** Deposits went into bank accounts tied to

Atlanta. Expenses paid from Atlanta. Prelisted Accounts Receivable were typed and sent to Atlanta by the end of each month with new accounts and canceled accounts noted.

- **Selling/rates:** Accounts were priced according to the estimate of cost. If cost was $105, then contract would be $200. No "rate card" was available, but costs were pretty much standardized. Materials shipped from Atlanta.

After 1946 an advisory or policy committee of district and home office managers began meeting with company officials regularly to help plan and determine overall company goals and guidelines. Initially, longtime managers like Kotler, Krawcheck, and Pressman overwhelmingly influenced the decisions. But as the number of districts increased, membership on the committee was rotated among the managers, with a different manager presiding as chairman. A representative from the company's general counsel, the accounting office, or tax consultants usually sat in on the committee meetings. To get an idea of what topics were discussed, consider this agenda for the May 9, 1950, policy committee meeting:

1) **Status of Orkin Company under new wage and hour law**
2) **Incentive pay plans**
3) **Insurance**
4) **Advertising proposal presented by Abe Weinstein**
5) **Termite control as applied to new homes and other construction.**

To his branch and district managers—and to the growing number of men and women in the field working as service and salespeople—Otto continued to be an inspiration and a mentor.

"I believe the early growth of the company can be directly attributed to Mr. Orkin's basic theories concerning service, sales, and collections. I believe he placed their importance in that order," remembered Don Holt, who started with Orkin as a serviceman in Norfolk, Virginia, in August 1949. "Early in my employment, he pointed out that when you lose one account, you must sell two to make an increase. Save one, and you need only sell one for the same result."

Apparently Otto never stopped his habit of calling branch managers in the middle of the night in order to question them about canceled accounts. Kolkana, who developed the Miami Orkin branch into one of the foremost income producers in the company, established his own way of handling these disconcerting late-night calls: he kept his canceled accounts by his bedside, so he could have an answer for his boss when he called at 2 A.M. and demanded to know why someone had canceled service. Years later, he still remembered

Otto's middle-of-the-night lectures: "When you lose an account, you could soon be out of business!" But Kolkana, who continued to advance in the Orkin ranks, claimed that Otto and his unconventional style taught him more about "business than I ever learned in college. When customers wake up every morning, they should give thanks for Orkin."

When Mr. Orkin visited his out-of-town branch managers, he almost always invited the managers and their wives out to dinner. But even dinner out was viewed by Otto as a business opportunity.

"Soon after I was employed as a manager of the Norfolk office, Mr. Orkin came to work with me one day," said Holt. "About five o'clock, he told me to call my wife to meet us at one of Norfolk's best downtown restaurants. As we were finishing our dinner, Mr. Orkin asked me if we served the account. When I said no, he immediately jumped to his feet and went to the counter asking to see the owner. Finally, after Mr. Orkin's pleasing but determined

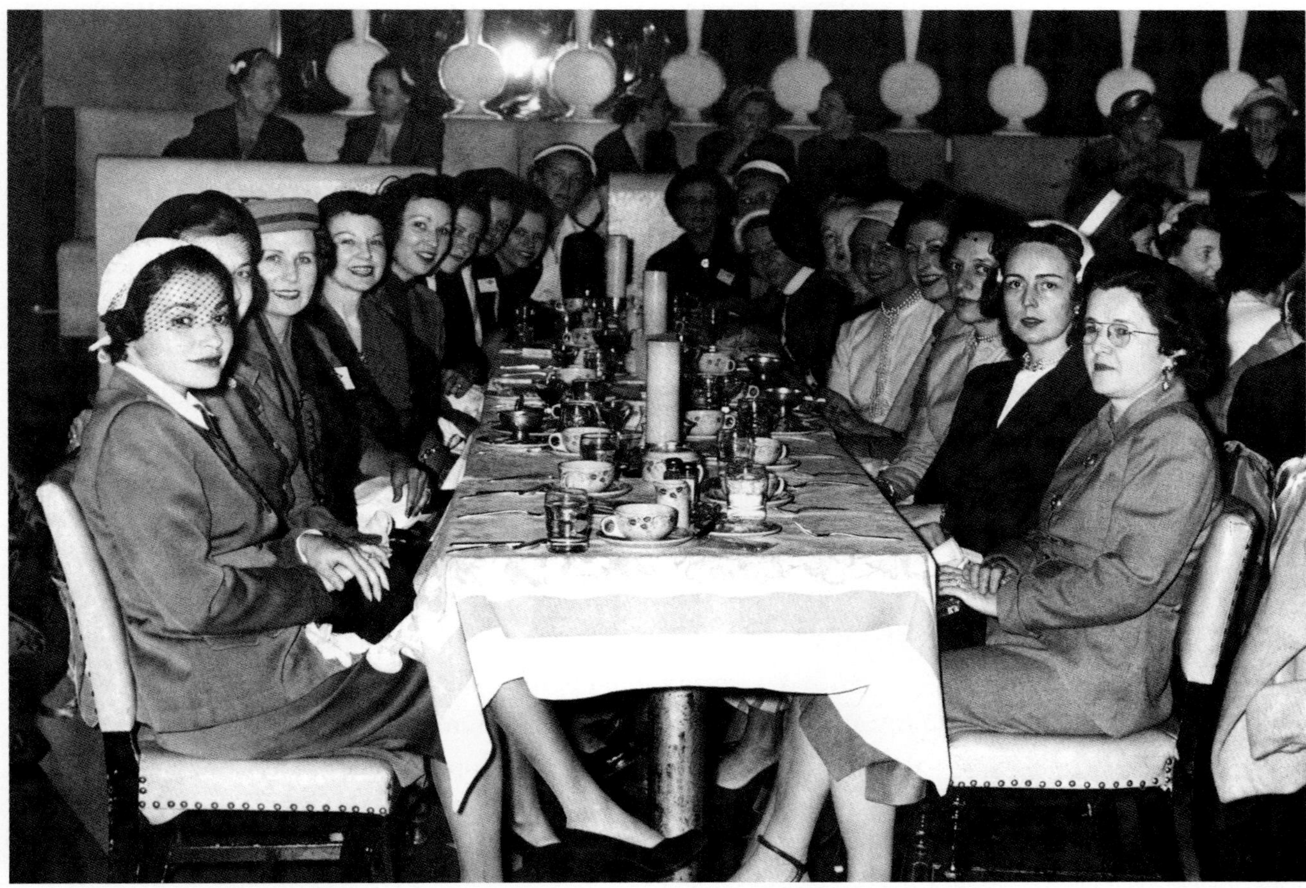

Otto always encouraged spouses to participate in conventions. Here (left to right) Mrs. Irving Kaler (Atlanta), Mrs. Murray Cooper (Atlanta), Mrs. Frank Aiello (Little Rock), Mrs. Carl Whitson (Little Rock), Ms. Micky Lubbs (Memphis), Mrs. Don Holt (Norfolk), Mrs. B. L. Holt (Norfolk), Mrs. J. O. Honeycutt (Birmingham), Mrs. C. W. Miller (St. Petersburg), Mrs. Pam Burion (Atlanta), Mrs. Joe Gurson (Atlanta), Mrs. C. E. Nixon (Gastonia), Mrs. John Hatcher, Mrs. A. B. Wright (Atlanta), Mrs. Gerald Ellerbee (Atlanta), and Mrs. R. J. Ellerby (Winter Haven) attend a luncheon in the Paradise Room of the Henry Grady Hotel in Atlanta in 1953.

insistence, the owner did come out, and after a nice conversation, the owner was assured that I would be calling on him from time to time.

"From the restaurant, the three of us walked up Granby Street. It was about 7:30 to 8:00 in the evening, and the stores were closed. We came to Baker's Shoe Store—the headquarters of the company being in Atlanta—and the manager was trimming the window and arranging the shoes. For door openers, Mr. Orkin cupped his face to his hands and called through the door: 'I have greetings for you from Atlanta.' Of course, the manager, thinking there was a message from his boss, hurried to the door and unlocked it and was greeted with: 'I am Mr. Orkin from Atlanta. Do we service your account? How is the service? This is my local manager who you can call any time with a problem.' The store manager was impressed with Mr. Orkin's interest in the service and to know he could call on me anytime he might have a problem."

Holt frequently told another story to illustrate how Otto's insistence on satisfied customers and good service paid off.

Around 1950, in the Norfolk branch, "One of our first termite jobs was sold for five hundred dollars—including repairs—and I thought we had a plum!" said Holt. "It was on an old church in Princess Anne County, being restored by the local Historical Society. We started to work on the job and found that all of the eighteen-by-eighteen sills in the church had to be replaced. Knowing Mr. Orkin's insistence on satisfied customers and good service, we replaced the sills, and I sent a lumber bill for over five hundred to Atlanta. I was never once criticized for my handling of the account. Now, for the reward for good service. The person in charge of procurement for the Fifth Naval District was interested in the restoration of that church. As a result of his satisfaction with our service, we subsequently were awarded an eighty-thousand-dollar termite job on the Little Creek Amphibian Base and many more termite and pest control contracts, all with the minimum of competition.

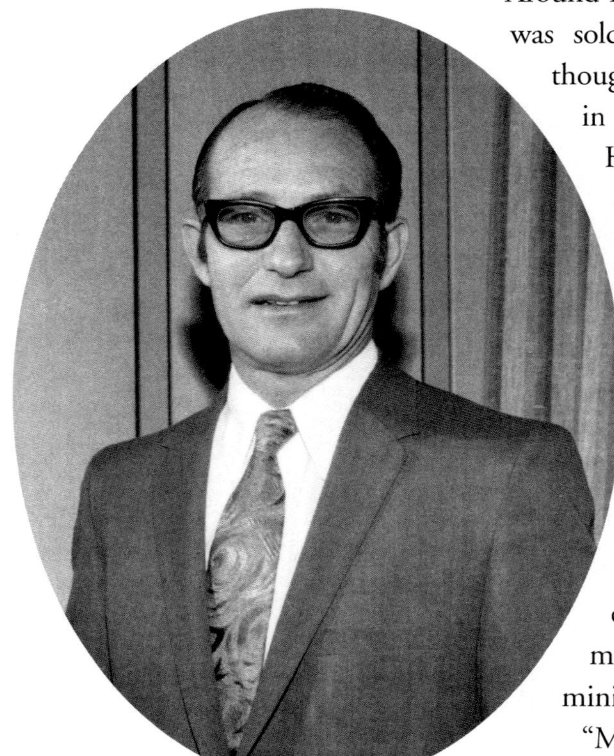

"No one has ever been more customer-conscious than Otto Orkin."
—Walt Helms

"Mr. Orkin . . . developed in all of us a sense of pride in our work and to value accomplishments. This pride was enjoyed by every person in every successful branch office. It continued year after year, and so did the progress."

The Orkin employees, though, never failed to recognize that their boss had his own peculiar way of doing things.

Whenever he visited the branch offices, the first thing Otto wanted to "go over was the Lost Business Report," remembered Walt Helms. "He didn't talk about sales. He would immediately ask why we didn't reduce the price to keep from losing the customer. No one has ever been more customer-conscious than Otto Orkin."

Remembered Red Tindol: "When he talked to a manager, [Otto] was always more interested in lost customers than in new sales. Nothing could make him madder than losing an account. Once a district reported excellent new sales with about seventy-five new accounts, but Mr. Orkin looked at the bottom of the report and expressed dismay over losing seven accounts."

Because the staff was devoted to Otto—or perhaps a bit afraid of him—they didn't question his idiosyncratic ways. When Walt and Ruth Helms moved to Kansas City in the early 1950s to expand Orkin's Midwest territory, Otto visited and asked to see their house. He even wanted to see the attic. After an inspection, he promptly told the couple that the house looked very nice, but that he had seen some cobwebs in the attic. "Now, if you take an old sheet and wrap around a broom and sweep through the attic ceiling and walls," Mr. Orkin announced, "the cobwebs would be gone."

Although census records show Otto was born in April 1887, he celebrated his birthday with George Washington on February 22.

Otto's other eccentricities were easily noted. After his second divorce in 1946, he developed a reputation as either a ladies' man or a lonely gentleman who didn't like to dine alone, depending on which stories you choose to believe. He developed a unique approach to celebrating his birthday: although all of the early census records report that Otto was born in April 1887, Otto began celebrating his birthday with George Washington on February 22. According to his son Sanford, Otto "never really knew when his birthday was. He picked a president's birthday because it made him feel important, I guess."

No one would dispute that Otto was extremely clothes-conscious. It was reliably reported that this son of a dirt-poor immigrant had two hundred suits and ordered his shoes by the dozen. The tailor shop located in the downstairs of his Atlanta apartment building kept his suits cleaned and ready; when Otto called for a particular suit, it was sent up with shoes and accessories to match. Sometimes Otto changed suits four or five times during the day, and he favored vests and tweed suits, and a gray overcoat with a felt collar. He loved fiery red ties, and he never went without a shoeshine and a manicure.

Ted Oser, apparently, emulated his uncle's penchant for fine clothes, only Ted preferred to dress in black, including black patent leather shoes and a black homburg, remembered David Kotler, Lou Kotler's son. For their tastes in expensive, flashy clothes, Otto and Ted "were referred to as the 'Bobbsey Twins' or the 'Gold Dust Twins.'"

As he grew in stature with the company, Ted was just as likely to be contrasted as compared to his uncle. In 1950, when he was vice president of Orkin and celebrating thirty-three years with the company, *Orkin Talkin* profiled Ted Oser and came to this conclusion:

> To a surprisingly large number of people, "Oser" is almost synonymous with "Orkin," and rightly so, because Mr. Oser is truly one of the pioneers of the company, and has played an important and decisive role in the remarkable development and growth of the Orkin Company in the past 33 years. . . . All those who have close contact with Ted Oser never fail to be impressed with his dynamic energy and drive, and those of us who are intimately associated with him in the company are continually amazed at his capacity for hard work and his unflagging devotion to the company and its affairs.

Many employees who worked at Orkin recalled Ted's aggressive, confident manner. "Ted would storm into my office, dressed to the hilt, big wide smile, and ask me to do him a little favor," said James Llewallyn from the Orkin print shop. "The favor meant he wanted me to stop whatever I was working on and get right on his project. He usually got his way. If you didn't know better, you'd think Ted Oser owned Orkin and ran the entire company."

Virginia C. Wood, who served as a personal secretary to most of the top Orkin executives, including Ted and Otto, believed that "Ted Oser has to be credited with a major part of Orkin's success. Ted was the PR man, but loyal to Otto. Otto was not a joiner; Ted kept the company before the public. Ted was gregarious and dealt with the managers, but he seemed to want Otto as the figurehead."

Neither Ted nor Otto ever lost sight of the fact that the servicemen were the frontline of Orkin's reputation. And both had amazingly good insights into generating good public relations for the company. From the beginning, Otto encouraged his staff to dress appropriately and professionally, and even his technicians wore ties to work. But in 1947, he took this one step forward and issued company-wide uniforms. Riverside Manufacturing Company in Moultrie, Georgia, was the first supplier of Orkin uniforms, with Orkin's diamond logo and identification on caps, jackets, and shirts. For Otto, the Orkin image was a package: crisp, professional uniform; immaculate truck with Orkin decals; and pride in a job that helped individuals fight disease and keep their homes safe and clean.

But Otto did more than provide uniforms and try to instill a sense of pride in his employees for a job well done. His random acts of generosity to his employees are fairly legendary. When one of the Kolkana children tragically died, Otto sent the grieving family a two-thousand-dollar check with a note, "Hope this helps." Said Kolkana, "Mr. Orkin had a big heart."

When James Llewallyn admired a leather sofa in Otto's office, Otto remembered and gave it to the print shop clerk when his office was remodeled. Mrs. C. E. Hundley, who worked for Orkin from 1942 to 1949, recalled that Otto "was a friend and ate many meals with my husband and children. Our son has osteomyelitis, an infection of the bone, and Mr. Orkin was a great friend to me." When Ed Fulford, a longtime termite supervisor in Albany, was accidentally shot during a hunting trip, Otto paid for Fulford, Fulford's wife, and Red Tindol to be flown to New York for Fulford's surgery and rehabilitation; the accident paralyzed Fulford from the waist down, but Otto found a job for him and kept him on the payroll as an office manager, working from his electric wheelchair. When Anita Ritchie, assistant advertising manager at Orkin, announced that she was pregnant, Otto got tears in his eyes, kissed her on both cheeks, and announced that she was to use the elevator, not the stairs, for the remainder of her pregnancy. And when Sally Robbins was in the hospital having a baby, Otto asked her husband, Lee, how she was doing. When Otto found out that she didn't like the hospital food, he arranged for the rest of her meals to be sent to her by the Progressive Club.

Otto did something else that contributed to the growth of his company and the positive attitude of his employees: he shared Orkin's wealth with those who helped him make it, by offering district managers and some servicemen a share of his company's profits. His profit-sharing deals were complicated and not always equitable, but they were a huge incentive for hard work and Orkin loyalty. Depending on their location, servicemen were paid either a basic salary or a percentage of the work they performed. At one time, Orkin also gave out additional commissions for any new work or leads that the servicemen developed.

For Otto, the Orkin image was a package: crisp, professional uniform; immaculate truck with Orkin decals; and pride in a job that helped individuals fight disease and keep their homes safe and clean.

"You make me money, and I'll make you money," James Hutto remembered Otto telling his servicemen and branch managers. "He always paid me more than he promised."

How much money? Many branch and district managers made double or triple what Otto paid himself, and Orkin enabled many dedicated employees to become millionaires. According to Robert Couhig, the branch managers were earning an amazing amount of money. "Kotler, Krawcheck, Pressman got 20 percent of gross profits," he said. "I got 5 percent in the 1950s, and I was making $180,000—while Otto was making $60,000." In twenty years Couhig opened, or took over the management of, twenty-three offices in Louisiana, Mississippi, and Arkansas. "The growth was phenomenal."

Lester Meis, who joined the Orkin Institute in 1952, agreed. "Otto brought in top-notch, highly qualified people, who, if you didn't know something, didn't mind sitting down with you and going over it," he once said in a magazine article. "The esprit de corps was tremendous because we were paid well and we were treated well."

The incentive programs clearly paved the way for a large portion of Orkin's expansion—from representation in twenty-one states in 1951 to twenty-eight states in 1956. But it couldn't possibly have accounted for all of the company's phenomenal growth in the 1950s; from 1951 to 1956 alone, Orkin's gross revenues more than doubled, from just over $7 million to $15.6 million. As Orkin celebrated its golden anniversary, the exterminating company that had already established the industry's first technical department, was the first to specialize in pest control for food-processing plants, and had developed the first nylon tent fumigation of drywood termites was about to embark on yet another industry first—one that helped explain Orkin's spectacular growth.

In one word? Television.

In three words? The Orkin Man.

THE ORKIN MAN

Imagine a woman standing on a couch, screaming her head off at the sight of a rat. That melodramatic image was the first Orkin television spot, produced by WSB-TV in Atlanta and aired briefly in March 1950. Though this real-life character was replaced rather quickly by such dubious cartoon characters as "Legs the Repulsive Roach" and "Rags the Ruinous Rat," the concept of advertising Orkin on television would succeed beyond anyone's initial expectations. And through this new medium, Orkin would introduce its most beloved and venerable trademark to date: The Orkin Man.

Otto had always believed in advertising and branding—dating back to his primitive skull and crossbones on a paper bag of rat poisons and to his first "Otto The Rat Man" ad in the 1912 Richmond telephone directory. He wanted placards, signs, and decals prominently displayed, and he loved to see the *Orkin* name emblazoned on all of his offices, on all vehicles, and on the servicemen's uniforms. Walt Helms remembered when Otto visited his Kansas City branch just after the new Orkin neon sign was installed over the office. Otto rode up and down the street, looking at that sign from every angle. "He was so proud of that sign," Helms said.

Originally, each branch or district handled its own advertising. But starting in September 1946, the Technical Department in Atlanta began directing all company advertising, ensuring that accurate and consistent information about the company's services was presented and that all ad information conformed to regulatory requirements. More direct mail fliers and pamphlets were designed, and new window displays and signage were prepared for the branches. Merle A. "Tommy" Thompson, who began handling Orkin's advertising in 1926 and was probably responsible for the familiar Orkin diamond, was one of the founding partners of the Bearden-Thompson-Frankel advertising agency that handled the placement of all Orkin advertising in telephone directories, newspapers, and trade journals throughout the country.

In March 1950 Orkin decided to test out a new advertising medium—television. After the company's first filmed television spots with the hysterical woman, the company recognized that television attracted more attention and comment than any other medium. Instead of real people, however, Orkin decided to use cartoon characters, apparently to reflect the company's policy of refraining from the use of scare tactics to entice customers. Orkin's assistant advertising manager, Anita E. Ritchie, used her experiences with her two-year-old son for inspiration and created cartoon characters called "Rags the Ruinous Rat," "Legs the Repulsive Roach," and "Toothy the Terrible Termite," writing short story scripts around them. Her inspiration for a hero of sorts, however, came from another source. Namely, the Orkin mailroom, where a bunch of scattered paper clips was about to make advertising history.

The Orkin Man after World War II:
James Hutto

In 1946 James Hutto wasn't really looking for a job. "After five and a half years in the army," he recalled, "I went to work for a grocery store. I saw this man come with a black box, flashlight, and dust bulb that squirted something behind cases and in cracks. I asked him what he was doing, and he said he was killing roaches, insects, and rats. I said I hadn't seen any roaches or rats, and he said that was because he was exterminating.

"I didn't believe him, so I kept my eyes open to find some pests. Then I saw a roach and followed it behind a drink box and saw hundreds of little feelers sticking out between the bottom of the wall and the floor. When the Orkin man came back, I showed him what I had found, and he shot his powder stuff from a bulb spray and hundreds of roaches came boiling out like a Sunday picnic. I started stomping on them, and he said that wasn't necessary. They just started dropping dead within a few feet. He said the store paid Orkin four dollars a month, and he went to about eight places a day. I knew I wanted to do what that Orkin man was doing."

It wasn't long before Hutto was hired as a pest control serviceman for Orkin in eastern North Carolina. In 1948, after two years as an Orkin Man, he was made manager of the Rocky Mount Orkin branch, where he remained for twenty years. It was Hutto who suggested and implemented the division of North Carolina into two districts—East North Carolina and West North Carolina. This division allowed managers to keep better track of customers and employees, which helped build their overall customer base and increase revenue. Hutto retired from Orkin on August 31, 1981, after thirty-five years of remarkable service.

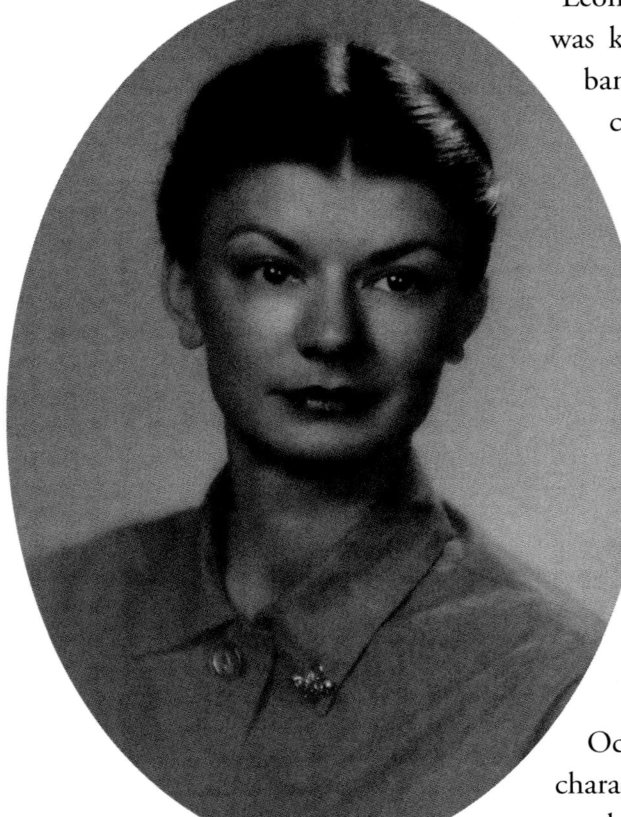

Anita Ritchie of the marketing department created the cartoon characters used in Orkin's early television advertising.

Leon Mims, a warehouse and mailroom employee at Orkin, was known for making objects out of paper clips, rubber bands, and bits of almost nothing. Gene Loyd, Mims's coworker and a longtime employee, would frequently place Mims's gadgets and paper-clip characters on Otto's or other managers' desks. One day in early 1950, Gene Abraham Weinstein, Orkin's first advertising manager, saw one of Mims's paper-clip figures and something clicked. He quickly suggested that Mims get some modeling clay and make the paper-clip image into a pesticide spray-can figure with arms and legs. In no time at all, Loyd recalled, Mims molded that clay into the final image of a tiny Orkin Man. But it needed something—a name. Jake Pressman, so the story goes, asked Otto Orkin if they could name the clay figure after him. And that's how "Otto the Orkin Man" was born.

"Otto the Orkin Man" was first introduced in the October 1950 issue of *Orkin Talkin* as the "energetic little character portraying Orkin's on-the-ball, dependable serviceman, who's always friendly and courteous." By 1951 Otto the Orkin Man was featured in the company's twenty-second television commercial being produced by Motion Pictures Associates in New Orleans. The animated pesticide spray can was portrayed as the hero in "stirring dramas of life and death in the insect world." The advertising creators dealt discreetly with the touchy subject of extermination by portraying the pests as villainous characters, doing their mischief, until Orkin's animated spray gun turns with his blast of smoke to mow down the repulsive thugs, and "Otto the Orkin Man" wins again.

Leon R. Robbins, who was appointed Orkin's advertising manager in 1953, once said that "Rags and Legs, while villainous and depraved, are nonetheless very lovable" and adored by Orkin fans. "Even though Otto always gets the best of them with his spray gun, and they're done away with at the end of each commercial, they always bounce back with new rascality in the next announcement. Our viewers like it that way."

In no time Otto the Orkin Man began to appear on every medium of Orkin communication—letterheads, envelopes, specialized mailings, proposal folders, pest control and termite booklets, decals, and every other conceivable promotional item, including company vehicles. And it wasn't long before Otto the Orkin Man had his own jingle at the end of every film, developed by Wade Creager of Atlanta and sung to the tune of "Popeye the Sailor Man":

I'm Otto the Orkin Man.
We kill all the pests in the land.
When Termites start swarming,
They better take warning.
I'm Otto the Orkin Man.

The public's reaction to Otto the Orkin Man was nothing short of remarkable. Overnight, the spray-can cartoon man became an American icon. In a direct repeat of dialogue they heard on television advertisements, children began calling the Orkin offices and shouting, "Orkin, come quickly!" before hanging up the telephone. Orkin offices received calls almost daily from youngsters who wanted to speak to Otto. One North Carolina physician called a competitive company to rid his house of termites, but his son kept asking, "Where is Otto?" The father finally called Orkin to bid on the work, and Orkin got the job.

"For some inexplicable reason, hoards of small fry are moved to rush to the phone, look up Otto's number, and call him," said Robbins. "Because of our TV advertising, many people think Otto the Orkin Man is our corporate name, so we're listed that way in telephone directories in TV cities."

At one point, Orkin conducted a survey to determine how customers first heard about Orkin. The most popular answer? That they listened to, and responded to, the jingle, which became one of only twenty-three sounds to be patented and carry a copyright. In a tribute to the power of advertising, children were often disappointed when the Orkin Man showed up as a human being rather than the spray gun character.

"When the Orkin truck appears, and we have the Otto character as well as the Orkin name in big bold lettering, the kids expect Otto to leap out and start spraying," said Robbins. "We've given serious consideration to equipping our local servicemen with some type of headgear in keeping with the TV trademark of Otto the spray gun to please the children."

When Orkin celebrated its fiftieth anniversary in January 1951, the "Otto the Orkin Man" advertisements were running in five major television viewing areas, and were scheduled to expand to eight in 1952. Clearly riding a wave of phenomenally positive public relations, the *Atlanta Journal* and *Constitution* wrote a story about the company's golden anniversary with this headline: "Want to Know Whether Democracy Is A Good System?—Ask Otto Orkin." The story reported how the "little black satchel expanded into a vast enterprise service in two thousand communities in twenty states. This man is a living testimonial to the success of the American free enterprise system."

The lavish anniversary event, designed to celebrate not only Orkin's fiftieth anniversary but also Otto Orkin's half century of service to the pest control industry, was held at the Ansley Hotel, where Orkin was just finishing the end of a three-day annual managers' conference for more than two hundred managers and supervisory personnel. In a room filled with an additional seventy-five or so government and educational leaders, Ted Oser served as master of ceremonies. On behalf of all of Orkin's employees, A. B. Billingsworth, manager of the Birmingham office, presented Otto with a testimonial book, hand-tooled in gold and bound in leather, carrying the names of all of Otto's one thousand employees. And in a sweeping and verbose tribute, Atlanta Mayor W. B. Hartsfield presented Otto with a gold plaque and pronounced, "This man is a living testimonial to the success of the American free enterprise system. And were it possible to televise these proceedings tonight and pipe them to Riga, Latvia, it would do more to impede the progress of communism than a dozen atomic bombs."

The next morning the newspapers carried the following description of Otto's response: "Mr. Orkin, a dapper, familiar figure about Atlanta, listened to these words of the mayor and heard the applause of his friends. And it was little wonder that his response to the presentation of a commemorative plaque was a brief, 'Thank you.' A man's emotions can stand just so much."

Otto the Orkin Man was first introduced in the October 1950 issue of Orkin Talkin. *He became the central figure of Orkin's advertising during the 1950s.*

The *Orkin Talkin* later reported that "Mr. Orkin was so completely overwhelmed with surprise and emotion, he could hardly utter words of gratitude. His voice choked and his eyes were filled with tears as he looked into the faces of the gathering of over 300 who were assembled to pay him homage."

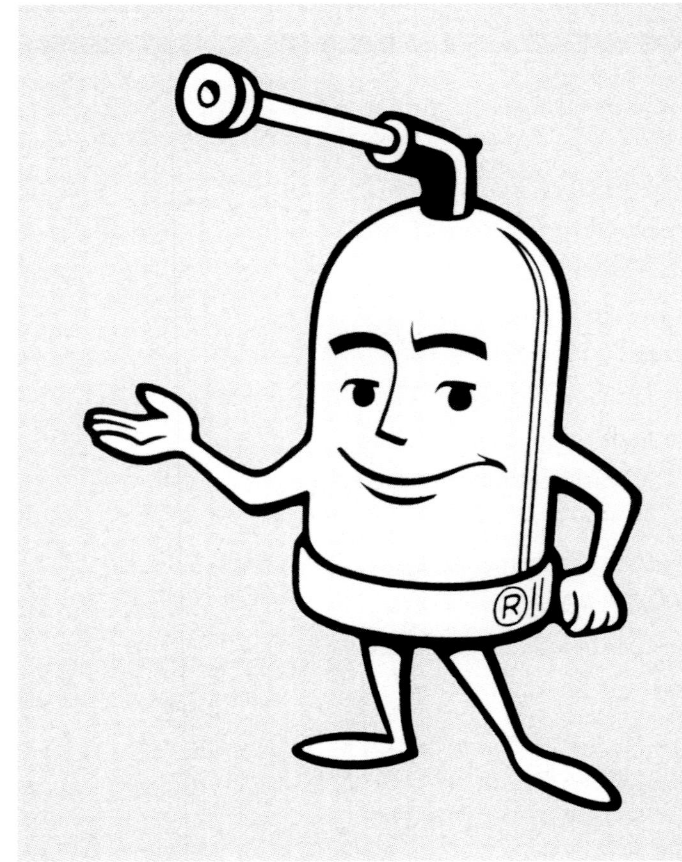

For the next several years, the public and the press couldn't get enough of "Otto the Orkin Man." Wherever Otto traveled, newspaper reports and columnists clamored to meet the "real" Orkin man, and Otto dutifully repeated his "rats to riches" story in newspapers and magazines across the country. Otto and his company had clearly been "bitten" by the public relations bug (pun intended). When the company moved in late 1951 to its new headquarters at 713 West Peachtree, every detail of the home office relocation was reported: the $225,000 price tag for the twenty-six-thousand-square-foot, two-story headquarters; the $60,000 spent for modifications; and equipment, furniture, and fixtures with a book value of $998,000. The headquarters contained the "beautifully

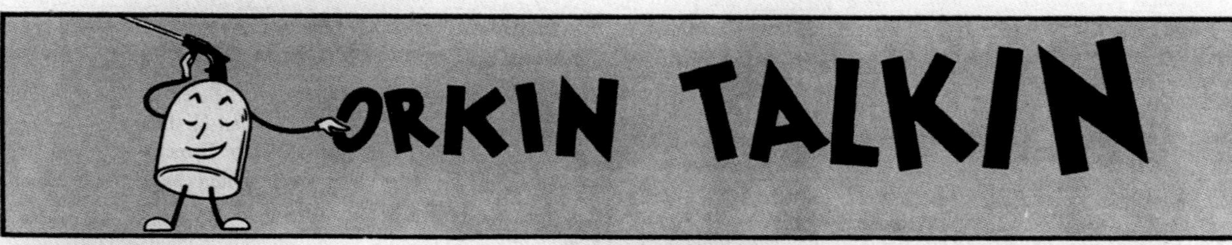

Volume IV, Number 1 "Of, By, and For Orkin Employees" Jan., Feb., Mar., Apr., 1951

Mr. Orkin Honored at Testimonial Dinner Marking 50 Years of Pest Control Service

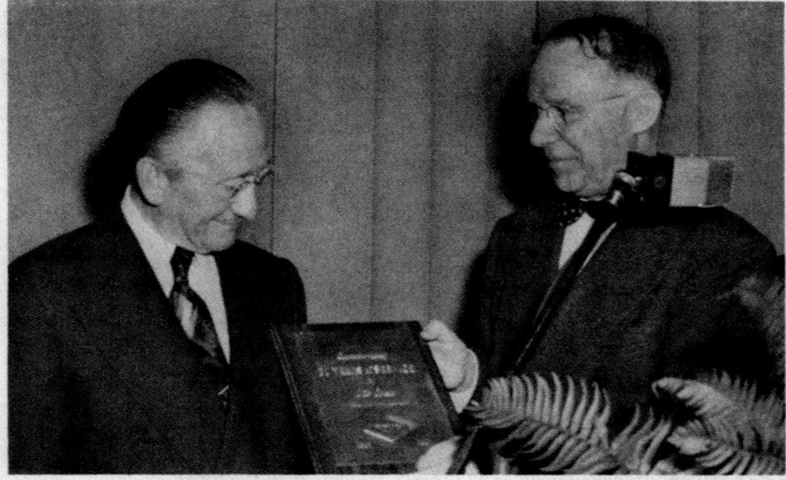

Mr. Orkin receiving 50-year plaque from Mayor Hartsfield of Atlanta.

"Modern Pied Piper" Presented Gold Plaque

As a fitting climax to the company's fifth annual managers conference in January, Mr. Orkin, our beloved president was honored at a banquet on Tuesday, January 9th. All of our company's principals, managers and salesmen, along with the mayor and other notables from Atlanta, gathered to commemorate Mr. Orkin's 50 years of service in the pest control industry.

Mr. Orkin, often called the "Modern Pied Piper," was presented with a gold plaque in honor of his golden anniversary as head of Orkin Exterminating Company. This presentation was made by Atlanta's Mayor Wm. B. Hartsfield.

He also received a testimonial book, hand tooled in gold and leather bound, which will eventually bear the names and congratulatory messages of all of his

(Continued on Page 8)

Annual Conference Acclaimed by Managers As Most Outstanding in Five Years

All Phases of Pest Control and Management Covered In Well-Planned 3-Day Meet

Orkin Exterminating Co., the world's largest pest control organization, gathered at the Ansley Hotel January 8th through the 10th for its fifth managers conference. This conference is an annual feature of the continuous and coordinated training program which keeps the Orkin Company as a leader in scientific pest control and surety-bonded termite control.

Under the auspices of the Orkin Technical Department, the managers, salesmen, and supervisory personnel of Orkin's 175 company-owned and operated branch offices serving twenty-one states, received three days of intensive instruction in all operational phases of pest control and termite control. Such specialized subjects as Food Plant Sanitation, Fabric Pest Control, Development of New Rodenticides, and Termite Control during Construction were highlighted with refresher courses of instruction being devoted to always-important operations as General Pest Control, Safety, General Management, Sales, Accounting and Branch Office Operation.

Prominent company officials participating in this valuable training program were Otto Orkin, President; Theodore Oser, Vice-President, and Herman L. Fellton, Technical Director, who organizes and administers the company's training program. Program Chairmen for the three-day session were A. B. Hollingsworth our Montgomery, Alabama Manager; Walter A. Helms, our Jacksonville, Florida Manager; Orvis B. Griggs, our Richmond, Virginia Man-

(Continued on Page 6)

Virginia Cook New Orkin Talkin Editor

Miss Virginia Cook, long-time home office employee, has been chosen as the new Editor of Orkin Talkin, it was announced as this issue went to press.

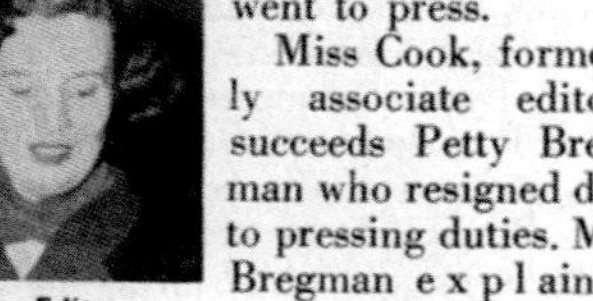

New Editor.

Miss Cook, formerly associate editor, succeeds Petty Bregman who resigned due to pressing duties. Mr. Bregman explained that he did not feel he was able to devote sufficient time to the responsibility of editor in view of the extra duties confronting him by Orkin's expansion program.

Also announced is the appointment of R. M. Russell as Associate Editor. Mr. Russell, assistant to the Technical Director, has been a constant contributor to Orkin Talkin, both with stories and photography.

1

A special issue of Orkin Talkin *covered Orkin's fiftieth-anniversary celebration.*

paneled and carpeted executive offices appointed with modern furnishings, central accounting and billing, advertising, sales promotion, and technical training departments, a laboratory for chemical analysis and insect identification, a print shop, the mailing room, an employees' kitchen, a large warehouse area including four 2,500 gallon chemical storage tanks, and adequate inside parking space of Orkin's fleet of 15 Chevrolet panel trucks and 20 three-quarter to one ton trucks used in the Atlanta district. One room alone is devoted to an elaborate Addressograph automatic biller that prints the customer's name and address, the amount of his monthly charge, dates the invoice, cuts it to size, stamps it ready to be mailed. The Orkin company services better than 69,000 general pest control accounts."

For the first time, *Pest Control* magazine reported that Orkin was, indeed, "the *world's largest pest control company*. In these days, when superlatives have become almost meaningless, a claim to be the 'largest' anything requires close scrutiny to justify or disprove such a position. The Orkin company's place in the pest control industry is verified by one of the country's leading credit rating services. Otto Orkin, president and founder, began 51 years ago as a one-man sales force selling rat powders in eastern Pennsylvania. Today, his company has grown into an organization that has 186 branch offices in 21 states and does a gross volume of business exceeding seven million dollars annually. . . . 'We've just scratched the surface,' Mr. Orkin told us."

To celebrate the opening of the new headquarters, Orkin staged an open house celebration the likes of which Atlanta had never seen. Over five thousand Atlantans turned out in a steady stream from 10 A.M. to 10 P.M. for the Orkin

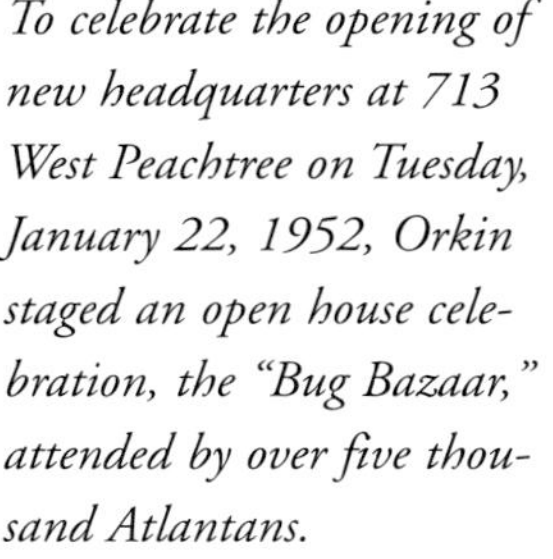

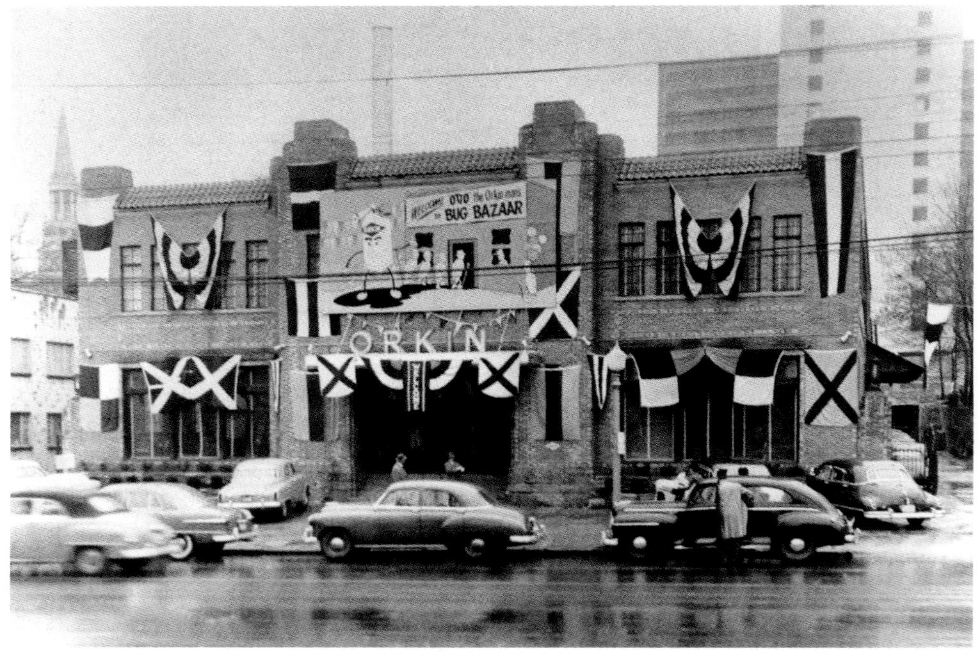

To celebrate the opening of new headquarters at 713 West Peachtree on Tuesday, January 22, 1952, Orkin staged an open house celebration, the "Bug Bazaar," attended by over five thousand Atlantans.

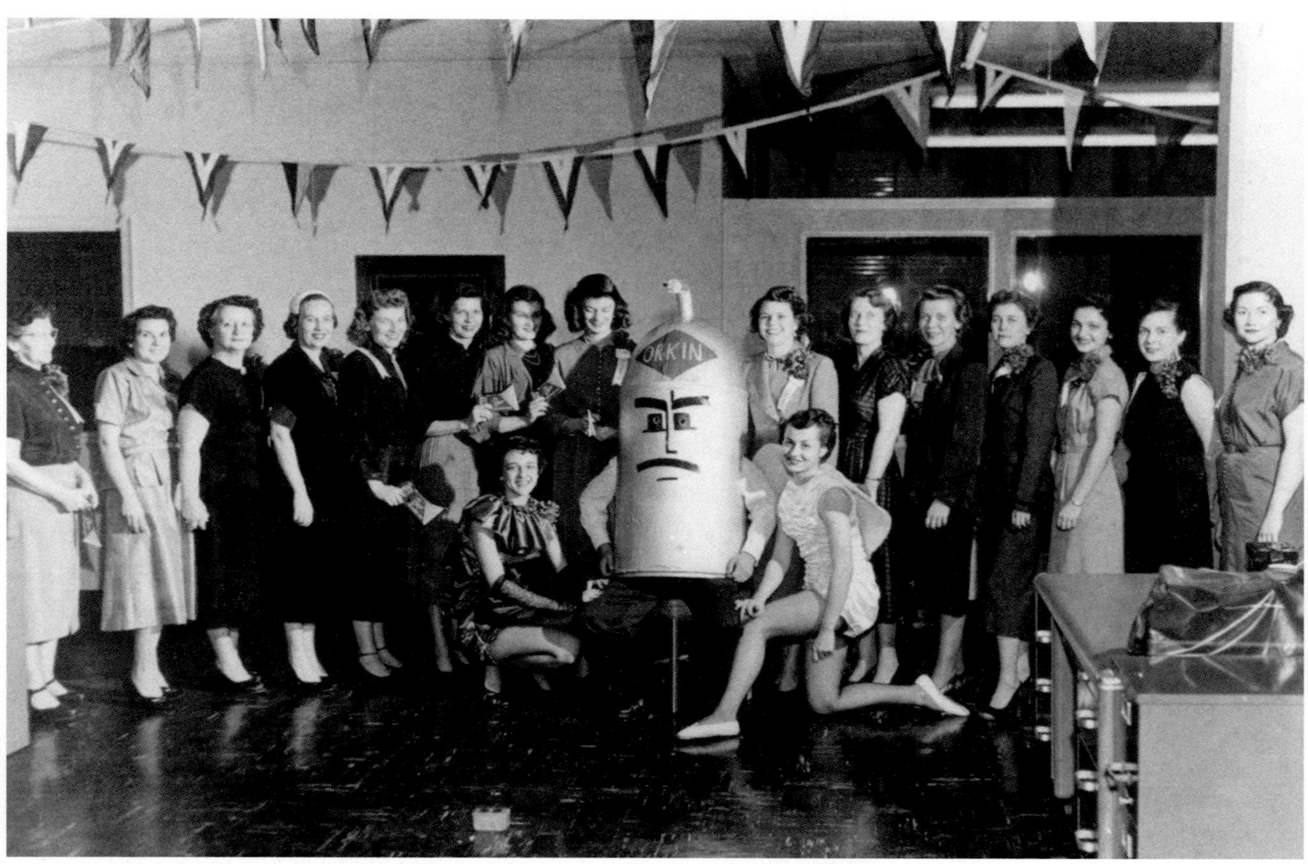

Hostessing the Bug Bazaar were the female employees of Orkin in Atlanta. Left to right: Willie Courtney (sales), not identified, Cora Wallach (Atlanta exterminating bookkeeper), Virginia Cook Wood (Ted Oser's secretary), not identified, Margie Thorsen (advertising), not identified, Anita Edberg Ritchie (advertising), Mary Campbell (Herman Fellton's secretary), Ethlyn Arotlin (accounting), Nita Talbot (technical department), Mary Helen Carter (Atlanta exterminating), not identified, Edith Morris (accounting), and not identified. Kneeling: Ann Marinos (secretary to Clyde Young) and Margie Moss (sales).

"Bug Bazaar" on Tuesday, January 22, 1952. "Probably never in the history of the pest control industry was there such a fabulous opening," one magazine reported. Standing next to Otto, Mayor Hartsfield officially started the ceremonies—not by cutting the ceremonial ribbon but by snapping a chain of mousetraps stretched across the front door. Upon entering, guests were treated to a variety of entertainment acts, exhibits of major household pests, two active termite colonies (with mirrors placed beneath them to show everything), a twenty-eight-minute video on how to identify and control termites, Max Isbill's prized international collection of insects (including his rare specimens of beetles with luminescent coverings), and exhibits from the U.S. Public Health Service that graphically displayed the geographical distribution of disease-bearing insects. Several Orkin secretaries dressed up as a black-widow spider, a clothes moth, and a June bug and welcomed guests throughout the day, encouraging them to enjoy the "Otto-Matic" souvenir pistols, gingerbread men shaped like Otto the Orkin Man, pink lemonade, cotton candy, popcorn, and hot coffee and—Gasp!—the Chamber of Horrors, where "fake" models of flies, mosquitoes, bats, and wasps dangled from the ceiling of a dimly lit room, while rats, mice, and termites "scampered" about on the floor.

The *Atlanta Journal* reported that "the thousands who visited the many entomological exhibits were entertained and came away with a new appreciation of just how big the urban and industrial pest control business really is."

As he walked among the crowds all day, it was clear that the sixty-four-year-old Otto Orkin—his dark suit impeccable and his straight dark hair now nearly white around the temples and combed straight back—was in his element. And why shouldn't he be? His company had just been declared the world's largest pest control company. In just six years, company sales had tripled, and all indications pointed to even higher gains in the future. And with an advertising budget of $180,000 for 1952 that included spots on 17 television stations, ads in 425 newspapers, and approximately 300 painted signs throughout his service areas, the eccentric Otto Orkin had literally catapulted himself and his company into the national spotlight. Just a few months after the Bug Bazaar, *Fortune* magazine included Otto Orkin in a collection of "100 Stories of Business Success," labeling Orkin the "Chain Store Exterminator." *Fortune*'s four-paragraph summary of Otto's career to date was chock-full of priceless details:

> Otto Orkin is the founder and president of Orkin Exterminating Co., Inc., Atlanta, a chain-store exterminator, largest in the business. His company has 190 offices, in twenty-two southern and southwestern states and he now proposes still further expansion. Surprisingly, Americans spend over $70 million annually for general pest control (agricultural insecticides excluded). These are the professional exterminators and of this market Otto Orkin gets almost 10 cents of every $1 spent, making Orkin the General Motors of this business. His company now has 69,000 contracts for monthly pest-control inspection. For $100, a house can be made termite-proof, for $20 he will rid a house of rats. These are considered spot jobs by Orkin, although important to him, and his real money comes from holding down the pest population on a contract basis. Among his large accounts are shipping lines, grain elevators, railroads, chain stores and textile mills. He also has the fly-control contract at the AEC's Oak Ridge plant.
>
> His employees exterminate every sort of pest from mites to snakes. The snake job is done in the home and is profitable work because southern snakes tend to be homebodies. Sixty types of equipment are used from hand sprays to thermal aerosol generators that cost $1,800 each. Each branch office stocks thirty kinds of chemicals, from arsenic to lindane (for DDT-immune flies). To kill rats his employees set out warfarin, a slow-acting poison, or zinc phosphide, which works faster but still takes several days. Both

> of the chemicals, though effective, are troublesome—the rats die in inaccessible places and decay slowly and odoriferously. The best rat poison, though extremely toxic to humans, is sodium fluoracetate: it kills a rat in his tracks. Termites are controlled by insulating the wood of a building from the soil, or by poisoning the soil around a house with, for example, sodium arsenite.
>
> Otto Orkin, sixty-four, came to this country from Latvia in 1893, began peddling rat poison at fourteen, set up his own shop in Richmond, Virginia, as "Otto the Rat Man" when he was nineteen. In 1926 Orkin picked Atlanta as a central location from which to expand his business and he has been expanding ever since. Last year Otto Orkin paid himself a $70,000 salary, met a payroll of more than $4 million for 1,150 employees and netted $299,498 after taxes on a gross of $7,032,489.
>
> This year the company's handsome new plant, consisting of offices, warehouse and laboratory, was formally dedicated when Atlanta's Mayor William Hartsfield snapped open a chain of mousetraps in tribute to one of the city's largest home enterprises.

During late 1953 the story of Orkin and its services received more national attention when it was broadcast on *Industry on Parade,* one of the popular weekly television features about various industries and how they grew. The program, sponsored by the National Association of Manufacturers and produced by NBC, attracted millions of viewers each

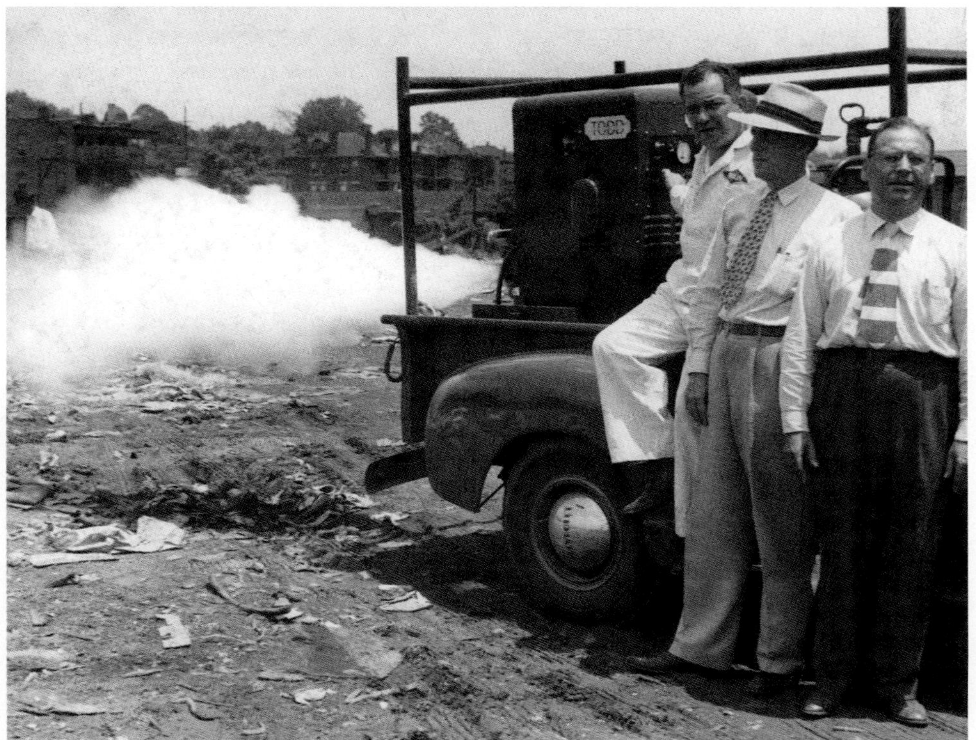

An early example of a fogging machine in action.

week from around the world. People in São Paulo, Havana, Copenhagen, Milan, Turin, Tokyo, Mexico City, Caracas, and Paris tuned in with Americans to see Otto the Orkin Man in action. The film also showed a house being treated for termite infestation, an Atlanta lake being fogged for mosquitoes, a service school in session, and a testing laboratory. In cities already served by Orkin, a twenty-second Otto the Orkin Man commercial followed the film clip, and sales spiked.

Approximately eighty-two thousand people passed the thirty-by-twenty-three-foot sign above the old Orkin building at 591 Peachtree Street every day when it was installed in 1954. The neon portion of the sign operated from 6:00 A.M. until midnight.

But the barrage of relatively new, international exposure didn't keep Otto from paying attention to business at home. Always the self-promoter, Otto approved when Leon Robbins designed a spectacular, thirty-by-twenty-three-foot neon action sign and placed it above Orkin's former office building at 591 Peachtree Street. The sign, which was later duplicated in other areas across the country, showed moving insects or rats; Otto's spray can nozzle would flash, and a puff of smoke would light up as each insect (or rat) was hit. The sign contained eight different action displays (depending on which pest was most prevalent during a particular season), and it was a huge success.

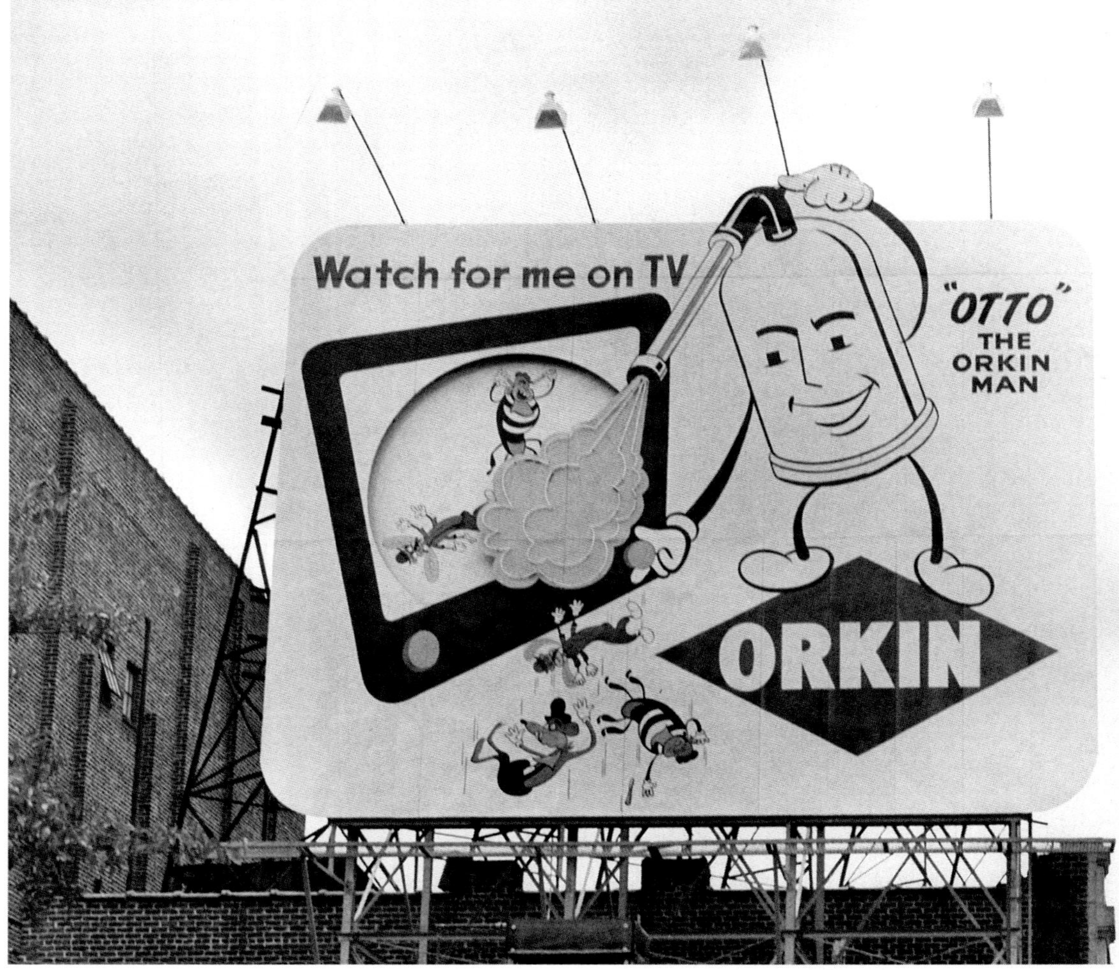

For all the accolades, national media attention, and neon signs that pointed his way, Otto continued to offer a fairly simple explanation as to why his business was so successful. When Otto Orkin was selected by *Look* magazine to be quoted in its "What They Are Saying" feature in 1953—along with Tallulah Bankhead and Salvador Dali—Otto's "quotable" would have been as easily recognized in 1901 as it was fifty years later: "Behind every door," Otto continued to say, "is a prospect."

And when Otto the Orkin Man was quoted in the November 1953 issue of *Orkin Talkin*, the message was equally simple and in keeping with Otto's lifelong business philosophy:

> Why is Orkin the world's largest pest control company? A business is successful only if it makes a legitimate profit. It can make a profit only if consumers buy its product or its service. Our business is service. Orkin has become the world's largest pest control company because it has provided the *best* service in its field. To maintain service leadership, Orkin holds annual service conferences to keep old-timers and newcomers up-to-date on the latest in scientific pest control methods. *We must never be satisfied with less than the best in service* if we are to secure our share of tomorrow's market. As long as the Orkin name remains the symbol of the best in pest and termite control service, we will be the world's largest in size—and in numbers of satisfied customers!

GROWTH, GROWTH, AND MORE GROWTH

From exposure to national advertising, television, and an amazing run of good public relations, Orkin sales soared in the 1950s. A look at straightforward statistics tells the story:

- From airtime on one television station in 1950, Orkin moved to 5 stations in 1951, 8 in 1952, 27 in 1953, 90 in 1954, 95 in 1955, 104 in 1956, and 115 in 1957. The company started with sixty-second commercials to get its message across; once established, Orkin shifted primarily to ten- and twenty-second announcements, all featuring Otto the Orkin Man in a cartoon melodrama played out against his bug victims.
- Orkin sales jumped from just over $7 million in 1950 to nearly $20 million in 1957. In 1955 alone, company executives reported that no month in the entire year made less than a 17 percent gain on the same month for 1954: May and June, for example, shot ahead more than 28 percent; August, 29 percent; and September, 32 percent.
- On May 1, 1952, Orkin Exterminating opened its first international office in Havana, *Cuba-Fumigadora Orkin.* Orkin's services included

members of the Institute of Sanitation, who served as consultants to Cuban hotels, sugar refineries, and rum exporters. Havana's first branch manager, Manuel M. Canle, was born in Cuba but had been a U.S. citizen since 1934.

- During 1955 more than thirty new offices were established throughout the United States, as Orkin moved in checkerboard fashion from state to state toward the Pacific Coast. In the fall of 1955 Orkin opened a branch in Pasadena, California, realizing Otto Orkin's dream of having his company span from "coast to coast." By 1955 Orkin counted 325 branches in twenty-eight states.
- In 1950 Orkin's advertising budget was $177,615, with just over $50,000 spent on television, over $10,000 on radio, nearly $85,000 on newspapers, and some $35,000 spent on telephone directories; in 1957, the budget had increased to $706,000, but the allocations had shifted dramatically, with television and telephone directories leading the spending: $333,000 was spent on television commercials and approximately $210,000 was spent on telephone directories.

In an interview with *Television Age* magazine in 1957, Robbins explained why nearly half a million dollars was spent on these two advertising tools: "We are strictly a service organization. Our point-of-sale is the telephone. That is, no one ever comes into our offices. We sell no products; we only perform a service. Therefore, we advertise in approximately one thousand telephone directories throughout our territory. Where we have been able to make concrete surveys, we have determined that 70 percent of our unsolicited business—coming in over the telephone—is a direct result of our television advertising."

People call for pest control service when they see bugs, but rarely before. Orkin struggled with how to promote pest control as a way to prevent bugs.

According to Robbins's magazine interview, every sale reported to the company's home office was accompanied by a notation on just exactly why the potential customer called Orkin. "Invariably," Robbins said, "the caller will say it was because of TV. However, if you explore the situation, you find that these people have been seeing Orkin on television for several years, but they only recently saw bugs."

Robbins's comment illustrated a continuing sales issue for Orkin, one as old as the pest control industry itself: people call for pest control service when they *see* bugs, but rarely *before*. In spite of Orkin's insistence on regular pest control service, the company's successful advertising campaign was still struggling to find a way to capitalize on Orkin's promotion of pest control as a way to *prevent* bugs from ever showing up in the first place. After all, the Orkin ads predicted, "as long as groceries are delivered to the kitchen, as long as there are water pipes, as long as food is kept in the house, as long as there are careless neighbors, there will be insects and rodents."

Through advertising, Orkin appeared to be making some important headway in getting this message across. In the early days of its television advertising, Orkin bowed to the seasonal nature of pest control; in other words, it sharply curtailed its advertising during the winter months, and juiced it up during the summer months for pests and during the termite swarming season from February to June. In the mid-1950s, however, the company maintained its regular television schedule during the winter and realized a 20 percent increase in business during this period. And when Orkin introduced a new service called Orkin-Tox, the effectiveness of television to sell termite control was finally documented.

Orkin-Tox was sold as a new construction pretreating system designed to control termites. Before a house was even built, the land around it was treated, and all of the wooden construction joints and sections within a certain radius of the ground were sprayed. Then a series of small aluminum pipes was installed in especially vulnerable areas beneath the house, in case it was necessary to treat the house after construction. When Orkin started advertising Orkin-Tox on television, it quickly noted an upswing in consumer demand and acceptance of the idea.

Orkin-Tox, introduced in 1953, was a construction-pretreating system in which aluminum pipes were installed beneath a house in case further termite treatment was required. Here Ed Elkins, then manager of the Knoxville, Tennessee, branch, is shown after inspecting the first Better Homes and Gardens 5-Star Plan Home to be built in Tennessee and treated by Orkin-Tox (1954). When Orkin started advertising the system on television, an upswing in consumer demand was immediate.

THIS IS THE 5 STAR PLAN NO. 2409
CONSTRUCTION BY
WADE KEEVER
Better Homes
Home for all America Program
ORKIN-TOX
TRIPLE PROTECTION
Against Termites-Beetles-Decay
ORKIN
SINCE 1901
THE NEW EXCLUSIVE PIPE SYSTEM
FOR SALE
WADE KEEVER
BUILDER & GENERAL CONTRACTOR
PHONE
2-8822
SEPT. 12th

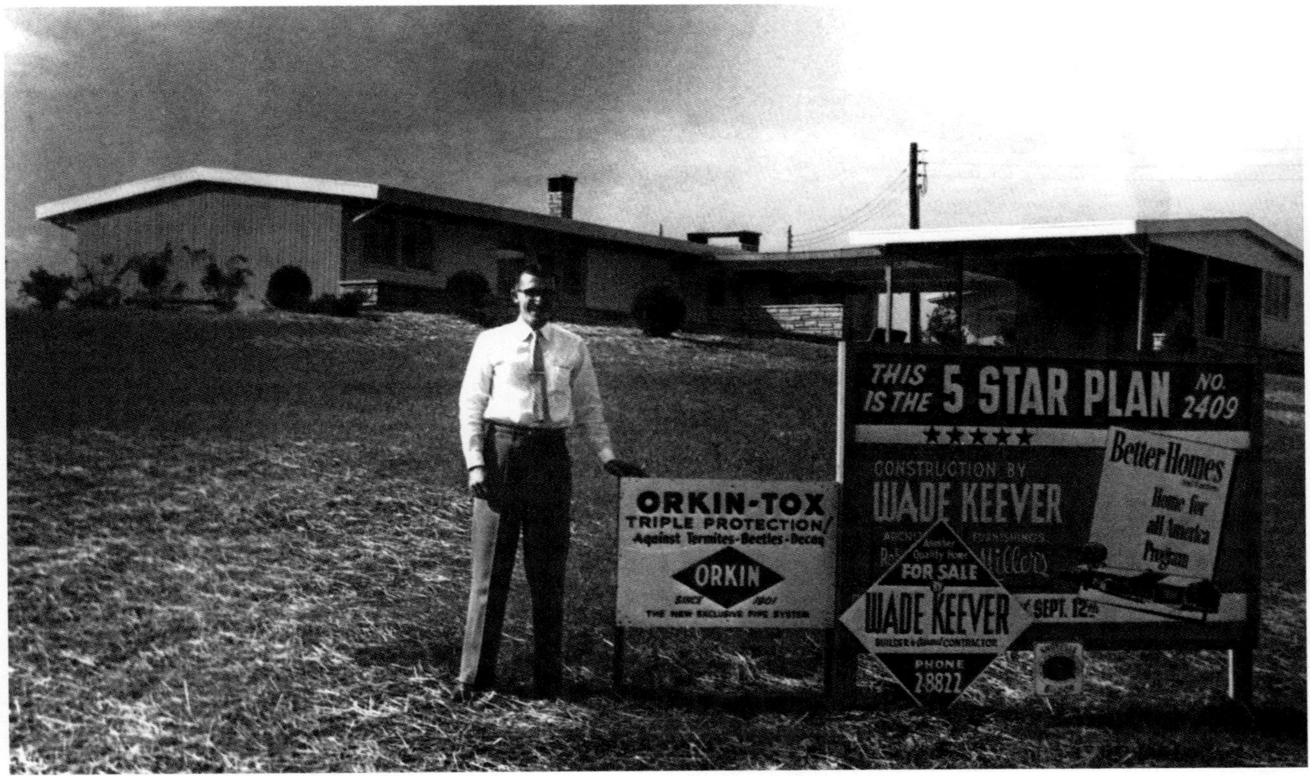

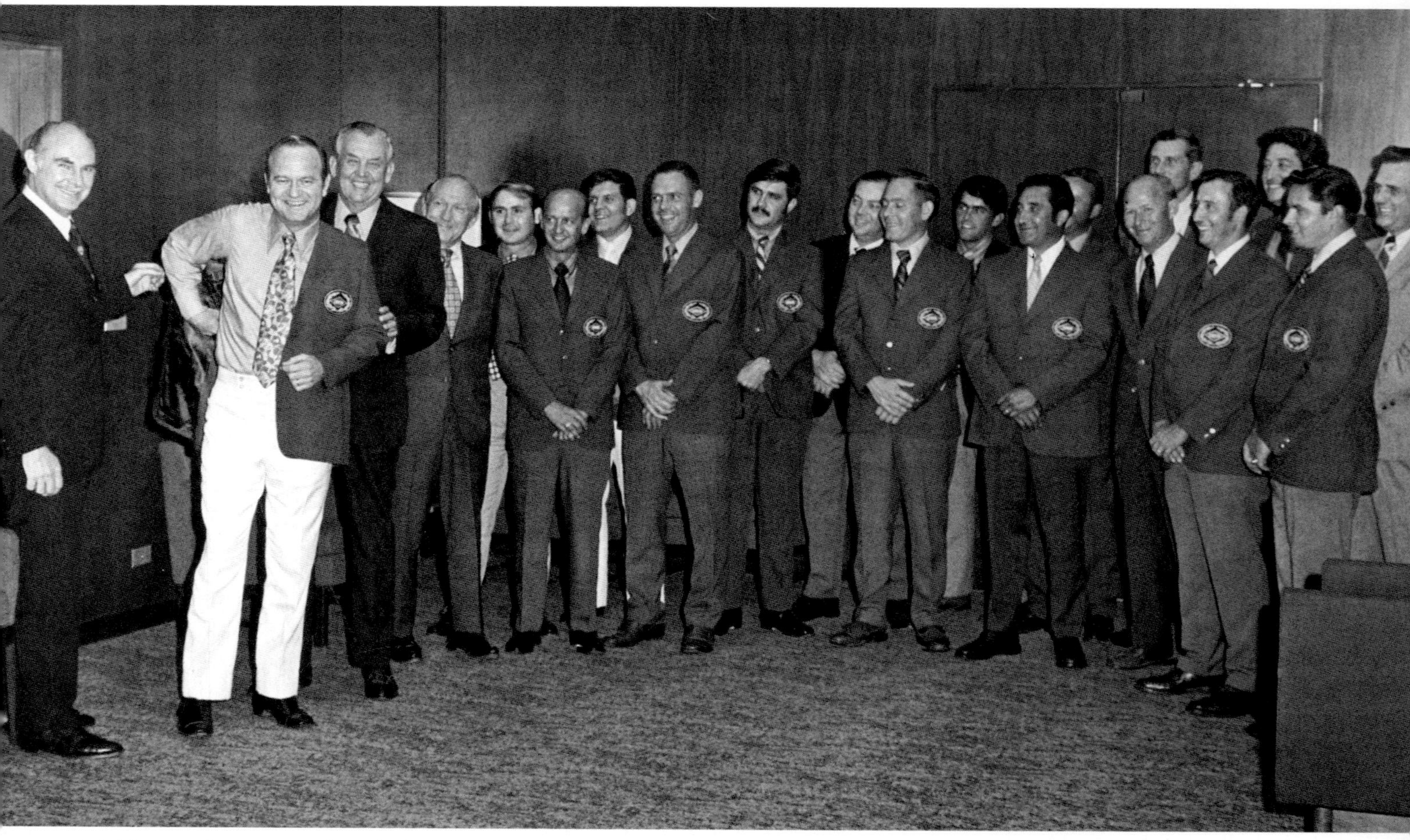

The Virginia district outperformed all other Orkin districts in the fiscal 1971 King Bee contest. Branch managers in the district, together with district office representatives, received a trip to Atlanta and red Orkin blazers for leading the division. District manager Ken Conners, who also won a trip to Europe, is pictured being helped into his blazer by Earl F. Geiger, left, executive vice president, and O. Wayne Rollins, third from left, chairman and president. Looking on are, left to right, front row, Bernie Kolkana, Southeast Region vice president; Buddy Laumann, Norfolk; Tom Cox, Roanoke; Joe Wilson, Louisville; Tom Taylor, Hampton; Ray Lasley, Charlottesville; Glen Pittman, Portsmouth; Bob Furlough, district service manager; and Sam Hayes, Richmond. Back row: Larry Spruill, Warrenton; Ralph DeVour, Petersburg; Jim Jett, Norfolk; Steve Drennan, Lynchburg; Kenny Haymore, Danville; Norman Smith, district sales manager; Fred Cliff, South Carolina district manager; and Paul Bowes, assistant to the executive vice president.

Throughout the 1950s newspaper and magazine stories about Orkin's successful use of television commercials projected the medium as a near godsend to Orkin in particular and the industry in general. Read the headlines: "Otto Slays 'Em on TV—Animated Cartoons Built Business for a Pest Control Firm," "Spot Removes a Stigma—Orkin helps solve its public-relations problem by heavy use of television," "Orkin of Atlanta did so well on TV—sales have doubled in five years."

But the headlines missed another story unfolding at Orkin, one that also contributed significantly to its sales growth. At Orkin, the district managers were experts in urging their salesmen and servicemen to knock on just one more door—a message that Otto and Ted had preached since opening the first office in Richmond.

Each district and branch devised its own programs to meet sales quotas. In the Carolinas, Pressman was an acknowledged expert in developing sales crews to solicit pest control and termite work in smaller towns. They would go as a group—managers, supervisors, everyone—and knock on every door. Pressman believed in recognition and monetary rewards, and free vacation trips for those who brought in the most sales. He always included recognition for his administrative support staff; without their diligent attention to details, Pressman argued, the sales representatives would have a harder time making their numbers.

Throughout the company, contests were often used in an effort to create a sense of camaraderie among the employees—as well as to keep each district more aware of what the other districts were doing. There were frequent sales contests with various incentives—such as the 1952 Sales Round-Up Catalog, offering merchandise ranging from refrigerators to house slippers to those who earned bonus points through increased sales. This particular contest was conducted during the late fall and winter season to increase sales during those slower months—with salesmen receiving points for any leads and new contracts they developed over regular quotas. The "King Bee" contest was another form of company recognition, which started with competition between fourteen districts in 1954. Points were awarded monthly for comparative standings in controllable profits, wages, materials and supplies, auto expenses, allowances, collections, and sales increases. Each district was made aware of how the other districts were doing; competition was keen. The face of the winning district manager was imposed on a cartoon body of a bee, and that manager was "King Bee" for the quarter. Alabama's Abe Krawcheck was the first King Bee, winning by a mere ten points over Bob Couhig's New Orleans District. During the fall of 1956, a "Selling Bee" contest challenged each district to bring in the "*bizzness.*" "The King Bee" contest was so successful that it remained part of Orkin's sales strategy for many years.

Throughout the company, contests were often used in an effort to create a sense of camaraderie among employees—as well as to keep each district more aware of what the other districts were doing.

In keeping with Pressman's belief in the importance of recognition, the secretaries weren't forgotten either. The first Secretaries Collection Contest, in 1953, brought fourteen winners to Atlanta for a two-day celebration. During the visit the group toured the Atlanta office and learned how the branch and home operations worked together. Among the winners was Charles Risinger, who had been hired in Columbia, South Carolina, one year earlier. Later Risinger would become the company auditor, a position he held until he

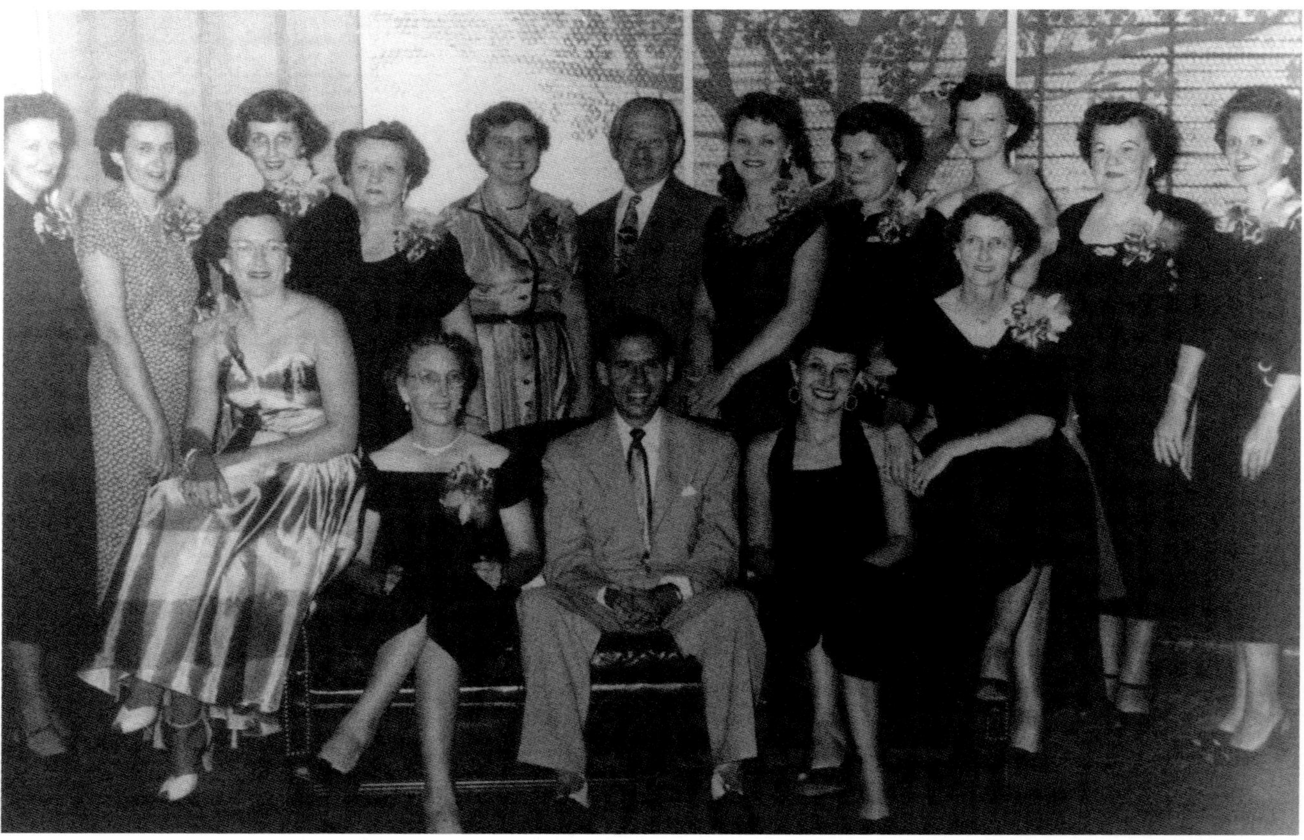

Fifteen winners of the Secretaries' Collection Contest enjoy their prize, a two-day holiday in Atlanta (August 27–28, 1953). Front row, left to right: Polly Eubanks, Tallahassee; Louise Gentry, Chattanooga; Charlie Risinger, Columbia; Helen Cutsinger, Nashville; and Nell Ballantine, Roanoke. Back row: Pearl Pennybaker, Little Rock; Earline Hendrickson, West Palm Beach; Grace Ellis, Fort Worth; Cora Wallach, Atlanta; Bettie Clemmer, Rocky Mountain; Otto Orkin; Charlotte Bush, Montgomery; Nancy White, Charlottesville; Dot Robbins, Birmingham; Bess Little, Houston; and Theresa Chrupcala, Jacksonville.

retired in 1984. During his tenure he worked in branch offices throughout the company, assuring that collections and record keeping were performed according to company policies.

By 1954 twenty secretaries were recognized for best collection efforts, including Dorothy Barrett of the Charlotte branch. The top prize in 1956 for the best collection record was a Red Nash Metropolitan automobile—won by Frances Jarrett in Tampa. There was only one problem: Jarrett, who had been with the company since 1936, didn't know how to drive (she took lessons).

And the home office didn't forget the real-life Orkin Man—those men and women who serviced the homes and businesses for protection against pests and termites. Orkin announced a Pension Plan in 1952, and later offered scholarship programs for employees and their children. With the advent of Otto the Orkin Man on television, the corporate office did everything within its power to ensure that the serviceman lived up to people's expectations. Emphasis was placed on personal appearance, and the Orkin Man's uniform was to be cleaned and pressed each day; trucks and service vans were expected to be immaculate. Each serviceman was trained to understand the importance of his relationship with the customer, and instructed to begin each visit with a cordial "Hello, Mr. or Mrs. . . ." every time he entered the house. Too much conversation was discouraged, but each serviceman was expected to engage in some personal conversation with the customer. Otto went so far as to encourage the Orkin servicemen to perform small favors for the customers—changing a lightbulb, moving a chair—that would endear him or her to the household. In 1953, Gerald Ellerbee, an Atlanta termite salesman, had to roll up four thousand pennies given to him by an Atlanta housewife as payment for the last forty dollars she owed for a termite job. Ellerbee was soundly praised for his cooperation—and featured in the next edition of *Orkin Talkin.*

In fact, the word went out from the home office: "No matter how good your service may be, if the customer does not have a personal liking for the man or men who do the work, the account can be lost more easily."

Orkin continued to do everything possible to promote the real Orkin Man and to develop the serviceman's impeccable image—through training, guidance, good driving records, and public relations. To promote their image of using only the latest technology, engineers and entomologists from Orkin's Technical Department reported on the company's use of Orkin-Aire, a new aerosol for treating pests, and for a "modern line of labor-saving devices—the Schramm Air Compressors and Air Hammers." Used to drill holes to facilitate termite treatment, the new air compressors worked better and faster than previous electric drills and could cut through concrete or difficult construction material in one-fifth the time.

The versatility of the Orkin Man was apparent when *Life* magazine reported that Orkin had completed the world's largest "tent" fumigation of the J. B. Hill Company in Fresno, California, in 1955. Dramatic magazine photographs showed how Orkin technicians successfully sealed and fumigated a series of mammoth grain elevators infested with khapra beetles through the use of nine and one-third acres of vinyl-coated nylon tarpaulins. The Orkin Diamond graced the top of the tarps, which covered three and one half million cubic feet. Proving that "no job is too large nor is one too small for Otto the Orkin Man," Orkin then advertised that "Orkin also had the distinction of completing the world's *smallest* tent fumigation"—on a dollhouse.

Orkin servicemen were encouraged to perform small favors for the customers—collecting the newspaper, changing a lightbulb, moving a chair—that would endear him to the household.

Orkin's appeal to housewives and women was never ending. Orkin was listed in the Buyers' Guide section of *House Beautiful* magazine in the 1950s—a not-so-subtle message that pest control was just one of many ways to keep your house looking spectacular. In November 1954 a female Orkin service technician appeared on *What's My Line?* dispelling the myth that women fear insects. Eventually, no less wholesome a representative than Bess Myerson, Miss America 1961, became a spokesperson for Orkin, appearing in a variety of commercial media, including cartoon spots with Arnold Stang of movie, radio, and television fame.

Despite the public's perception of Orkin as a company with unlimited successes, this time of great growth and achievement by Orkin brought with it some special challenges—not only in pest control but in home office management.

Increasingly, pests were developing resistance to chemicals. Flies, for instance, had developed immunity to DDT, and Orkin had begun treating them with lindane (which would eventually be taken off the market, along with DDT). By the late 1950s, flies had also developed resistance to malathion and diazinon. "Roaches," read an Orkin memo, "in all probability, will be next. We are insisting that you discontinue using diazinon except when absolutely necessary. We have outlined the use of 933 and pyrocide for maintenance sprays in technical bulletins and service schools. Some offices continue to use chlordane routinely both inside and outside. The excuse offered is that the use of chlordane is for control of American roaches. This constant and routine use can also be damaging and service methods should be altered to make use of alternates which are also effective in American roach control. Please acknowledge, by return mail, that you are following recommended resistant roach procedures by using Diazinon on cleanouts and then switching to pyrethrum formulations for maintenance."

This time of great growth and achievement by Orkin brought with it special challenges—not only in pest control but in home office management.

On the management front, problems surfaced. Within the pest control industry, Orkin made a controversial decision: it withdrew from the membership of the NPCA in a dispute over dues and membership requirements.

As the pest control industry became more complicated and subject to more federal regulations, the Orkin Man in the field no doubt began to sense some tensions brewing in the leadership of the home office. In fact, the changes taking place in Atlanta were absolutely shocking—not only to Orkin employees but also to the outside members of the pest control industry. Herman Fellton, who had trained hundreds if not thousands of Orkin men over the years, left Orkin in 1953 and later sued the company, charging that officials of the company had conspired to break his contract and then prevent him from going into business for himself. In 1956, after twenty-five years of service with Orkin, Abe Krawcheck was discharged and given a ninety-thousand-dollar settlement, payable over a five-year period. By now, no less an Orkin pioneer than Ted Oser had grown disenchanted with Orkin's management and its decision to pull out of the NPCA; in early 1957, after forty-one years with the company, Ted was discharged on short notice and given only minimum benefits.

To the outside world, it appeared that the Orkin management team was in complete chaos. But those inside the company knew exactly what was happening, and why.

OTTO ORKIN AND HIS FAMILY—THE FINAL YEARS

At Orkin, the company's executive management structure had become increasingly more complicated over the years as Otto tried to introduce a new element to his long-standing executive team: his sons and his sons-in-law.

Within a matter of years, four ambitious young men entered the Orkin organization, all with exceptionally close ties to Otto: Perry Kaye, who was married to Otto's older daughter Bernice; Petty Bregman, who married Otto's younger daughter Gloria; Sanford Orkin, Otto's oldest son, who graduated with a business degree from the University of Georgia; and William Orkin, Otto's youngest son, who attended Purdue University. These young men clashed with many of Otto's longtime managers—Pressman, Krawcheck, Russell, Tindol, Oser, and others. As time went by, Otto grew to appreciate Petty Bregman's style of management, while Sanford and William favored Perry Kaye's fairly ruthless and demanding manner. It didn't require a complicated management flowchart to understand that the family would eventually become polarized, a twist that would one day break the family in two and leave Otto without the company he founded.

Son-in-law Perry Kaye joined the company first, opening up the Fort Worth territory in 1946. Reviews of his performance as a branch manager were mixed, and he moved into the home office to become assistant secretary in 1951. From there, he climbed up the ranks of his father-in-law's company's management team very quickly. He joined the board of directors in 1955 and was named vice president and operations manager from 1958 to 1964.

Otto's sons—who remembered working as servicemen and termite inspectors during summers growing up in Atlanta—joined the company one year apart. William joined Orkin in 1952, one year after graduating from high school, and worked with employee initiatives but little else until he became a board member in 1955, with the title of executive vice president. After graduating from college, Sanford joined Orkin in 1953 and was named an executive vice president and board member in 1955. Quiet-spoken like his father, Sanford became president of Orkin in 1961, a position he held until 1964.

Son-in-law Petty Bregman joined Orkin in 1949 as editor of *Orkin Talkin*. In 1950 he served as secretary and then assistant to Otto Orkin until he, too, was named an executive vice president in 1955. From the beginning, he was aligned with Otto, and he left the company in mid-1956 when many of Otto's long-term executives were also asked to leave or were forced out.

The young men's rise within the company was astounding to those who watched: In 1952, for instance, a flowchart of the company lists Otto as president; Petty Bregman as executive vice president; Ted Oser as vice president of sales; Herman Fellton as vice president of technical operations; C. M. Young as secretary; and Perry Kaye as assistant secretary. Two years later, by 1954, the slate had changed dramatically: Otto, the founder, was still president; Perry Kaye was first vice president; Sanford Orkin was vice president; William Orkin was vice president; Ted Oser was still vice president of sales; and C. M. Young was secretary.

The family members were often in conflict with Otto's managers—his "lieutenants," as someone once referred to the group made up of Pressman, Krawcheck, Couhig, Tindol, Kotler, Oser, Russell, and many others. Initially, the group disagreed about their payment plans: the long-term executives wanted to continue on the lucrative compensation plans set up for them by Otto; the sons and sons-in-law wanted the plans rewritten. As members of the old guard began to leave the company, the reasons they gave resonated like a chorus throughout the industry: "Atlanta management was not satisfactory." To many, however, it was crystal clear that more important issues were at the heart of the dispute. In short, what was happening to Otto and the company?

By 1956, the sixty-nine-year-old Otto appeared to be a mere figurehead at the company he had founded and directed for over fifty-five years.

According to company observers, Otto Orkin was already locked in a battle with his children for control of the firm. Long-term employees like Louis Kotler not only confirmed the controversy, but also fell victim to it. In 1956, Kotler, who had worked for Orkin for thirty-three years and had risen to be vice president, was summoned to the executive office. "Bill Orkin, then only twenty-three years old, called me in and fired me," Kotler told a newspaper in Memphis. "He told me there would be no more vice presidents outside the family. That's when the fight really began."

By 1956, apparently, the sixty-nine-year-old Otto was a mere figurehead at the company he had founded and directed for over fifty-five years. He no longer had an office to himself on the coveted "mahogany row" in the Peachtree Street headquarters; in fact, his desk had been moved to William's office, at the end of the hall on the second floor. In this office, Otto continued his favorite obsession of pouring over canceled accounts. Each month, every office was required to send in a list of new accounts and of contract cancellations, among other records, to the Atlanta office. Otto kept long green sheets to tally his "Lost Business Accounts" forms, and would spend hours calling managers, customers, and district managers about these accounts. His conversation always started out pleasantly, but got progressively more intense, especially if Otto found out someone had not tried to save the accounts. "Do you realize how important our customers are?" Otto would say.

Still physically fit, Otto regularly embarked on visits to various branches around the country, always on hand to open a new office or ready to give an interview to any reporter who was curious enough to meet the "real" Otto the Orkin Man. Granted, Otto was one of the company's most valuable public relations tools; but to many observers, the routine branch tours offered a convenient way of keeping Otto out of the home office.

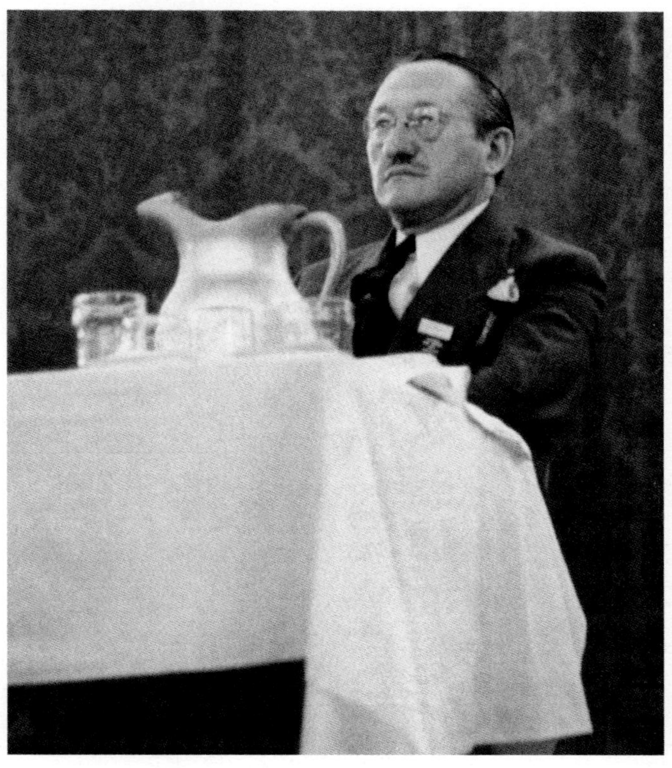

At some point Otto became a figurehead in his own company, which was run by his sons and his son-in-law.

The question, then, becomes "Why?" Why would a family who had so benefited from their father's hard work and expertise seek to diminish his role in the company and dramatically change the way the company was managed?

Granted, Otto was eccentric. "I first met Mr. Orkin in 1957," said Joe Judge, a longtime Orkin employee who lived next door to Otto at the Howell House. "We were coming out of our apartments at the Howell House in Atlanta to walk the one block to the Orkin office on West Peachtree Street. It was 6:45 A.M. Mr. Orkin was properly dressed in suit, coat, tie, shined shoes. I was in the uniform of a termite treater—coveralls, old shoes, and baseball hat. Mr. Orkin was always a kind and gentle person. Soft-spoken in public, polite, and of course, always the salesman, he saw me and quietly said, 'Son, do you work for me?' I said, 'Yes, sir, I do.' I recognized him from photos. He said, 'I like that very much. I am proud to have you working for me.' I later found out that he was pleased that I said, 'Yes, sir.'

"As we walked down the hill, I noticed that I was walking on the pavement and he was walking on the grass. I didn't want to say anything, so I just continued to walk beside him to the office. When I came to the front door, I held it open for him to go first. After entering, he stopped, turned to me and said, 'What is your name?' I told him and he said, 'I like you, Joe. And I will repay you for your kindness.'

"Not long after, I met Starky Thomas, the termite supervisor, and Jimmy Farrar, the pest control supervisor. I asked Jimmy about Mr. Orkin's walking on the grass. And he said, 'You're going to find out Mr. Orkin does some unconventional things. He walks on the grass to save shoe leather.' A few days later, I met Mr. Orkin again at 6:45 A.M. Again, we walked and talked. This time, we got on the subject of food. He implored me to stay away from fattening foods. Then he said to me, 'Joe, someday you must come to lunch with me at the Progressive Club. I have one lamb chop, boiled, and for dinner a piece of fish.' To a young person like me, that diet was not very appealing. But Mr. Orkin was trim and glad that he had cautioned me about my diet.

"The Tuesday before Thanksgiving, November 1957, I was calling Pest Control cancellations for John Hatcher, the PC manager, when I was called to Billy Orkin's office. Billy called me over and gave me an airline ticket so I would be home with my family for the Thanksgiving holidays. Here I was, a one-month employee, hardly yet a productive person for the company, shown an extraordinary bit of kindness. Is it any wonder I worked hard for the Orkin family? Is it any wonder I was loyal?"

That December, Otto called Judge into his office—and presented him with not only a plane ticket home but a twenty-five-dollar Christmas gift. "To me, their kind expression of faith in me as a person left me lost for words."

Walking on grass . . . saving shoe leather . . . showing kindness to new employees . . . fussing over lost accounts . . . fanatically staying trim and eating healthy—it's hard to imagine that these activities worried Otto's sons so much that they believed he could harm the company enough for them to want him out of the business. It was particularly hard to make that argument as Otto continued to travel to the branch offices and give interviews to reporters.

For instance, when he stopped in Richmond to visit the original Orkin office at 819 West Broad Street in the late 1950s, Otto was described as "vigorous as in the years when he first was winning a reputation as a modern pied piper. Reflections of youth twinkle in his eyes. His words, hung on the solid accents of his homeland, carry a staccato excitement. Otto still has the manner of a young man in a hurry. 'Quit?' he said. 'I should say not. I've never been sick a day in my life. My business is what keeps me healthy—that and walking five miles every day.' He interrupted himself to stand, do a little jig, and pump himself on the chest. 'Quit? Why I'm going to expand into the other twenty states within the next six or seven years!'"

Newspapers around the country described Otto as trim and alert, five feet seven inches tall, and 122 pounds. Granted, he was exceedingly thin. But was he confused? Incoherent? Were his actions hurting the company and putting the jobs of thirty-six hundred employees at risk? Back home, Joe Judge recalled that "Mr. Orkin had a sharp mind. He never forgot my name, and he would remember our walks to the office and then remind me about my food consumption. His tone of voice was always pleasant, and I got the impression he really cared." Otto would often stop by the stockroom to talk with Gene Loyd or James Llewallyn in the nearby sign office. "I was his sign man," recalled Llewallyn. "He often came downstairs to visit with Gene Loyd, who was in charge of the stockroom, next to my little office. He seemed to enjoy visiting with Gene and finding some little something to fuss about. Maybe a ream of forms that was opened and not closed properly or not straight on the shelf."

Rumors persisted that Otto was increasingly confused and paranoid, unable to function in the home office on anything but the most basic level—making phone calls, straightening supplies on the shelf. At one point, Otto supposedly called Jim Farrar, Orkin's service manager, to "drop whatever he was doing and come to Otto's apartment because someone was trying to poison him." Other unfounded but persistent rumors painted his sons and son-in-law as the problem, suggesting that William, Sanford, and Perry Kaye were eager to exaggerate Otto's condition in order to take control of the company. Often referred to as the "Family Troika," the three young men were considered by many to be too impatient and inexperienced to handle smoothly a transition in corporate governance. Many of the longtime managers and employees resisted the new management's moves to centralization, and didn't want to give up their power and autonomy. As much as anything, Otto was said to be devastated when many longtime employees or relatives left the company or were fired.

Unfounded but persistent rumors said Otto's sons and son-in-law exaggerated his eccentricities to try to take control of the company.

In spite of their disagreements, the sons continued to use their father's venerable and valuable image to sell new products. In 1959, when Otto was seventy-one years old, the company put Otto's likeness on new advertisements to introduce the company's new termiticide called Orkil—"A dramatic Scientific Triumph in Termite Control, backed by an unmatched termite guarantee." At the time, Orkin promoted Orkil as the most effective termiticide available, backed by "the world's strongest surety bonded guarantee against future termite damage."

But Orkil was the last Orkin product Otto was ever associated with at the Orkin company. In a soap opera–like saga that was played out weekly in the press, Otto's two sons and his son-in-law Perry Kaye had Otto hospitalized and declared incompetent on May 16, 1960—shortly after the elder Orkin had transferred 51 percent controlling stock in the corporation to his two sons and one daughter, Bernice Kaye, Perry's wife.

With the help of Ted Oser, Petty Bregman, and his daughter Gloria, Otto successfully fought to have his competency status restored. A Fulton County lunacy commission ruled in August 1960 that the seventy-two-year-old Otto Orkin was sane and able to manage his own affairs; the commission ruled that "Mr. Orkin is suffering from a form of mental illness which is called cerebral hardening of the arteries." According to newspaper accounts in the *Atlanta Journal,* the commission said that Mr. Orkin "possesses a strong and determined intention to preserve his own interest in the face of opposition. His judgment in business and personal affairs is at times sharp and perceptive and reflects the use of his long experience in conducting business affairs. However, the commission added, certain memory defects may stand in the way of Mr. Orkin's engaging in major business transactions."

In spite of what the commission called "a warmth of feeling for all of his children," Otto eventually filed a $5 million lawsuit against William, Sanford, and Perry and Bernice Kaye, charging that they had conspired to unlawfully put him in a hospital and have him declared of unsound mind in order to take over the business. Daughter Gloria joined him in the suit. In November, however, Otto gave up the fight and agreed to a settlement. He sold his remaining interest in the company for $5.35 million, and Gloria sold her interest for approximately $750,000. In a move that made every headline read like it came straight from the tabloids, Otto also quickly announced that he was going on a honeymoon—with his thirty-nine-year-old bride. "Orkin Sells Out, Weds Ex-Secretary." Otto had married for the third time, to Eva Claxton, a former Orkin employee.

Employee morale was exceptionally low as the company began to adjust to its new leadership after Otto reluctantly sold his remaining interest in the business.

The painful and embarrassing scandal was over. No one at the company—including Sanford, William, or Perry—ever talked publicly about what happened. Within Orkin, the demise of Otto Orkin and his legendary association with the company that he founded was considered tragic, unnecessary, or inevitable—depending on whom you talked to. And decades later, when asked about the decision to have his father declared incompetent, Sanford Orkin stated: "We relied on doctors from Emory University, and other very prominent doctors, to tell us that he needed to not be there. It became a very difficult time. On the one hand, you want emotionally for your father to be there. But at the same time, you know that in the best interests of the business, it wasn't the right thing to do. It made it very difficult for us. But we had to make some decisions, if we wanted that business to survive."

MOVING FORWARD

The controversy clearly took a toll on Orkin, and the period from 1958 to 1961 was in many ways a troubled one for the Orkin Company. Servicemen continued to encounter serious pest resistance to insecticides, particularly with cockroaches and houseflies. Despite significant improvements in Orkin's termite control procedures and in the guarantees it offered the public, sales personnel were reporting a low percentage of closures on calls and leads. In a dispute over growing regulations, the company had gone to court to have the state pest control law of Georgia declared unconstitutional—even though the Georgia law was one of the first state laws ever passed and considered a model for subsequent legislation in other states. The papers carried the story of the death of one child and the critical condition of two others due to a cyanide fumigation by the company in Fayetteville, North Carolina. In 1959 the company was slapped on the wrist for "alleged misuse of 1080." Two more long-term employees left the company—Bob Russell and Red Tindol—only to join competing pest control companies.

And in 1960, for the first time in its history, Orkin reported a drop in net earnings after taxes from the previous year, down from $2.054 million on gross earnings of $26 million to $1.92 million on gross earnings of $29.7 million. The general morale of the employees was exceptionally low as the company began to adjust to its new leadership: Sanford, thirty, was named president and treasurer of Orkin and all its subsidiaries; William, twenty-nine, was given the title of executive vice president; Perry Kaye, thirty-eight, was the new vice president and operations manager; and Stuart Bohacheck continued as secretary.

Perry Kaye gradually emerged as the individual who ran the company on a daily basis. He was bright and ambitious, but those around him said that Kaye also had a quick temper and an arrogance he couldn't hide. He endeared himself to no one when he started a form of communication called "Immediate Action Memos." As their name implies, the memos were typically missives from an angry or frustrated Kaye about something he wanted corrected or changed immediately. They nearly always contained exclamation points, and a note on the top of each memo reminded the reader that the content was confidential and that it "MUST be placed in a three-ring binder."

Some highlights from these Immediate Action Memos show how Kaye set a tone for the company, as well as what he emphasized and tried to change:

> **January 23, 1958**—For your information, the company is trailing—profit-wise—in year-to-date figures over the previous year. I need not tell you the importance of reversing this trend promptly. In spite of numerous bulletins, letters, phone calls and—on occasion—visits to Atlanta, there are still a number of managers who are lax in primary operational phases which determine the profit or loss in a branch office. Now is the time to demonstrate and exercise your managerial capabilities. DO SO!

October 2, 1958—You received Action Bulletin #2, dated 3/12/58, concerning Petty Cash. Evidentally [*sic*], some managers and/or office personnel are not sufficiently impressed with the necessity of complying with its contents. *This bulletin will be the last reminder to certain offices to familiarize themselves with Action Bulletin #2 dated 3/12/58 concerning Petty Cash!*

June 17, 1959 [an unusual Immediate Action Memo from William Orkin]—Most food processors are subject to inspections by the U.S. Food and Drug Administration. Many food manufacturers are hiring sanitation consultants to audit their operations and show them how the plant can meet the regulations. . . . WE HAVE LOST several long-standing accounts to these consultants simply because we were not providing sanitation inspection and consulting services together with our pest control. In almost every case, the fact that ORKIN can provide consulting and inspectional services had never even been mentioned to the account so he had *gone elsewhere to find a service which we offer. Gentlemen, let me warn you now that we are not to lose another account because of such a situation.*

November 25, 1959—The bad debt column for Fiscal 1959 totaled a staggering $308,980.72. This figure represents the largest sum of bad debts in the company's history. The realization of the seriousness of this fact and its effect on the company is better illustrated by remembering that in order to obtain a profit of $308,980.72, the company must have a volume of business of approximately THREE MILLION DOLLARS!!!!!!!!! We very definitely must reverse the bad debt trend, and in some cases attitudes, toward this phase of the company's operation.

April 22, 1960—[In the height of termite season, Perry was incredulous that the company was reporting the "almost unbelievable low of 36% closures from leads to sales." He highlighted one salesman's weekly sales reports for thirty days, where he reported seventy-two leads and twenty-six sales.] It is obvious that some sales personnel are "clock watchers" who at 5 P.M. stuff their remaining leads in their shirt pocket and head for home. This practice must be stopped immediately. Some salesmen are not making the required evening calls to meet with the husband of the household to present the results of their inspection in the form of a completed proposal, sitting down to discuss with him the work required to correct the problem and to justify the price of being asked, to explain our surety bonded guarantee, our financial stability, the quality of our workmanship, and of course to close the sale. [Kaye then chided all branch managers who are leaving at 5, and daring to close the doors at noon on Saturday.] Give your sales personnel an incentive to work after office hours.

June 9, 1960—COLLECTIONS ARE LAGGING! IMMEDIATE ACTION IS EXPECTED!

In 1961, with the family scandal behind them, the new management appeared to regain its footing somewhat. The company opened 44 new offices, bringing the total count to 578 offices and call offices in 29 states and the District of Columbia. A total of 18 district offices were in operation, including new

ORKIN EXTERMINATING CO.
1901
The world's largest pest control company has a new home. Contains enough concrete to pave two and one-half miles of six lane highway. Enough lumber to build fifteen houses. A mile and one-half of water pipe. Takes 6,000 light bulbs to light the offices. Everything in it is designed to serve you better. How did all this come about? Simple. People from coast to coast say we kill bugs better than anybody else.
1963
ORKIN
ORKIN
call Orkin
for the sake of your home
ORKIN EXTERMINATING COMPANY, INC.

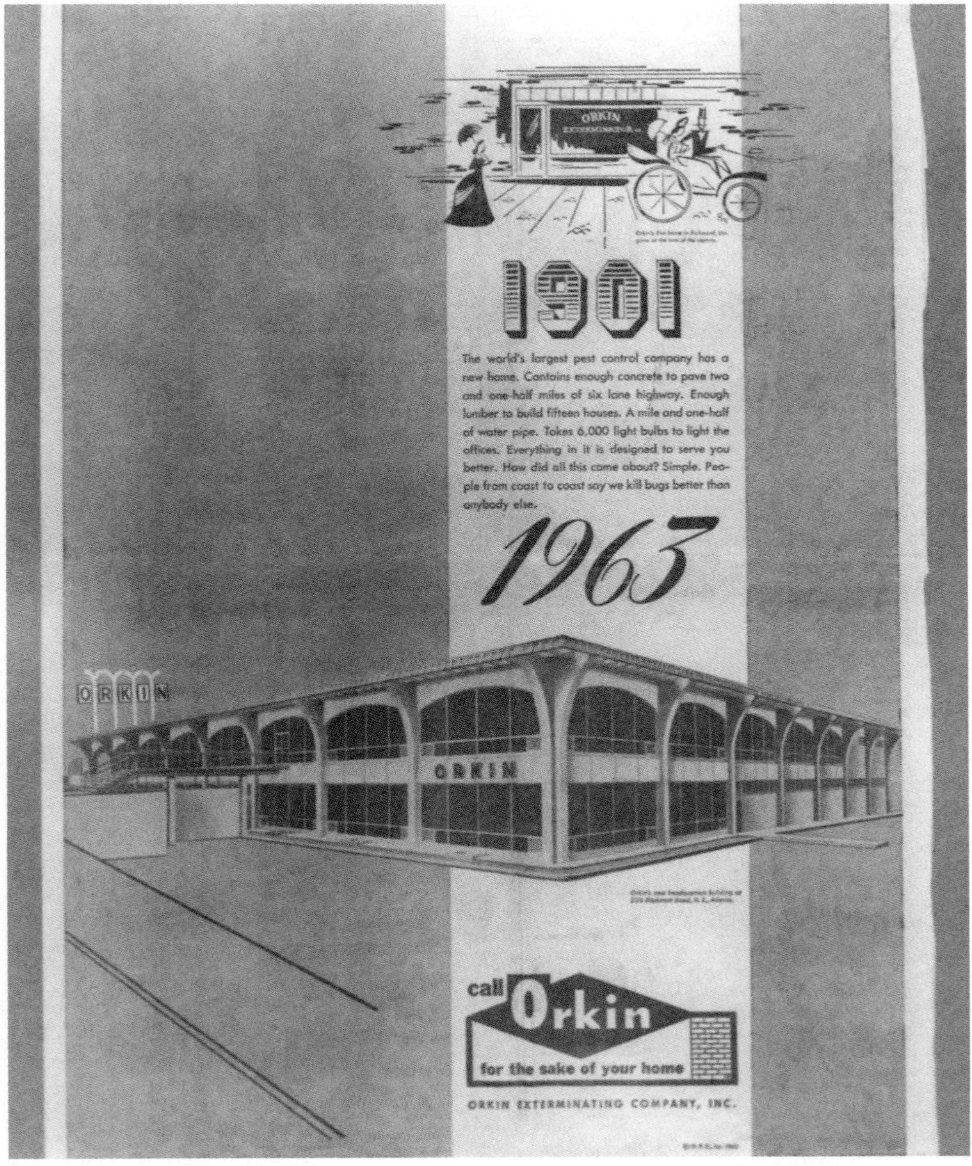

At the time Orkin completed its new $1.8 million headquarters at 2170 Piedmont Road, it was considered to be in the suburbs. The Atlanta Journal and Constitution *for September 15, 1963, touts the new Orkin headquarters building as containing a mile and a half of water pipe, six thousand light bulbs, enough concrete to pave two and a half miles of six-lane highway, and enough lumber to build fifteen houses.*

divisions in California and Kentucky. Nearly thirty-six hundred people worked for the company—with twenty-four hundred in service, five hundred in sales, five hundred in clerical, and two hundred in administration and management.

In August, after sixty years of private ownership, Sanford, William, and Bernice Kaye sold 360,000 shares of the company to the public at $24 each ($9.36 million) "in order to diversify on a personal basis." The three Orkins still retained about 85 percent of the 2.4 million shares outstanding—which made the public over-the-counter (OTC) shares available pretty thin. The company issued its first Annual Report to Stockholders, with a letter from Sanford H. Orkin as the company's new president. In the annual report, Sanford noted that net revenues for the year were over $31 million, with net profits after taxes of $2.4 million. "Not only were these profits the highest in the Company's history, but they also represented a 27 percent increase over the previous fiscal year.

"In keeping with our policy of financing growth and expansion as far as practicable through reinvested earnings, your Board of Directors deemed it advisable not to declare a dividend. Increased cash reserves are required to continue the Company's fleet replacement program and for construction of a new home office building which is scheduled to begin in 1962."

The headquarters building on Piedmont Road was considered very modern with its two-story lobby.

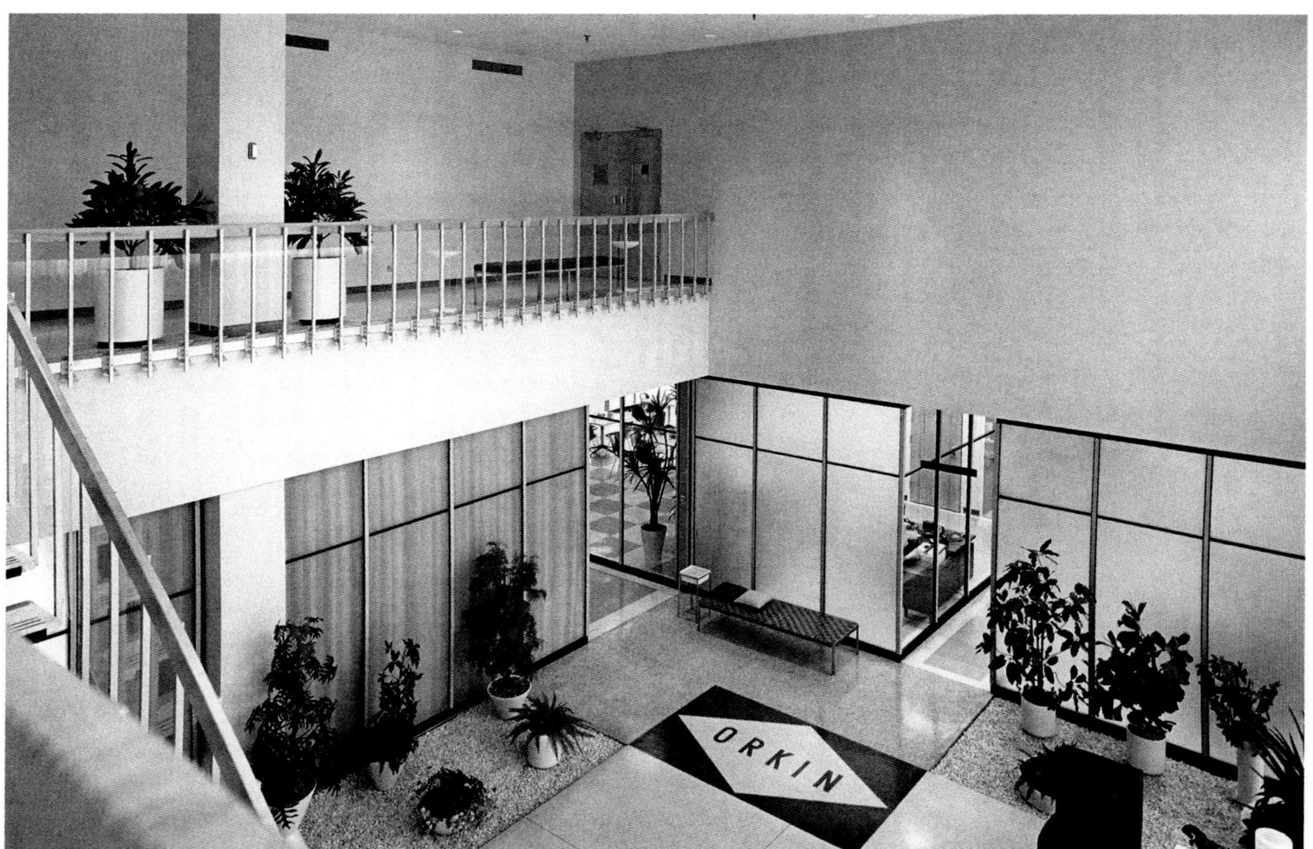

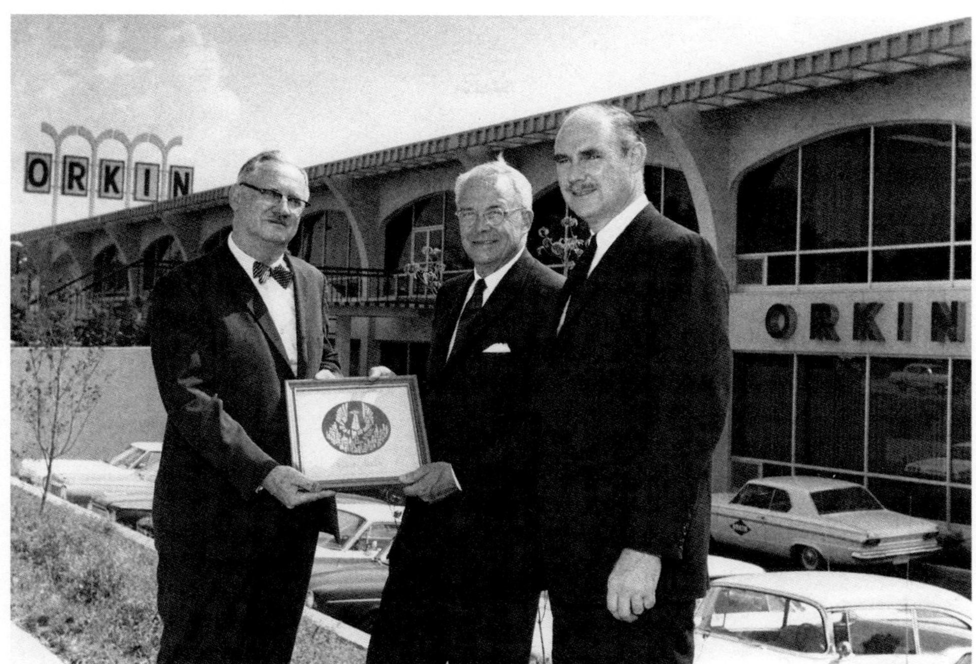

Herbert C. Millkey (left), the architect who designed the building, and Earl Geiger (right), Orkin's executive vice president, accepted an award from Atlanta mayor Ivan Allen Jr. on behalf of the Atlanta Beautiful Commission. The new building at 2170 Piedmont was cited for its outstanding contribution "to the increasing beauty of the city."

The Orkin headquarters was scheduled to move again—this time to 2170 Piedmont Road. On five acres of land acquired several years before, Orkin planned to build a $2 million state-of-the-art headquarters for the home office staff, the Georgia district offices, and the Atlanta operating branches. The two-story building, with its decidedly modern columns and arches, featured an unusual two-story lobby, with an Orkin diamond inlaid in terrazzo on the lobby floor.

When the company moved into its newly completed headquarters in July 1963, business seemed exceptionally solid. Both revenues and net earnings had set new records in 1963, with the company reporting a high of $37.3 million in revenues and $2.98 million in net earnings. Kaye's appointment of Earl Geiger, formerly Atlanta and New Orleans branch manager, to be the company's new vice president in charge of sales was applauded. Collections were up, and the company reported some 253,000 customers for its pest control services and around 275,000 surety-bonded guarantees in force in its termite control services. Through the efforts of Taft Pierce, one of Orkin's most respected field managers, Orkin rejoined the NPCA after a four-year absence.

And Sanford was beginning to make a prediction that Otto Orkin once made: "In time we hope to cover all the states, but it will be at least ten years before we attain national operation," he said "We can't say enough about the potential of this business."

Within the next few months, the Orkin executives would be heard saying a lot about the "potential of this business." After all, there was a new rumor going around about Orkin. The entire company, it turns out, was up for sale.

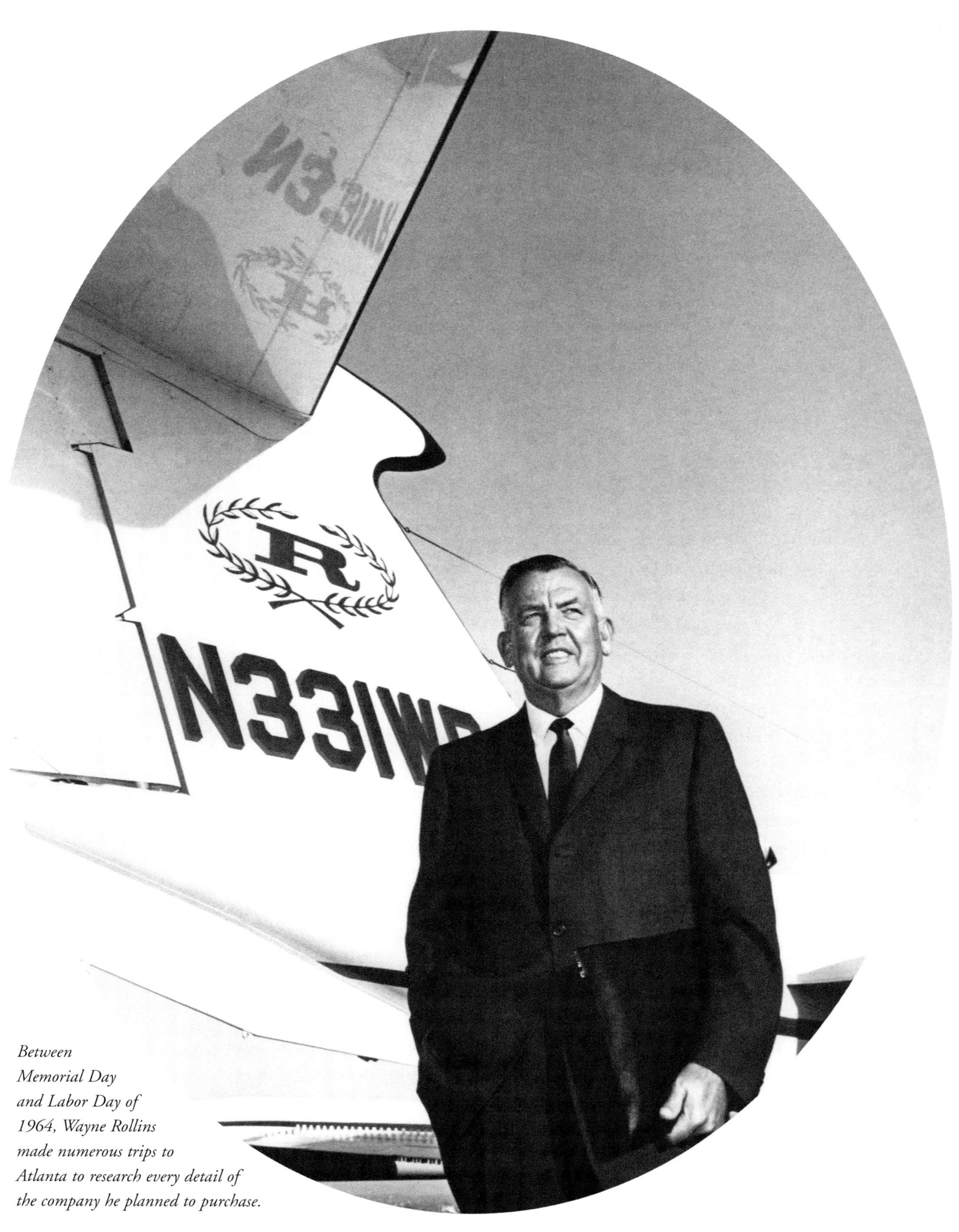

Between Memorial Day and Labor Day of 1964, Wayne Rollins made numerous trips to Atlanta to research every detail of the company he planned to purchase.

Chapter 4

1964: Rollins Buys Orkin

In April 1964, when O. Wayne Rollins heard that Orkin was for sale, his first question was right to the point: "What kind of price are we talking about?" When the $62.4 million price tag was floated, Wayne Rollins's immediate reaction was equally direct. "No. I'm not interested. I can already tell you that," he said, convinced that Orkin was too big and that he didn't have enough knowledge about the pest control industry to evaluate the deal effectively.

Over the next four months, however, as Wayne studied and researched every facet of this potential opportunity, he began to envision the transaction that would make business history.

The background was somewhat complicated. By the time Wayne Rollins heard that Orkin was for sale, many details of the deal had already been worked out. The Orkin family had earlier accepted a proposal from a New York investor named Lewis B. Cullman, who was an Orkin shareholder. Cullman had agreed to buy Orkin for $26 a share ($6 above the market price at that time), for a total of $62.4 million. In order to finance the deal, Cullman, whose family fortune came from the Philip Morris tobacco empire, had first persuaded Prudential Insurance Company of America to invest $40 million in the deal, and he then began to search for someone to provide the remaining equity. To clear that hurdle, Cullman brought in George T. Weymouth—a close personal friend of Wayne Rollins and a financial broker who had tried unsuccessfully to help Wayne purchase three Dallas media companies in April 1964. Weymouth was president of an investment banking firm based in Wilmington called Laird & Company, a member of the New York Stock Exchange. He was considered an adroit dealmaker with considerable business connections, due not only to his own professional accomplishments but also to his marriage into the well-respected DuPont family of Delaware. At one time they were thought to be potential investors in the Orkin deal. Weymouth agreed to help Cullman. With the help of a close associate named Martin Fenton, Weymouth quickly put together a new company called the Kinro Corporation that was organized solely as the vehicle to acquire Orkin, then resell it to a qualified buyer for a substantial fee. "Kinro," in fact, was simply a new word derived from all five letters in "Orkin."

After months of hot and cold negotiations, a tentative agreement was reached for the sale, but the DuPont investors became nervous. What if they couldn't find a buyer? Who would operate Orkin, since the founder's family wanted out? At this point, Weymouth mentioned the Orkin proposal to Wayne Rollins. After a Memorial Day meeting with Sanford and Billy Orkin and Perry Kaye in Atlanta, Wayne was convinced that he should continue to study the deal. Weymouth arranged for Earl F. Geiger, the Orkin vice president and general sales manager, to meet with Wayne in Wilmington at the offices of his media company Rollins Broadcasting. The two men instantly hit it off. "I want to know all I can about Orkin," Wayne told Earl, "as a possible acquisition." They started talking and didn't stop for two hours.

Earl Geiger outlined the potential of the pest control industry to Wayne Rollins: "The obvious penetration has to come from changing the casual user into a habitual user."

It turned out that Earl Geiger was one of the most valuable individuals ever hired by Perry Kaye and the Orkin brothers. Smart, ambitious, and a true promoter, Earl was a New York native who had served with the U.S. Army from 1944 to 1949, first as an intelligence officer and later as an executive officer for the Army Advisory Committee, First Army Headquarters in New York. After leaving the army with the rank of captain, he signed on as a salesman with a small Manhattan exterminating company called Bliss Exterminator Company. He advanced to operations manager of the New York firm but became frustrated when he and his employer couldn't agree on how to expand the company. "Any time your ambitions are greater than your employer's, you have the wrong employer," Earl once said. So he quit, joining Orkin in 1956 as a manager trainee and then branch manager in Atlanta. In 1959 he became New Orleans branch manager and then was promoted to vice president of sales, the highest position for anyone outside the family since Ted Oser had exited.

During his first two-hour meeting with Wayne, Earl outlined as much as he could about the exterminating business. "It's a remarkable business," he said, "You have a minimal amount of accounts receivable and you have no inventory. What inventory you have is in the form of your service staff, which you can increase or decrease according to the demand. You have no such thing as a stagnant inventory. A small percentage of households habitually use pest control, whereas a large number of households casually use pest control. So the obvious penetration has to come from changing the casual user into a habitual user."

The chemistry between Wayne and Earl was good from the start. Earl appreciated Wayne's ability to listen and ask the important questions; Wayne, in turn, felt a similar admiration for Earl's ability and enthusiasm and instantly recognized that Earl Geiger was the kind of man who could assist him in developing a sound evaluation of Orkin. When the meeting ended, Wayne agreed to take a closer look at Orkin. For the next two months, Wayne, along with Rollins Broadcasting executive Henry Tippie, traveled extensively between Wilmington and Atlanta, eventually staying for a week at a time instead of a few days. He also retained a leading management consulting firm, McKinsey & Company, Inc., to conduct a study of the pest control industry as a whole and of Orkin in particular, and the result confirmed what he already suspected: Orkin's growth could be accelerated. "It is our overall conclusion that the Orkin Exterminating Company has a strong position in a growing industry. The Company has a few important but correctable weaknesses, and with the correction of these weaknesses, Orkin's prospects for growth appear to be excellent."

The McKinsey report, one of the first independent reviews ever conducted of the Orkin Company, offered five major reasons to support this conclusion. And it gave Wayne Rollins a window into the company that would help him not only buy the business but decide how to run it.

First, McKinsey noted that the market for pest control services was large and offered untapped potential. With an estimated seven to eight thousand existing pest control companies accounting for some $480 million in business, McKinsey anticipated the "potential for total industry sales in the next five to seven years at about $1.1 billion."

Second, according to the report, "Orkin's strengths make it unusually competitive"—a conclusion McKinsey reached after analyzing Orkin's size relative to its competition and its branch-level organization. While the average pest control company had sales of fifty thousand to seventy-five thousand dollars, Orkin had sales of almost $40 million. Key to this, McKinsey concluded, is the "strong motivation that Orkin has achieved at the branch level." The report noted that Orkin "has some unusually competent field managers. We were impressed with the ability and the imagination of several of the branch and district managers with whom we worked."

And in a nod to Otto Orkin's tireless efforts to promote his company and create brand appeal, McKinsey noted that Orkin "is probably the best-known structural pest control company in the southeastern United States. Because the company has been established for many years, spends substantial amounts on advertising and has a large number of servicemen, trucks and offices, it would seem certain that Orkin is better known than any other competitor in its home marketing area. And in an industry where the quality of services is difficult to evaluate, such recognition is clearly a strong asset."

The report's third and fourth summary points reflected what McKinsey called Orkin's "few important but correctable weaknesses." The company's top management, according to the report, "is not exercising sufficient leadership over field operations. . . . While this system of management has certain advantages, its disadvantages are more pronounced: Atlanta does not have sufficient first-hand information about the districts to offer detailed guidance or to evaluate district performance; company policies are frequently not carried out at the branch level and in many areas, districts have established their own operating policies and procedures, which vary substantially in quality, as do the districts' operating ratios; prices set by Orkin's salesmen are not adequately controlled, and branch and district managers are not aware of the major impact of small price differences on profits." In addition, the report pointed out that the company's personnel development was so poor that "in the first six months of 1964, over a third of Orkin's salesmen and pest control servicemen either resigned or were discharged. Obviously, the turnover rate is too high." Another management shortfall involved the company's marketing plan—or, rather, the lack of one. "Orkin's marketing planning consists almost entirely of arbitrary sales goals set by district managers. No factual information is being developed on which to choose among alternatives for new branches or districts or to evaluate performance. Formal goals are not being set for factors—other than sales—that affect Orkin's position. No action programs are being developed to achieve district sales goals."

But it was probably the report's fourth summary point that caught Rollins's attention. "Orkin's percentage rate of growth has slowed; its dollar growth has not. In all but three of the last eleven years, the Company has increased its sales by $2 million to $4 million. But while sales have been increasing, the company's percentage sales gains have been generally declining. Still, the 1963 sales dollar gain was $2.82 million, slightly above the average 1952–1963 sales dollar gain of $2.59 million. Orkin's growth throughout this period has probably been somewhat retarded by certain top-management policies. However, there is no indication to date, either in the absolute sales gains or in Orkin's prospects, that the Company's growth will stop."

The fact that Orkin was inconsistently managed and financially underachieving was not a deterrent to Wayne Rollins. He loved a business challenge, and he often looked to purchase properties that he could improve. Since 1948 Rollins Broadcasting had specialized in buying radio or television stations that were either losing money or not meeting market expectations. With each one, Wayne pledged to make the stations profitable in a year or less, depending on their financial status when he bought them. His ability to buy stations with excellent potential for growth and profits reflected a decision at Rollins Broadcasting to devote 40 percent of its time to operations and 60 percent of its time to market research activities. With this strategy, Wayne developed a talent not only for finding good markets but avoiding the bad ones. From 1950 to 1963 Rollins Broadcasting purchased ten radio stations and three television stations throughout the country, becoming the only broadcaster other than CBS and ABC networks to have radio outlets in the nation's three largest markets—New York, Los Angeles, and Chicago.

"Rollins's superior record is attributable to management's ability to acquire broadcasting properties serving growing areas of the country but not being operated at their full potential," Weymouth's Laird & Company once wrote in an analysis of the Rollins company. "These properties have been bought at prices that have not reflected their latent value, and the potential has subsequently been realized by an infusion of Rollins's managerial and marketing ability, and occasionally, the capital required to upgrade physical plants. When a station is acquired by Rollins, programming is altered to conform to what the company's study of the market indicates will draw the largest possible audience. This new programming can be expected to draw a larger audience, which in turn permits higher rates (and revenue for Rollins).

The fact that Orkin was inconsistently managed and financially underachieving presented an interesting business challenge to Wayne.

"In other words, Rollins's initial success with its broadcasting properties has been the result of purchasing undervalued properties that have been upgraded by the application of more aggressive management and market research capabilities."

As Rollins reviewed the Orkin situation, the question on everyone's mind was not whether Wayne Rollins understood the minute details of the exterminating business or whether he knew the difference between drywood and subterranean termites. The question, rather, was whether this businessman could transfer the business principles he had perfected in the media business and impose them on a service company. In short, could Wayne Rollins once more purchase an undervalued business property and upgrade it through the application of more aggressive management and market research capabilities?

Armed with his professional experience and the new McKinsey report, Wayne was determined to answer that question. He began to spend even more time at Orkin, talking not only with Orkin family members but often meeting at length with Orkin managers and employees like Earl Geiger. He realized quickly that while the district and branch managers really knew their jobs, they worked essentially like independent contractors—a situation Wayne knew would have to change. As the McKinsey document clearly stated, the Orkin style of long-distance management was an impediment to the company's growth and profitability. The district managers needed specific annual goals and uniform operating procedures related to "pricing, development of sales leads, use of servicemen in selling activities, securing of termite renewal income, use of special sales incentives, method of compensating salesmen, determination of minimum equipment and internal office administration. In some instances, district procedures or policies differ only in emphasis. But in many cases, procedures differ clearly in both kind and quality. The impact of these policy and procedural differences is undoubtedly reflected in the range of district performance. In some instances, the best district performs twice as well as the worst."

As Wayne saw the company's management shortcomings firsthand, he also realized that the organization was essentially strong and that it could survive until changes could be made. He began to dig deeper. What was wrong with the company? Wayne began to wonder, and he surprised Earl with a series of questions. "What's wrong with the deal, Earl? What could go wrong with Orkin?"

First, they debated the changes that loomed in the pest control industry—including additional restrictions and attempts to ban the most effective

Otto Orkin: *His Final Years*

Otto Orkin was eighty-two years old when he died Sunday evening, February 11, 1968. The entrepreneur who started the world's leading pest control company—whose name was synonymous with quality and dependable services—died quietly in an Atlanta hospital, a mere shadow of the man who transformed selling rat poison into a multimillion-dollar business.

In the end, his life was a dim reflection of his life's work.

For one thing, it seemed that Otto was never really happy after he sold his interest in Orkin to his family for $5.35 million in 1960. His third marriage to a former Orkin secretary was short-lived. By 1962 he had married for a fourth time and was living in a modest, brick ranch house near Smyrna when he decided to protest the conditions of a trust that controlled his money. According to newspaper reports, Otto filed suit in Fulton Superior Court to have the trust set aside, and filed further amendments to the suit in 1964. Both times, courts upheld the trust, which was now estimated to be worth around $2 million. A Cobb County court declared Otto Orkin incompetent in 1964.

Two years later, lawyers for Otto were back in court, arguing that disagreements between Otto's two guardians had so dramatically reduced his monthly income that he and his wife, Ann, had been forced to apply for welfare. When word got out that the original "Otto the Orkin Man" was on public assistance, sympathetic letters and cash contributions were mailed to the *Atlanta Constitution* from readers across the country. In court, Otto was described as being totally dependent on others to approve his expenses and pay his bills. Without adequate income, Otto's wife Ann testified that Otto could no longer eat in restaurants, visit his club in Atlanta, or enjoy long car rides with his chauffeur. He apparently spent most of his time watching television or taking an occasional walk in his backyard. His telephone service had been disconnected, and his wife argued that she couldn't afford to take him to the dentist. In February 1967 a ruling by Georgia Supreme Court Judge Ralph Pharr demanded that the elderly Otto receive $4,000 a month from the trust. The order noted that Otto had been limited to an annual income of $21,750, an amount the judge clearly found

pesticides. After all, the year was 1964, only two years after the publication of Rachel Carson's *Silent Spring,* a book that alerted the public to the abuse and dangers of chemical pesticides like DDT and other long-lasting chlorinated hydrocarbon insecticides. In words that reverberated around the world and sparked the nation's first widespread environmental movement, Carson cautioned that while shorter-lived pesticides could be used responsibly, it was important to determine their effect on both

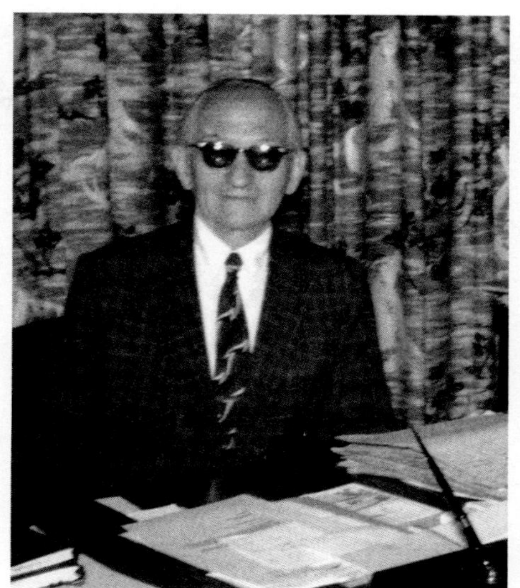

In a soap opera–like saga that was played out weekly in the press, Otto's two sons and his son-in-law Perry Kaye had Otto (right) hospitalized and declared incompetent on May 16, 1960. Orkin had earlier transferred 51 percent controlling stock in the corporation to his two sons and his daughter Bernice Kaye, Perry's wife.

disgraceful. Judge Pharr noted that while Otto had been determined incompetent by the court, "He still has the capacity and desire to enjoy some of the pleasures and comforts of life to which a man who, by his own efforts, has acquired substantial wealth is justly entitled."

Almost exactly one year later, Otto died. In his final days he had many hospital visitors, including his estranged oldest son, Sanford. "I was at peace by going there," Sanford remembered, years later, "though he was only partially aware of what was going on around him."

In honor of Otto, Rollins ran an advertisement in the Atlanta newspapers that acknowledged his contribution to the company: "On the Passing of Mr. Otto Orkin, Founder of Orkin Exterminating Co., Inc., the Management and Employees of Rollins Inc., Acknowledge His Contributions to the Community, the Industry and Our Company."

When Otto Orkin died, barely eight years after his departure from a $64 million business he created from scratch, not one obituary listed his accomplishments to the industry, or his many contributions to the Atlanta community. Instead, the melodrama of his last years overshadowed his life's work and his amazing success story, and the legend of Otto Orkin seemed in danger of being forgotten.

In the years to come, however, Gary Rollins, who never met Otto Orkin, would help reestablish both the man's dignity and his place in business history. As lasting tributes to Otto, Gary Rollins helped develop the O. Orkin Insect Zoo, located inside the Smithsonian Institution's National Museum of Natural History, and the Smithsonian/O. Orkin Insect Safari, an educational insect zoo that toured around the country from 2001 to 2002 celebrating the company's one hundredth anniversary. And as president of Orkin, Gary Rollins campaigned successfully for Otto Orkin's induction into the Pest Control Hall of Fame.

To former Orkin employees like Anita E. Ritchie, Otto Orkin deserved nothing less. As Ritchie once said: "There are people who possess tenacity, who are undaunted by obstacles, and Mr. Orkin was certainly one of them. He had a singleness of purpose, a goal he never lost sight of, and he worked tirelessly and diligently to achieve that goal. His was the epitome of the American Dream we hear so much about. His contribution to the industry is inestimable."

humans and the environment before they were used. The impact of Carson's book on the industry was immediate: by the end of 1962, over forty legislative bills had been introduced in various states in an effort to regulate the use of pesticides. Could this issue damage Orkin and its prospects for the future? Wayne wanted to know.

Earl was not overly concerned. "It doesn't make any difference whether DDT or chlordane is banned," he said. "Banning them won't make people invite rats, mice, and roaches in as household guests. You'd just have to do whatever was necessary to get rid of them, and people will pay for it."

When Rollins bought Orkin, the market for pest and termite control was unsaturated, with plenty of room to grow, both by adding new customers and by offering more services to existing customers.

The management consultants at McKinsey agreed. "As a result of public concern raised by the publication of *Silent Spring* and the more recent poisoning of fish in the Mississippi River, legislation on the use of chemical agents is increasing. But most of the recent legislation has been at the state level and aimed at chemical manufacturers and outdoor pest control operators (e.g., crop dusters). Most structural pest control authorities (like Orkin) believe that the public's concern will lead to *increased* interest in the use of professional structural pest control companies and that any restrictive legislation will only drive out the marginal structural pest control business. This judgment makes sense to us. Restrictive legislation would probably favor the larger, established companies that could afford to take the steps to comply with the law. The major risk Orkin runs from legislation is that some of the effective chemicals the Company now uses might be taken off the market. To the extent replacement chemicals were not available, the Company's service would become less effective and therefore require more frequent and more expensive service."

Translated? As the largest pest control company around, Orkin could actually benefit from the public's scrutiny of pest control operators and market its expertise to its advantage; people would pay for the best. And Orkin would have the financial resources to invest in more expensive chemicals, if traditional products were banned or taken off the market.

Second, what about competition? Sears had recently entered the pest control business, one of the reasons the Orkin family wanted to sell their company. But together, Wayne and Earl concluded that Sears could not successfully operate a service business along with its retail business—there was just too much difference in the two types of businesses. And Orkin, it turned out, was larger than its next ten competitors combined. Its closest nonfranchise competitor was Arwell, Inc., a Waukegan, Illinois, firm with sales of about $5 million, compared to Orkin's sales of $37 million. As the McKinsey

Report had noted, "The average pest control company has sales of $50,000 to $75,000, and only a handful of companies have a million dollars in sales. Thus Orkin, with sales of almost $40 million, is truly a giant in its industry, and is able to: support a local sales effort with a company advertising budget of $1.5 million; afford supervisory and technical personnel to maintain the quality of its services; utilize its favorable image and pay well enough to attract and recruit high-potential personnel; and add personnel, offices and equipment and sustain these investment expenditures until they can fully pay their way."

The McKinsey study acknowledged that one of the "persistent questions throughout this study has been: What would happen to Orkin if another giant with established householder contact entered the industry? . . . It seems to us that Orkin is not seriously vulnerable to large, new competitors because of its relatively small market share in any given area, its pest control work, the quality of its services, and the customer franchise it has built up in its marketing area."

And third, though everyone agreed that Orkin was poised for growth, how much? Even Wayne was surprised by the answer presented both by the McKinsey Report and his own research into the Orkin records. When he analyzed its customer base, Wayne realized that 53 percent of all the accounts were concentrated in only five states. If Orkin conducted as much business in other states as it was already doing in Georgia and Florida, "then we would double our business," Wayne told Earl. His enthusiasm was contagious.

"Orkin is really in its 'embryonic stage,'" said Earl. "The market for pest and termite control is unsaturated, with plenty of room to grow, both by adding new customers and by offering more services to existing customers. We can build this company into a hundred-million-dollar business within the next ten years. There's no reason we couldn't make it a billion-dollar company!"

"Let's make it a hundred million first," Wayne cautioned. But he was sure of two things. One, he was ready to sign a "letter of intent" to buy Orkin, an action he completed and announced in a June 19, 1964, press release that was distributed by the Orkin family to the staff. And two, he had concluded that he needed Earl Geiger to stay and run the company. In an unusual move, Wayne Rollins made Geiger's continued employment a condition of the sale of Orkin by requiring Geiger to be a signatory, thereby guaranteeing that Geiger would remain with Orkin after it was acquired by Rollins.

By all accounts, Geiger was delighted. He joined an inner circle of Rollins executives that reflected one of Wayne Rollins's leading business maxims: surround yourself with good people. "If you're going to build a business as well as you'd like, you ought to surround yourself with people who, on particular things, are smarter than you are," said Wayne. "And I don't hesitate. That doesn't bother me a bit." Those good people included not only Geiger and Wayne's brother John Rollins but also a circle of Rollins Broadcasting executives that included Russ Chambers, Henry Tippie, Tim Crow and Jim Roddey, Albert R. Lanphear, George BarenBregge, John R. Wilson, and Wayne's older son, Richard Randall Rollins. And over time, Wayne's trusted associates would include his younger son—Gary Wayne Rollins.

O. Wayne Rollins: "If you're going to build a business as well as you'd like, you ought to surround yourself with people who, on particular things, are smarter than you are."

As Wayne studied the Orkin deal, Randall's role in Rollins Broadcasting was expanding through the recent acquisition of two new outdoor advertising concerns. Under Randall's supervision, the purchase of a General Outdoor Advertising subsidiary in Mexico and the purchase of General Outdoor's business in Philadelphia and Washington, D.C., made Rollins Outdoor one of the largest outdoor advertising companies in the United States. And though Gary was not yet officially involved in the family businesses, the young college student was getting an introductory business education nonetheless. In the second semester of his sophomore year, Gary left college in Tennessee, and Wayne made sure his younger son went to work. He quickly dispatched Gary to Fort Pierce, Florida, where the family had extensive property holdings, including an orange grove in Okeechobee County. Here, Gary was assigned to learn about citrus production; Gary even enrolled at nearby St. Lucie Junior College for a course in citrus management. "Dad was determined that this wasn't going to be a vacation," his younger son remembered.

But Gary's destiny was not orange trees or citrus groves, or radio or television broadcasting. His father's actions during the summer of 1964 would lay the foundation for a career that Gary had probably never imagined. Gary, as it turned out, was destined to be an Orkin Man.

✦ ✦ ✦

On Memorial Day, Wayne had made his first trip to Atlanta to see what he thought of Orkin. On Labor Day, he purchased it. During the three long summer months in between, the challenge of financing the $62.4 million purchase occupied nearly everyone involved with what would become known as the nation's first leveraged buyout. There were many times, Henry B. Tippie later recalled, when he thought "the deal could have fallen apart. I think that Wayne's sense of humor, or on occasion a story of his, assisted in getting things back on track and allowed it to eventually move on down the pike to conclusion."

Whatever tensions surrounded the Orkin deal, they did not reflect the transaction's historical significance. Why? Because no one knew or thought about the fact that they were making history.

"We were very calm about it," recalled Henry Tippie, Rollins's top financial executive and a member of the Rollins board of directors since 1960. "Our deal consisted of a thirteen-column, green accounting pad, which I fixed up in pencil, and each column was year 1, year 2. We went out 15 or 20 years on it, and looked at different levels of growth, like no growth, 5 percent, and then 10 percent. We looked at the interest expense and principal payments to see whether all of this would work. That's how we always approached everything.

"We never thought about it being a leveraged buyout. From our standpoint, it wasn't anything new because we bought everything with very little or no money. Radio, television stations—you have to understand that everything that we had bought basically up to that point was either a bankruptcy or a money-losing situation. We operated on the basis of starting with almost nothing, and building from there. Anytime you make an acquisition, the real work starts the day after the acquisition."

Perry Kaye, left, and Sanford Orkin, center, listen to advice from George Weymouth at the closing of the deal to sell Orkin to Rollins Broadcasting, Inc.

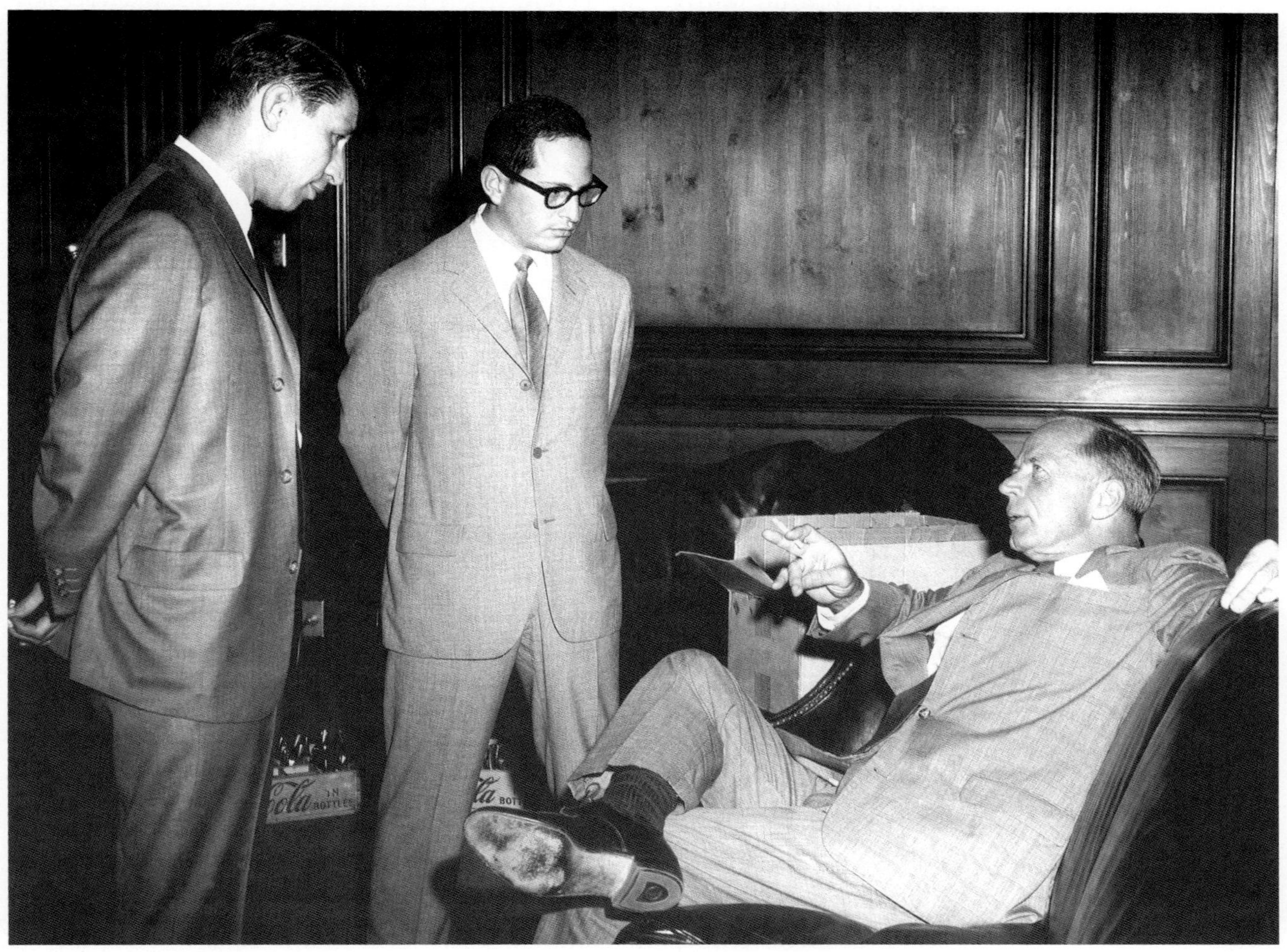

Randall agreed. "Dad didn't know that buying Orkin was the first leveraged buyout," he said. "He was just making a deal."

And the deal was so unusual for its day that there was no initial special business coverage of the event or any announcement that a leveraged buyout, or LBO as it became known, was in the works. In 1967 John W. Aber Jr., a student at the Harvard Business School, completed a case study of the Rollins-Orkin deal under the direction of Professor Charles M. Williams "for a class discussion rather than to illustrate either effective or ineffective handling of an administrative situation." But the concept of LBOs was not widely understood until the 1980s, when the transaction became rather widespread.

"It's not as complicated as most people think," said Dr. Jim Rosenfeld, associate professor with the Goizueta Business School at Emory University in Atlanta. "The [buyers] are putting up next to nothing and they are heavily leveraged. After the transaction, most companies try to pay down their debt by selling off assets that don't fit into the core of the business. It's the old classic business transaction—you are borrowing other people's money. And when you carry that much debt, one bad year could wipe you out, and that's the danger you run into. In the 1980s, when LBOs really took off, one of every five went bankrupt."

Though Dr. Rosenfeld hadn't specifically studied the Rollins-Orkin LBO, he did point out one interesting fact that made the deal unique even in leveraged buyout circles. In most documented LBOs, the companies borrow against their assets. But Wayne Rollins only borrowed $10 million against the assets of his media company; the Prudential deal was based on Orkin's earning stream. With this move, Wayne demonstrated confidence in his predictions that Orkin would not only grow but also grow dramatically; plus, he did not want to encumber the broadcasting company. When his assumptions proved correct, Rollins would use the additional assets to pay off the LBO debt at an accelerated pace, which made the deal more profitable for nearly everyone involved.

Without ever mentioning the words "leveraged buyout," the various parties worked throughout the summer of '64 to bring the deal to the proverbial table. One of the main issues involved Prudential Insurance Company, and how it was going to be compensated for assuming so much of the deal's financial risk. Executives at Prudential, who had first been lured to the deal by Weymouth when the DuPont family was interested, concluded early on that if they agreed to provide the $40 million loan, their company should receive some incentive beyond the interest return; the elements of risk inherent in this type of investment, the experts agreed, should be compensated. Prudential argued successfully that the compensation could be provided by making $2.5 million of the senior debt convertible into common stock of the new company.

During the negotiations, Wayne's ability to stay focused on an issue—and to see the larger picture unfolding around it—amazed his peers. As Lewis Cullman once said, "I've met every illustrious man in the United States, and Mr. Rollins was the only man I've ever met who had a zoom lens mind.'"

Earl Geiger agreed. "He did have that ability. He could focus on the broadest concept or the smallest detail with equal clarity. 'A zoom lens mind.' That was the best description I've ever heard of his mental prowess."

By the end of August, the contracts for the sale were being drawn up in various offices throughout Atlanta. Wayne and Henry Tippie represented Rollins. At other times, John Rollins, Earl Geiger, and George Weymouth joined them, as well as representatives from George's firm. Wayne had only one attorney—Jack Killoran of Wilmington.

The Prudential Insurance Company had many attorneys present, as did Chase Manhattan Bank and Equitable Life, the institutions that would also help finance the acquisition. The Orkins—Sanford and Billy Orkin and Perry Kaye—relied on counsel from two law firms. Or as Henry Tippie put it, "They had platoons of attorneys." Their lead attorney was Allen Post, a former Rhodes scholar whose antics alternately amazed and annoyed Wayne and the other Rollins representatives. In scenes Wayne thought worthy of Shakespearean drama, Post would get up on his desk, he would cry, he would get down on his knees, and even lie on the floor to drive home a point for his clients.

On the final day before the September 1 closing, the negotiations became increasingly difficult. According to Post, there were at least eight items in the contract that "would ruin" the Orkins. Three came up more often than the others: how the accounts receivable would be handled, what liabilities the sellers would assume, and Rollins's insistence on reserving the right to offset the deferred portion of the purchase price against any undisclosed expenses that emerged after the closing—a provision that stirred Allen Post into melodramatic anguish. "Oh, my Lord! We can never do that!" he almost sobbed, holding his head between his knees. "We can't do that! It'd ruin us! It'd absolutely ruin us!"

Henry Tippie: "We never thought about it being a leveraged buyout. From our standpoint, it wasn't anything new because we bought everything with very little or no money."

Wayne refused to budge. For one thing, the provisions of the contract were standard. He knew it was imperative that the offset in expenses be agreed upon; otherwise, Rollins could be left holding the bag with undisclosed expenses. As the clock ticked toward ten o'clock that night, exactly twelve hours before the scheduled signing of the contract, Allen Post issued a final warning. "If you insist on these provisions," he said, "we can never agree."

And the meeting adjourned.

"I wouldn't give a nickel," Wayne said to himself on the way back to the hotel, "for our chance of closing tomorrow morning."

At breakfast the next morning, John Rollins and Jack Killoran wanted to know if Wayne had changed his mind on any issues. "I favor just staying where we are," Wayne declared firmly. "I think we've been over this. These are basic things, and I think we've got to insist on them."

The Rollins group soon left for the closing, scheduled at the First National Bank for ten o'clock Tuesday morning, September 1, 1964. Wayne was braced for another harangue from Allen Post, and prepared for the closing to be postponed. But O. Wayne Rollins was *not* prepared for what actually happened as the parties gathered around a large conference table. Without a word of objection from Allen Post or the Orkin family members, the formal signing of the documents began. Rollins Broadcasting was about to acquire Orkin for $62.4 million.

Harvard Case Study: *The First Leveraged Buyout*

In 1967 Harvard University business professor Charles M. Williams asked a young doctoral student named John W. Aber Jr. to be his research associate. The two-year appointment meant that Aber would develop case studies for Williams to use as teaching tools for a course called "Management of Financial Institutions."

For his first case study, Williams asked Aber to review a business transaction that had fascinated the Harvard professor for several years—the 1964 purchase of Orkin by Rollins.

To this day, Williams, who taught hundreds if not thousands of case studies at Harvard and is now retired and a Harvard professor emeritus, remembers the Rollins-Orkin case study as "one of the more interesting ones to teach." And Aber, now professor of finance at Boston University School of Management, still recalls that "a note of mystery was sounded when the deal was announced. It wasn't clear to anyone why Rollins would have anything to do with Orkin. It was a very famous transaction at the time."

For the case study, Aber focused primarily on the role of Prudential Insurance, which approved a loan of $40 million to finance the $62.4 million transaction. He met as many as four times with Prudential representatives from the company's Bond Department in order to discuss the case and develop the study. "They were on the forefront of leveraged buyouts," Aber recalled. "They were very innovative at the time. It was certainly something of a maverick deal when it was announced."

Williams, however, recalled that he "was not thinking in terms of a leveraged buyout" when he asked Aber to develop a case study. "We were thinking of looking at why someone would pay a sizable price for what some would call a flimsy company," he said. "There was no security, really, with a pest control operation. You can't make people continue to buy your services. And it was a service company and a company that had virtually no assets. Given the extent of the debt incurred to make the purchase, we talked a great deal about the absence of solid assets and the reliance on cash flow. However, there was a

By all accounts, it was an amazing deal for Wayne Rollins and one of the biggest coups ever seen by Wall Street. Rollins Broadcasting's revenues for its fiscal year ending April 30, 1964, were $9.1 million with net income of $894,000, compared to Orkin's revenues of $37.3 million for its fiscal year ended October 31, 1963, and net profits of $3 million.

As finally agreed upon, the $62.4 million buyout was financed from the following sources: $40 million senior debt from Prudential (over twenty years at 5.75 percent interest); of which $2.5 million was convertible by Prudential into 19 percent of Kinro Corporation equity; $10 million capital contribution from Rollins, which was borrowed; $10 million subordinated note payable to the Orkin sellers (over fifteen years at 4.5 percent); and $2.4 million paid to the sellers upon closing from Orkin's cash position.

Under this arrangement, Rollins borrowed a total of $60 million (with $10 million from the sellers) and used the excess cash of Orkin to pay the

lot of cash flow that could service the debt. I remember that there was a good bit of discussion, however, about how vulnerable the company would be to economic downturns. I don't remember, though, where we came out on that issue. But I think there was a feeling that the company was not as vulnerable as we at first believed."

During his two years as a research associate, Aber wrote many case studies, working alongside other research associates from desks tucked into a garretlike space on the third floor of Harvard's Sherman Hall. Aber organized his first case study into two parts: first, he described Prudential's role in putting together the financial package that was approved by the company Bond Department in late May 1964; second, he described how Rollins executed the deal and used the loan to buy Orkin. The case study includes extensive charts and graphs to document the transaction, as well as proposed loan terms and debt payment schedules. Throughout the thirty-one-page document, Rollins Broadcasting is referred to as the "Payne" Broadcasting Group, and Orkin is referenced as the "Pestmort" Company. The names of important individuals are changed, too. Wayne Rollins is known as "Harold Payne"; Otto Orkin becomes "Max Burgher."

"I'm not sure that the interested parties insisted on a disguise, but I preferred it. That was our requirement," said Williams, who claims that he invented the name 'Pestmort.' He laughed. "I was rather pleased with myself for coming up with that. It's better than 'Orkin.'"

But Aber recalls that in the real world of pest control, the Orkin name definitely worked. "Orkin had quite a brand franchise," he said, "When we studied it, it was just one of those instances where someone like Rollins comes out of the blue and takes over what was then a really successful business."

The case study was apparently a success, too. Aber noted that Williams "probably taught it thirty or forty times. He used the case extensively in his courses—not only at Harvard but in a great deal of executive teaching in banks throughout the country and the world."

remaining $2.4 million of the purchase price. To finance its own capital contribution of $10 million, Rollins borrowed $15.5 million from two financial institutions: $4 million at 5.25 percent from Chase Manhattan, and $11.5 million at 5.75 percent from Equitable Life Assurance Society of New York. After contributing $10 million to buy Orkin, the remaining $5.5 million was used to pay off Rollins's existing indebtedness.

Rollins began the complex transaction by acquiring Kinro Corporation for 55,000 shares of Rollins common stock. Then, Kinro, the original company created solely as a vehicle for the transaction, actually borrowed the $40 million from Prudential, with $2.5 million convertible by the insurance company into 19 percent of Kinro equity. As its equity kicker, Prudential also was granted a warrant to purchase 115,000 shares of Rollins stock at $22 per share, the price at which it was selling on June 11 before the sale was made public. However, when a press release about the agreement for Rollins to purchase Orkin was issued on June 19, the stock price started rising and was up to $40 in July. By the time the deal was closed on September 1, Rollins stock was selling at $61.25.

The $62.4 million transaction was a done deal. Rollins owned Orkin.

In his annual report to Rollins shareholders published on June 16, 1964, O. Wayne Rollins explained the complicated transaction in very simple terms:

> In June 1964, after the close of the fiscal year, the Company negotiated with Kinro Corp. to exchange 55,000 shares of Rollins' stock for the entire stock of Kinro. Kinro has an agreement to purchase all the assets and business of Orkin Exterminating Co., Inc. for $62.4 million. . . . Rollins has made arrangements with financial institutions, on a long-term basis, to permit the Company to make a $10 million equity investment in Kinro Corp. Kinro has arranged to borrow $40 million at 5 3/4 %, on a 20-year basis, from an insurance company, with $2 1/2 million convertible by the insurance company into 19% of Kinro Corp. equity. The insurance company will receive an option on 115,000 shares of Rollins' stock at $22 per share, which was above the market at the time of the negotiations. The sellers are receiving $10 million of 4 1/2 % long-term notes from Kinro, and the balance of payment will be from certain available cash to be received at the closing and returned to the sellers.

For its investment, Rollins acquired 100 percent ownership of Kinro, which in turn held 100 percent of Orkin's stock. The deal allowed Rollins to acquire Orkin with an outlay of only $10 million—and even that $10 million was borrowed based on Rollins's assets.

Kinro, now a wholly owned subsidiary of Rollins, was liable for the remaining debt of $50 million. Under this structure, the debt was not carried on the Rollins books, thus freeing the company's assets for more acquisitions. What's more, Rollins did not guarantee the underlying loan and felt there was no great risk. Even if something bad had happened, Rollins had enough earning power to service its own debts.

Under the agreement, the Orkin family would be paid 45 percent of Kinro-Orkin's net income after taxes and depreciation annually until the $10 million debt was retired, but no payments would be due until 1968, when a lump sum would be paid for the preceding four years. The bottom line? This arrangement allowed Rollins to retain the use of $10 million of relatively cheap money.

For Prudential, it was a windfall profit. Ray Charles, who handled the financing package for the company, called it the best deal Prudential had ever made. Ultimately, the company would reap not only the interest paid on the loan but a profit of $22.5 million when Rollins bought back all of Prudential's $2.5 million conversion feature before the insurance company converted it. Indeed, the "equity kicker" had paid off handsomely for the company when Rollins paid Prudential a premium for their warrants.

In the end, Rollins didn't even pay cash to their investment brokers. Rather, the company made a $10 million equity investment in the Kinro Corporation. And in all, 55,000 shares of Rollins stock were distributed to the organizers of Kinro: George Weymouth and Lewis Cullman's group.

At the closing table, Wayne signed one check for $52.4 million—the largest check he had ever signed in his life. The remaining $10 million needed to close the transaction came from the subordinated note payable to the sellers. The $62.4 million transaction was a done deal.

Rollins owned Orkin.

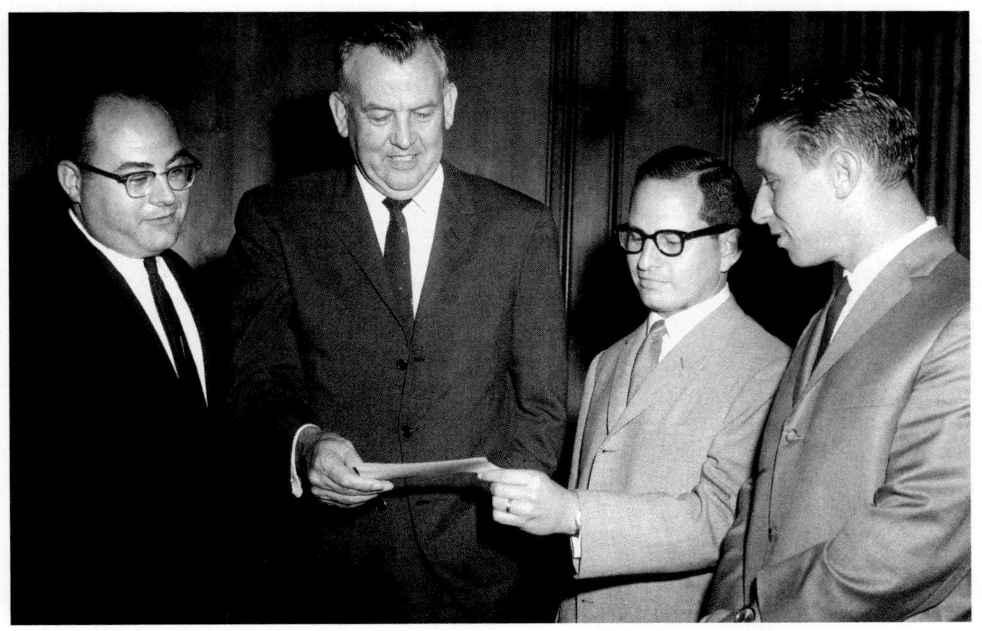

William Orkin, left, and Perry Kaye, right, look on as O. Wayne Rollins, second from left, hands Sanford Orkin, second from right, the check for the purchase of Orkin Exterminating Company.

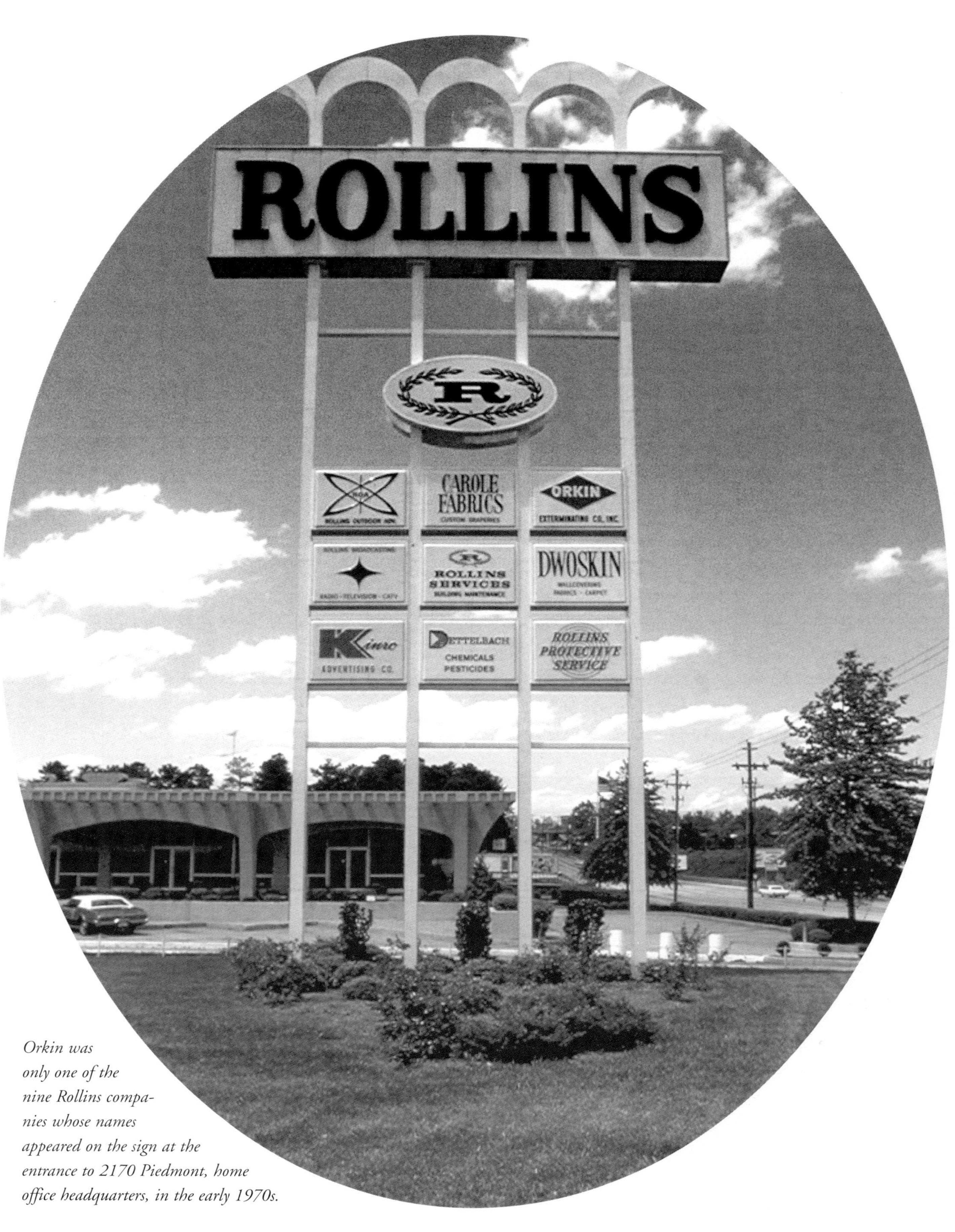

Orkin was only one of the nine Rollins companies whose names appeared on the sign at the entrance to 2170 Piedmont, home office headquarters, in the early 1970s.

Chapter 5

1964–1989: The Rollins Years

Under the leadership of O. Wayne Rollins, Orkin became the crown jewel of Rollins, Inc., now one of the largest service companies in the world. Rollins swiftly "Rollinized" Orkin — through professional management principles, acquisitions, innovative new products and services, and groundbreaking advertising techniques. Revenues and stock prices soared as Orkin expanded to be the company that Otto Orkin had only dreamed was possible. Gary Rollins, Wayne's son, charted his career path through the organization, starting out as an Orkin Man and ultimately rising to the executive office. Along the way, Gary guided the company through a tumultuous series of company reorganizations and industry challenges, emerging as a nationally recognized leader in the pest control industry. And gradually, Orkin emerged as the core business of Rollins, Inc., and the world's best pest control company, anchoring one of the nation's largest consumer service companies and servicing 1.4 million residential and commercial customers.

Though Orville Wayne Rollins often referred to himself as "a Georgia farm boy," he was relatively unknown in the Atlanta business community when news leaked out that Orkin had a new owner. Wilton Looney, then chief executive officer of Genuine Parts Company in Atlanta, had never even heard of Wayne Rollins. "The first time I ever heard of Wayne Rollins was when they came and bought Orkin. And I remember what they paid for it. And what they owed on it," said Looney, who became friends with Wayne Rollins and was elected to the Rollins, Inc., board of directors in 1975. "I remember it shocked me, because I was a small country boy businessman who didn't believe in owing money. I said to myself, 'This is really something.'"

Even those who knew the fifty-two-year-old Wayne Rollins must have found the deal astonishing, particularly his neighbors and cousins who lived just a few hours away from Atlanta in the rural community of Smith Chapel in the northwest Georgia mountains. But looking back, perhaps remembering the young boy who was determined to be successful at whatever he did, it probably wasn't too difficult to comprehend that Wayne Rollins would be a part of business history.

Wayne was born in 1912, the oldest of two sons of Claudia and Henry Rollins, a schoolteacher and a farmer who lived in the rural community of Smith Chapel, just outside the town of Ringgold in Catoosa County. They were loving but demanding parents, who insisted that Wayne and his younger brother John help out on the family farm as soon as they were old enough to handle chores. Sleeping after 4 A.M. was considered "sleeping in." From his parents, Wayne often said that he learned the values of perseverance, frugality, religion, and family, but he credited his grandmother with teaching him the foundations of good management and business organization. "That lady was the best manager I ever saw," he often began, telling one of his favorite stories. "She lived on a farm and the house was way up on a hill. She would keep lines of pails outside the house, and every time any one of us went to the bottom of the hill, we would take down two empty pails and bring back two full ones when we returned later. This way, she never did have to send anyone down to the spring for water."

After a hailstorm destroyed his family's crops and any chance O. Wayne Rollins had of going to college and pursuing his dream of being a lawyer, he got a job at a textile mill working ten hours a day, six days a week, for ten dollars a week.

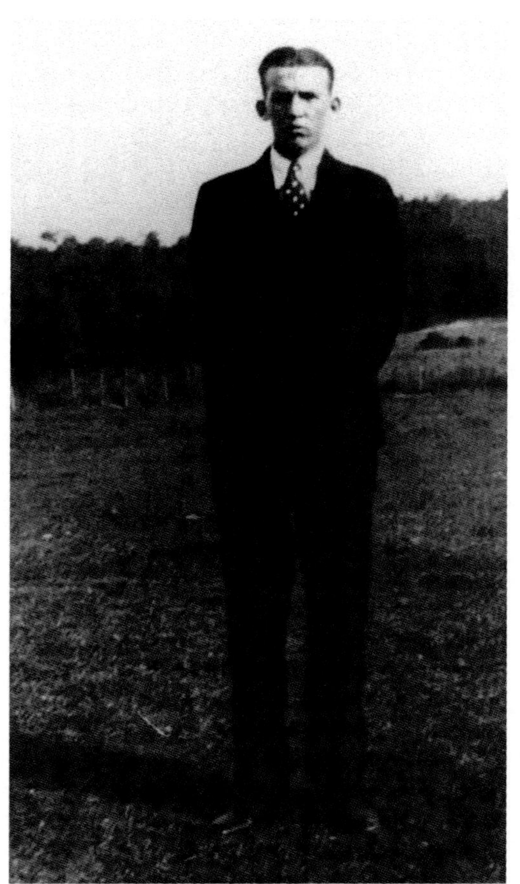

From the first time he set out for the one-room school near his home, Wayne Rollins was a driven young man. "I spent my life competing against the average in whatever it was, not being satisfied, constantly wanting to be better than the average," he often said. Perhaps it was the poverty around him that inspired Wayne Rollins to want something better than average. Or the stories from the Horatio Alger books that Claudia Rollins read out loud to her sons while sitting by the fireplace. Or a mother's unwavering faith in her two sons' abilities, and her oft-repeated message that they could achieve anything they set out to do. "I thank God my boys are leaders," Claudia Rollins once said, "and not followers." In 1930, when the gangly, six-foot-two Wayne Rollins graduated as valedictorian from the high school in Ringgold, his graduation speech reflected his ambitions and clear determination. "If we are willing to put forth the effort to do the things that are right, we will succeed," he said. "Our success will be according to how much effort we are willing to put into it."

When a hailstorm destroyed both the family's crops and any chance Wayne had to go to college to pursue his dream of being a lawyer, the nineteen-year-old left Ringgold to accept his first job at Standard-Coosa-Thatcher, a textile mill in Chattanooga, Tennessee. In the beginning, he worked six days a week, ten hours a day, for ten dollars a week. He learned early that the greatest job insurance he could find was to make his boss's job easier, and he would often handle up to four different jobs at once to show how invaluable he was. When others were being laid off, Wayne was promoted to supervisor of the plant's dye and fabric division. After ten years, he joined the Hercules Powder Company in Chattanooga as a TNT supervisor. But in 1945 he returned to Ringgold with his wife, Grace, and his two sons: Randall, a teenager, and Gary, just a toddler. Here, Wayne, Grace, and John Rollins bought an old mineral springs resort called Catoosa Springs in Catoosa County. With $10,900, the trio purchased 280 acres, seventeen houses, and twenty-two cottages that made up the heart of the resort, and the mineral springs that were still vital. As he phased out of his work at Hercules, Wayne devoted more time to rebuilding the resort, renting the properties, and selling the mineral spring water door to door. But the physical demands of loading and delivering the five-gallon mineral water bottles took its toll on Wayne; in the summer of 1947, he was diagnosed with two ruptured discs in his back. While forced to rest on a three-quarter-inch plywood panel positioned on his bed, Wayne developed a new strategy for his future that involved his brother John and radio. In 1948 they applied for a license to open a radio station WRAD in Radford, Virginia, ostensibly to give John an economical way to advertise his automobile dealership in the area. Why should they pay so much for advertising, the brothers reasoned, when they could own the station and get it for free? And this was the beginning of Rollins Broadcasting, Inc., the company that only fourteen years later would purchase Orkin.

O. Wayne Rollins: "I spent my life competing against the average in whatever it was, not being satisfied, constantly wanting to be better than average."

"The only thing I knew about radio at the time was the name of the microphone, but I employed people who knew the business," Wayne liked to say. "I made a commitment to them: if you will teach me about radio, I will teach you how to work."

In many ways, the two brothers made perfect business partners. Wayne was the more reserved, studied brother who used his considerable business instincts and knowledge to meticulously analyze every deal before jumping in; John was gregarious, an idea-a-minute man who provided the bravura and the energy that made business deals seem worth the risk. "John really did want to buy everything, and he never did think about what it cost or anything like that," Wayne said of his younger brother, who by the early 1950s was already dabbling in politics and would later be elected lieutenant governor of Delaware. "I'd regularly ask him, 'Where are you going to get the money?' And he'd say that kind of thinking would just ruin his deal."

In the middle of the two brothers stood, literally, a man who brought harmony to both personalities and order to the sometimes chaotic Rollinses' financial records: Henry B. Tippie. An accountant from the Midwest, he offered a much-needed balance to the brothers. He passed Wayne's first business challenge when he made it from Des Moines to the brothers' new headquarters in Rehoboth Beach, Delaware, without asking for directions. And he agreed to a pay cut in order to work for Rollins, a second employment factor that Wayne imposed to judge how much someone wanted to work for him. From their first meeting, Henry Tippie admired the force of the brothers' ambition and the sheer will of their very different personalities. He sensed an opportunity for great potential with Rollins, and he signed on.

By the time Tippie joined the company in 1953, Rollins Broadcasting was poised for a growth spurt. When the first radio station proved to be successful, Wayne and John began looking for a larger consumer base. They found it in Fayetteville, North Carolina, where they bought a second station and began to develop a practice now known as "niche marketing"—programming tailored to specific community segments, in this case the military markets associated with Fayetteville's Fort Bragg. After achieving success in smaller markets, Wayne Rollins moved into more sophisticated and competitive New York markets, a move that prompted the always story-rich Rollins to tell one of his favorite tales. "When we first moved into the New York market, all the people who were supposed to know said we were making a mistake. They told us we should stay where we belonged, in the smaller markets. But I'm like the bumblebee. He isn't supposed to be able to fly, but doesn't know it and flies anyway."

True to its track record, Rollins Broadcasting quickly took the New York station, which had lost $1.5 million the previous year, and put it in the black in the first year. Rollins continued to acquire radio stations, and in 1956 Rollins Broadcasting entered the television field by buying the first of its three television stations. Eventually, the company would own ten radio stations (though they regularly sold off some stations to stay within FCC ownership guidelines), four television stations, and four cable television systems comprising of about thirty-five individual franchises, along with nine outdoor advertising plants. By 1964 the company that came calling to buy Orkin had revenues of just over $9 million and was listed on the American Stock Exchange; it held the fourth-largest U.S. outdoor advertising company through its Rollins Outdoor Advertising division; and it was the only broadcaster other than the CBS and ABC networks to have radio outlets in the nation's three largest markets.

"The Orkin deal put us in the big leagues," admitted Wayne, who had emerged as the leader behind the brothers' broadcasting and outdoor advertising ventures while John assumed the leadership role in what would become his own separate vehicle leasing, environmental waste disposal, and bulk-hauling trucking company under the banner of Rollins International, Inc. "But without outdoor advertising, and the radio and television stations, we wouldn't have had the management to handle such a project."

A CHANGE IN TEMPO

When Rollins Broadcasting bought Orkin, it seemed natural to attempt to identify the similarities between the two entrepreneurs who had founded these rather extraordinary family-owned businesses. After all, both Wayne Rollins and Otto Orkin grew up extremely poor on their respective family farms, without one legitimate business connection to their names. They both wanted better lives than their backgrounds would seem to predict, and they believed that hard work and determination would help them realize those dreams. Once established, they both demanded hard work from their employees, and they always put the needs of the customers first. They were both inspiring individuals, with the ability to motivate others. And oddly enough, they both shared a taste for fine clothing, which as much as anything else separated them from the sheer poverty of their humble beginnings.

Wayne Rollins never proposed a deal or an expansion that he didn't thoroughly understand himself, and his high school education belied an inquisitive mind that bordered on genius.

But here the similarities end. Though an important figure in the company and an industry innovator when it came to expansion and advertising, Otto's power was diminished as soon as he gave too much authority to the branch managers. And while he was hardworking, Otto was virtually uneducated. He was extremely bright and intuitive and was absolutely devoted to pleasing his customers. And while he had the business sense to hire people who knew more than he did, he found it difficult to converse with them and be a part of their world; at one point, his associates joked that he couldn't even pronounce "entomologist." Initially, he hired family members because they were family and not because they were necessarily capable of handling their responsibilites. His lack of insight into his own profession hurt his credibility with his employees, who in the end focused less on his contributions to the industry and more on his personality quirks, his zealous exercising and eating habits, and his absentmindedness. His family life, which included four marriages, could be described as nothing less than a soap opera.

Wayne Rollins, on the other hand, never proposed a deal or an expansion that he didn't thoroughly understand himself, and his high school education belied an inquisitive mind that bordered on genius. He delegated authority and hired excellent people to carry out his instructions, but he didn't suffer fools gladly: if someone wasn't pulling his or her weight, they were gone. He once told Earl Geiger, "You know, Earl, I have enough relatives in Georgia that we could fill every position in the company with one of them. But if you hire one, it's your responsibility, not mine." His management style was hands-on, but he knew when to step back and let someone make his or her own mistakes. "The job of management is to make people more productive," he said. "People want more, so they work harder. They become more productive for the company, for themselves, and for their families. The only way to earn more is to become more productive." He often said, "I would rather have a person with 75 percent ability working at 100 percent capacity than a person with 100 percent ability working at 75 percent capacity." And while he accumulated a lifetime of remarkable achievements, he believed that his greatest accomplishment was having two sons who worked just as hard as he did, right by his side. "My biggest contribution, as I see it," he once said of his entire career, "is that I've been fortunate to have two sons who are interested in the business."

From the moment Wayne Rollins stepped into the executive suite at Orkin's Piedmont Road office, his management style and emphasis on productive employees was crystal clear. As the new chief executive officer of Orkin, Wayne named Geiger, formerly vice president and general manager of sales, as Orkin's new executive vice president; Taft Pierce, formerly Geiger's assistant, was named as the first vice president of operations. Overnight, it seemed, the Rollins top management set a standard for the work ethic in the company: Wayne Rollins worked six and seven days a week and the executives did the same. "We are all created equal in the sense that we all have twenty-four hours in a day," Orkin employees soon heard Wayne Rollins say. "It is what we do with this time that determines our success."

Randall Rollins: "When Dad took over, Orkin was a large company in comparison to our little company, and everything in Orkin seemed to get done later; next week or next month, or next year. . . . Dad wanted it done now."

The new mood was apparent right away. "When Rollins came in, there was a change in tempo," said Glenn Martin, who had worked in Orkin's mailroom since 1960. "I felt things were more secure when the Rollins family got the company. You had more supervision, and they expected you to work more. The only one you really ever saw often was Mr. Henry Tippie. He always wanted people working and not standing around. He was like a troubleshooter, always walking around. If you weren't busy, you're weren't needed."

Joe Cantrell, who was hired by Fred McColl in 1958 as general accounting manager, never forgot Wayne Rollins's first meeting with Orkin's department managers, shortly after acquiring the company. "Mr. Rollins called the meeting for 9 A.M., and he called on each manager to make comments and suggestions. The meeting lasted until every manager had his turn to talk, and Mr. Rollins listened attentively to and observed every person."

It wasn't long before placards printed with this three-letter word began to appear in all of the Orkin offices: "NOW." Randall Rollins explained why. "When Dad took over, Orkin was a large company in comparison to our little company, and everything in Orkin seemed to get done later; next week or

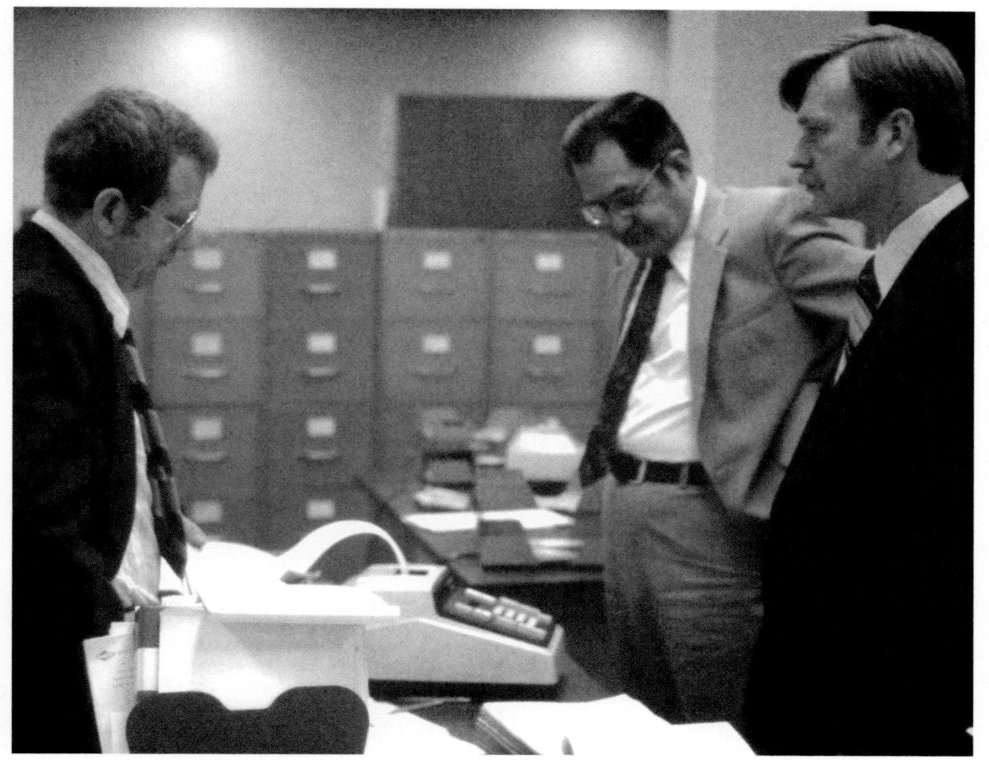

An unidentified coworker, left, discusses one of the many reports produced by the accounting department with general accounting manager Joe Cantrell, center, and Allen Meadows, right, then one of his accountants.

next month or next year," remembered Randall. "And we were used to doing it now. Dad wanted it done now."

From the beginning, Wayne's mission at Orkin was to accelerate the company's growth, provide more services to the existing pool of four hundred thousand clients, and to expand the company. In other words, he wanted the predictions of the McKinsey Report—"Orkin's prospects for growth appear to be excellent"—to come true sooner rather than later. He told everyone who would listen that he wanted the "NOW" strategy applied to something as simple as returning a customer's phone call the same day as well as to something as complicated as planning a new service treatment. And Wayne didn't rely on Immediate Action Memos to get across his message and new corporate philosophy; he delivered the message in person. For nearly thirteen weeks after the Orkin purchase, Wayne Rollins, Earl Geiger, vice president of operations Taft Pierce, and marketing manager James Llewallyn crisscrossed the country to visit every existing Orkin district in twenty-nine states and the District of Columbia.

In meetings with branch, district, and regional Orkin management, Wayne outlined his business goals: improved productivity, aggressive selling, meeting higher customer service expectations, and improved profit margins. As he started to explain how they were going to reach these ambitious new goals, Wayne Rollins was just as simple and direct as his "NOW" placard.

"We'd have a breakfast meeting with district and regional people, then we'd bring in the branch managers," said Geiger. "The basic field structure of

Orkin, at that time, was districts and branches. We'd sit down and talk to them about the transition to Rollins and how we expected them to carry on and what they could do better than they had been doing, how to increase sales, how to increase profit margins. Mr. Rollins always had some wonderful stories that reinforced those principles. The more management books you read today, the more you would understand how sound Mr. Rollins's business principles were in terms of what is taught in these sessions. I think that's true of every great entrepreneur. The instinct—they have the instinct for what is practical and logical."

Through instinct, experience, and his extensive business acumen, Wayne developed, and never hesitated to share, his favorite business principles, especially with the new people in the Orkin organization:

YOU PURCHASE SUCCESS WITH EFFORT,
THE SAME WAY YOU PURCHASE GROCERIES WITH MONEY.

YOU HAVE GOT TO PAY THE PRICE. AND THE PRICE IN THIS CASE IS EFFORT.

IF YOU WAIT UNTIL YOU'RE READY, YOU'LL NEVER DO ANYTHING.

ALWAYS LOOK BEHIND GOOD NEWS.

TAKE CARE OF THE LITTLE THINGS.
THE BIG THINGS WILL TAKE CARE OF THEMSELVES.

FIFTY PERCENT OF ANY JOB IS GETTING STARTED.

PEOPLE NEVER ACCOMPLISH MUCH WITH NEGATIVE THINKING.
AND IF THEY DO ACCOMPLISH ANYTHING, IT'S AN ACCIDENT.

MY MATERNAL GRANDMOTHER TAUGHT ME THAT IF THE AVERAGE PERSON WORKS EIGHT HOURS A DAY AND YOU WORK TWELVE HOURS, YOU ARE 50 PERCENT BETTER THAN THE AVERAGE. THAT'S BEEN MY WORK PHILOSOPHY FROM THE VERY BEGINNING. I'VE NEVER FOUND ONE BETTER.

He offered assurances to those employees who had been skeptical of the Orkin sale: "We're glad to have you, and we'll work with you. Our philosophy will not be to make any big changes, but to add to the growth of the company."

From discussions with the Orkin employees, Wayne heard in laymen's terms what his own personal research report had already confirmed: that in many instances, the branches operated mostly differently from one another; that some managers were paid on a percentage of sales while others were not; and that some managers ran private businesses in addition to their Orkin operations. Wayne Rollins knew that to operate efficiently, Orkin management needed to be standardized and streamlined. And all Orkin managers needed to devote all of their time to managing Orkin.

Gradually, Wayne won the loyalty of the Orkin people around the country. Walt Helms, the Midwest district manager in Kansas City, Missouri, saw in Wayne someone who was always a step ahead, who would listen, who possessed an unusual ability to communicate and make good decisions. Vince Stevens, then an Orkin route man from Columbia, South Carolina, came from a coal-mining family in West Virginia and immediately found common ground with Wayne's references to farming; Vince was impressed by Wayne's ability to reach every worker. In Oklahoma City, Orkin district manager Ed Elkins Jr. welcomed Wayne's businesslike approach and his desire to make the company grow. And though John Wilson was really shocked when Rollins bought Orkin, this district sales manager from Tennessee was impressed with Wayne's talent for assessing potential and his steadfast desire to promote from within the Orkin ranks. Gordon Crenshaw, who had started with Orkin as a pest control technician just a year earlier in Memphis, Tennessee (Crenshaw's initial claim to fame was being Elvis Presley's Orkin Man), felt after meeting Wayne that his chances to advance in the company were unlimited. In fact, Helms, Wilson, Crenshaw, Stevens, and Elkins would one day be vice presidents of the company, and Elkins would ultimately become president; Crenshaw would one day head two new Orkin divisions.

Wayne Rollins objected to anyone justifying an expense or a process because it had "traditionally" been done. "We don't traditionally do anything."

Wayne Rollins restructured Orkin's management—organizing regions under vice presidents, with districts reporting within those regions. It wasn't always easy. Some branch and district managers, and many of the technicians, had grown accustomed to sharing a large portion of the company's wealth; under new management, they would soon become salaried with a reasonable incentive bonus instead of commissioned employees, a move that reduced their excessive income and demanded more accountability.

"That was part of the turmoil," said Paul Hardy, who joined Orkin in 1961 as a part-time technician and was named termite service supervisor in Jacksonville in 1963 under Frank Hackett. "The district managers and the technicians—they never quit. Some district managers had gotten pieces of the Orkin pie, and they really had bank manager images. Mr. Rollins started to change that arrangement."

Hardy first met Wayne Rollins in Jacksonville as he made his tour of the district, and he remembered the "NOW" signs and the man behind them very well. "He was towering. He intimidated people. He believed in 110 percent scheduling—in order to get almost 100 percent done," said Hardy, a valued Orkin employee for over forty years. The new management, he said, didn't make wholesale changes overnight, but everyone knew that changes were inevitable. Gone were the days when branch managers could be paid 30 percent of the deposits; technicians would soon be on salary, not commission. "It was chaos," said Hardy. "We started forcing productivity, keeping to schedules. Otto would encourage the serviceman to hang out laundry, pick up eggs—anything to keep the customer happy and develop a relationship. Now we had new route management techniques, where management became more aware and began to dictate what technicians did. And we started our price increases, once or twice a year."

Gradually, the corporate changes became part of a process known throughout the company as "Rollinizing" Orkin. The term came to represent the many steps taken by the new management to bring business sophistication, marketing principles, and cost reduction discipline to service delivery, sales practices, budgeting, planning, and expansion. "Rollinizing" Orkin also meant that the employees got to learn exactly what their new boss wouldn't tolerate. Wayne Rollins objected to anyone justifying an expense or a process because it had "traditionally" been done. "We don't traditionally do anything," Wayne Rollins was known to argue. "We do things for a purpose, but not traditionally."

Together, Wayne Rollins, Earl Geiger, and Henry Tippie orchestrated many of the Rollins changes, with the assistance of Atlanta home office people like Charles Skypek, the Orkin treasurer, and Ray Minchew, Orkin's controller. These initial Rollinizing steps reached into every part of the company, like building blocks that would gradually lead to excellence:

- In September 1964, Wayne Rollins launched the Orkin Acceptance Corporation (OAC). Establishing this company-owned finance company was one of the key methods identified as a way to accelerate the growth of the company. Since the $150 to $200 termite treatment was at the time relatively expensive, some branch managers had been offering payment terms to their customers to make the purchase easier; but collecting these payments was precarious and sloppy without the structure of a finance company to handle the transactions. With OAC established, Orkin launched a special campaign enabling new customers to use OAC financing during the termite swarm season in 1965. The financing arrangement, which allowed customers to pay a small amount down and spread the remaining costs over six, twelve, or eighteen months, gave the termite salespeople a wonderful new tool for closing a sale. And it was a definite advantage over the competitors who couldn't provide financing.
- Orkin's billing, accounting, and record keeping were very labor intensive when Rollins acquired the company—manual typewriters, ten-key

adding machines, and all of the individual customer ledger sheets were posted by hand. Termite guarantees and renewals were prepared on manual typewriters by home office employees like Carolyn Harrison, who started with the company in 1961. The payroll was put on IBM punch cards with keypunch machines, and the billings statements were still processed by the company's Business and Addressograph (B&A) system that Otto Orkin so proudly displayed during the Open House Bug Bazaar on West Peachtree Street. The Addressograph equipment was so massive that it required fifteen to twenty people to operate and it was so loud that it sounded like a printing factory. It physically shook the building. The equipment processed the separate pest control and termite accounting records, printing stacks and stacks of customer statements that were forwarded to the appropriate branches, where they were verified for accuracy before the bills were mailed to the customers. For many years, these "Accounts Receivable Reports" were referred to as the "B&A."

Rollins executives immediately saw that Orkin needed a more sophisticated accounting system. As H. Tim Crow, Rollins's public relations director, put it, "We bought the largest company in the industry that was not computerized. But we knew that when we bought it, and we knew that it was going to be an investment in time and dollars to get to the point where we could grow faster, and it did just what we thought it would do. It grew just like topsy."

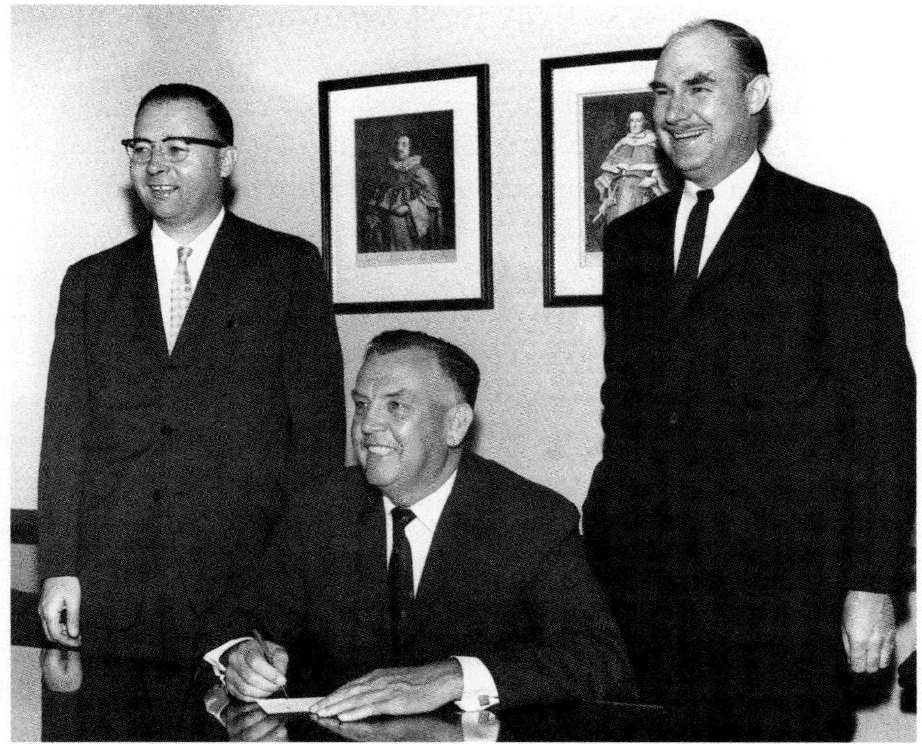

Henry B. Tippie, executive vice president–finance and treasurer, Rollins, Inc., left, and Earl Geiger, executive vice president, Orkin, right, look on as O. Wayne Rollins, chairman and president of Rollins, signs a check for $52.4 million, the major portion of the Orkin Exterminating Company purchase.

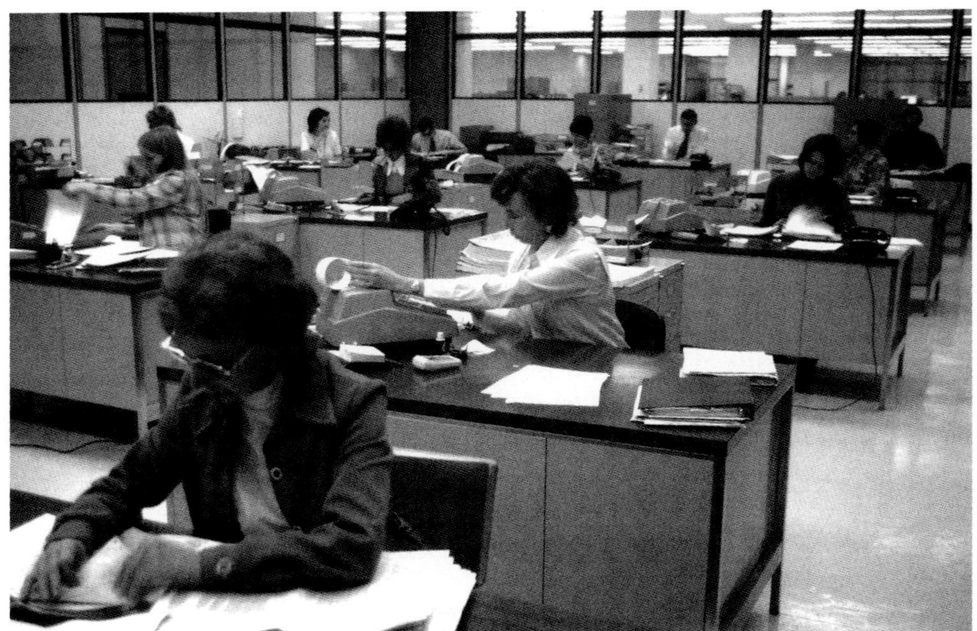

When Rollins acquired Orkin, the company had to improve the old manual posting system. The company was growing at geometric proportions, and the old system couldn't keep up.

Rollins was willing to provide "whatever we needed to improve the manual posting system," Allen Meadows recalled. "Orkin was growing in geometric proportions, and the old system just couldn't keep up." In the winter of 1966, Rollins established its own Electronic Data Processing (EDP) department, utilizing state-of-the-art IBM computers that were upgraded regularly. Crow admitted that in the beginning, "We didn't know beans about computers. We made a lot of mistakes." The company's data processing team began to develop its own programs not only to create profit and loss statements for Orkin but also to deal with accounts payable and payroll, central billing, and tax processing.

- On December 1, 1964, just three months after the Orkin purchase, Rollins bought an 80 percent interest in Dettelbach Pesticide Corporation, the major supplier of pesticides and rodenticides to Orkin. The company was created in 1952 by Louis L. Dettelbach to supply Orkin with termiticides when Orkin developed its Orkin-Tox pipe termite control system. In addition, the company supplied Orkin with rodenticides, insecticides, and pesticides, and many had trademarked names associated with Orkin: Orkil termiticide (chlordane and heptachlor), Orkin Aid (Diazinon), Orkinban (Dursban), RD-98 roach powder, and Orkin-Aire aerosols for controlling airborne bacteria, unpleasant odors, and flying insects. By 1967 Rollins would own 100 percent of Dettelbach Pesticide Corporation, which continued manufacturing and supplying Orkin with its chemicals. Eventually, as federal laws became more restrictive, Dettelbach stopped formulating chemicals and became a distributing company supplying pesticides to Orkin nationally and other pest control companies in the Southeast.

The fact that these initial Rollinizing steps were successful was in part responsible for the positive attention coming from Wall Street. The price of Rollins Broadcasting stock soared to $65 by the end of October following the acquisition—more than four and a half times the price six months earlier before the acquisition was announced. On November 23, 1964, the price of a Rollins Broadcasting share on the American Stock Exchange climbed to $76, an ascent that would continue until the stock reached a high of $80 1/4 and ultimately closed at year's end at $76 1/4 on December 31, 1964.

On November 24, 1964, the Rollins Board of Directors approved a three-for-one stock split (a move that sent the stock price up to $156 a share prior to the split; the stock settled at $52 a share after the split, which was effective on March 31, 1965). Wall Street applauded this move, because the relatively small number of outstanding company shares available before then had hampered more active trading. The board of directors also announced another important change: No longer did the name Rollins Broadcasting adequately portray this diversified company, which now stretched from coast to coast with facilities in thirty-five states and Mexico, a company that not only offered radio and television and outdoor advertising but also pest control services second to none. In recognition of the family that made it happen, the new corporate name would be simply Rollins, Inc.

POISED FOR MORE GROWTH

It was a good time to be in the exterminating business. By the end of 1964, Ralph E. Heal, then executive director of the National Pest Control Association, predicted that homeowners would spend a record $350 million for the services of pest control experts—an increase of nearly 15 percent over the year before and far bigger than the annual average increase of 7 to 10 percent since World War II.

Why? Several factors.

First, insects, including cockroaches and flies, were developing a resistance to the family of pesticides called chlorinated hydrocarbons, such as DDT; in response, the industry had switched to a newer group of organic phosphates, which, unlike the older, more toxic pesticides, were not as effective over long periods after the initial application, requiring repeat visits from exterminators to keep homes pest-free.

Second, it had been an unusually warm spring. Translated? Lots of bugs, including termites. The bedbug was making a roaring comeback from extinction in New England; roaches were worse than they had been for the last thirty years in Atlantic City, New Jersey; Boston officials reported a "soaring" rat population and called its seasonal termite swarming "almost explosive."

And third, in words that would have delighted Otto Orkin, the *Wall Street Journal* reported that "Americans are far less loath to call in an exterminator than they once were. In some areas now, a pest control truck is something of a status symbol."

"Man's conquest of the creeping, crawling sub-world of insects, rodents and other pests, far from being complete, seems actually to be slipping back at some points," reported the *Journal.* "The continuing battle, in fact, is bringing record business to a little known service industry—the professional exterminators."

In 1965, the year after acquiring Orkin, Rollins, Inc., continued to expand, primarily under two distinct business umbrellas: the media business (represented by radio, television, and outdoor advertising) and the service industry (represented by Orkin and its professional exterminators).

In early January Rollins paid $2 million for the L. P. Martin Maintenance Corporation, a provider of building maintenance in ten southern states. Renamed Rollins Services, the company provided janitorial, guard service, carpet care, building management, and consulting services. Elsewhere in the company, Rollins Broadcasting acquired a new FM radio station in Norfolk, Virginia; announced plans to build a cable television system serving the Wilmington, Delaware, area; sought FCC approval for cable television franchises in Connecticut, New York, and West Virginia; and applied for a UHF television channel allocated for Delaware.

Former Arwell owner Wellington W. Scott, front right, shown here with Orkin vice president Earl Geiger, remained a consultant to Orkin until 1967, when he chose to retire.

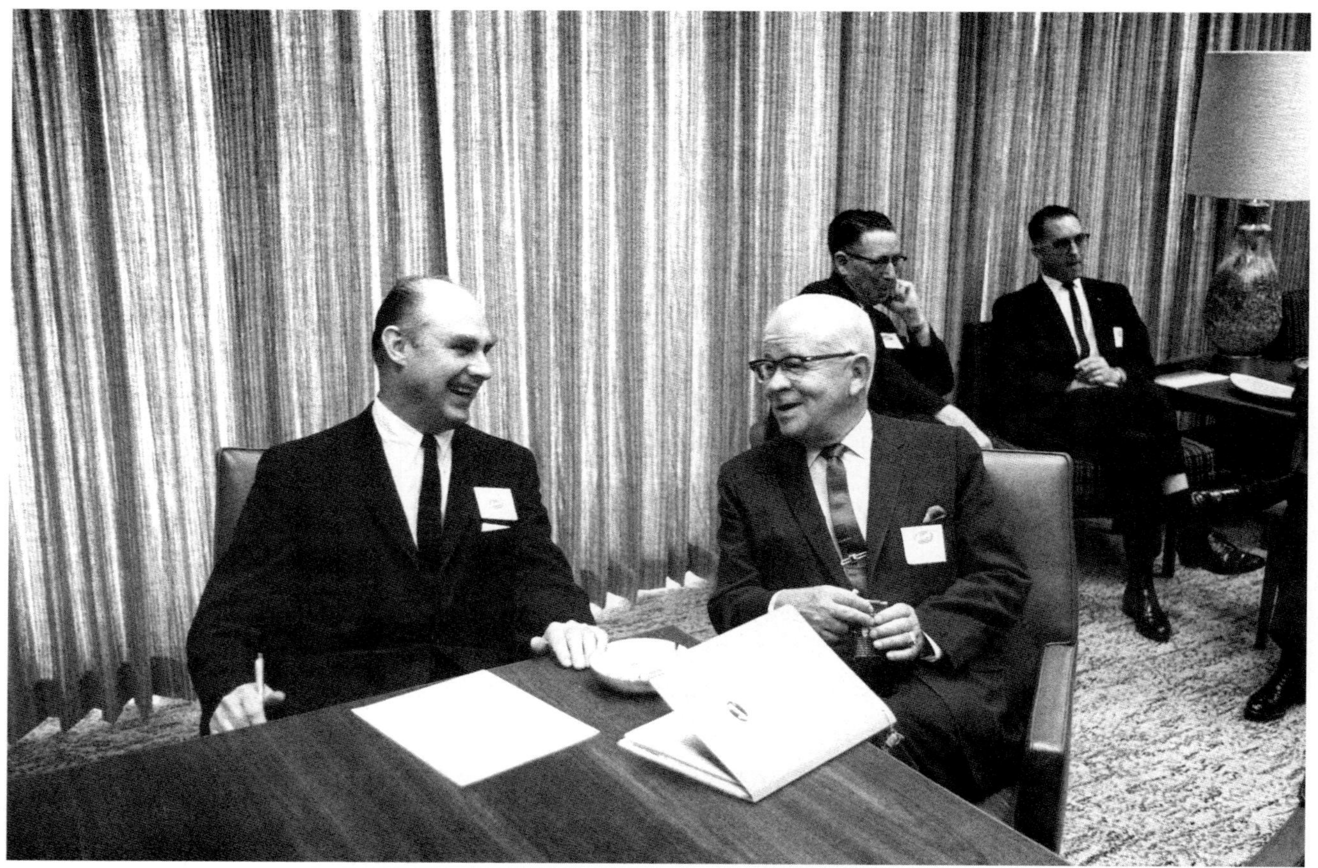

And on Tuesday, April 20, 1965, the business press reported a development that had a tremendous impact on Orkin, one that no doubt reflected how desirable expanding the exterminating business had become: Rollins had agreed to acquire Arwell, Inc., a major midwestern pest control and termite company based in Waukegan, Illinois.

"Arwell has enjoyed outstanding growth," Wayne Rollins said after the acquisition was made public, and "will most certainly complement our present business interests and will broaden our base as a service company. We will apply our financial resources and merchandising experience to accelerate the growth of this excellent company."

The news of the transaction, however, disappointed many of the loyal Arwell employees, who would have preferred to be part of an employee-owned company in what they referred to as "Arwell-Land." Rollins and Orkin executives, however, quickly welcomed the new employees into their company. When Arwell representatives visited the Orkin headquarters in Atlanta that spring, a large banner suspended over the telephone switchboard announced, "Otto Says Welcome Arwell." The company name changed gradually: Arwell Division of Orkin, then Arwell-Orkin; followed by Orkin-Arwell, then finally Midwest Region of Orkin Exterminating Company. At one time the Arwell name was displayed in the Orkin diamond logo.

Many of the Arwell veterans settled into important positions at Orkin.

- Arwell's former owner Wellington W. Scott remained a consultant to Orkin until 1967, when he chose to retire.
- Dorothy Wirta, who was one of only four females working for Arwell when she started in 1948, continued as secretary to the first six Orkin Midwest regional vice presidents after Orkin bought the company—Bernard Kolkana, Taft Pierce, Harvey Massey, John Wilson, Joe Wilson, and Steve Billmyer—before retiring from her job as customer retention manager for the Illinois Region in 1995.
- Charles Hubbell, a distinguished Arwell employee in southern Wisconsin since 1949, continued with Orkin as a district manager until his retirement in Phoenix, Arizona, in April 1989. Active in the state's Pest Control Association and an expert in wood-destroying organisms, he was asked by the Wisconsin Department of Agriculture to write the state certification exam required by the Federal Insecticide, Fungicide and Rodenticide Act for pest control operators. (FIFRA, as the legislation was known, was considered the first real national pesticide regulation when it was enacted in 1964.)
- Emmet Champion, a graduate of Columbia University, joined Arwell in 1952 and later became managing director of Orkin's National Institute of Industrial Sanitation. Champion, who stayed with Orkin until the mid-

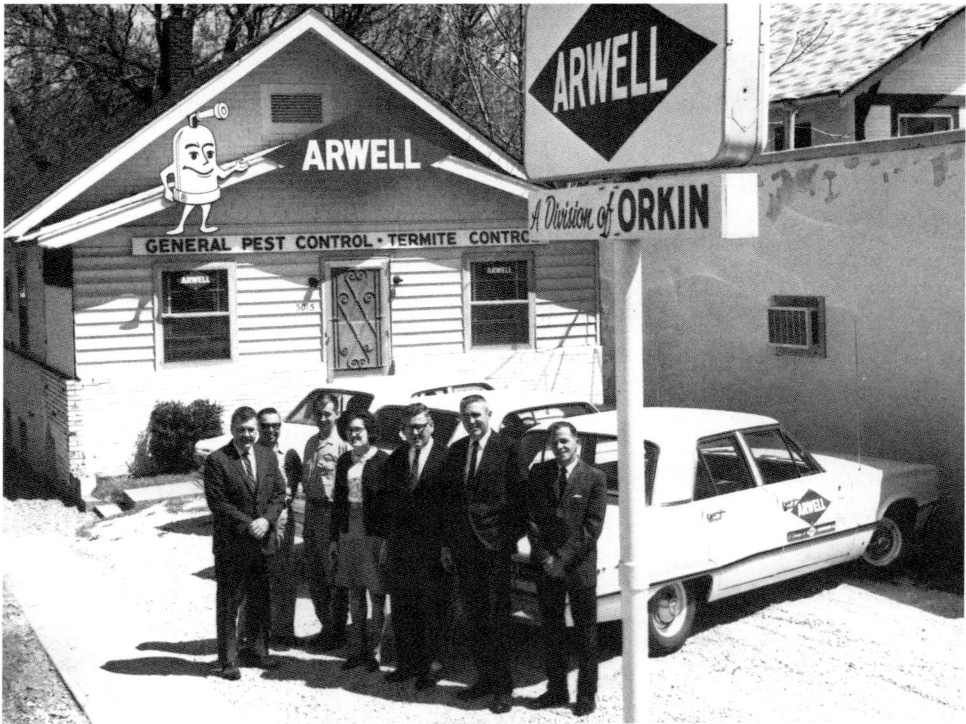

For a while after Orkin bought Arwell, the Arwell name was retained, but designated as a division of Orkin. In this 1967 photo of the Des Moines, Iowa, branch, the Arwell name still has more prominence. Left to right: District manager Clair Wiltgen, D. Traner, E. Karley, S. Treloar, D. Abshire, Tom Lonergan, and R. Pike.

1970s, was a registered professional sanitarian and was admitted into Britain's Royal Society of Health in 1969.

- Frank Zawin was a route technician for ten years after joining Arwell in 1953 and then moved to Waukegan to be service manager. In 1971 he became Illinois District service manager before moving to the same position in LaSalle, Wisconsin, where he concluded more than thirty-five years with the company.
- Joseph P. Irvine, a nephew of Wellington Scott, grew up in the Arwell Company and progressed from termite treater and pest control serviceman to Arwell vice president. After Orkin bought the company, he moved to Atlanta as Orkin's marketing manager and was promoted to vice president of Orkin's Marketing Department. In December 1967 he was named director of Kinro Advertising Company, the advertising and marketing arm of Orkin, a position he held until 1969.
- Ray Lochner joined Arwell in 1954 as a route technician in Lake Geneva, Wisconsin. He stayed with the company for thirty-eight years, as manager of the Wisconsin district, sales manager, region sales manager, region administrative assistant, and eventually Illinois region service coordinator.

- Ray Bateman was tired of traveling for his previous employer when he joined Arwell in Red Oak, Iowa, in 1963. Little did he know! After Orkin acquired Arwell, Bateman was assigned to open branches simultaneously in Sioux City, Iowa, and Omaha, Nebraska. On Mondays, Wednesdays, and Fridays he worked in Omaha; on Tuesdays, Thursdays, and Saturdays he worked in Sioux City. He was later named district manager of Wisconsin and then district manager of Michigan, where he spent five years opening seven new branches in Michigan and northern Indiana. In 1977, Bateman moved to Atlanta and continued with Orkin in the home office for another nineteen years, was one of three key people involved in Orkin's reorganization in the late 1980s. At the time of his retirement, he was assistant to the president.

Ray Lochner joined Arwell in 1954 as a route technician in Lake Geneva, Wisconsin, and stayed with the company for thirty-eight years in a variety of positions, winding up as service coordinator for the Illinois region.

Bernard Kolkana was the first Orkin Man to take charge at Arwell when he was named general manager and director of sales for the Arwell-Orkin divisions in September 1965. The company, which had grown accustomed to the comfort of routines and patterns established after decades of family-owned management, must have thought a Midwest tornado had blown through the business. After moving into Scott's back office, the first thing Kolkana did was

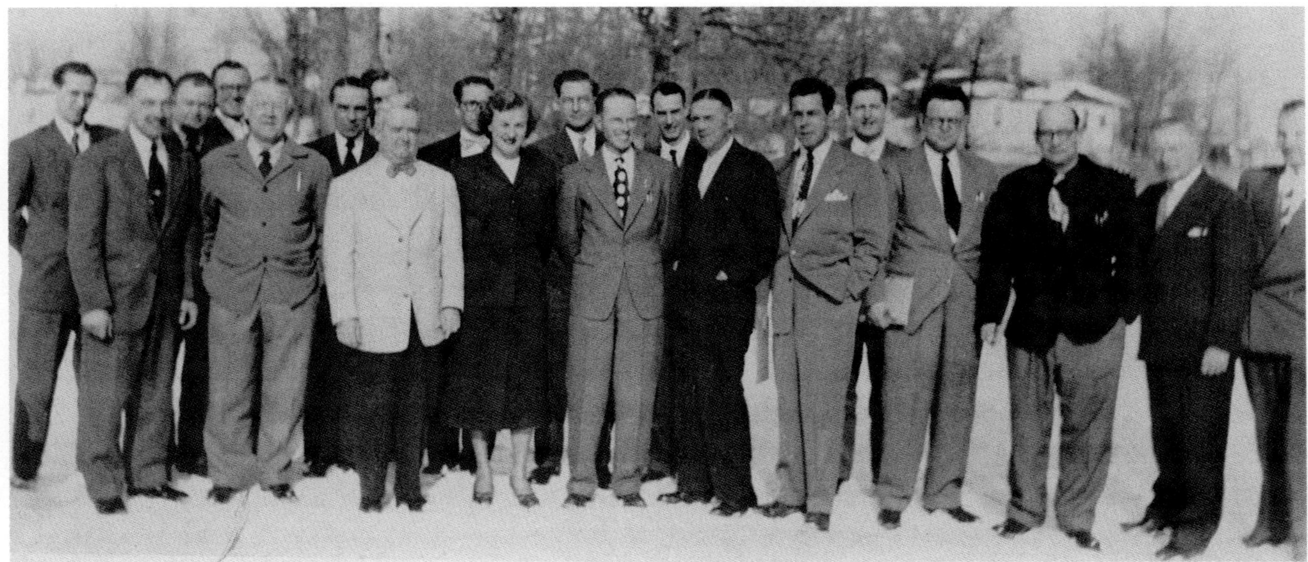

Dorothy Wirta, front row, fourth from left, was one of only four females working for Arwell when she started in 1948. At many of the early meetings she attended, she was the only female present, as was the case at this supervisors' meeting in 1951. Front row, left to right: C. Meyer, W. Kohn, J. McNeill, D. Wirta, G. Mulloy, E. Knudson, B. Lemmons, J. Kendrick, C. Peterson, H. Smith, and S. Bernard; (back row) R. Mulloy, J. Matthews, P. Cummins, H. Sherwood, I. Haggerty, C. Anderson, J. Mock, H. Gleason, and F. Smith.

establish a sales department and begin training salespeople, since Arwell did not have a full-time sales staff. Next, he established price increases for Arwell-Orkin services (up to 25 percent), something the Arwell customers hadn't seen for a few years. As Orkin's advertising and marketing programs were initiated—another step toward "Orkinizing" Arwell—leads began pouring into the branches for residential as well as commercial service, something Arwell had not pursued before Orkin. Teams of Orkin technicians and salesmen were brought in to train the Arwell staff on how to service residential clients since their experience had primarily been with commercial customers. Through the sales efforts and price increases he initiated, Kolkana raised the Arwell pest control revenue so much that Wayne Rollins told him, "In the three years you have been here, you have more than paid for this company."

Under Kolkana, the former Arwell sales and servicemen moved from working out of their homes (Kolkana remembered seeing sales contracts stacked on the floor) to a structure of standalone Orkin branches. For nearly two years, Kolkana opened various branch offices; in some cases, Dorothy Wirta would go to the location before it was opened to coordinate painting or repairs, while

Arwell, Inc.

In 1965, when Rollins purchased Arwell, Inc., a major Midwestern pest control and termite company based in Waukegan, Illinois, Earl Geiger called it "the most successful acquisition I thought we ever made." Why?

Arwell opened up the Midwest for Orkin. At the time, Orkin operated Midwest branch offices in Illinois (3), Indiana (4), Kansas (10), Missouri (9), and Ohio (7). Arwell, on the other hand, operated in nine Midwest states with sixty-eight locations: Illinois (24), Indiana (2), Iowa (11), Michigan (9), Minnesota (1), Nebraska (1), Ohio (1), South Dakota (1), and Wisconsin (18). In no city did Orkin and Arwell compete against each other.

Arwell also gave Orkin an important entry into the commercial pest control industry. Family-owned and managed, Arwell was primarily a commercial pest control company, specializing in industrial and grain storage pest control, mosquito control programs for towns and resort areas, and rat control in city dumps. It performed only a modest amount of household pest control but was recognized as the "Cadillac" of commercial pest control services in the Midwest.

The Arwell acquisition, which was seen as a bold move by Rollins so soon after the Orkin deal, represented a switch from Orkin's typical growth pattern, which until then had been accomplished almost entirely by the previous Orkin management through internal growth. Before 1964, there had only been several minor acquisitions: in one, Orkin bought Orkin Exterminator of Norfolk, Virginia, which was operated by Otto Orkin's nephew, so that the Orkin name could be used by Otto in Virginia. Under the new expansion model established by Rollins, growth by acquisition represented a means of rapidly expanding markets that were already predisposed toward Orkin or were accessible through Rollins media services. Instead of "Rollinizing"

Bob Reynolds and Wally Sorensen helped operate the new branch offices until everyone understood Orkin's operations, policies, and procedures. Administrative employees were brought into Waukegan and trained before being placed in the branch. Through the help of J. D. Burger and Allen Meadows in Orkin's home office, all of the accounting and payroll procedures and administrative changes went smoothly. "We integrated Arwell into Orkin very well," said Meadows.

Kolkana's role in "Orkinizing" Arwell was remarkably successful. But as the change agent, Kolkana had to be both demanding and relentless, and he was not the type of manager who relished the small details or became personally involved with his management decisions. In 1968 Taft A. Pierce replaced Kolkana as region vice president, responsible for the Arwell-Orkin operation and for establishing the first region office outside of Atlanta. Pierce would be vice president of the Midwest Region longer than any other vice president, from 1968 to 1974. Before that, he had a distinguished career as a branch manager in Tampa and Miami, the company's largest branch. And according to Orkin legend, Pierce once inspired his Miami servicemen and

Orkin, the Orkin team could now begin "Orkinizing" the various pest control companies acquired by the home office.

The Arwell acquisition had actually been set in motion shortly after Rollins had purchased Orkin, when Arwell's owner, Wellington W. Scott, first contacted Earl Geiger about selling Arwell to Orkin. The two men already knew each other; Geiger had once approached Scott about working with Arwell, but the kind and paternalistic Scott had advised him to explore the possibilities with Orkin because there was no open position at Arwell worthy of Geiger's talents. Geiger brought Arwell's offer to Wayne Rollins, and the negotiations quietly began. The deal was sealed on May 1, 1965, when Rollins acquired Arwell, Inc., of Waukegan, Illinois, for $3.14 million. At the time, Arwell reported $4 million in revenue with earnings before taxes in excess of $475,000. In addition to the promise of increased revenue, the Arwell acquisition also included about $1 million in assets consisting of marketable securities in publicly owned companies. Henry Tippie remembered counting them at the closing. "We didn't get just revenue, but also marketable securities," he said, further highlighting the transaction's benefits for Rollins.

Arwell, founded by Scott nearly forty years earlier, had nearly three hundred employees. Those who knew Scott understood that he took great pride in his company and its people, but he felt that everyone would be better served by having Arwell join a nationwide company with a solid reputation. Apparently, he never considered selling to anyone other than Orkin. In a letter to his employees shortly after the acquisition, Scott assured them that they would become a part of the Orkin operation. In the summer edition of Arwell's *News 'n Views*, the company newsletter for "Arwellmen and their families," the headline read, "ARWELL JOINS ORKIN!"

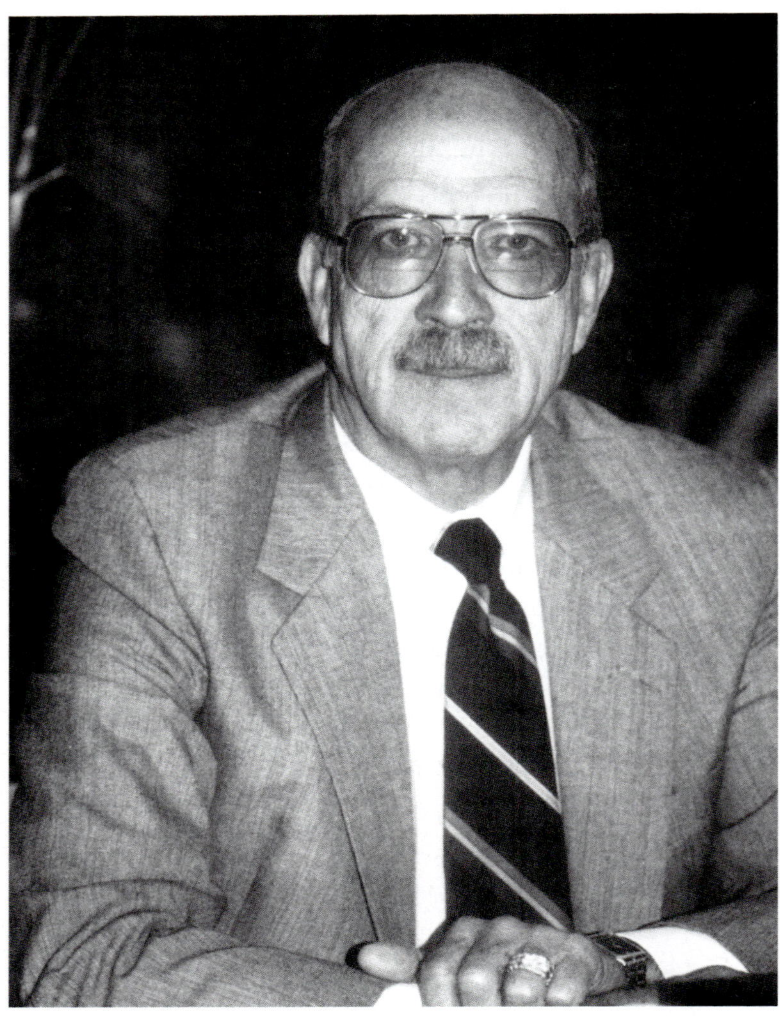

Ray Bateman was working for Arwell when the company was acquired by Orkin. He spent nineteen years in Orkin's home office in Atlanta and retired as assistant to the president.

technicians by taking his chair out of his office and putting his desk up on concrete blocks. "I'm not going to sit down," he reportedly said, "until this branch is successful."

Chair antics aside, Pierce was considered a consummate teacher who did everything by the book. He brought district managers to Waukegan for two days, where he explained each paragraph of Orkin's policies and procedures to help ensure that every aspect of Orkin's operations was implemented in their branches. "He wanted things done right," remembered Gary Rollins. "He showed a lot of people that you didn't have to cut corners or be deceitful. That you could accomplish things by doing things right. He had such high regard for his staff, and he could often get people to do so much more than they thought they could do. They felt that if Taft believed they could do something, then maybe they could. But he could be really hard if he thought you were taking advantage of him or doing something behind his back."

TWO CAREER PATHS

By now, Gary Rollins had been privy to many stories about Orkin—and not just because he had dinner regularly with the company president. Though Wayne Rollins never intended to develop two different business interests for his sons, the divisions of the company offered two natural career paths for them. Because of his previous experience, Randall, thirty-three, was naturally directed to the media business, represented by radio, television, and outdoor advertising; later, he would head the company's interests in the oil services businesses, as well as its protective services and burglar alarm business. Randall was appointed executive vice president of Rollins, Inc., on January 25, 1965—the same day Rollins Broadcasting shareholders met in Wilmington to officially approve the board of directors' vote to change the company name and to approve a three-for-one split of the common stock. Randall was now responsible for all of the media interests—in addition to the company's Florida citrus operations. The media division at the time consisted of seven AM radio stations, three FM stations, and three television stations, with outdoor advertising operations in the Northeast, Texas, and Mexico, including such cities as Mexico City, Monterrey, and Guadalajara.

Gary, it turned out, was drawn to the service industry side of Rollins, represented by Orkin and its various divisions. In 1965 Gary's decision to work for Orkin was a deliberate one. When he returned to the University of Tennessee–Chattanooga from his summer in the Florida orange groves, Gary decided not only to buckle down and successfully complete his last two years of college but also to go to work for the company. The only branch of Rollins that was in Chattanooga was Orkin. "The thing that really motivated me," Gary still

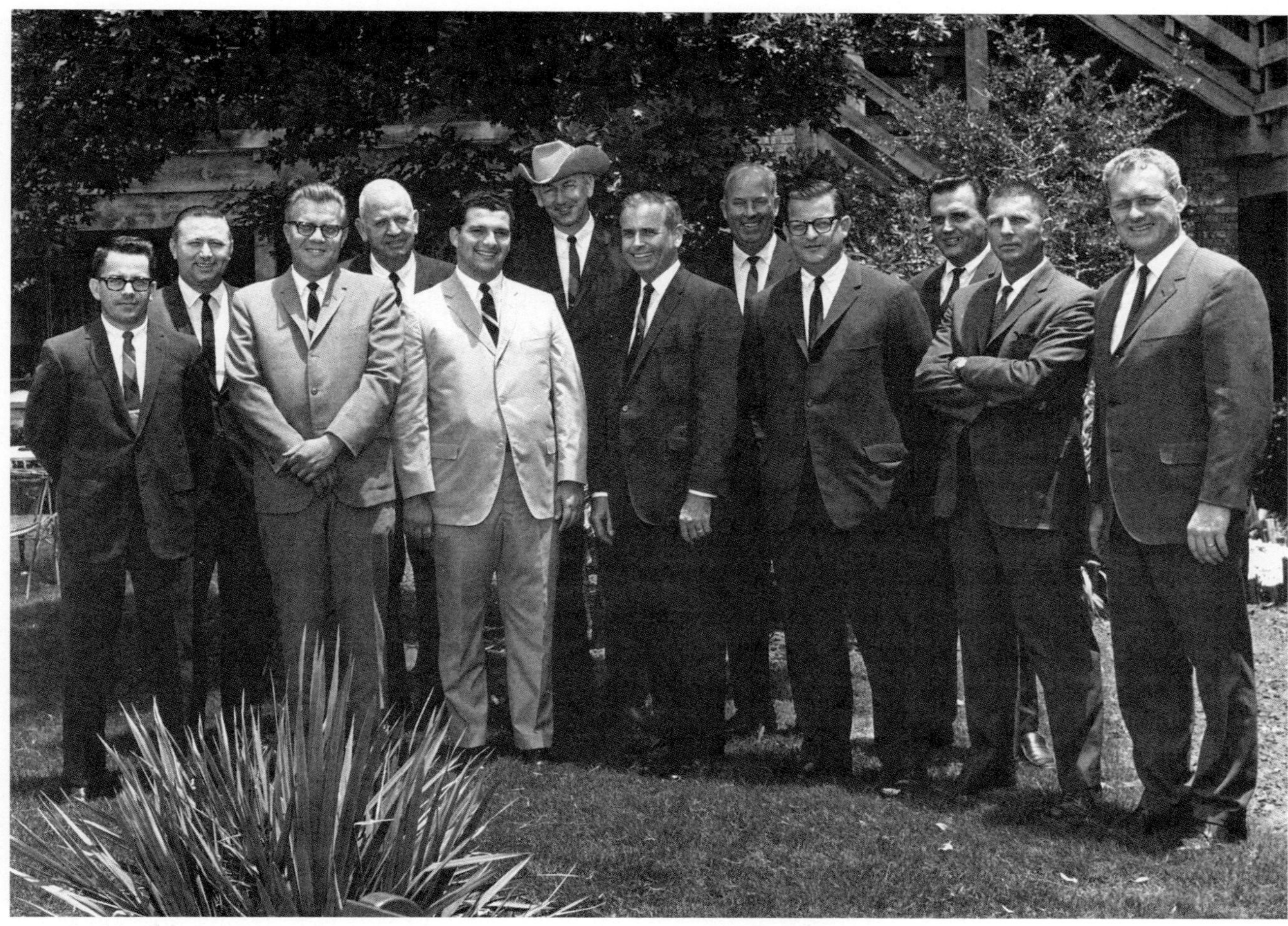

Two regional offices were established in 1966 to direct the operations of Orkin. The Eastern Region was headed by Jack Dorris, former Georgia district manager, and the Western Region was under the direction of Taft Pierce, vice president of operations. District managers from the Western Region were, left to right: Bob Shaw, Oklahoma district (sales); Bob Elkins, Arkansas district; Russell Bull, Oklahoma district; Don Holt, Kansas-Missouri district; Norman Goldenberg, California district; Taft Pierce; Elwood Cahill, Indiana district; Bill Booth, South Texas district; Rene Bourgeois, Southwest district; Paul Bowes, Louisiana district; Bob Russell, North Texas district; and Jack Edwards, Mississippi district.

remembers, "is that Orkin was there." In 1965 he married his high school sweetheart, Ruth Magness, in Chattanooga, "and it was time for me to get serious." Though Gary had worked for several summers in Wilmington, Delaware, at Rollins Broadcasting and Rollins Outdoor during high school, that wasn't possible in Tennessee. "So what better thing was there for me to do than to make my stake with Orkin? I arranged my schedule so that I could go to school in the morning and at night, and work at Orkin in the afternoon. I loved it. And I developed a grass-roots understanding of the bug business."

Gary Rollins: "I arranged my schedule so that I could go to school in the morning and at night, and work for Orkin in the after-noon. I loved it. And I developed a grass-roots understanding of the bug business."

"Gary began by crawling under houses, looking for termites," recalled Tim Crow, then corporate vice president and secretary. "His father worked him just as hard as he did anyone else, and he expected more out of him."

And from the beginning, from the corporate suites to the field, anyone who met Gary was impressed more by his hard work and dedication as an Orkin Man than by the inherent privileges associated with his last name. "He was out every day, working in the field in khaki uniforms, just like everyone else," said the mailroom's Glenn Martin. As he moved through the company and up the corporate ladder, Gary realized how valuable his early experiences really were. "One of the good things that I always had was the credibility of being 'an Orkin Man.'"

These experiences taught him as much about the human side of the business as the technical. During the spring, when termites were swarming, Gary, as a salesman, was called to make an inspection at a house near the airport. Based on consumer research, company policy at the time dictated that the Orkin salesperson must include the husband in the presentation to explain how a home would be treated for termites. Though women bought pest control services for inside the house, at that time men typically bought termite service. On this particular day, Gary had to go to the nearby Farmers' Market to find the husband, a disheveled-looking farmer. Gary explained the situation and quoted a price of $350 to treat the house—a substantial price, Gary thought to himself, that this farmer could never afford the treatment. Within minutes, the farmer had reached into a pocket and pulled out the biggest wad of bills Gary had ever seen. Gary was so startled, he blurted out, "You don't have to pay me until the work is complete."

"Well, are you gonna do what you said you were gonna do?" he asked Gary. "And you're gonna supervise it and make sure that everything is right?" Gary replied that he would.

"Well, there's no need for me to hold on to this money. I might as well give it to you." Gary accepted the money and took away two lessons from his encounter: first, never judge a person by his appearance. Second, by being shrewd, the man had guaranteed Gary's personal interest in the job, which virtually guaranteed an excellent termite treatment.

One year after buying Orkin—and in the same year that Arwell, Dettelbach, and L. P. Martin Maintenance Corp were acquired—Rollins reported that revenues had increased 369 percent in 1965, up from $9.13 million in 1964 to $42.814 million in 1965, which also reflected a 94 percent gain in net earnings, totaling $1.738 million compared to $894,254 a year earlier. By the spring of 1966, Rollins, Inc.'s revenues had increased 65 percent and net income 140 percent for the year ending April 30, 1966. Leading the growth was Orkin, now the crown jewel of Rollins.

In October 1966 *Forbes* magazine profiled Wayne, emphasizing his spectacular success with Orkin while acknowledging problems in keeping all the Orkin representatives on their toes. One incentive Wayne offered was a cash bonus for the employee who didn't lose a single customer in a month. "If you believe in yourself, that's what makes it in the service business," said Wayne. "The product is your service. I hate to lose a customer, and I think you have to feel that way in the service business. You've got to really bleed when you lose a customer.

"And to really have a great service business, it's got to start at the top. You have to be service-oriented. I take a service call or complaint ahead of every other call. Because if you have a customer and that customer has a complaint and you take care of it, you have a more loyal customer than one who never had a complaint. So you turn that into an asset."

In the winter of 1966, Wayne introduced a new company magazine called *Rollins Today*, which reinforced many of his business expectations and created a new sense of community for long-term Orkin employees and those who were relatively new to the company:

> This is the first issue of "Rollins Today," a company magazine, by which we hope to increase the general understanding of our Company, our people, our services, products, and policies.
>
> Rollins is considered one of the largest service companies in the world. . . . Our Company is widespread and diversified, and we expect to continue to enjoy the unusual growth and expansion that we've had in the past.
>
> In order for us to realize our anticipated growth, we shall attempt to build buildings, buy machinery, hire people to produce the products and services we sell, and earn a profit for our shareholder.
>
> We have invested in this Company magazine to help accomplish these objectives. The philosophy of our publication is based on the premise that what is good for the Company is good for the employee and that as the Company succeeds, so the employee succeeds.

> We have attained our present respected position in the industry with the help of hard-working, loyal men and women who today number about 9,000. And in our opinion, of all the goals to which our Company aspires, none is more important than security and opportunity for all our employees.

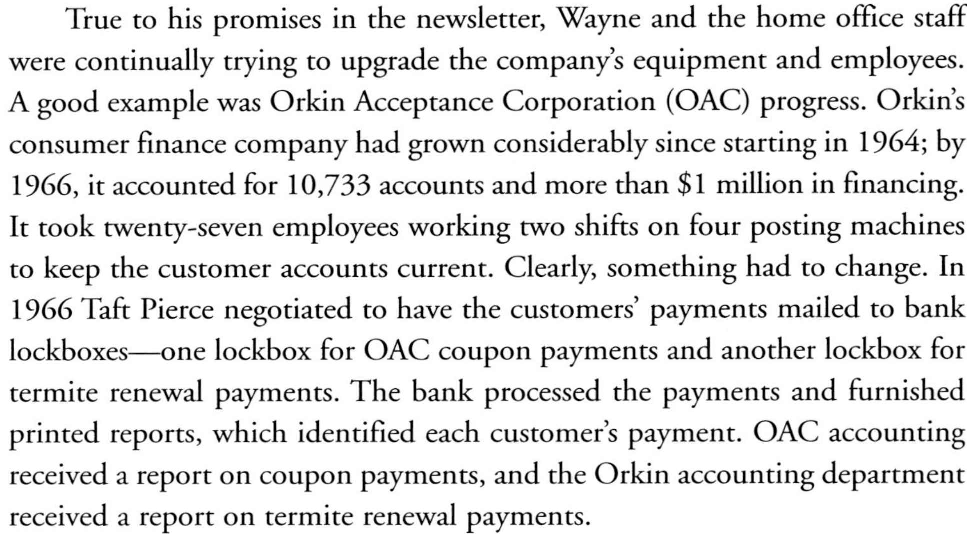

True to his promises in the newsletter, Wayne and the home office staff were continually trying to upgrade the company's equipment and employees. A good example was Orkin Acceptance Corporation (OAC) progress. Orkin's consumer finance company had grown considerably since starting in 1964; by 1966, it accounted for 10,733 accounts and more than $1 million in financing. It took twenty-seven employees working two shifts on four posting machines to keep the customer accounts current. Clearly, something had to change. In 1966 Taft Pierce negotiated to have the customers' payments mailed to bank lockboxes—one lockbox for OAC coupon payments and another lockbox for termite renewal payments. The bank processed the payments and furnished printed reports, which identified each customer's payment. OAC accounting received a report on coupon payments, and the Orkin accounting department received a report on termite renewal payments.

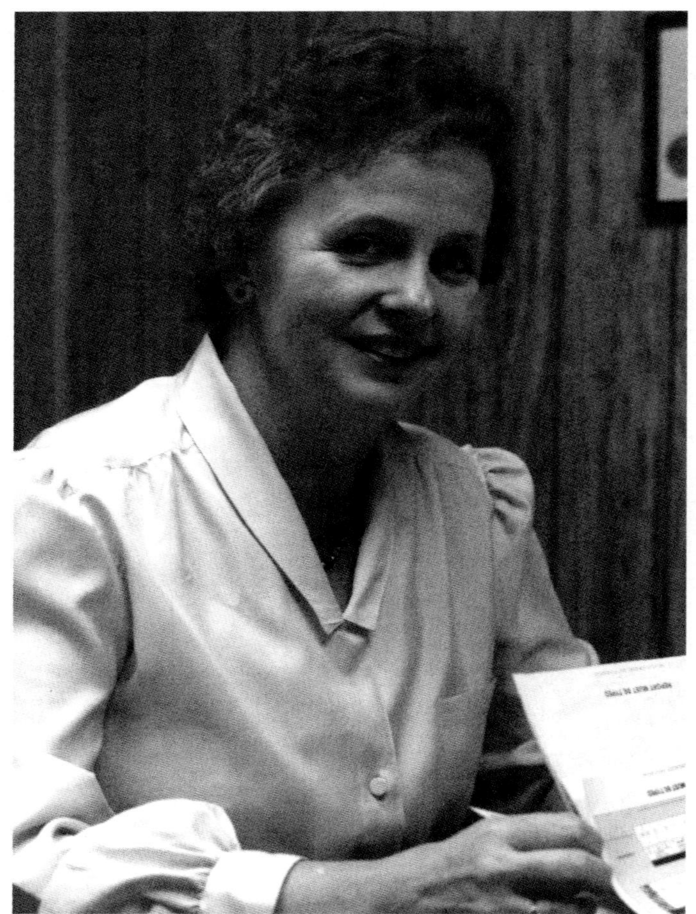

Hilda Brady Pennington, who retired from Rollins Acceptance Corporation in 1997, was in charge of the Orkin Acceptance Corporation administrative staff in its early years. In 1967 she and her team transferred approximately 36,900 customer accounts worth over $4.25 million to a new computer system.

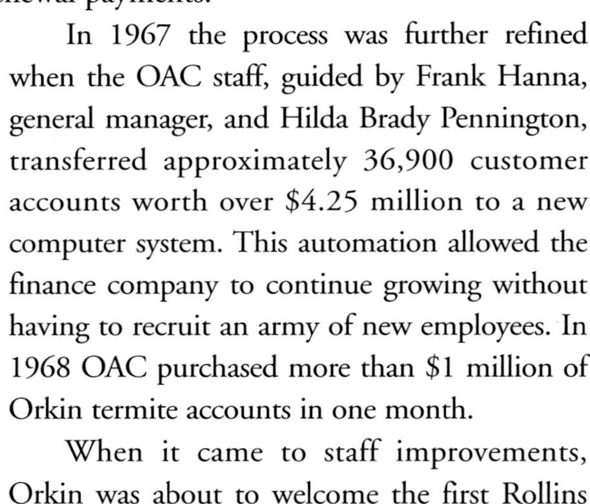

In 1967 the process was further refined when the OAC staff, guided by Frank Hanna, general manager, and Hilda Brady Pennington, transferred approximately 36,900 customer accounts worth over $4.25 million to a new computer system. This automation allowed the finance company to continue growing without having to recruit an army of new employees. In 1968 OAC purchased more than $1 million of Orkin termite accounts in one month.

When it came to staff improvements, Orkin was about to welcome the first Rollins family member to work full-time at the home office. After Gary graduated from college in 1967 with a bachelor's degree in business administration, he convinced Ruthie that they should move with their infant son, Glen William, to Atlanta. "I convinced her that in Atlanta, I would not have to be in anyone's shadow, and that it would be good to have a family member at Orkin who understood the business," Gary said. "It was really a great bridge between Rollins and Orkin."

Two months later Wayne Rollins announced he was moving the corporate Rollins headquarters from Wilmington, Delaware, to Atlanta, and would relocate at the Orkin offices on Piedmont Road. "My first reaction was, 'Gee, that's great,'" Gary remembers. "My second was, 'What do I tell Ruthie?' She would later teasingly say that I double-crossed her to get her to move to Atlanta."

The entire Rollins family and seventeen high-level executives moved to Atlanta in 1967. "There is nothing as good for a business as the footsteps of the owner in the hall," said Wayne. Russ Chambers, head of the company's engineering division, stayed in Wilmington, though he traveled to Atlanta so frequently that he also had an office there. Within a year, Gary was appointed administrative assistant to Earl Geiger, who would continue as Orkin's executive vice president and division head until 1974. And with renewed interest, Gary watched carefully as the company expanded its foreign operations by establishing Orkin International, Inc., in Panama, the base for entering pest control markets in Central America and Mexico.

By now Wayne Rollins had slightly shifted his sights from termites and other insects to the most dangerous and repulsive of pests, the rat. His interest

In 1967 O. Wayne Rollins moved the corporate headquarters of Rollins, Inc., from Wilmington, Delaware, to Orkin's headquarters at 2170 Piedmont Road in Atlanta.

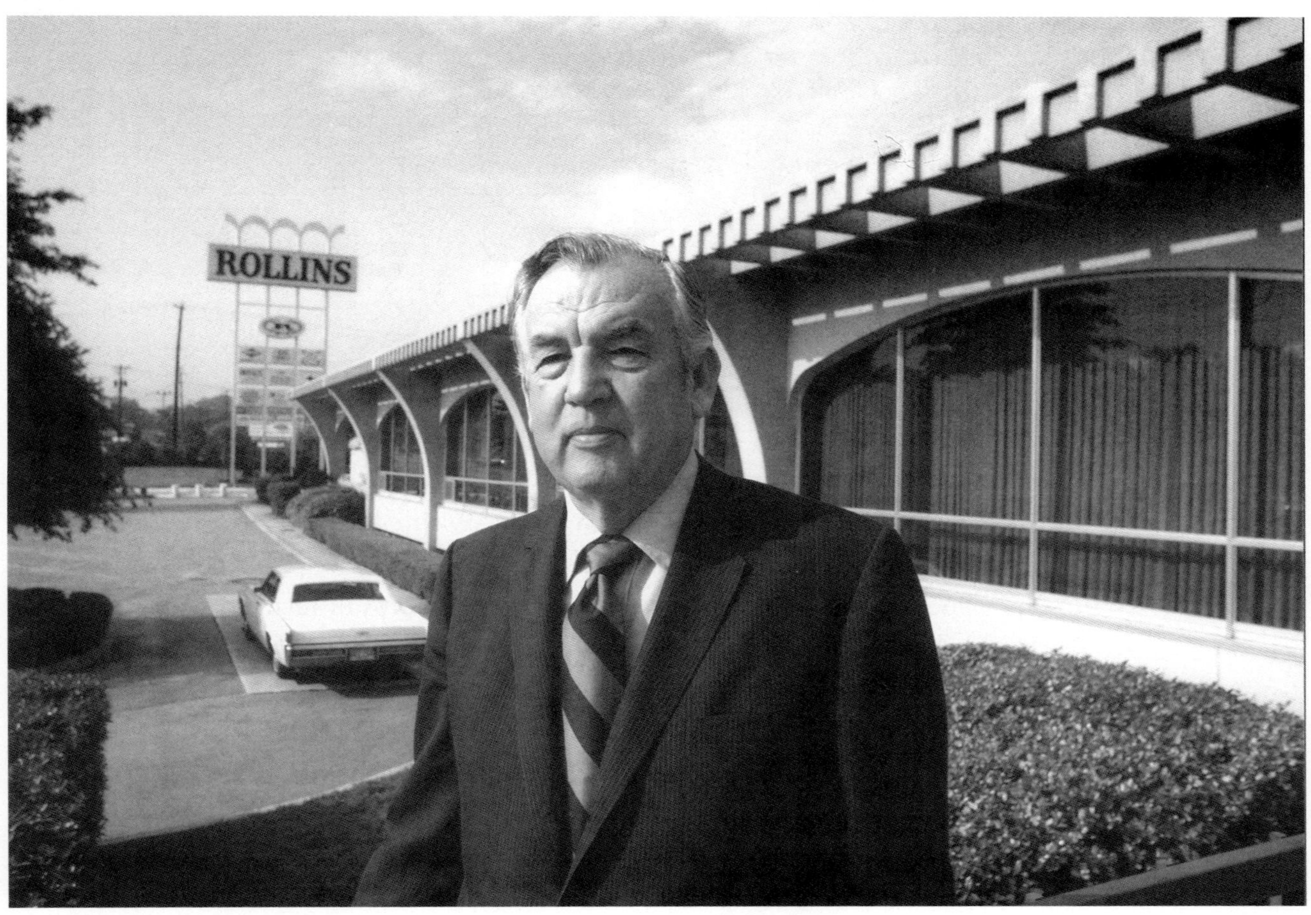

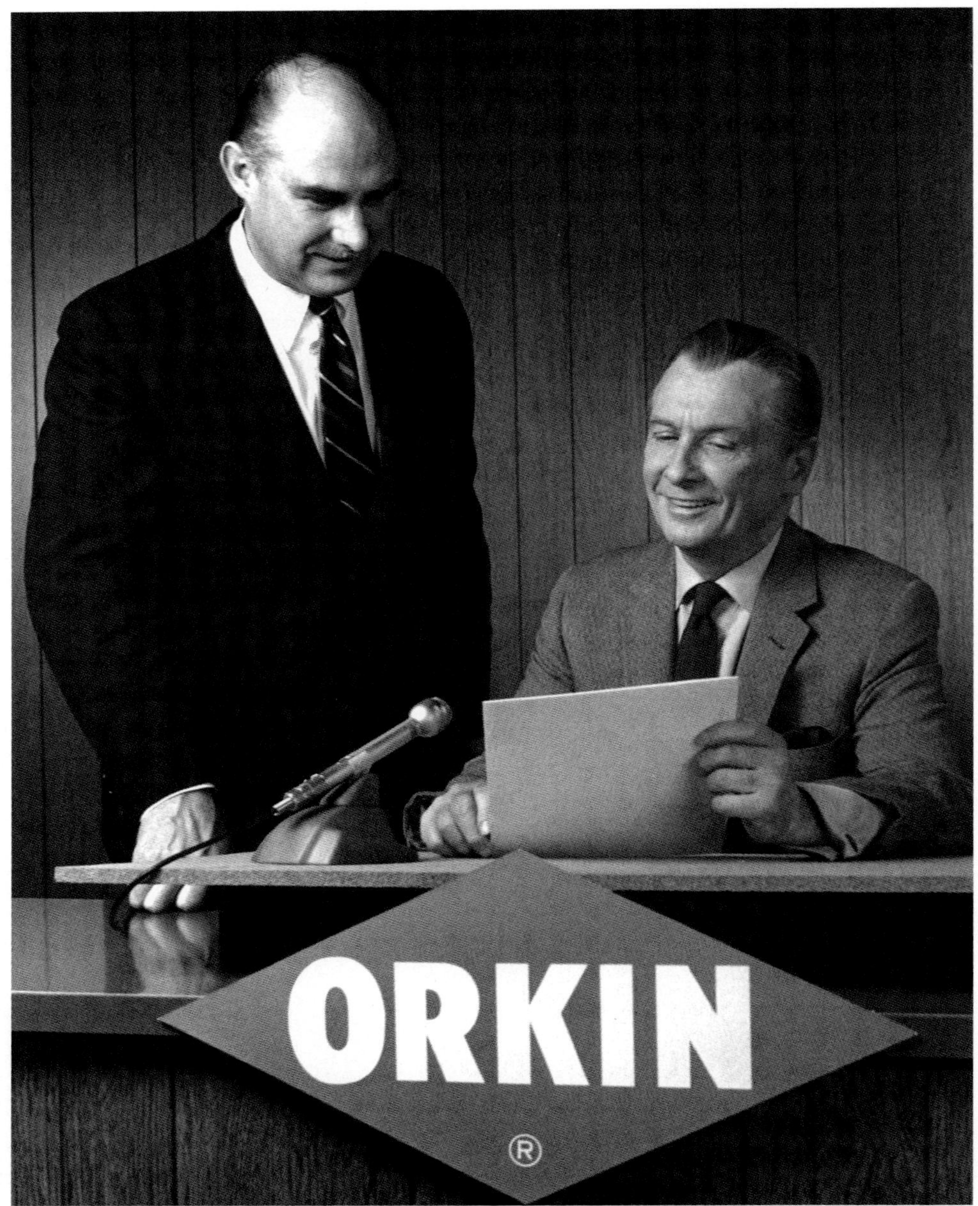

Orkin executive vice president Earl Geiger, left, and John Cameron Swayze, at one time the country's most famous news personality, look over the script for a television commercial Swayze did for Orkin in 1968.

was kindled by the $40 million Rat Control Bill enacted by Congress and aimed at fighting rats in urban slums. Wayne believed the principal benefit of the initial federal effort would be to develop public awareness because the money alone would not be enough to rid slums of rats. That job would fall to cities, landlords, and tenants. "It will be a matter of control," he told a journalist. "We will never be able to exterminate all the rats. They reproduce in thirty days."

At a conference in the Waldorf-Astoria Hotel in New York in October 1967, Orkin reviewed its national program to get rid of rats in cities around the country. Clearly, Orkin intended to claim its share of the rat control business—just as it continued to claim the lion's share of the nation's pest exterminating business.

Six-month earnings at the end of October 1967 were up 23 percent from the previous year. Rollins common stock split again, a five-for-four multiple, with an increase of 25 percent in the quarterly dividends pre-split. By January 1, 1968, Orkin had expanded from three regions to five, with operations in thirty-five states and the District of Columbia, Mexico, Guatemala, and Panama.

In the spring of 1968, John Cameron Swayze, arguably the country's most popular television news personality, starred in the company's new full-color TV commercials introducing the Orkin "12" plan for termite control and the OrkinGuard program of pest control protection. "It costs no more to have the best," advised Swayze in a commercial that proved highly successful in generating new leads. And though the television cameras weren't present, there were plenty of flashbulbs going off when Rollins, Inc.—"ROL"—was listed for the first time on the New York Stock Exchange on August 12, 1968. It had been nearly two months since Rollins had applied to list 4,626,291 of the shares of Rollins common stock with the exchange; Wayne Rollins held 1,698,220 shares, or 36.7 percent, and John Rollins owned 502,470 shares, or 12.6 percent. On August 12, watching from the floor of the stock exchange, Wayne and John broke into smiles when the electronic tape first rolled "ROL" on the Big Board. The price was 65 1/2.

The company's growth continued as shareholders received another stock dividend, a two-for-one split, plus a 20 percent pre-split increase in the dividend. The stock split was the third since 1961. When the books were closed for the fiscal year on April 30, 1969, Rollins, Inc.'s revenues hit $106.3 million. For the first time, the company's revenues exceeded the $100 million goal that Wayne had set when he first talked with Lehman Brothers executives about taking Rollins Broadcasting public in 1960.

But one of Wayne Rollins's favorite sayings—"Look behind good news"—would echo through the Piedmont Road home office hallways as the Orkin executives tackled some important issues—namely, employee retention and the creation of the Environmental Protection Agency.

POLICIES AND PROCEDURES

At one point, Gary Rollins admitted that the Orkin organization reminded him of the Wild West. When the Rollins family took over, there were few manuals and standardized procedures to help branch managers or district managers coordinate the services offered in the existing thirty-five states. There was no concentrated effort to coordinate vehicles and service trucks and drivers; when Gary moved into his position as vice president of Orkin operations, one of his first assignments was to review the inventory in the fleet department and match it up with designated drivers. "We helped to identify two thousand surplus vehicles, and none of them was missed," Gary said.

There were few written codes of conduct, few budget procedures and controls, and few branch standards. "What did I bring to the party?" Gary once reflected: "We took a pretty disjointed but wonderful business and started putting structure to it, putting some legs under it. It took about five years after Rollins purchased Orkin, but it became very clear that we were going to have law and order. That people who misrepresented the company were going to be terminated. A rogue employee would no longer make money at the expense of our company and customers. We started building the business up from the guy with the uniform and epaulets, putting in controls and balances at every level of the organization."

Porter Thompson, right, shown here accepting an award from Gary Rollins at Rollins's fiftieth-anniversary celebration, handled electronic data processing, the termite renewal department, Orkin Acceptance Corporation, payroll, and Rollins fleet and supply at various times during his service to the company.

Even *Pest Control* magazine noted in an article about Orkin that the "new emphasis of management . . . seems to be placed on organization and efficiency." At the home office, cleanliness, organization, and higher levels of commitment and productivity were the order of the day under the parent company. The building, offices, and furnishings were routinely inspected to ensure that everything was clean and properly organized. There were rules: desks had to be cleared every night; no coffee or drinks were allowed outside the break rooms and cafeteria. A home office dress code was enforced to ensure a professional appearance by all personnel. Under a system developed by Randall Rollins, policies and procedures for all functions were produced. Managers were expected to use an organizational method called the Lee List to prioritize their weekly tasks. Fred McColl began compiling and organizing the Orkin policies and procedures into the General Office Procedure Manual and the Pest Control and Termite Procedure Manuals, to name a few. Within several years, Rollins would create an official position for a "Policy and Procedures Analyst," later filled by such highly experienced and field-savvy individuals as Linda Morton, Barbara Ladner, and Cindy Bordes. In many ways Orkin and Rollins were

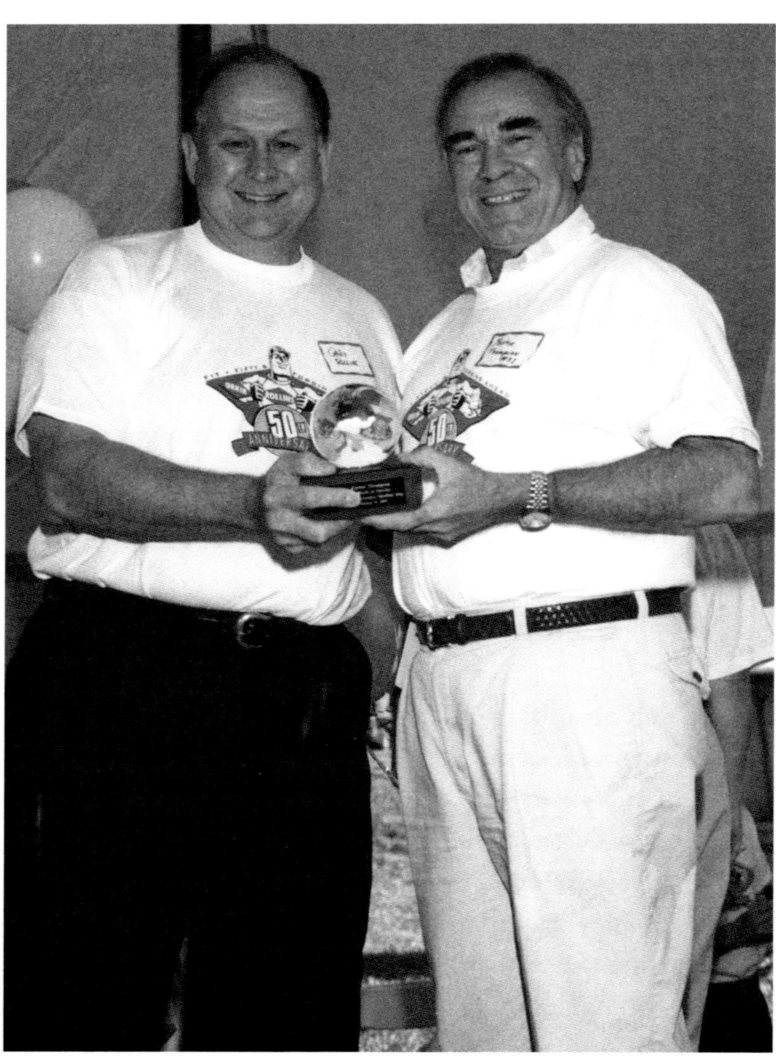

pioneers in their attempts to standardize procedures while making employees accountable and their efforts measurable. The value of measuring staff performance—which would be referred to as "human capital metrics" in about thirty years—was just beginning to surface in organizations and industries across the country.

Porter Thompson, a longtime Orkin employee who moved from data processing to be staff assistant to Randall Rollins before being named a home office vice president, used the organizational systems he learned at Orkin for the rest of his career. But he admitted that the early changes were difficult for many in the company to accept.

"There was a much higher level of accountability," said Thompson. "The Rollinses wanted you to make money, but they also wanted intense control and accountability over the process—two elements that were very difficult for a lot of people to accept willingly. With the first signs of cost cutting, some of the managers realized that they were not going to continue making the big money they had made before, and they felt threatened that the freedom and opportunities they had before were diminishing. In addition, we had to keep everything organized and clear our desks every night. This was quite different from my days with Orkin in the old West Peachtree location, where the place was not well maintained and the desks were hardly ever cleaned. In the Rollins structure, we would be inspected to ensure that things were clean, that everything was organized properly, that people were doing the right things, and that we were abiding by the rules. Some people found it very difficult to go along with this new structure."

Gary Rollins: "We took a pretty disjointed but wonderful business and started putting structure to it. . . . It took about five years after Rollins came into Orkin, but it became very clear that we were going to have law and order."

At the Orkin level, a heightened sense of organization was imposed, one deemed necessary not only by the ongoing acquisition of additional pest control companies but also by the growing magnitude of the original Orkin company. To help impose order and accountability, Orkin decided to switch from three to five regions, each headed by a vice president who reported to executive vice president Earl F. Geiger: Northeastern Region, Bernard Kolkana; Southeastern Region, Jack Dorris; Western Region, Walt Helms; Midwestern Region, Taft Pierce; and International Region, Louis Dettelbach. Within each region, districts were led by a manager, a sales manager, and a service manager. Within each district there were branch offices, staffed with a manager, a clerical staff, a sales force, supervisors for termite and pest control services, and service technicians. Like the distinctive uniforms worn by the Orkin Men, a standardized building design—with a revolving Orkin Diamond sign out front—was developed for all new branch locations. And under Orkin's new National Service Department,

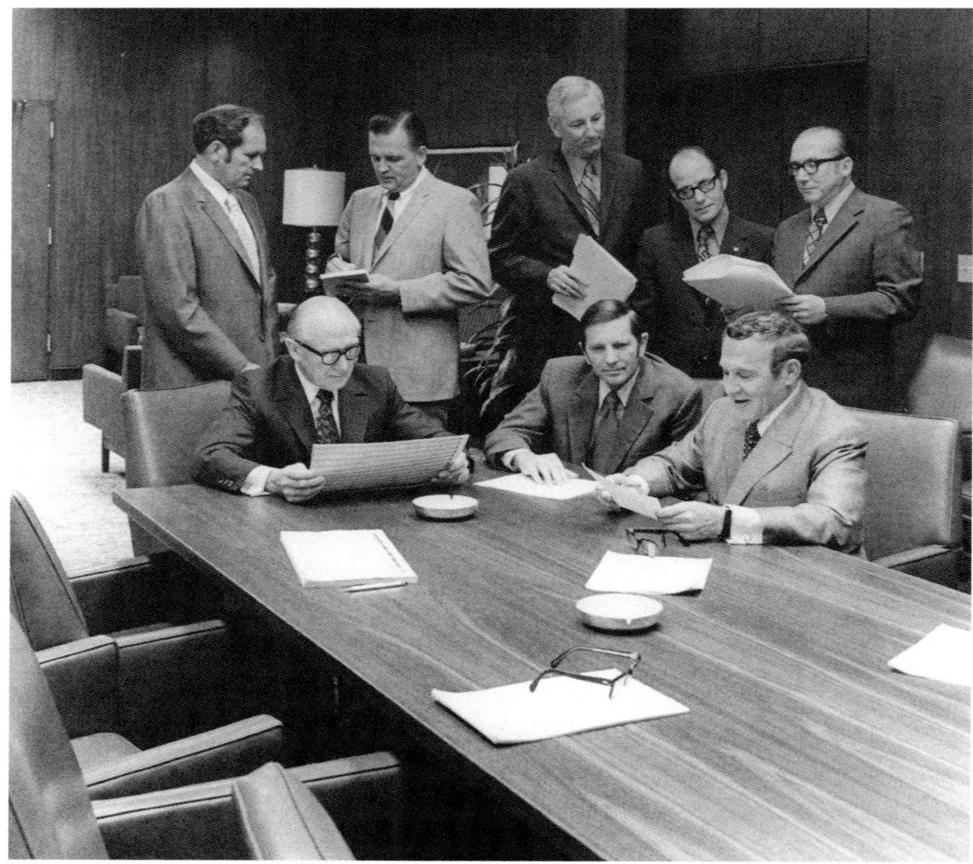

The management team during the late 1960s, left to right, standing: Jack Dorris, Paul Bowes, Taft Pierce, Walt Helms, and Ed Elkins; seated: Bernard Kolkana, Bob Russell, and Louis Dettelbach.

employees at almost every level received standardized technical training. Bob Russell, vice president, standards and training, headed up this new department, assisted by C. W. "Doc" Marshall, technical director, and Glenn Burkhalter, training director. Though training had always been emphasized by Orkin, the National Service Department pushed standardized company-wide training to a new level—through training to service personnel in branch offices, regional training conferences, and managers' training schools conducted at the home office. In addition, the National Service Department designed and developed treatments for all Orkin insect, rodent, and other pest control services, and selected equipment, insecticides, and methods of application for these services.

These new levels of organization did not bring order to Orkin immediately. In fact, the change from old to new, from flexibility to accountability, created chaos in the field. By some estimates, there was 60 to 80 percent turnover among the company's pest control service technicians in the late 1960s and early '70s, when Orkin restructured the pay schedule and removed commissions (often as high as 25 to 30 percent of production) from technicians, converting them to salaries. In many areas, pest control routes were reduced due to the loss of technicians. As the company continued to reorganize and downsize, some people lost their jobs.

Paul Hardy managed to survive. To this day, his office is filled with books on pest control technology, management techniques, entomology reference materials, and various scientific textbooks. John Neal, the sales representative in the Leesburg office in 1961, told Hardy what book to buy first—*Truman's Scientific Guide to Pest Control Operations,* published by Purdue University, which cost Hardy seventeen dollars on a forty-five-dollar weekly paycheck. This book opened up the pest control world to Hardy, and tapped an intellectual curiosity that this high school dropout didn't even know he had. "As I began to flip the pages and read, I got more and more interested in the subject, and I ended up outlining the book into an easier, understandable form and preparing review questions from each chapter. That was within my first ninety days of employment with Orkin. Then I found out about *The Mallis Handbook on Pest Control,* which is about two and a half inches thick. I outlined the entire *Mallis* and prepared questions from the chapters that I felt were relevant to the pest control business. In fact, those outlines became part of the study materials I used to train other people to take the state certification tests."

The new levels of organization did not bring order to Orkin immediately. In fact, the change from old to new, from flexibility to accountability, created chaos in the field.

When Hardy knew all the answers in the training classes taught by Doc Marshall and Bob Russell, they suggested that he start teaching. From 1964 to 1988 he assisted in teaching classes for state exams in Florida, Georgia, Mississippi, Tennessee, and South Carolina, often running branches at the same time (his passing percentage in Florida was 90–100 percent). Earlier, after serving as a termite technician and a pest control technician in Orlando and Cocoa Beach, Hardy went to Jacksonville in 1963 as a termite service supervisor, then on to Waycross as branch manager in 1966, then to Gainesville as manager in 1967, and finally he was named district service manager for north Florida–south Georgia in June 1969. In 1970 Kolkana sent Hardy to Tallahassee as a branch manager. By May 15, 1971, Hardy was driving a company-owned Chrysler New Yorker, a company credit card was in his wallet, and there was a new title beside his name: Paul Hardy, Southeast Region Service Manager. His first assignment was to bring accountability and standards to the branches, using a "Branch Check List" system that still exists. Paul was an excellent example of opportunity coming from all the changes that were taking place.

With the "accountability" message now coming from inside of Orkin, rank and file began to settle down. Toward the end of fiscal year 1968, Orkin had introduced new sales programs for management and sales personnel that were designed to increase Orkin's share of what was then a $700 million pest control market, which was expected to double by the early 1970s. The company began test-marketing a new automated aerosol system—Orkin-Aire—designed to control bacteria, flying insects, and odors.

But in reality, the yin and yang of order and chaos were actually the watchwords for the company for the next several years. Employee turnover remained high, even as management sought to impose order and formality. Customer retention was up and down, though sales continued to grow dramatically. New services and innovations came and went as fast as state and federal government regulations could be typed up and presented to the field. Pesticides that had been used for thirty years would suddenly be phased out, and technicians and servicemen would require new products, new training, and new messages to communicate to an anxious public.

At Orkin no one escaped the whirlwind of change, not even the bookkeepers. "Taft Pierce was a great person for changing methods, procedures, and ways of doing things," said Lowell Buckingham, an auditor in the south Florida region. "We used to say he was next to God in creation because he would always be inventing forms and making changes. I remember one time he got after me because I must not have liked making a change, and he said, 'Lowell! You've got to stop fighting change! Change is good. Sometimes it's what we need.'"

ACQUISITION AND DIVERSIFICATION

After six years of ownership, the order that the Rollins-Orkin executives tried to impose on their organization no doubt flew in the face of the overall evolution that would soon confront both the pest control industry and Orkin nearly every day. And ironically, it was often in contrast to the exciting, sometimes surprising, news coming out of Rollins headquarters. From the late 1960s to 1990, Wayne Rollins and his company were on an acquisition and business-building roll that would leave other companies breathless. Rollins was about to enter into a new era of diversification, a time when company revenues would climb from $106 million to $500 million in just thirteen years. For the men in the field, perhaps, it was proof positive that their new boss, O. Wayne Rollins, meant what he said when he first stopped by with his "NOW" cards and gave them all this message: "*If you wait until you're ready, you'll never do anything.*"

First, there was Dwoskin, Inc., the country's largest wholesale distributor of wallcoverings and a leading supplier of fabrics and carpets for the decorator, and one of the South's top painting and interior decorating contractors—acquired by Rollins on January 1, 1968. Then, in 1969, Rollins developed and introduced the first affordable wireless security systems for burglar and fire alarms; two years later, a new Rollins division called Rollins Protective Services (RPS) began marketing and servicing these monitored electronic security systems in homes and businesses. By the end of 1969, Rollins received FCC approval to begin operating its cable television system in Wilmington, Delaware, while its building maintenance company, now called Rollins Services, continued to be one of the largest in the Southeast and Southwest. By 1970, Orkin offices in thirty-five states, the District of Columbia, and Mexico serviced more than one million residential and commercial accounts.

A five-year phase-in period for the EPA to apply and enforce the FIFRA laws produced some of the greatest changes in the history of the pest control industry from 1972 through 1977.

When Rollins Protective Services (RPS) was formed, this division would also need customer financing; the name of Orkin Acceptance Corporation was changed to a more generic name, State Fidelity, to provide customer financing throughout the company. In 1977, the name of the finance company would change again—to Rollins Acceptance Corporation, or RAC.

With such growth, new services, and company-wide expansion, it's little wonder that Rollins set all-time record revenues and earnings by the end of fiscal year 1971—with revenues over $127 million; net earnings after taxes of $10 million; and per share earnings up from $1.18 in 1970 to $1.25 in 1971. Through this financial success, Orkin retired the first half of its convertible debt from the Orkin deal to Prudential Insurance Company for $11.25 million. Exactly one year and one day later, Rollins, Inc., retired the second half of Orkin's convertible debt for another $11.25 million, paying off the indebtedness without having it converted into Orkin stock ownership by Prudential. Reclaiming the stock had been one of Wayne's key goals when the company bought Orkin.

As the Rollins corporation continued to grow, factors beyond its control would influence the company. In 1970 the Environmental Protection Agency (EPA) was created as the federal enforcement agency for FIFRA legislation. There was a five-year phase-in period for the EPA to apply and enforce the FIFRA laws, and that period from 1972 through 1977 produced some of the greatest changes in the history of the pest control industry. Bob Russell, who had returned to Orkin in 1965 as technical director and was eventually promoted to vice president of government relations, became the company's expert in government regulations and legislation that affected the industry. For Russell it was familiar territory; in the 1960s Russell had worked diligently to understand the regulatory agencies and congressional committees in Washington, and he had reestablished Orkin's once fragile liaison with the NPCA while working with governmental agencies for both Orkin and the industry as a whole. Both Russell and Gary Rollins began attending the annual meetings of the National Association of State Departments of Agriculture (NASDA) and the Southern Association of State Departments of Agriculture (SASDA); Orkin was regulated in most states by the Department of Agriculture, so developing relationships with these southern and national associations' members was very important. When the EPA took over enforcement of FIFRA regulations, representing the start of one of the greatest periods of change in the pest control industry, Russell was at the forefront, working to reach agreements on less restrictive regulations and a more commonsense approach.

"The early issues with the EPA concerned where you could spray, how often you could spray, and the chemical you could use," Russell said. In his lobbying efforts, Russell often worked with Congressman Richard Ray from Perry, Georgia, a former pest control operator who had sold his Ray Pest Control to Getz. "The formula for working with the bureaucracy is, first, they have to get to know you," said Russell. "Second, they have to get to like you and respect you. Then, third, they *may* do something for you."

One of Russell's most successful agreements involved the problem of overlapping regulations. For instance, the state could penalize a company for a violation, and the EPA could immediately impose another penalty for the same violation. Or as Russell put it, "When EPA started, the state would zap you, and EPA would come along and they would zap you." Through his Washington contacts, Russell worked to encourage fair and appropriate legislation that gave the state "primacy of regulation"; the EPA would serve only as backup regulator if a state failed to handle the situation appropriately.

With their extensive pest control backgrounds, Bob Russell and Paul Hardy—as well as Doc Marshall, Bud Snyder, and Eddie Faircloth Jr.—often collaborated on developing equipment for Orkin with the assistance of equipment companies like B&G Equipment and Black & Decker. According to Hardy, the evolution of modern exterminating equipment can be traced back to the early 1960s, when the liquid organic phosphates and new pesticides became available and the use of dust products decreased. From traditional hand dusters and atomizers, servicemen began to use spray devices like the custom-designed stainless steel compressed air sprayer B&G developed with Orkin's name on the side. Everyone in the industry knew that such spray devices had to meet two criteria: first, when it came to application, it had to be precise; and second, when it came to chemicals, the goal was to use as little as possible while still providing effective pest control.

For termite treatments, Orkin technicians also needed a reliable drill—but most standard drills would not hold up for termite servicemen, who had to be able to drill continuously, often in cramped quarters. The Skil 736, a pneumatic hammer developed by Skil in 1967 to drill cement floors and porches, was humorously referred to as a "man killer," Hardy once said, because it was so hard to work with; the equipment manufacturer worked with Orkin on several different models before dropping that line of equipment in the late 1970s.

As the new EPA regulations and protocols were being developed, Orkin worked with Micro-Gen to design a small commercial misting application unit to treat large spaces with the least amount of chemicals to control harmful pests in commercial accounts. Little did anyone know that a Micro-Gen unit, carried overseas by an Orkin Man, would soon get an amazing amount of publicity when, in 1972, the Orkin branch office in Washington, D.C., got a call for help from the American Embassy in Moscow: roaches, it seemed, had taken over the embassy. Within three weeks, Orkin entomologist Glenn Burkhalter, the company's training director, left for Moscow, where he found a heavy infestation of both German roaches and Oriental roaches in the U.S. Embassy. Glenn worked for twelve days to get rid of the roaches. And before he left, he trained a Russian national employed by the embassy to make the necessary monthly follow-up treatments.

In addition to overseas roach control, there were a few more surprises in store for Orkin and its parent company in 1972. In May Rollins acquired

The equipment commonly used in the early 1970s included, bottom row, left to right, a flashlight, a dust applicator, a service kit, the B&G one-gallon pressurized sprayer, along with, top row, the Orkin-Aire aerosol dispenser, a granule hand applicator, a fogger, and a hand pump duster. Service manager Jerry Adams demonstrates the B&G.

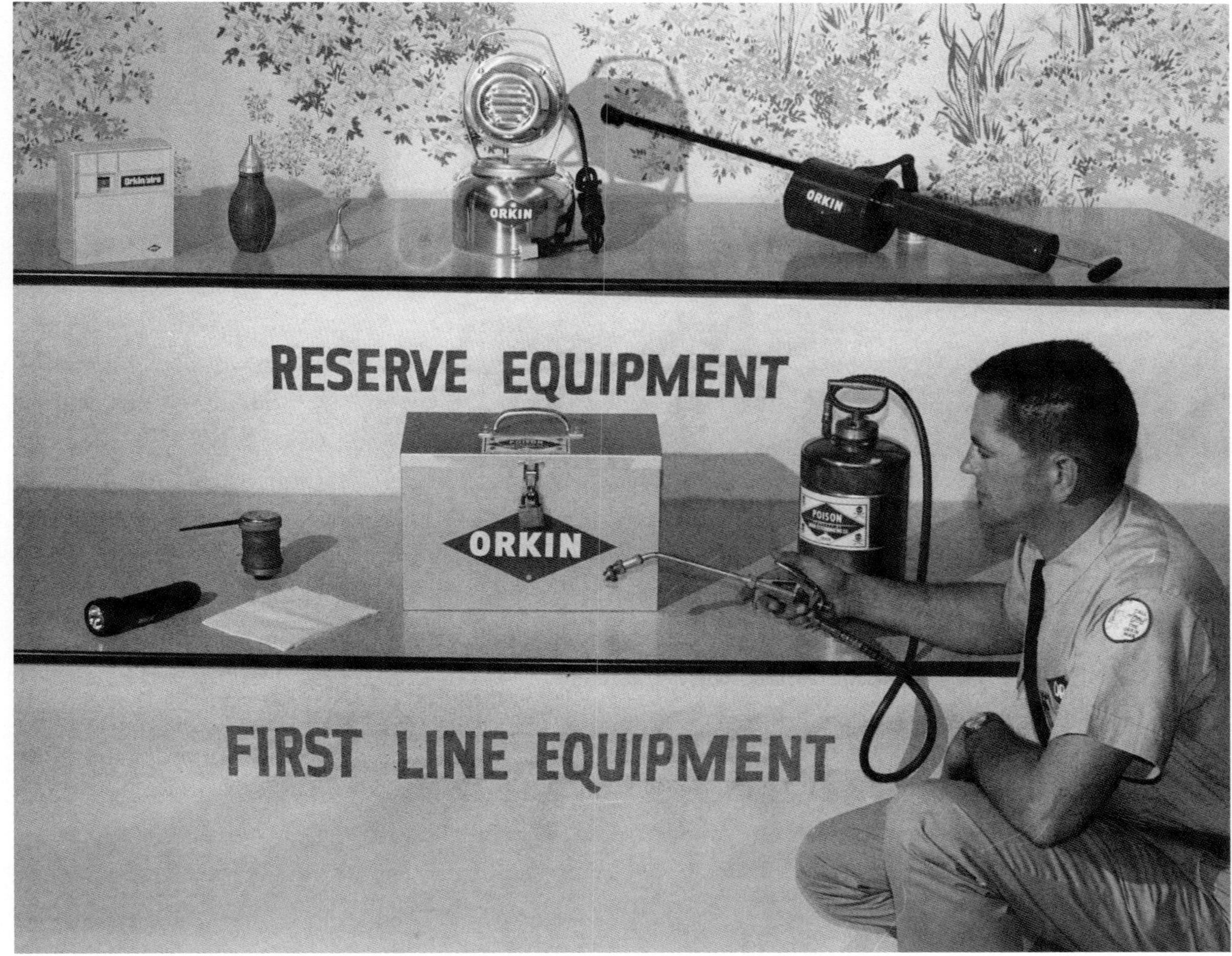

United Buying Service of New York, the leader in the consumer buying field with discount prices on everything from furniture to furs, cars, cameras, appliances, stereos, eyeglasses, and travel. On the media side of business, Rollins Outdoor Advertising was experiencing strong growth and had made several acquisitions: Alford Outdoor Advertising Company in Austin, Texas; Dixie Sign of Ocean City, Maryland; and ABS Advertising Co. of Corpus Christi, Texas. Rollins Broadcasting sold a few properties and began cable TV operations in three more Delaware towns.

In 1972, Gary Rollins had worked himself up to manager of the Marietta, Georgia, Orkin branch. "I totally enjoyed my job. Branch manager is one of the best jobs in the company."

But the company's biggest announcement in 1972 involved Gary Rollins. After five years with Orkin, Gary had worked his way up to be branch manager in Marietta, Georgia, the fifth-largest branch in the company; after Gary took over, revenue grew and profits in the branch had increased about 30 percent. Gary's boss was Ed Elkins, whose path would cross with his again in the future. "I totally enjoyed my job," remembered Gary, then twenty-eight, married, and the father of three young children. "Branch manager is one of the best jobs in the company."

One day, unexpectedly, Gary was called into the Rollins home office executive suite. "How would you like to go into Dwoskin?" Wayne Rollins asked his younger son.

"I could not have been more startled," Gary remembered. For one thing, he liked what he was doing at Orkin and the progress of his branch. And he knew that Dwoskin, Rollins's wall-covering distribution division, had serious problems; this low-margin, inventory-intense, undisciplined business was the exact opposite of the low-inventory, strong-margin, low-capital business he had grown accustomed to at Orkin. Dwoskin's computer programs, once expected to be the finest in the industry, "were just a disaster," Gary knew.

Despite Gary's misgivings, Wayne Rollins convinced his son that he could handle the challenges, and he named Gary general manager of Dwoskin. At the same time, the Rollins Board of Directors elected Gary as vice president of Rollins, Inc. For three years, he worked to unravel Dwoskin's operating problems and put the business on a solid fiscal footing. It wasn't easy. The process, said Gary, was "almost like trying to bail out a rowboat when someone's in the back with a brace and bit boring a hole." Numerous inventory problems existed. In fact, at one point, he discovered a theft ring in the large Atlanta distribution center and engaged an undercover agent to catch the thieves. For the first time in his career, Gary was working under Randall, and he routinely had the opportunity to seek advice from his father and his brother on management problems while searching for solutions to the company's habitual cash flow shortages. The Dwoskin experience, Gary eventually realized, was probably equivalent to attaining a master's degree in business administration. Gradually, he developed policies, procedures, and systems, initiated management recruiting to replace inadequate employees, established controls (many of which were taken from Orkin), worked with suppliers, and organized the sales force. Randall, Gary, and their new team helped instill discipline especially in the area of overstocking new lines of inventory and, with Randall's assistance, assembled a solid management team. And he began to realize that he had developed his own management and decision-making style. The sons used to tease their father that his management style involved seeing the big picture, following his instinct, and finding the right people to fill in the details. Randall's approach was to study the details of every conceivable angle of a situation thoroughly, developing reports and summaries of data before he felt comfortable making decisions. Gary realized that he was "somewhere in the middle" of these two styles. He would listen to arguments from both sides, gather enough but not too much information, and then make his decisions after weighing what everyone had to say. Randall, at one point, called him an "equalizer."

By 1975 Dwoskin turned a profit. With the threat of a recession looming, however, Rollins decided that it was time to sell the nation's largest wallpaper distributor. Fortunately, a subsidiary of Reed Paper, Ltd., of Toronto, a division of the world's largest paper manufacturer, was a motivated acquirer and purchased Dwoskin for $9 million. "It was an exit with a certain amount of—'glory' would be too strong of a statement—but we went out of it with our head up," said Gary. "Our biggest supplier bought us, and although I can't say we got rich with the business, it was a favorable sale on our behalf. And one of the real positives of the Dwoskin experience is that I got to work with my brother."

Only after the Dwoskin sale did Gary dare ask his father this question: "Why did you put me in that job? Do you know how close I came to just wanting to throw in the towel, being overwhelmed with all the internal and external forces?"

"Well, for one thing," Wayne Rollins replied, "I thought you could do it. For another thing, I knew I could trust you and that I wouldn't get so mad that I would fire you."

From his unique vantage point, Randall Rollins, who was elected president and chief operating officer of Rollins, Inc., in October 1975, enjoyed watching his father and brother interact. As he would later say, "Gary has a lot of Dad's characteristics. I think that Dad had a charisma about him. I think Gary has that, too. They both have good people skills. He's a quick thinker. There's thirteen years difference in our ages and while I've never thought of Gary as anything but my brother, I'm as proud of him as a son. And I've said many times that he'll be a lot better in business than I am. I really believe that. I just think that he's taken some of my qualities and taken some of Dad's, and that's a good mix."

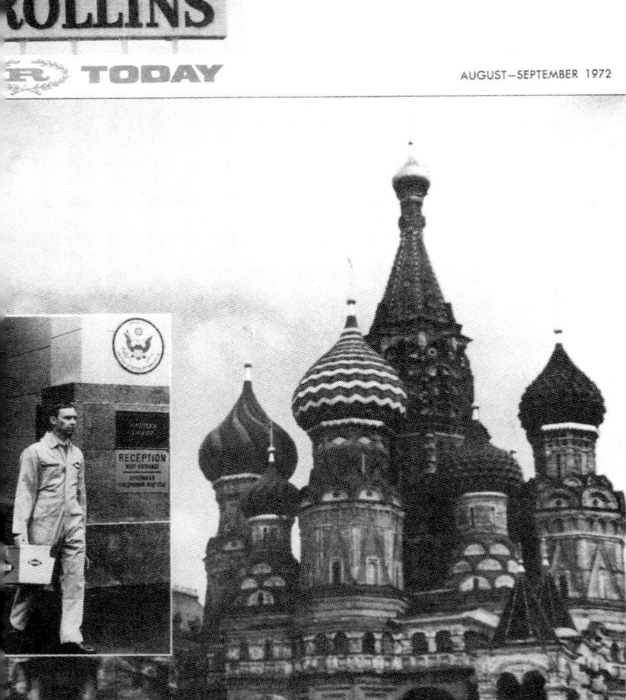

The fact that Wayne trusted Gary to handle the Dwoskin challenges gave the Rollins chief executive the time he needed to focus on the other business deals on his corporate plate. In 1973 the company took a bold leap and entered the oil and gas services business when it purchased Patterson Companies of Houma, Louisiana. Patterson, a family business founded in 1945, fit the Rollins concept of a service company: it provided trucking and equipment rental to oil and gas companies and crews operating in seven southern and Gulf Coast states, serving many offshore

Orkin entomologist Glenn F. Burkhalter, the company's training director, flew to Moscow to get rid of a heavy infestation of German and Oriental roaches in the U.S. Embassy. Glenn worked for twelve days to rid the embassy and some forty apartments leased by the embassy of the roaches.

Glenn Burkhalter

It's been called the "longest known service call in the history of the pest control industry"—an eleven-thousand-mile round trip made by an Orkin Man to combat roaches at the American Embassy in Moscow. And by the time it was over, Glenn Burkhalter, the Orkin Man in Russia, was like a hero to the Russian citizens who met him.

It began like most Orkin customer relationships—with a call for help. In the spring of 1972, the administrative officer of the American Embassy in Moscow wrote to Orkin offices in Washington, D.C., asking for guidance because roaches were taking over the entire embassy. There was no pest control industry in Russia; the government service called upon to get rid of the prolific pests couldn't even begin to cure the problem. The letter made its way to the home office in Atlanta, and Orkin quickly agreed to study the situation and provide the service free of charge. At Orkin's request, the embassy sent over two sets of specimens: German roaches, it turned out, had invaded the embassy.

To handle the extermination assignment—which included eliminating the roaches in the embassy building, the ambassador's residence, and some forty staff apartments—Orkin tapped Glenn Burkhalter, an entomologist and training director for the Orkin division. Married with two children, Glenn had worked for Orkin since 1961. He considered the Russian assignment the "experience of a lifetime" when he boarded a Pan Am–Delta Flight in Atlanta on June 7 and arrived in Moscow some seventeen hours later. For twelve days, Glenn worked to "debug" the buildings, using materials that he had shipped over and cleared in advance. For a lot of the work, he used the compact Micro-Gen, a small motor-powered unit designed to apply pest control chemicals at ultra-low-volume (ULV). Under the ULV method, the liquid pesticide is broken down into minute particles that, Orkin research showed, provided quicker and enhanced contact as compared to other applicators. And everywhere he went, Glenn was dressed in his crisp Orkin uniform, and carried his supplies in a tool kit that sported the Orkin Diamond.

Throughout the embassy, Glenn discovered not only German roaches but some of an Oriental species. And in

drilling installations. When the gasoline shortage hit in early 1974 and prices at the pump climbed dramatically, the newly acquired Patterson Services saw its earnings rise sharply. The oil price escalation, however, could hurt a business that depended heavily on vehicles—like Orkin. Bulk fuel tanks were placed at the large Orkin branches and at the home office, tanks in some cases that held up to thirty thousand gallons of gasoline. And though the Orkin servicemen strongly objected, the Orkin fleet of full-size American pickups was replaced with small Japanese-imported trucks in order to conserve gasoline and oil.

RENEWED FOCUS ON ORKIN

After the sale of Dwoskin, Gary Rollins returned to Orkin as vice president of operations under Earl Geiger. His three years with Dwoskin—which Gary often referred to as his "baptism by fire"—had given the young executive a sense of cautious confidence. Exactly like his father, he even started telling stories and jokes to illustrate business principles, finding just the right

a quirk of entomology lore, Glenn pointed out that while there was no known Russian species of roach, the Oriental roach was known in East Germany as the Russian roach.

During his stay, Glenn became something of a hero to those around him, working effectively and efficiently to stop the roach infestation and to train a Russian maintenance employee named Alexander to do the follow-up work when he left. The Orkin Man also found time to keep a diary and do some sightseeing—writing about his wonderful experiences at the circus and on a three-hour riverboat cruise; having dinner on the twenty-first floor of the Rossiea Hotel, overlooking the Kremlin; finding time to ride the subways; and shopping for an antique Russian samovar to give his wife, Carolyn, for her birthday in July.

His mission accomplished, Glenn returned to the United States on June 21. An avalanche of publicity greeted him. Everyone, it seemed, wanted to know about the trip that wiped out the roaches at our Moscow embassy. Glenn was interviewed on the NBC *Today* program by Barbara Walters and Frank McGee. Then he appeared on *What's My Line?*—a syndicated program with Arlene Francis, Anita Gillette, Jack Cassidy, and Soupy Sales. He proudly wore his Orkin Man uniform when he appeared on *To Tell the Truth,* another national television show, and *Today in Georgia,* a local show on WSB-TV. A picture of Glenn in his Orkin Man uniform, walking into the U.S. Embassy, made a big splash in the Rollins 1972 Annual Report.

Though the trip of a lifetime was over, Glenn always remembered one special moment during his trip, when he was tired and hungry but happened to enter the embassy commissary late in the day, near closing time. The American clerk told him he had only one minute to get what he needed—but changed her tune when someone yelled out, "He's the Bug Man!" Glenn recorded the moment in his diary. "She yelled down the aisle, 'I'm sorry. If you're going to get rid of our bugs, you take all the time you want.'"

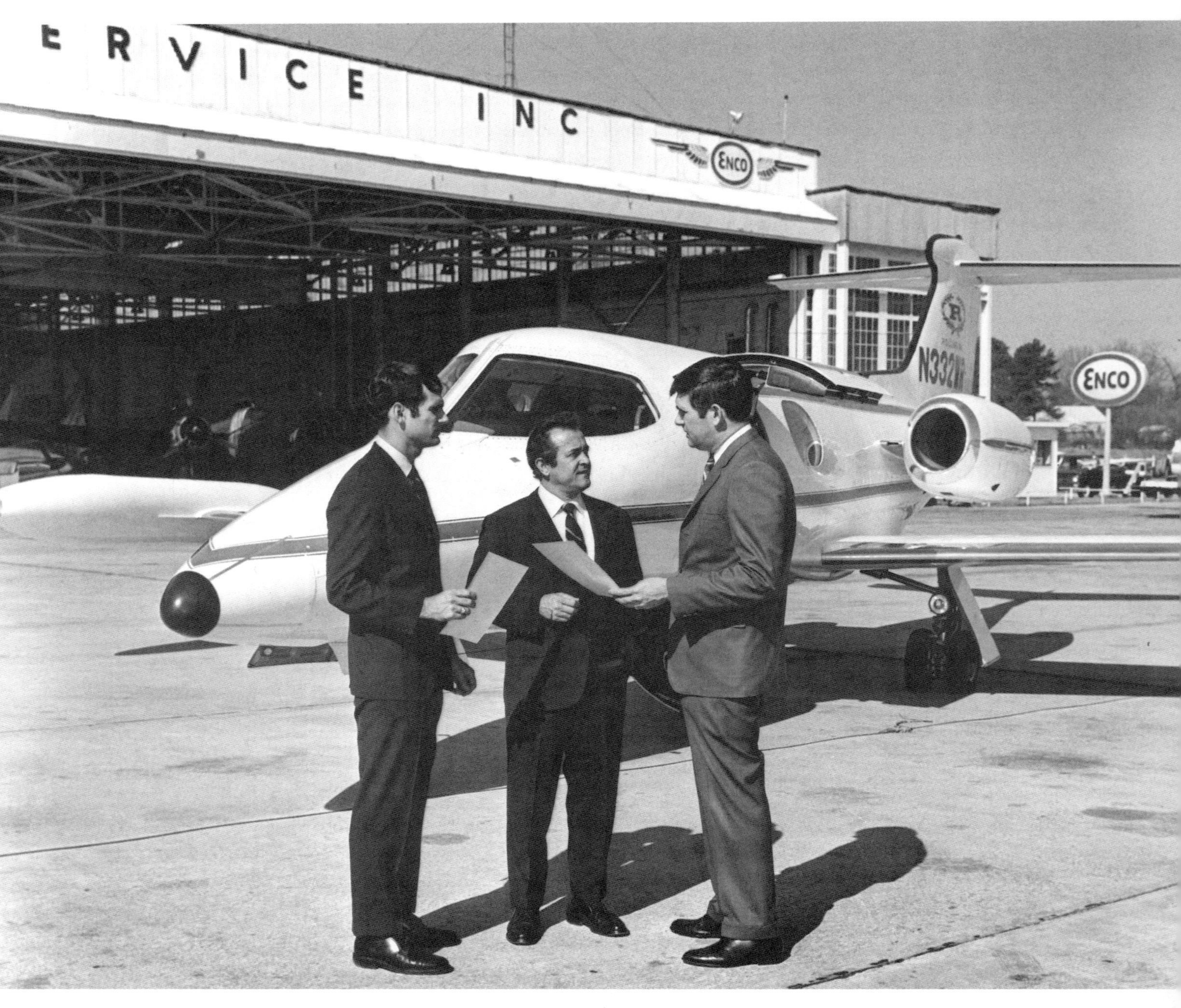

With Rollins, Inc. holding a variety of companies with locations all over the country in the early 1970s, company executives used the corporate jets to cut down travel time. Left to right: pilot Charlie Campbell, chief pilot Joe Anastasia, and Randall Rollins.

tone to deliver the message: "I heard this story about a fella who listens to just one radio station: W-I-I FM. 'What's in it for me. . . .'" Those around Gary noticed that he was clearly a bit tougher around the edges, and less naive, now that his work world was larger than pest control. But he stayed grounded in his own past, always sensitive to the demands of the frontline Orkin Man, an aspect of Gary's rise through the organization that always guaranteed him a vital connection with employees.

Though Orkin had made a dozen acquisitions of smaller pest control companies around the country while he was away, Gary felt back at home in no time. Aware of the rapidly changing world of environmental regulations, he quickly created a Government Relations Department headed by Bob Russell to become more involved in federal and state regulatory and industry matters, and assisted in establishing numerous code-of-conduct initiatives to properly describe appropriate sales and service behavior. He continued to push for the standardization of operating policies, procedures, and equipment for Orkin from coast to coast. John Raymond, a former branch manager in six locations, was tapped by Gary in 1976 to be his first director of administrative operations. That same year, Gary, with Randall's encouragement, led the transition from using Kinro, Orkin's in-house advertising agency, to hiring an outside advertising agency, J. Walter Thompson (JWT), and designating that a certain percentage of the previous year's revenue be routinely spent on advertising. At the time, the agency had no way of knowing that it was beginning what would become one of the longest-running client-agency relationships in the world of advertising. JWT's first national Orkin campaign—"Big Number One"—rolled out in 1977 and became a national award-winning campaign.

Orkin hired J. Walter Thompson as its advertising agency in 1976, beginning one of the longest-running client-agency relationships in the world of advertising.

In a short time Orkin management focused on two more issues. They wanted to improve the company's position as both a residential and commercial pest control operator, and began working on plans to expand the company's commercial business.

Rollins Lawn Care, a new division designed to provide fertilization, aeration, and other related lawn services to homes, was introduced. The service, which had originated with an Orkin lawn care service offering in Florida, fit well with the protective and exterminating home services provided by the company. It promoted the basic premise that a business could perform the lawn care work as cheaply as the homeowner—while eliminating the owner's work and related time. Orkin executives recognized that it even had an advantage over Orkin's pest control treatments. Namely, a lawn could be treated when no one was home. And with the introduction of Rollins Lawn Care, Rollins and Orkin now had a bundle of services they could sell to the same consumer.

In spite of these many changes and improvements, Wayne Rollins was not satisfied with Orkin's performance. Granted, Orkin was still the cash cow for Rollins, bringing in triple the revenues of any other division. But in Wayne's opinion, it wasn't meeting its potential and performing as well as it should. As Gary Rollins described it, "The train came off the track."

Though the company's 1977 revenue of $138 million was up 6 percent from the year before, the increase was dismal when compared to Rollins's oil and gas operations (a 34 percent increase in revenues) and media operations (a 16 percent increase in revenues). To top it off, Orkin was the only Rollins division to report a drop in earnings that year. The 1977 Annual Report noted that the "severe winter and much cooler weather than usual in early spring" was largely to blame for the lack of significant growth in revenues and a decrease in earnings. But from the chairman's perspective, there was more to blame than the weather. When he looked at Orkin, he saw a company that had grown stagnant and flabby, one that appeared more interested in sales, sales, sales than in customer service and retention. His goal was to move Orkin to the next level, to refocus the company's efforts on basic business elements. This time, he didn't turn to Earl Geiger for advice or leadership. He turned to Randall to help him make it happen.

From January 25 to February 1, 1978, Randall Rollins convened one of the most unprecedented executive lockdowns in Orkin history. In a Hilton Hotel near the Memphis, Tennessee, airport, Randall and Gary Rollins and their top Orkin regional vice presidents did nothing but eat, sleep, and drink Orkin—a marathon review of every conceivable Orkin policy and procedure in order to figure out how to improve the business, increase revenue, and get earnings back on track. Randall's reputation for detail left nothing to chance—manuals, equipment, and boxes of documents were flown in for the meeting. But he forgot one thing. He failed to mention to the regional VPs that they'd be staying in Memphis for as long as it took to get the job done, and the eight Orkin executives summoned on January 25 honestly believed they would be away from homes and offices for an overnight meeting. Instead, they stayed for seven long nights and eight days, coping with decidedly lean wardrobes by washing out socks and underwear in the hotel sinks when they finally got back to their rooms each night.

In 1977, Orkin was the only Rollins division to report a drop in earnings. Wayne Rollins looked at Orkin and saw a company that had grown stagnant and flabby.

"Randall set the stage," recalled Harvey L. Massey, then regional vice president for the Central states. "We were going to look at every policy, every procedure, every system we had. And we were going to change anything that needed changing—administrative or operational. We argued and we hollered, all in order to find consensus and reach agreement. It was heated at times, but there was a bond. Our goal was to identify the five most important things that needed to be done and then go and do them."

Remembered James E. Cotton, then vice president of the Northeast Region: "We were isolated, we were sequestered, we were there for over a week. Tempers flared. People were pretty forceful putting their opinions across. I remember one exchange between Massey and Randall, where Massey had commented that a million dollars was not a lot of money, in relation to what the company was trying to achieve. And that upset Randall. 'It may not be a lot of money to you, but it certainly is a lot of money to me, Bud!' It's a wonder we didn't kill each other. But I honestly think they felt that once they got this Orkin animal harnessed, that it could do great things. And it *did*."

And there was another thing that Joe Wilson, then vice president of the midwestern region, never forgot about Memphis: "It was a meeting to affirm that Gary was indeed going to be in charge. Randall was running this meeting, but Gary was about to take over and run the company. For Gary, this meeting really taught him the business. It was like someone handed him the bicycle without the training wheels."

When the Memphis meeting adjourned, Randall immediately sent an unusual executive "thank you" to spouses of those who had unexpectedly been away from home so long; he gave each wife a deluxe Cuisinart, a kitchen appliance that was so innovative and much-coveted at the time that many wives later joked that Randall could kidnap their husbands whenever he wanted.

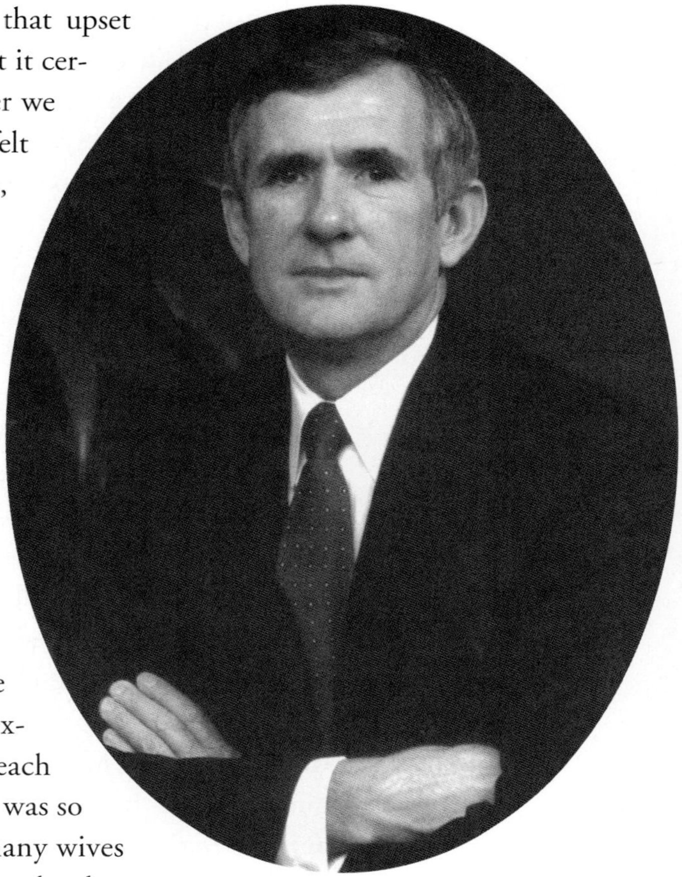

Early in 1978, Randall Rollins convened a meeting with Gary and the Orkin regional vice presidents at the Hilton Hotel near the Memphis airport. The purpose was to change anything operational or administrative that needed changing in order to take Orkin to the next level.

Then Randall, Gary, and the vice presidents traveled all over the country to explain the new policies and procedures to Orkin management—a commitment that took until the end of March. They held firm to their five top principles: grow the business, service the business, collect money, control expenses, and promote people. Said Massey, who later left Orkin and is now president and CEO of Massey Services, Inc.: "Regardless of what you hear, Orkin created the management template for the industry, and the groundwork was certainly done during those eight days in Memphis. The procedures, the policies, how to hold people accountable—Orkin created all of that. To this day, they created a standard for management that you can use to run a great service company."

The Memphis meeting was something of a watershed moment for the Rollins family and its management of Orkin. Because Earl Geiger was not invited to participate in the Memphis meetings, any ties to the old Orkin management style were clearly broken. For Randall, the Memphis meeting represented his first involvement with making management decisions for Orkin, because his areas of expertise had always been with other Rollins divisions; though no one knew it then, this meeting foreshadowed a unique working relationship between the two Rollins brothers, one in which the success of the business was far more important than marking off executive turf. For Gary, who was then vice president of Orkin operations, the Memphis meeting was a crash course in everything he would one day need to manage the company. And that day came sooner rather than later.

In July 1978, in a major restructuring of the Rollins executive offices, Gary Rollins was named president of Orkin. In the new corporate alignment, William Alias was named president of Rollins Protective Services; James C. Roddey, president of the media division; and Fred W. Rowley, president of both Rollins Building Services and Rollins Lawn Care, with all four reporting to Randall. When Gary was appointed president, former Orkin auditor Charles Risinger couldn't help but remember the words of advice he had given to the future company president the first time he met Gary at the Gainesville, Georgia, branch: "If you work hard, you're going to amount to something!"

In reality, Gary Rollins was the first new Orkin president since the Rollins family purchased the company in 1964. Until then, Earl Geiger, who now became vice chairman of the parent company, had always held the title of executive vice president and division head, but never president. After three years of directing Orkin's field operations, the new president found himself in charge of a company whose profit margins had been rapidly deteriorating. Immediately, Gary set out to follow the principles set forth in the Memphis meeting, working to streamline the business, reduce its excessive workforce, and increase what Orkin charged for its services. He was the first executive to initiate a company-wide annual price increase program for pest control and termite services, as well as rate cards specific to various regions of the country.

In order to explain his new policies—and perhaps to soften the blow of so many changes—Gary started his annual field "Road Shows" and "Halftime" conferences for branch and region managers. First, he told them, "We're going to have fewer people but better-paid people." Second, he admitted that the company cuts were still "a very bitter pill to swallow, but our loyalty must be to the employees who stay and to making our company healthier." Third, with fewer people, everyone was going to have to work harder. "The average calls per day for an Orkin pest control technician was ten. We figured it should be fourteen," said Gary.

But instead of focusing on the past, he tried to convey the company's future plans and how the reductions would eventually benefit those who remained. "One of the things that I told them is that we work for a company and that how well the *company* does depends on how well *they* do and how hard *they* work. I promised them that if we all worked hard, they wouldn't have to read in the newspaper about their company closing down or laying off more people. I told them that we were blessed in that there are bugs and rodents out there, and they're multiplying twenty-four hours a day. And the Japanese can't import what we do. I think this commitment gave our employees a sense of security, that as long as they do their job and do it well, they're going to have a job. And one of the things that I try to convey to our folks is that there's no preordained decision that a 'Rollins' has to run this company. So if you really want a job or a job like mine, then go for it."

Harvey L. Massey: "Orkin created the management template for the industry. . . . The procedures, the policies, how to hold people accountable—Orkin created all of that."

Together, Randall and Gary demonstrated that they were not averse to trying something new, to in essence "go for it." In January 1979 Randall decided to take one branch aside and set it up as a developmental branch—a laboratory of sorts to try out new ideas, new procedures, and new techniques in order to improve the bottom line. They chose the Decatur, Georgia, Orkin branch, which had one of the company's most dismal records and exceptionally high employee turnover. Ed Strickland, who joined Orkin in 1977 as head of customer services, was asked to run what he eventually called the Decatur project, and he started with one premise: "We weren't going to hurt it. It had so many problems, we didn't think that we could mess it up."

First up, new and improved uniforms and a stronger work ethic for the branch employees. Ed cut nine routes down to five and increased productivity and earnings, with each route technician increasing from eight customers a day to sixteen. Second, the branch tackled its end-of-the-month allowance problem, created when the customer was scheduled for a service but the technician couldn't gain access. The problem stopped when Orkin instituted an incentive program for the technicians—the more you collect, the more you get paid. "We decided to pay them based on collections, to give the technician an incentive to work harder to collect the money each month," said Ed. "From 1979 to 1984, we doubled our productivity, and we were able to maintain it."

The Orkin Decatur project produced a solid record of service and sales initiatives that resulted in numerous changes throughout the company. Something as simple as premeasured chemicals created greater control over inventory for the company and more standardized treatments for the customer. Other service changes involved the Orkin Men; if a pest control technician was six or more accounts behind schedule, he automatically worked on Saturday. And every salesman and saleswoman would follow the 10-4-1 program: ten calls equals four presentations and one sale. Wrote Ed, "Even a 'no-sale' is getting us closer to a sure sale."

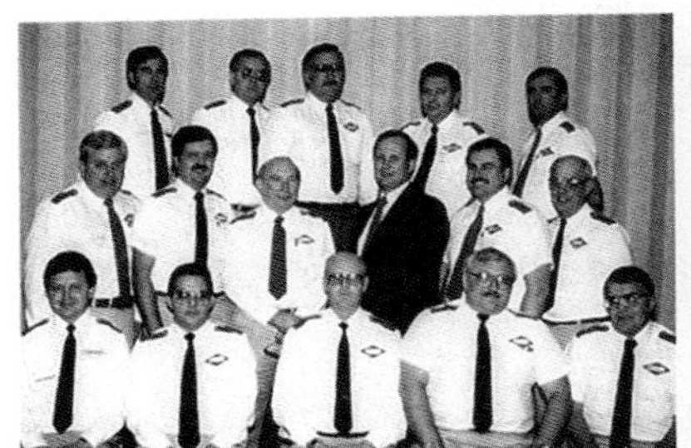
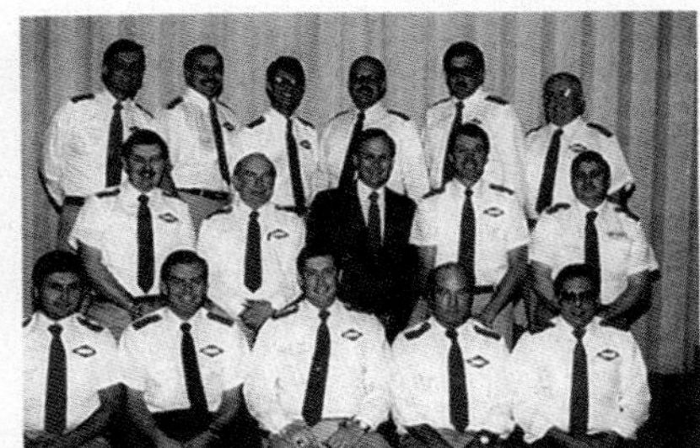
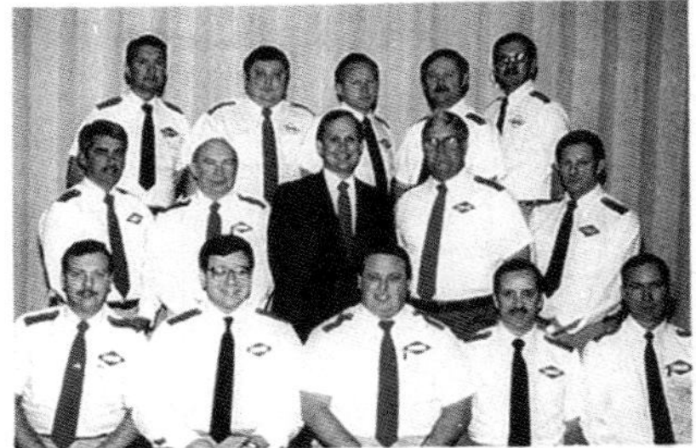
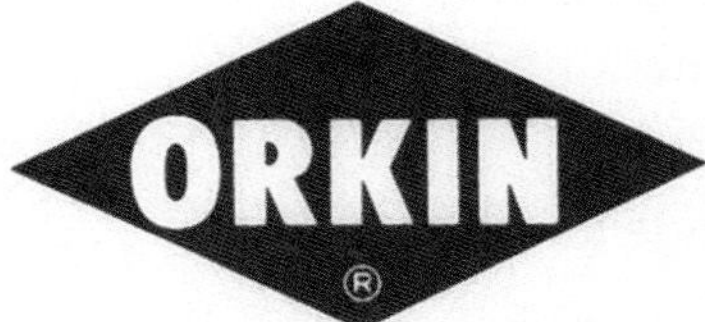

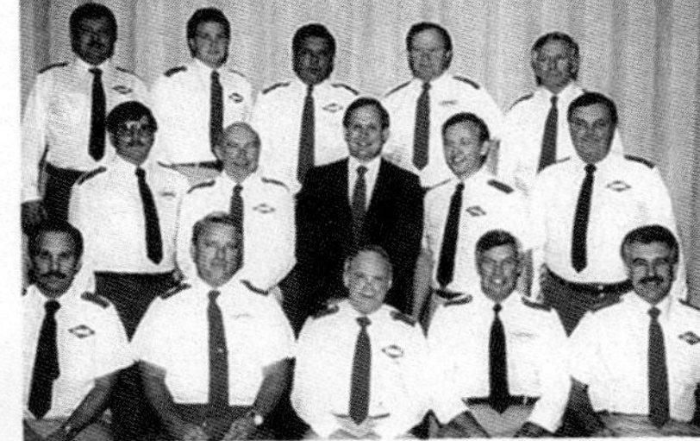
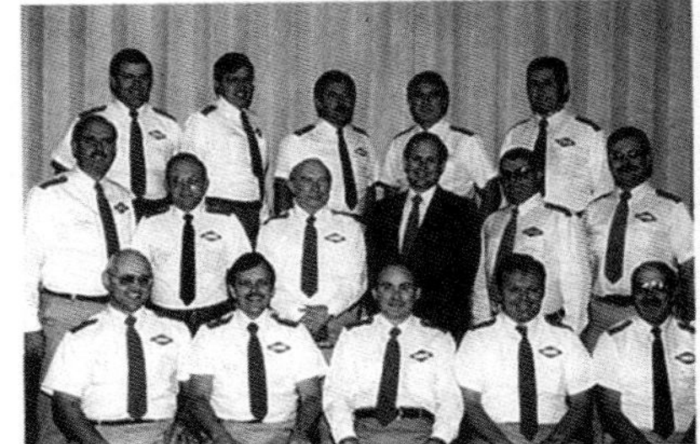
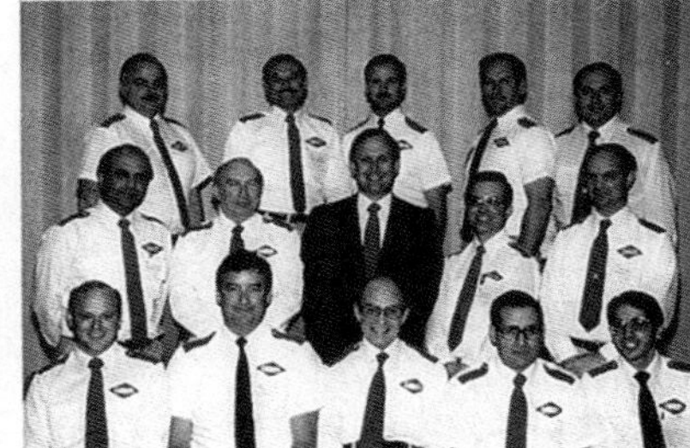
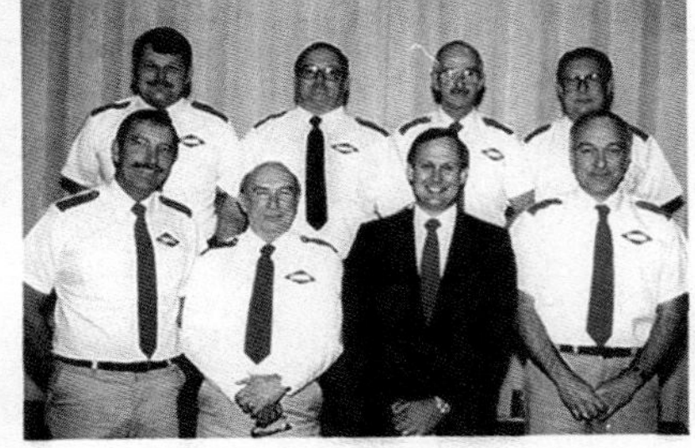
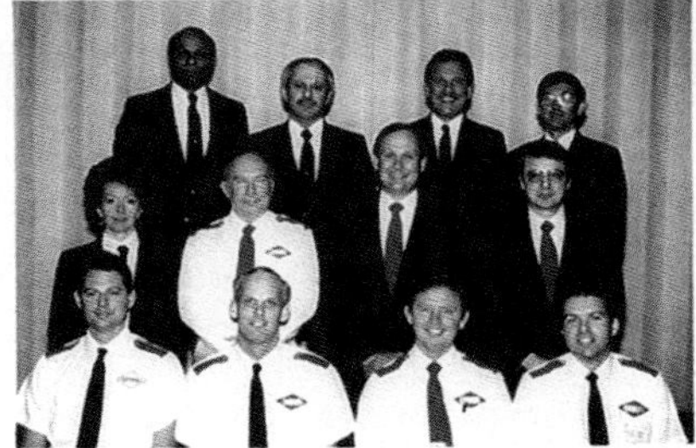

HALFTIME 1985

Halftime Conferences for branch and region managers helped top management explain new policies. These photos are from the 1985 Halftime Conference.

The Decatur branch was reassigned to the Atlanta region around 1984, and Ed eventually left Orkin to work for Randall at Rollins Protective Services. But he remembered the Decatur project as a successful experiment. "If we could improve a branch operation and come up with ideas that could be implemented throughout Orkin, that was our goal," he said.

Though no one knew it at the time, the Decatur project wouldn't be the last time that Randall and Gary dared to try something new on a smaller scale before launching new initiatives throughout the company. In hindsight, the two brothers set the stage in Decatur for a more ambitious business experiment nearly two decades later.

GROWTH AND CHANGE

When the Decatur project began in 1979, Orkin had more than a million active accounts in thirty-eight states and Washington, D.C., supervised by forty-five district offices in six regions: Northeast (headed by Ed Elkins); Western (Clyde Cobb); Midwest (Joe Wilson); North Central (John Wilson); Central (Vince Stevens); and Southeast (Taft Pierce). And when the numbers were all added up, the restructuring efforts and drives to increase profits had worked. Orkin's improving margins were part of the positive financial picture painted by Rollins during the 1979 fiscal year. In October 1979 the company's strong performance sparked rumors that Rollins was the target of a possible takeover. The stock rose from the mid-teens to about $20 a share before Rollins could issue a statement declaring that the firm was not involved in discussions concerning a sale of the company.

On June 20, 1980, Rollins, Inc., reported its twentieth year of record sales and uninterrupted earnings growth with net earnings of $35 million, almost one hundred times the $375,000 net profits in 1960. The record placed Rollins, Inc., third among the nation's multi-industry companies in *Forbes* magazine's thirty-third annual "Report on American Industry." In profits and sales growth, Rollins ranked ahead of such giants as General Electric, American Brands, RCA, Bendix, Sperry, and Westinghouse. The company's five-year return on equity was 21.7 percent, and its five-year sales growth rate was 12.9 percent. Gary Rollins was especially gratified to report Orkin's strong recovery of earnings and improved profit margins after three years of decline. The company's impressive performance didn't go unnoticed. One investment banking firm's report credited Rollins management with pursuing "a well-conceived and executed strategy to transform its business base from the cash-generating, mature pest control and broadcasting businesses to the faster growing oil and gas services and cable divisions." The communications and oil and gas services divisions now accounted for 66 percent of the company's operating income.

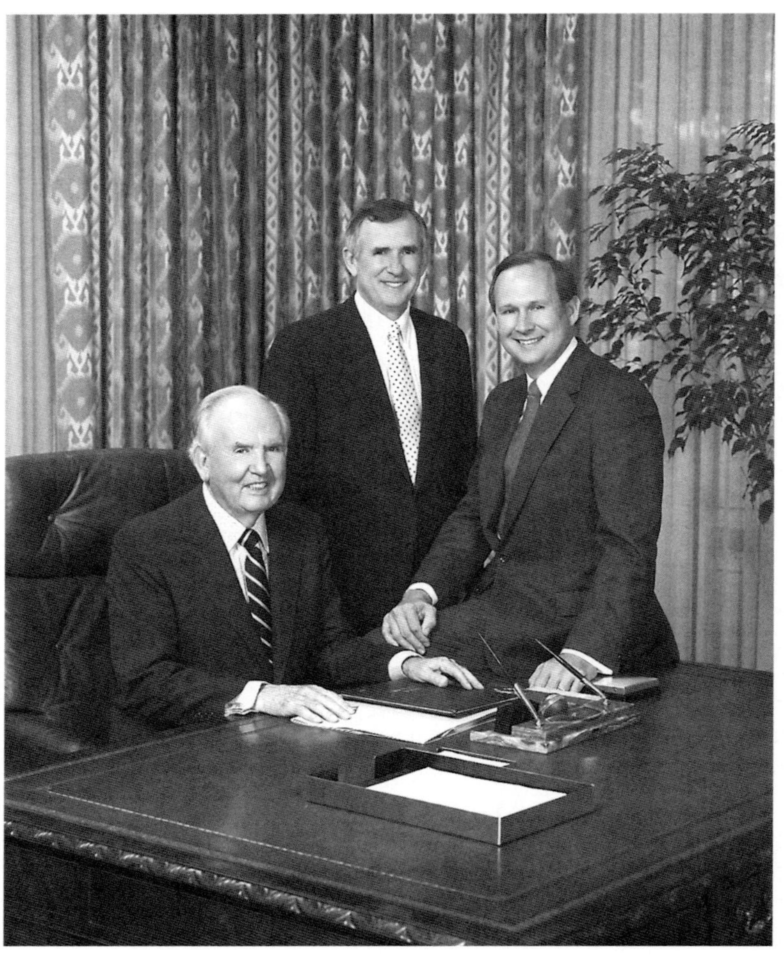

Photographic portrait of O. Wayne Rollins (left), Randall Rollins (center), and Gary Rollins (Gittings, 1985), which hangs in Gary Rollins's office.

Wayne, Randall, Gary—all three Rollins executives had each always encouraged their employees to take initiative, to make suggestions. In 1981 longtime employee J. D. Burger took them at their word and proposed that Dettelbach sell products to an outside market. Over time J. D. helped build the company from twenty-five initial customers to a multimillion-dollar company. "We were competing with well-known companies, so we had to upgrade our inventory and school ourselves in various chemicals—not just those used by Orkin," Burger said. "Joyce Barrow and I worked the company by ourselves, developing a product catalogue and joining several state and local trade associations. And I took to the road. We displayed our products at trade shows to make ourselves known. We had to blaze the trail and learn from trial and error, trying something, then analyzing and making refinements. We sell termiticides, rodenticides, and pesticides."

When Rollins, Inc., surpassed the $500 million revenue mark in 1982, it lay claim to twenty-two years of uninterrupted annual earnings and dividend increases. Revenues reached $526 million, while earnings edged up slightly to $46 million. Orkin's performance was no exception: for the second consecutive year, Orkin reported record profits and improved operating margins, its best performance since the mid-1970s.

In a move that reflected Henry Tippie's business adage that "the best business is the business on the books," the company continued to focus on increased customer retention. His efforts resulted in the "Customers Are First" Campaign, which included the solicitation of customer needs and special employee incentives to encourage prompt action to service those needs. To combat the company's continual problems with customer retention, new early morning and evening service hours were established in order to fit pest control services into the increasingly busy lives of Orkin's customers. In an effort to reduce employee turnover, Orkin management adopted a new pay plan for pest control technicians and a bonus program for service managers. The

Orkin President's Club, which had formerly been for sales employees, was expanded to include the President's Management Council, another way to honor branch and region managers who had excelled throughout the company. And Orkin initiated its first move to a branch computer system, with John Raymond in charge of the project.

"We had procedure manuals, but we had to ask the branch employees what they really did" in order to figure out what kind of computer system the branches needed, said Raymond. "In LaFayette, Louisiana, there was a lady named Jenny, and she pulled out this black book she had worked up to keep track of the salespeople, recording payments, chargebacks, etc. to make sure they were paid correctly. It was a 'how-to' book, and 'Jenny's Black Book' became a buzzword to find out what was actually being done and what the best practices were."

Orkin hired a consultant company, Corstar, to put together a computer system that could better manage customer accounts receivable records and summaries and that had the capacity to schedule and track service status from the various branches. Eventually, Sam Sharara was hired to do a feasibility study from the perspective of data processing, while Raymond explored every angle pertaining to Orkin's needs. The process got a little complicated for a while, when the solution proved more expensive than anyone originally anticipated. Randall Rollins was very involved in Orkin's early computerization and once again used the Decatur branch to test new processes and software packages. Eventually, however, the PCS software system was purchased and

This customer communication piece from 1976 shows that customer service has always been important at Orkin. Left to right, first row: Sue Howard, Merrilyn Clark, Jan Bell, Anna Del Valle, Marge Gehman, Pat Butler, and Phyllis Burton; second row: Janie Messina and Jackie Stafford; third row, Jan Wilkie, Barbara (last name unknown), and Carolyn Harrison; back: Ron Kimbell.

we are YOUR people at ORKIN
WE WORK FOR YOU!
If we
can help you,
please CALL us.
ORKIN
CUSTOMER SERVICE
404 873-2355
or write H. Tim Crow, Vice President, Rollins, Inc., P. O. Box 647, Atlanta, Ga. 30301

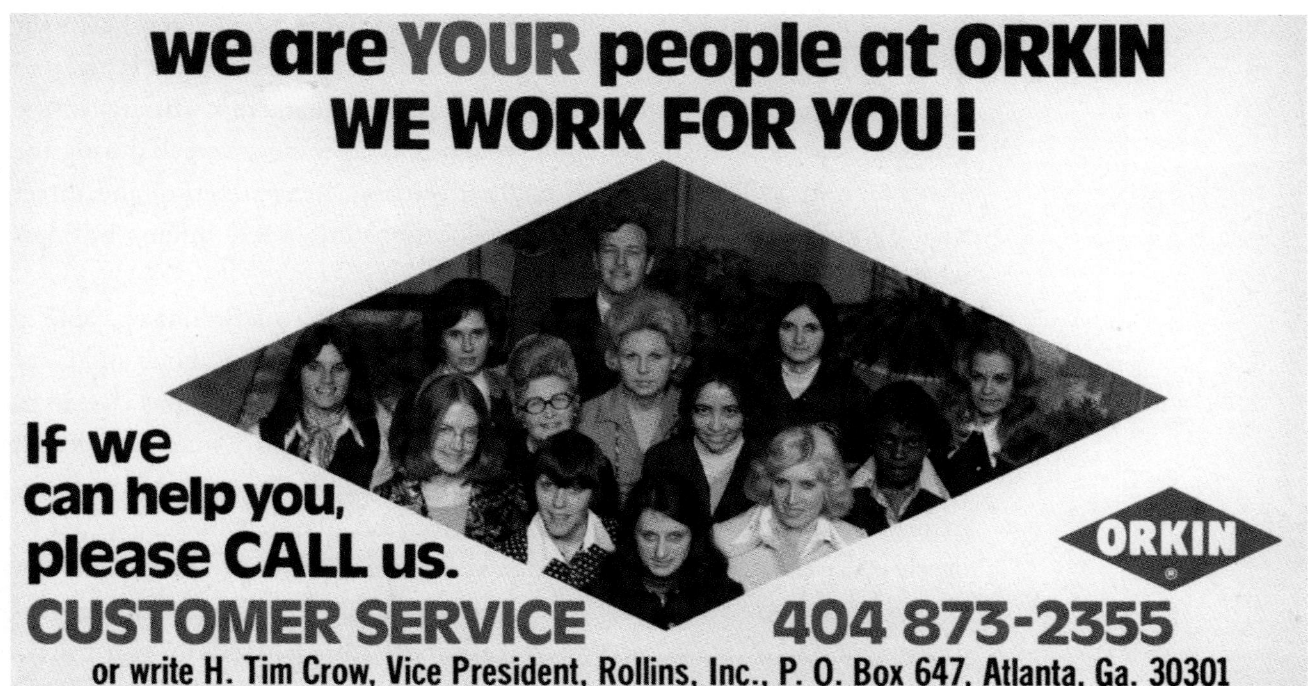

installed and all branches became fully automated, with regular computer updates becoming the norm. This was a major step for Orkin and its bookkeepers. Now, Raymond was free to move to another project Gary had in mind for him: Orkin Lawn Care.

In reality, Orkin had done lawn care in Florida since the 1950s, and in 1976 the parent company had attempted to start a Rollins Lawn Care division. But the Rollins division just hadn't performed very well (five years after it started, it was only doing five hundred thousand dollars worth of business annually in five locations), and John Raymond was asked to handle the merger of Rollins Lawn Care into Orkin and acquire additional lawn care companies. Gary simply couldn't give up on the idea and thought the Orkin hookup could make a positive impact. After all, it made so much sense to cross-market the services. The market for lawn care at the time was estimated at about $2 billion annually and was likely to grow even larger as homeowners put more of a premium on their leisure time. Orkin's brand name should give the business a huge advantage, not to mention access to existing pest customers. The lawn service was provided on a contractual basis, with a specified number of annual treatments of fertilizer and weed control specific to the area. Gordon Crenshaw, who had a degree in agriculture, followed Raymond as head of this division. Future acquisitions included Amcare, with twenty-four branches in New England and the Midwest; Easy Lawn, Village Green, Year-Round, with eight branches on the West Coast, just to name a few. Crenshaw concluded that telemarketing could help the lawn care business grow faster, and he was correct; at one point, Orkin had eight telemarketers working in the Tucker, Georgia, branch, averaging selling 350 customers a week during the season. From 1984 to 1990, through advertising, telemarketing and direct mail, Orkin Lawn Care grew from five locations into a $30 million business with seventy-two branches.

Rollins Lawn Care was merged into Orkin to take advantage of the Orkin name and cross-market to existing pest control customers.

With Orkin Lawn Care successfully launched, Wayne Rollins was able to fulfill another one of his goals. In late February 1984, both Randall and Gary accepted new positions within Rollins, Inc. Randall, fifty-two, was elected to the newly created office of senior vice chairman. Gary, thirty-nine, was elected president and chief operating officer of Rollins, Inc. Wayne remained as chairman of the board and chief executive officer. Ed Elkins, who had served in nearly every capacity with the company since the days of Otto Orkin and was Gary's former boss, was elected president of Orkin, in charge of the day-to-day operations of the company's three hundred branch locations in thirty-eight states. In Ed's thirty-eight years with the company, he had been a service

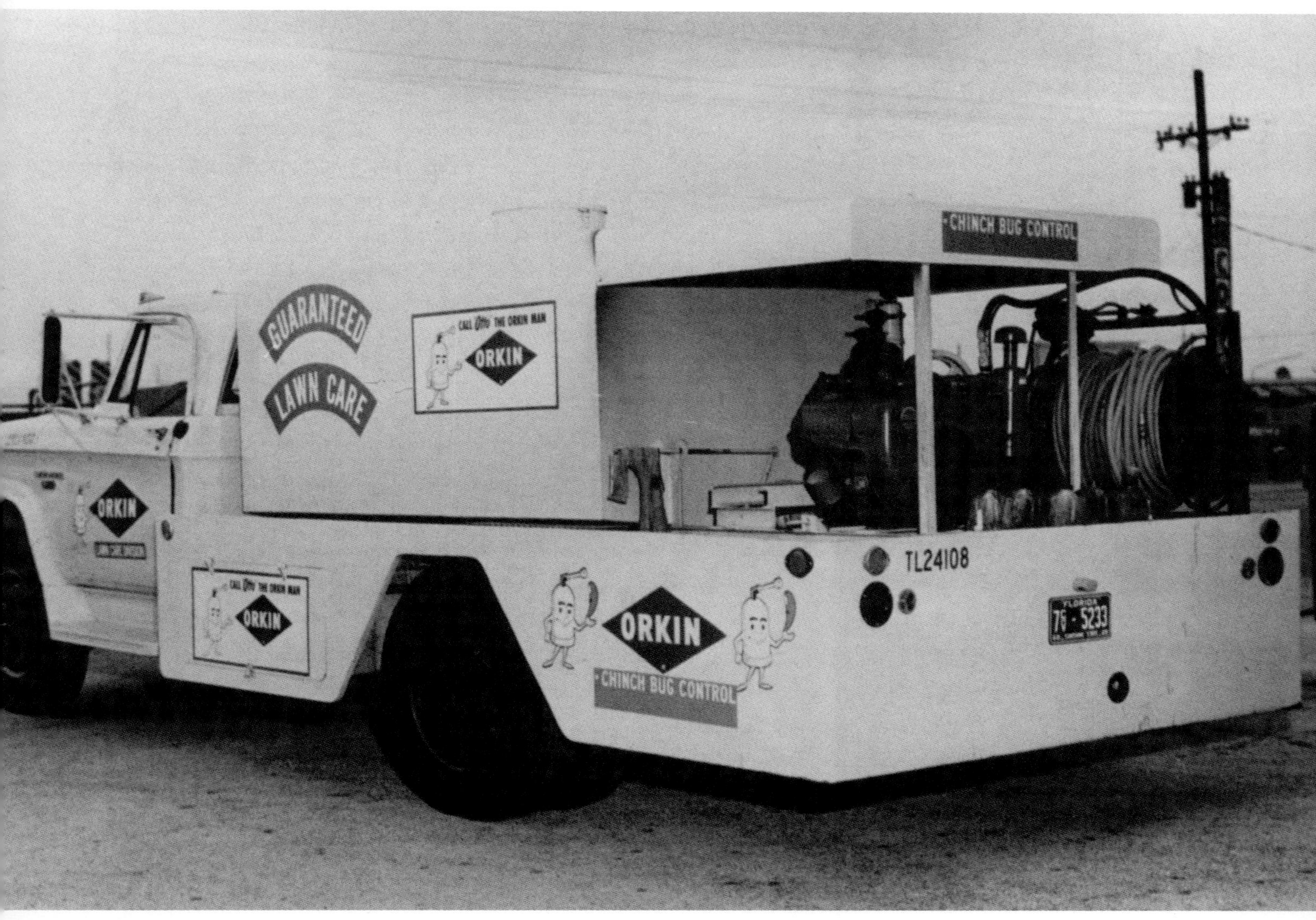

technician, a salesman, a branch manager, a district manager, a region vice president, and vice president of operations.

Orkin had done lawn care service in Florida since the 1950s. In 1976 Rollins started the Rollins Lawn Care Division, and the business would go the full cycle by returning as Orkin Lawn Care in 1983.

As Ed settled into what would be his last and highest executive position for Orkin, the Rollins Board of Directors decided in 1984 that the diversified Rollins, Inc., was in reality three different companies. Wayne Rollins had been concerned about the company's investor profile, despite the company's portrayal of itself as a total service company. "We had a problem with analysts understanding our business when we were in oil, communications, and exterminating," he said. "We were involved in so many things that no one wanted to follow us. The analysts had to learn too many industries to effectively follow the company. Also, separating the companies would avoid the possibility that one company's performance could adversely affect the entire enterprise. And finally we believed that the sum of the parts would be worth more than the whole."

The solution? Rollins, Inc., would spin off two new companies to its shareholders: a new Rollins Communications consisting of radio, television, cable, and outdoor advertising, and RPC Energy Services with the oil and gas services businesses. Orkin (including the lawn care business) and Rollins Protective Services would continue under the Rollins, Inc. banner. On June 12, 1984, the two new companies were listed for the first time on the New York Stock Exchange, and flashed on the Big Board: Rollins Communications, Inc. (symbol ROC on Wall Street, referred to as RCI at Rollins headquarters), and RPC Energy Services, Inc. (symbol RES). Apparently, it was the first time in the history of the NYSE that two Georgia companies with common ownership had been spun off and listed simultaneously on the Big Board.

Rollins spun off two new companies to its shareholders in 1984, Rollins Communications and RPC Energy Services. Orkin and Rollins Protective Services continued under the Rollins, Inc. banner.

As the stock prices for the three companies began to climb, the wisdom of the spin-offs became apparent. In less than a year, Rollins, Inc., stock grew by 53 percent from its offering price of $8 to $12 1/4. By March 1985 Rollins Communications' stock stood at $20 per share, an increase of 29 percent from its offering price of $15 3/8 per share. RPC Energy Services rose 9.5 percent to $4 1/4, up from $3 7/8 per share for its launch date the previous summer. A company whose stock a year before the spin-off traded at 18 5/8 with a shareholder value of $453.519 million now had a combined shareholder value of $615.81 million, a gain of almost 36 percent.

For Rollins, Inc., there was more good news. In 1986 *Forbes* acknowledged the company as the "Nation's Best Performing Service Company," a remarkable achievement that the company would earn and keep for seven consecutive years. In its annual report, both Gary and Wayne Rollins gave a nod to those who made the recognition possible: "Our employees are our most important asset and are dedicated to achieving our goal of being the NATION'S BEST SERVICE COMPANY." Interestingly enough, the coveted distinction came during a year when Orkin reestablished a service guarantee that was always a point of pride for the company founder, Otto Orkin: namely, if you aren't completely satisfied with your service, you get your money back. Orkin's new money-back guarantee for household pest control promised the customer a refund of the last monthly payment if the customer was not happy with the service. "In effect, we have removed all risk for the customer and increased the value of our service," Gary announced in the annual report. "Initial results clearly indicate our sales are growing and customers are retaining our services longer."

The "Nation's Best" recognition came just as the company said farewell to two prominent people who "contributed significantly to the growth and

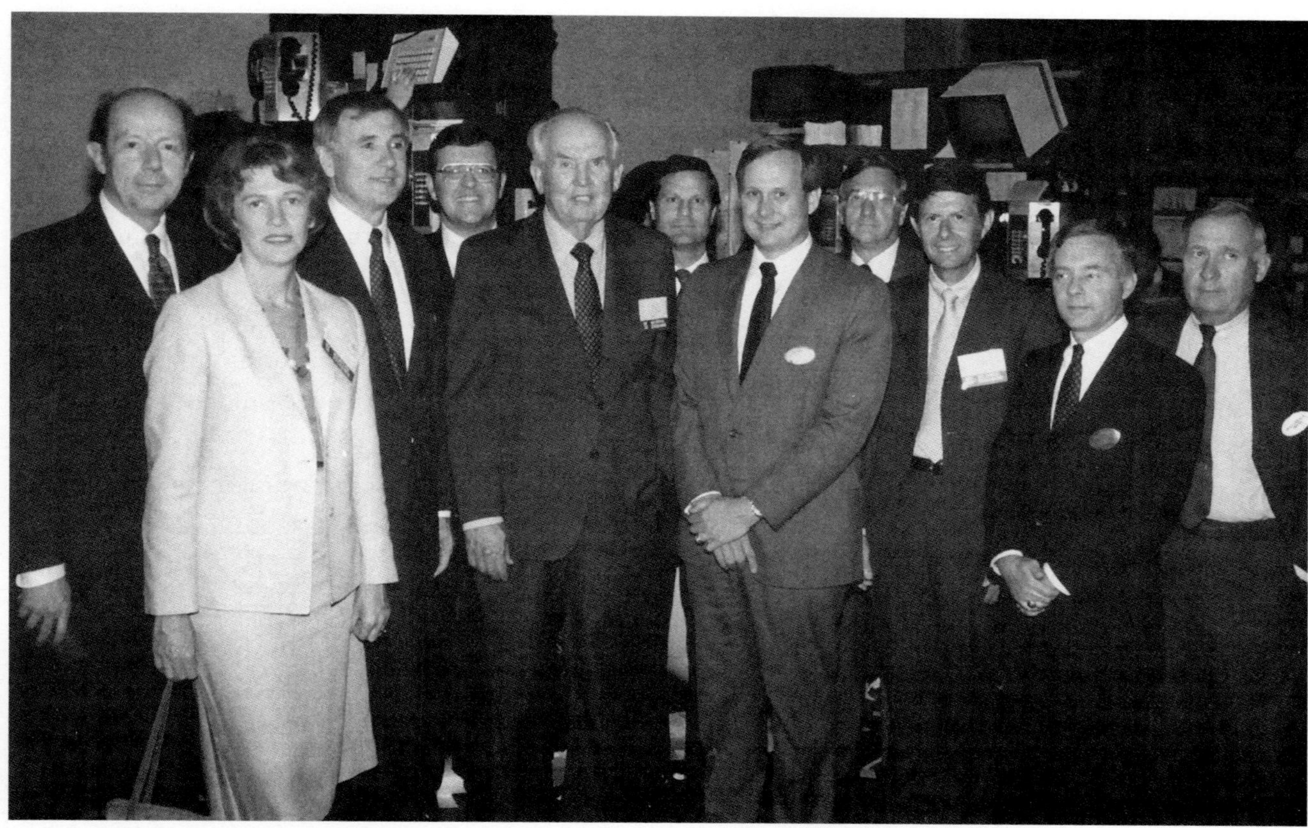

On the floor of the New York Stock Exchange for listing ceremonies for Rollins Communications and RPC Energy Services are, left to right, Tim Crow, Linda Graham, R. Randall Rollins, Michael E. Higgins, O. Wayne Rollins, Harrison Jones II, Gary Rollins, James Hicks, Bill J. Dismuke, Richard Hubbell, and Justus Martin, president of Robinson-Humphrey, the brokerage firm that helped facilitate the spin-off.

success of the Company": Earl F. Geiger, vice chairman of the board, and H. Tim Crow, vice president and secretary, retired early in the year. The two men were among the first to call with congratulations, however, when Wayne Rollins received the Horatio Alger Award in May 1986, an award given annually to outstanding Americans who exemplify the rags-to-riches stories told so simply in the old Horatio Alger books. In Houston, Texas, Wayne was presented his award in this annual gala by his brother John, a previous recipient of the award. As they stood together before a large crowd of business, civic, and religious leaders and over a hundred family members and friends, it was the first time that two brothers had ever won this prestigious award since it was first initiated in 1947.

In 1986 circumstances developed that resulted in the sale of Rollins Communications. Obviously, Wayne Rollins, now seventy-four, had an emotional attachment to the media business; it represented the very beginning of his remarkable business career and his success, starting with his first radio station in Radford, Virginia, thirty-six years earlier. But as Wayne himself

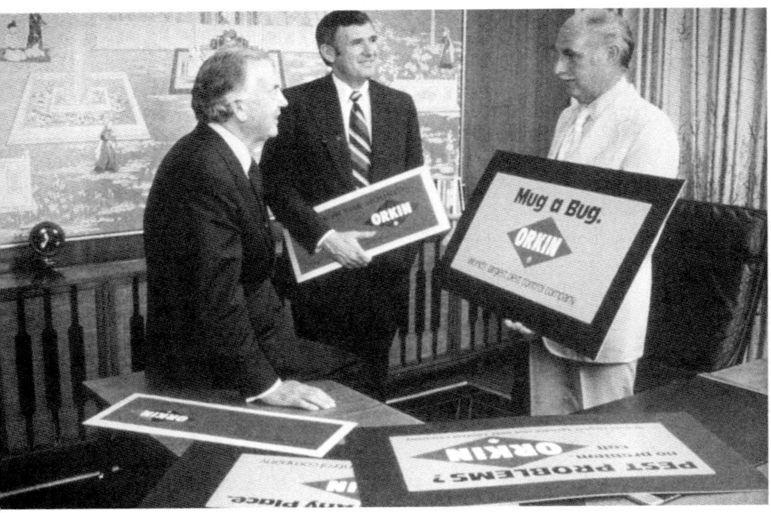

O. Wayne Rollins, left, and Randall Rollins, center, discuss an advertising campaign with Earl Geiger.

believed, business instincts should trump emotion every time. In 1986 broadcast stations, cable systems, and outdoor advertising businesses were commanding premium prices in the marketplace. Wayne knew that the time to sell was in a time of strong demand. "I have always found that when someone wants to buy, it is a good time to sell," Wayne noted. "And if you've got more than one person who wants to buy something, then it's a really good time to sell."

Rollins Communications was purchased in 1986 by Heritage Communications Inc., headed by chairman and chief executive James Hoak. Hoak had given up a law practice in 1971 to start his own cable television company in Des Moines, Iowa, and had progressively expanded to become a major player in the media industry. The deal was completed for a total price of $608.1 million (5.4 times

Advertising through the Ages: *1965–1989*

After Rollins purchased Orkin, Rollins's in-house advertising agency, Kinro, managed Orkin's advertising campaigns through the late 1960s and early '70s. Beginning in 1967, Orkin used an actor who portrayed a scientist to counter the launch of Raid bug spray. Through the early 1970s, Orkin changed advertising themes numerous times in order to generate new leads; one commercial, known as the "Underminers," which took viewers into the tunneled world of termites, capitalized on the science fiction craze that was started by the movie *2001* and the *Twilight Zone* television show.

But the company's first big breakout campaign—one that would set the advertising standard for the next few decades—actually began when Orkin moved its marketing responsibilities to the J. Walter Thompson agency in 1976. Within a year, the national advertising company had launched Orkin's award-winning "Big Number One" campaign, with the instantly memorable tune, "Orkin. We're Number One. We get the job done. We're Orkin!"

"Orkin was the first pest control company running ads on television," Mark Simonton, senior partner and management director at J. Walter Thompson, said in an interview when Orkin celebrated its hundredth birthday. "The 'Big Number One' campaign solidified that perception in the minds of the public. Back when the ad ran, the world was full of fly-by-night local PCOs. The standardization of Orkin was different and compelling for consumers. Being first on the scene with clean-looking diamonds, epaulets, advertising, clean uniforms, and trucks allowed Orkin to set itself apart and build a reputation that continues to be unmatched."

Steve Danuser served as vice president of marketing for Orkin between 1984 and 2002 and helped Orkin earn numerous advertising awards—including the Silver

the company's revenue), with the Rollins family stockholding valued at approximately $270 million. When asked later about the day's post-closing events, Randall was somewhat surprised. "We never spent any time celebrating or crowing. We sold the communications business in the morning and we returned to focusing on our business problems that very afternoon. It was just business as usual."

At Orkin, "business as usual" for its 1.3 million customers involved some of the most challenging issues the company had ever faced. In 1987 Gary Rollins made an unusual public step within the industry when he and Robert Russell began to negotiate the voluntary removal of chlordane from the pest control industry. For over thirty years, chlordane had been one of the most successful termiticides ever used by the pest control industries, but recent mouse studies had begun to question its safety. Prompted by the growing media and political attention given to pesticides and chlordane specifically, Orkin had already been testing alternative termiticides—even though they continued to believe that chlordane was a safe, effective product. Gary could see that a voluntary withdrawal action on the part of chlordane's only

Effie. He still believes that "'Otto the Orkin Man' was sheer branding genius on Otto Orkin's part. The personification of the Orkin Man was one of the smartest marketing moves ever. Because the objective of our advertising for our services is to get the consumer to call Orkin AND keep Orkin. We want leads. The foremost purpose of our advertising is to get the consumer to call, which enables us to tell them about our service."

After the award-winning "Big Number One" campaign, JWT launched the company's "Orkin Army" campaign in 1982, which likened Orkin's services and expertise against pests and termites to an army of experts that literally invades your home and wipes out pesky invaders. The message was a bit softer in 1984, when JWT featured children in the Orkin television, radio, and billboard spots with this message: protect what you care about. One television commercial called "Ice Cream" featured a little boy named Jason, who sees his Orkin man outside an ice cream store. The commercial reminded viewers that Orkin protects them from pests even beyond the boundaries of their own home. The softer message, however, didn't generate the customer leads that Orkin anticipated, so the "Orkin Army" theme returned during 1986 with the message, "All the protection you'll ever need." And it worked; the campaign generated 24 percent more termite leads in 1986.

A very hard-hitting "Facts" campaign ran from 1987 through 1989, with the television series featuring facts and pictures about insects and the problems they can create. At this point, Orkin included not only termites but also ants, fleas, and roaches. These nonemotional, "just the facts, ma'am" presentations were extremely effective. In fact, the "Cost from Termite Damage" fact campaign was awarded the advertising industry's most prestigious recognition when it received a Silver Effie Award.

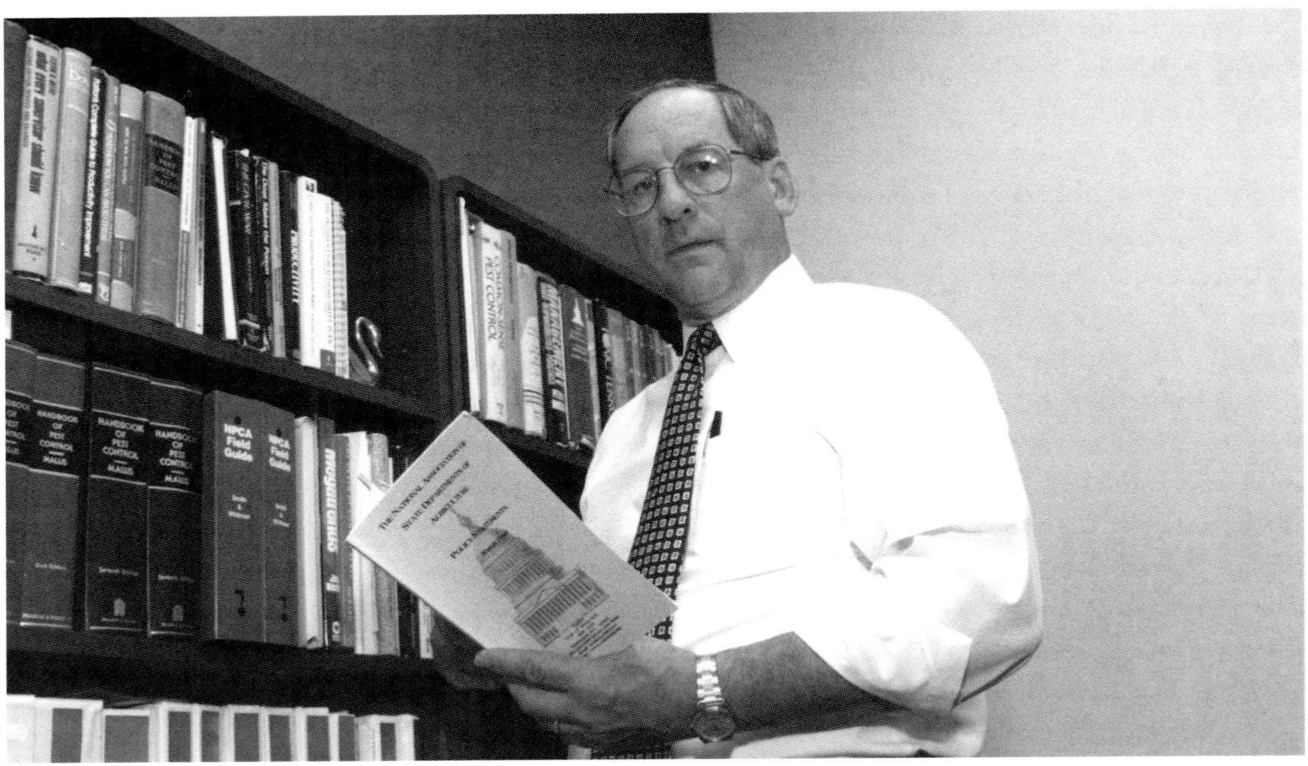

Tom Diederich, then director of safety and training, prepared a statement explaining to employees the reasons for discontinuing the use of chlordane.

manufacturer, Velsicol Chemical, rather than a forced government ban would greatly decrease the likelihood of litigation and product liability lawsuits. More than one expert had predicted that PCOs all over the country would be inundated with consumer suits if the EPA ruled that chlordane posed an imminent hazard to the public and demanded that it be removed from the market. More than anything, Gary wanted to avoid an industry liability situation similar to the one that had resulted with asbestos. His reasons, perhaps, were both professional and personal: Orkin's own Herman Fellton was credited with introducing the use of chlordane in 1946, under the code identification of "1068"; it seemed ironic that Orkin would be responsible for the entry and exit of this product.

Throughout the spring and summer of 1987, Bob Russell and other NPCA representatives met repeatedly with EPA officials to try to negotiate a solution. The two Orkin men created a formidable team, a unique blend of power and credibility: Gary Rollins had the name, experience, and business savvy; Russell had years of experience dealing with various government agencies and was, as one industry expert said, "the right person, in the right place, at the right time."

During these critical summer months, Orkin also sought to calm the fears of its own employees, who in some cases were starting to have concerns about chlordane and the related health risks. In a message to all Orkin employees in June, Tom Diederich, director of safety and training, wrote the following response:

"Even though chlordane is an effective product to use against termites, what about the health risks? Orkin would not want to continue to use a product—however effective—if there was a possibility of a health risk to our employees or the customers whose property we protect. So the big question is: is chlordane a human carcinogen? The answer is a resounding NO. Studies of humans who work with chlordane give no grounds to conclude that occupational exposure to chlordane causes cancer in human beings."

The voluntary withdrawal of chlordane from the market by its manufacturer rather than a forced government ban—a compromise brokered by Orkin—is thought by many to have saved the pest control industry.

After orchestrating a meeting with the EPA head and the president of Velsicol Chemical, Gary Rollins and Bob Russell were able to help forge an agreement. On August 11, 1987, Velsicol Chemical and the EPA jointly announced that Velsicol was voluntarily withdrawing the product from the market, while it evaluated several modified application techniques designed to reduce potential chlordane exposure. This compromise brokered by Orkin is thought by many to have saved the pest control industry. The news, long anticipated by Orkin, confirmed the company's earlier decision to switch from chlordane to Dursban and other new termiticides.

For Gary Rollins, chlordane's voluntary withdrawal from the market and his role in those negotiations would always be one of his proudest accomplishments. And it was clearly one of the crowning achievements for Russell. When Russell completed his term as the president of the National Pest Control Association in October 1987 (an organization that would eventually change its name to National Pest Management Association), *Pest Control Technology* named him Professional of the Year, and the NCPA issued a glowing press release that clearly stated the issues both Bob and Gary Rollins had been up against:

> 1986–87 President Bob Russell served his association during one of the most turbulent episodes in the industry's history. He was faced with directing a course for the association and the industry that would not discredit the service and products the industry provides, while at the same time acknowledging the media attention, anti-pesticide group protests, state and federal government intervention and increased litigation. It was apparent that our side of the chlordane issue was going to be ignored. With the assistance of the NPCA staff and his key contacts in government and industry, Russell helped forge a settlement that was acceptable to all parties concerned.

The resolution of the chlordane issue always remained something of a mystery to Russell, who soon retired as vice president of government relations. The EPA "was making noises about the use of chlordane, but there were questions about their scientific procedures," he said. "There were questions about whether these tumors would further develop into cancer. Was that particular strain of mice just very susceptible to tumors? Were they force-fed large doses of the chemical? Would the tumors develop into cancers or remain as tumors? Nevertheless, the EPA jumped on the results of that particular study and ruled that we had to get rid of chlordane. They never really took it off the market, but Velsicol withdrew it, and that's where Gary Rollins talked them into making a retreat rather than just cut it off. They never tried to complete the conditions that would have allowed them to put it back on the market because they realized it would have been impossible."

The chlordane experience had reinforced Orkin's belief that "no pest control company is an island unto itself." The company's participation in national, state, and local industry organizations reflected Orkin's "strength in numbers" philosophy, long removed from the days when the industry giant had temporarily pulled out of the national organization. Gary Rollins's insistence that the reputation of one company in the industry ultimately affects the whole industry was not lost on pest control providers during the chlordane debate. And as the entire industry faced further challenges and litigation over practices, the support of the industry-wide leaders would be vital.

As the company moved to put the chlordane issue behind it, Orkin launched into four major initiatives that reached into virtually every corner

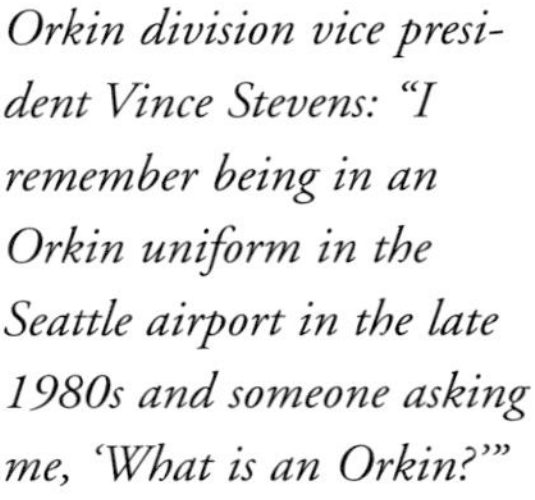

Orkin division vice president Vince Stevens: "I remember being in an Orkin uniform in the Seattle airport in the late 1980s and someone asking me, 'What is an Orkin?'"

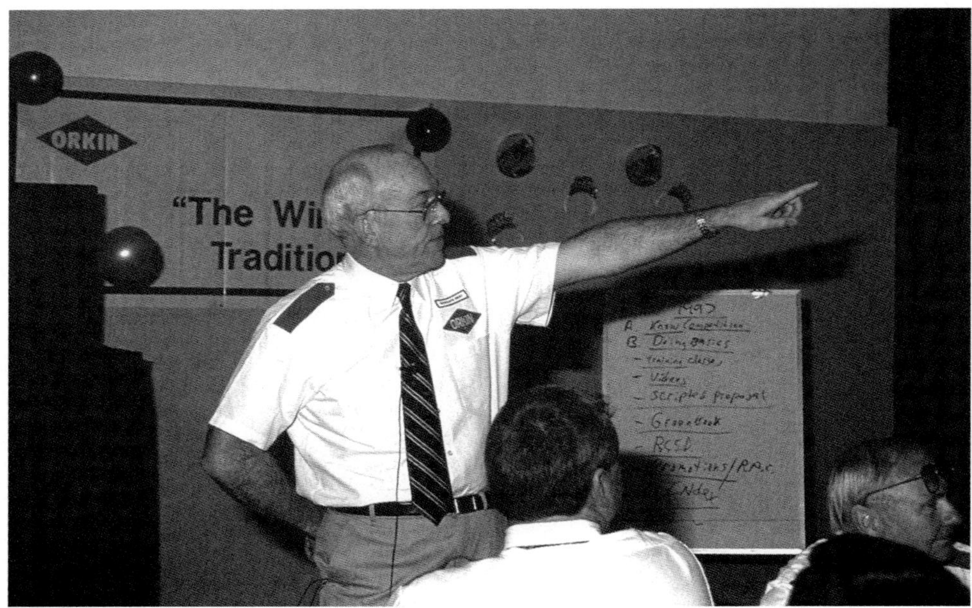

of the company: public relations, new products, advanced training, and finding a new president.

With a newly reorganized marketing department, Orkin moved to showcase its company, services, and products on television, cable, radio, and other media outlets. The Orkin Exterminator Robot made its national advertising debut, a hulking Orkin Man of armor and steel, who promised to eliminate any pest control problems. Additionally, within months, eighty male models posing as "real" Orkin Men were on hand in Atlanta to shoot a new television campaign to promote Orkin's new outside pest control service called the Perimeter Defense System (PDS). Paul Hardy and Steven Danuser, Orkin vice president of marketing, watched carefully as the actors lined up side-by-side in front of a brick colonial home, creating a wall of Orkin Men in uniform guarding the perimeter against pests and termites.

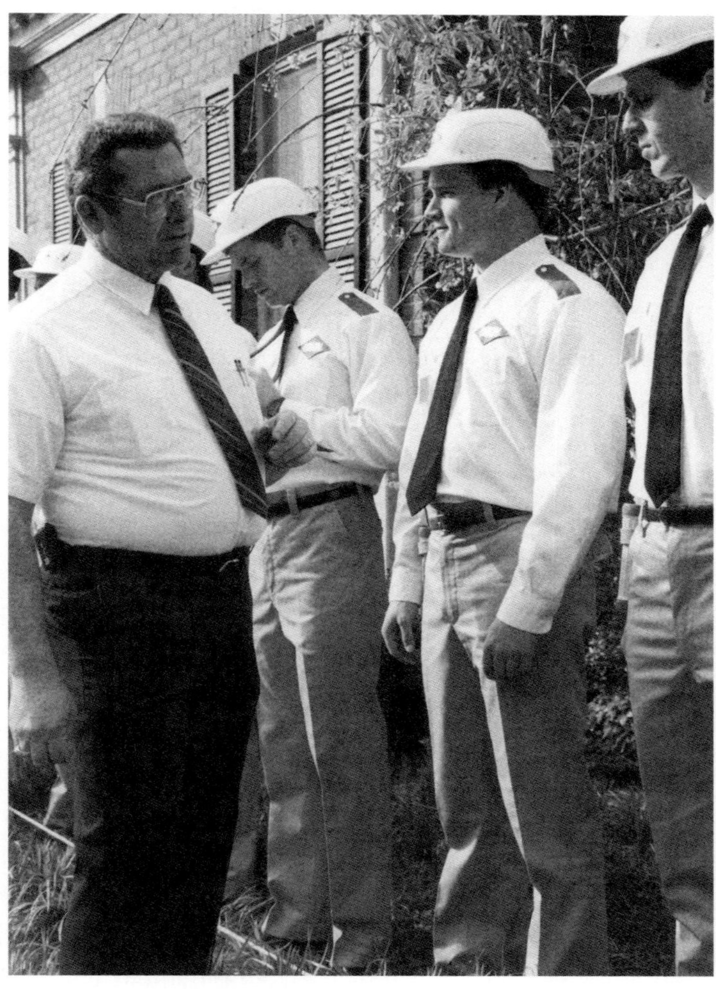

Technical director Paul Hardy, left, provides technical advice during shooting of the Orkin "Perimeter Defense" commercial during the late 1980s.

A public relations push also included many Orkin managers, who fanned out into different elementary schools across the country to deliver the unique Orkin mantra: "We love bugs, but we don't like the ones that hurt you, your family, and your property." The new advertising and PR initiatives extended throughout the country, and Vince Stevens, the new West Coast vice president, was especially grateful for the PR push and Orkin's efforts to keep promoting its brand. Said Stevens: "I remember being in an Orkin uniform in the Seattle airport in the late 1980s and someone asking me, 'What is an Orkin?'"

Before he retired in 1987, Ed Elkins expanded the training department staff and increased the time Orkin Men devoted to training. The company invested in new branch video equipment for training purposes, and expanded training programs through regional seminars and training sessions for all levels of the organization. What's more, Orkin began developing close relationships with leading entomological universities such as Purdue, Virginia Polytechnic Institute, the University of Florida, the University of Georgia, Texas A&M, and California Polytechnic—building relationships that would prove to be invaluable in the future.

When Ed Elkins retired, Gary Rollins knew that there was "no heir apparent" to fill the position of Orkin president. For the first time in the company's history, the position would be filled not by someone from within the Orkin ranks but by an outsider. After an executive search, Bob Mercer, an executive with twenty years of experience in the propane gas business, was hired to run the nation's largest PCO.

Gary Rollins, returning to the presidency of Orkin in 1989 after serving in other capacities for five years: "I feel like an old fire horse they keep hooking up to the wagon."

In an interview with *Rollins Today,* Mercer acknowledged that "Orkin has a very strong, knowledgeable management team, mostly developed and promoted from within. However, many of the managers have had no opportunity to observe how other companies do things. I think the idea was to find someone who had varied experience in a large multi-location service organization and attempt to apply some of that experience to positive improvement at Orkin."

Immediately, Mercer saw three challenges: the need to reduce employee turnover, the need to reduce customer cancellations, and the need to make some organizational changes to give more responsibility and authority to district and branch management. Mercer reasoned that there would be fewer cancellations and less employee turnover if technicians were better trained—echoing a theme that both Gary and Ed Elkins had put forth before. "Most people want to perform well in their jobs," Mercer said. Many of the frustrations that, in the past, had led technicians to resign during the early months of their employment could be eliminated by making sure the technician is thoroughly trained before he is expected to meet production goals and before he starts providing service to the customer. And, Mercer argued, more competent and confident technicians would result in more satisfied customers, particularly if the same technician provides the service from month to month.

As he worked to increase training programs, personnel, and incentives, Mercer began to revamp the Orkin organization. With the assistance of Ray Bateman, Mercer worked to reorganize the field operations and the home office reporting responsibilities, looking to give the organization a larger span of control and reduce some top-heavy management positions. In an effort to understand the organization, Mercer and Bateman traveled unannounced to branches in order to study branch operations; they worked with Human Resource data to determine optimum staffing levels and began planning the reorganization from the branch up; and according to Bateman, they often worked "secretly nights and Sundays with a wall map of the United States" which was removed before the work day began.

The result? In 1989 Mercer announced a new field reorganization that reduced the five Orkin regions to three new and much-expanded divisions with three reassigned vice presidents: Northern, led by Clyde Cobb; Central, led by Steve Drennan; and Southern, led by Vince Stevens. According to Gary Rollins, who approved the plan, "Mercer consolidated the forty-three districts and merged them into twenty-eight regions. We went from eight or nine branches per district to ten or twelve branches in what was now called a region, which enabled us to take marginal district managers and put them in big branches, and use about half the money we saved with the reorganization to add regional sales directors and service directors."

The change was drastic and, initially, not very popular.

"It was the kind of wake-up call the company needed," said Gary, somewhat in defense of the difficult changes. "Some of the people who had been complacent hit another gear. The people who had earlier been promoted over their head were put back into a job where they could be more successful. And the additional staff people we put in the larger regions would make a contribution, and for a couple of years, things looked pretty good. Mercer was very service-oriented. In retrospect, we didn't continue the emphasis on service improvement to the extent we should have. However, when you look at the statistics, the allowances and cancellations have continued to improve, although we still have room to do better."

As the company approached its tenth decade of business, Mercer stepped down, and Gary Rollins agreed to return to Orkin as president while keeping his title as president and chief operating officer for Rollins, Inc. He jokingly admitted, "I feel like an old fire horse they keep hooking up to the wagon." But when he stood before the Orkin management team, the collective sigh of relief was real, not imagined. Their own Orkin Man was back. Said Gary, "I got them all together when I went back, and all I had to say was, 'Hey, guys, we don't need any honeymoon here, we just need to get right down to the nitty-gritty.'

"And we did."

In an industry full of mom-and-pop businesses, Orkin ads in the 1970s focused on the standardization that comes with a big organization.

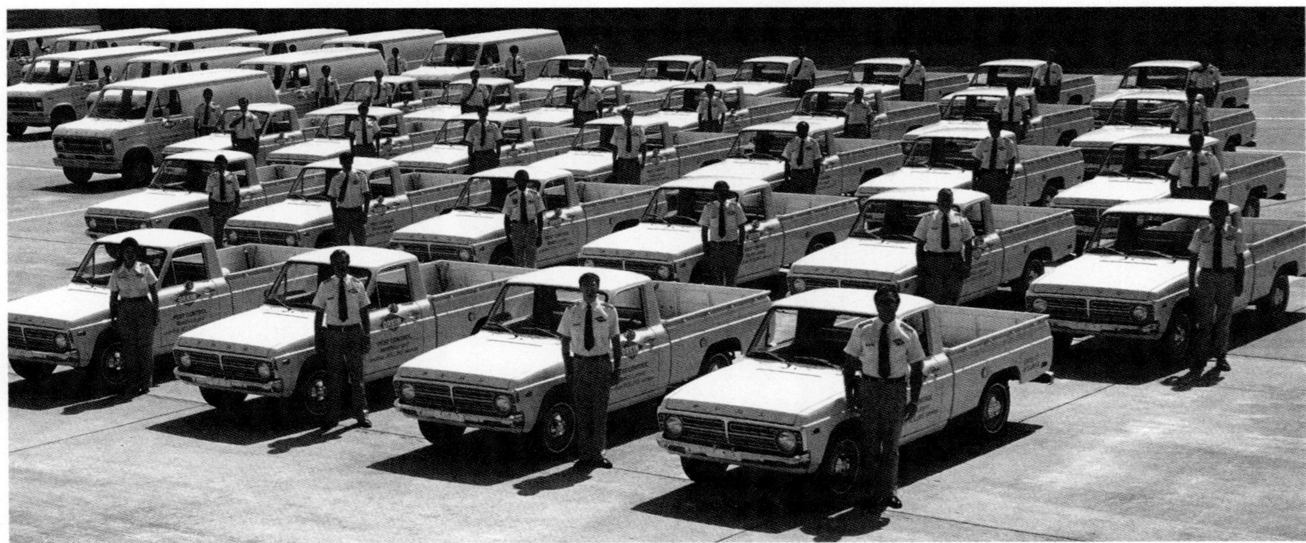

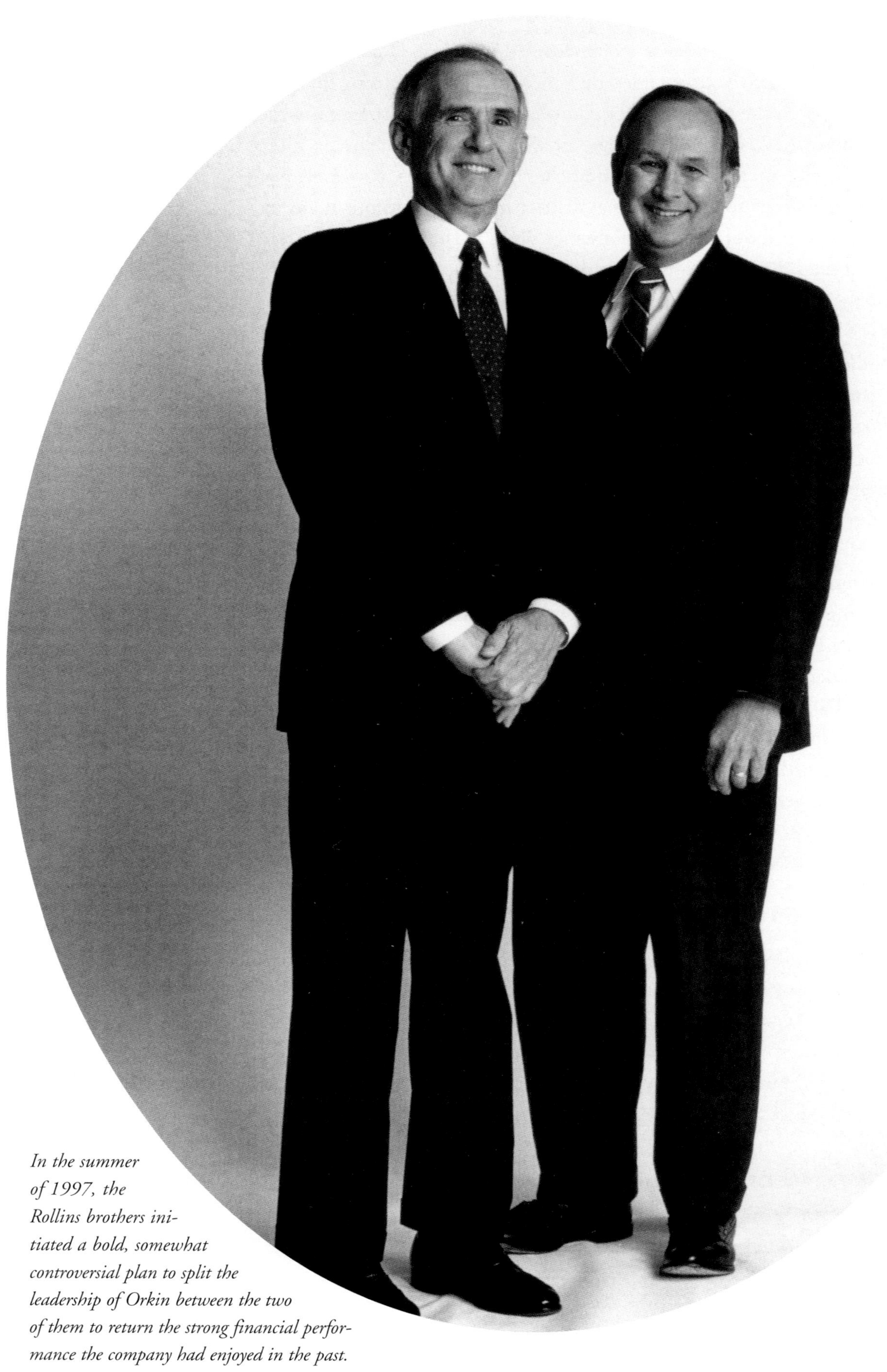

In the summer of 1997, the Rollins brothers initiated a bold, somewhat controversial plan to split the leadership of Orkin between the two of them to return the strong financial performance the company had enjoyed in the past.

Chapter 6

The 1990s: Challenge and Innovation

As Orkin moved closer to celebrating a century of service, the nitty-gritty issues faced by the pest control company and its returning president would define the company's agenda for the next decade and reflect the very essence of the turbulent pest control industry. Government regulations and restrictions continued to challenge the use of certain chemicals for pest control, and Orkin would respond with innovations and techniques that would lead the industry through the post-chlordane era, though not without its share of termite claims, retreatments, and lawsuits. In addition, Orkin would refine its termite services, the way treatments were delivered, and its customer guarantees. In the late 1990s the company would launch an every-other-month residential pest control service, begin to franchise its operation through a new branch franchising program, and discontinue its lifetime termite guarantees—three critical, strategic changes that might have traumatized company founder Otto Orkin, but that were seen as progressive steps by the current management. And Orkin would continue to expand its residential and commercial pest control services throughout the United States and Canada, with a renewed emphasis on commercial services.

In several bold and aggressive public relations steps, Orkin took its name to the hallowed halls of the Smithsonian Institution and into nearly every corner of the country through a traveling exhibit, publicly declaring that "we love bugs—but not the ones that hurt you and your home and property." And when Rollins responded to a skeptical financial market and downsized its corporate makeup in order to concentrate on Orkin Pest Control as its core business, the strategy worked. As profit increases resumed, financial analysts, who had stopped following the company for over five years, would once again consider Rollins as a "BUY."

THE CONTINUUM

As Gary Rollins and his team struggled to improve the company's employee turnover and customer retention rates, he welcomed the third generation of the Rollins family into the Orkin fold. In 1990 Glen W. Rollins, Gary and Ruthie Rollins's oldest son, joined the company as a full-time employee. By nearly every account, he was a welcome breath of fresh air at the ninety-year-old company. A graduate of Princeton University, Glen had dabbled in starting a venture capital business on the West Coast after college before returning to the family business. Like his father, Glen started out in the field; in fact, he first wore an Orkin Man uniform in 1979 when, as a fourteen-year-old, he spent his summer as a termite technician helper in the Atlanta area. In future summers, Glen worked as a pest control route manager and sales inspector, learning the business the same way his father had—literally from the ground up. Once he committed to the family business, he moved quickly through the company, as service manager, sales manager, branch manager, region sales manager, assistant region manager, and region manager in various field locations in Georgia, Texas, Virginia, and North Carolina. He was considered exceptionally intelligent and ambitious, yet gracious enough to acknowledge that his rise through the corporate ranks was fortuitous. "I've had so much help," he once said in an interview. "I feel like I was born on third base, and I think I can get home. I've had help the whole way from the terrific people at Orkin."

One magazine article speculated about Gary Rollins at the head of Orkin: "Everything he does will be measured against his father's record, a difficult if not impossible standard to meet."

Those Orkin people included not only his father and uncle but also his grandfather. "I feel like he has confidence in me," Glen said in an interview in 1991, when asked about his relationship with O. Wayne Rollins. "He just always acts that way. You can imagine what a boost that is. He has often said to me, 'Glen, what you have to do will be in many ways a lot harder than what I had to do because, for me, there were no expectations. You are going to have a lot more so you have a lot harder thing ahead of you.' When I was working on starting the California business and having these ideas and going through all this, sometimes he would say, 'I understand. You probably don't think I do. But I was a lot more like you when I was your age than you might ever realize.' And when he and I were going through all these discussions, we were never disagreeable. I would say, 'Can I come talk with you?' I would come in there and two or three hours later, we'd still be talking. He never said, 'I've got this to do or this is more important.' He had unlimited time for me. He and I have a real love for business."

As Wayne Rollins maintained his role as chairman of the Rollins, Inc., board and watched his sons and grandchildren assume leadership roles within

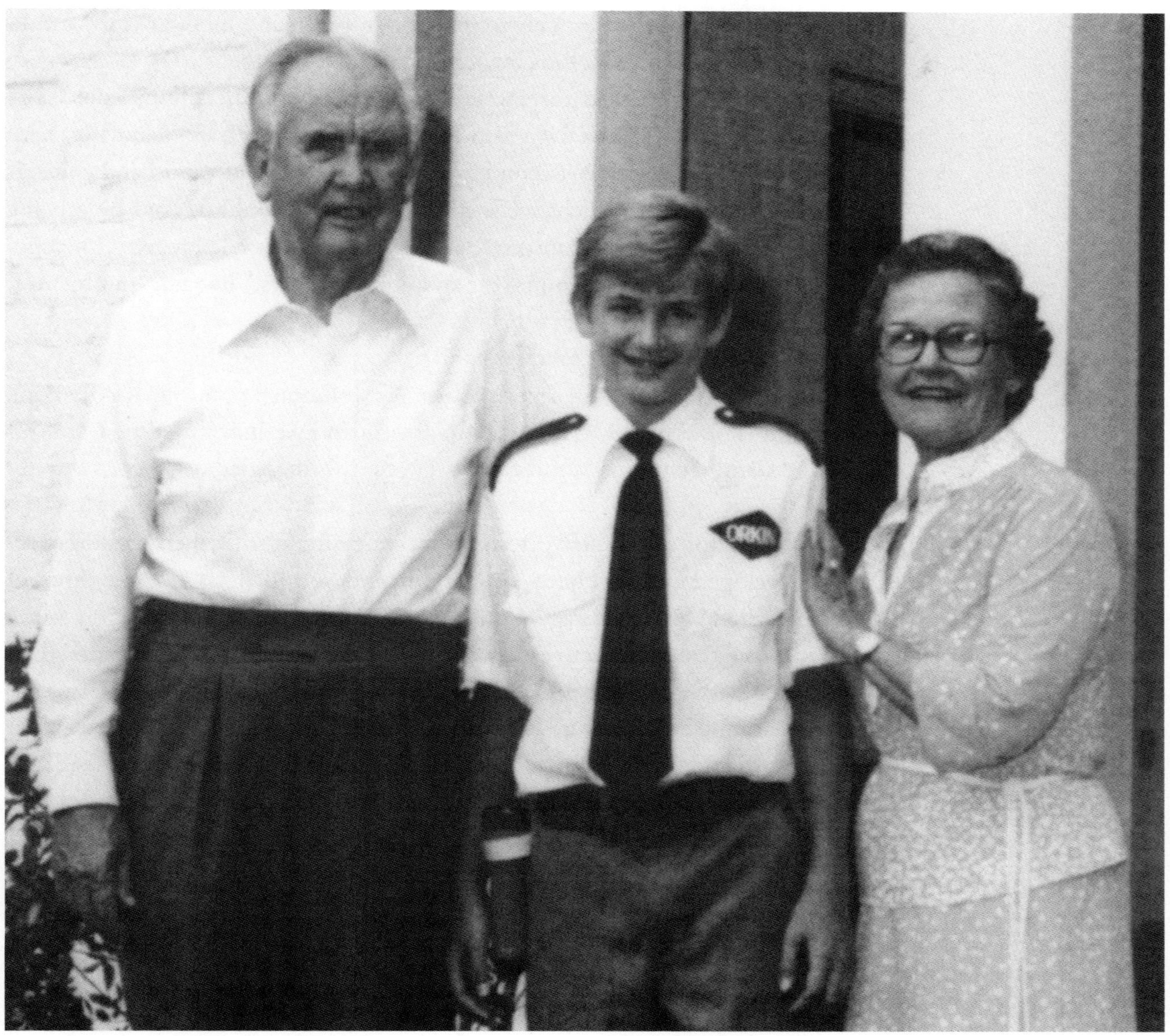

the company, the press often had a field day, speculating on their chances of success. "Family company at a crossroad," read one magazine article, speculating that "the company is Gary's to lose. Everything he does will be measured against his father's record, a difficult if not impossible standard to meet." Still others speculated that the company could not survive without Wayne Rollins, predicting that the company would be bought out, even though half of the company's eight directors were family members and in 1990 controlled approximately 40 percent of the company's stock. Articles pointed out that while Orkin accounted for over 90 percent of the entire company's operating income, the pest control company's growth had slowed to about 7 percent annually. With only 20 percent of all homes in the country using pest control services, Wall Street analysts reasoned that Orkin should be more aggressive in

Glen Rollins, center, who eventually became president and COO of Orkin, held his first job with Orkin when he was fourteen. Here he is shown with his grandfather, O. Wayne Rollins, and his grandmother, Grace Rollins.

capturing more of the pest control market and realizing more growth. Could the next generation of Rollins owners meet the challenge?

The skeptics seemed to embolden the Rollins brothers, especially Gary. Described in the press as a "down-to-earth guy," a very "private man with a very public job," he stayed focused on his business objectives at Orkin and concentrated on what he could change instead of what he couldn't. And he put the company's chance for success squarely where he thought it belonged. "Our success is determined by our employees and our customers," he said, "not by me."

INNOVATIONS AND NEW DIRECTIONS

Following its successful role in Velsicol's voluntary removal of chlordane from the market, Orkin continued to introduce innovative pest control products and techniques. In the early 1990s, this included:

- The use of an exclusive termiticide-carrying agent called OrkinFoam. Developed by Paul Hardy, Eric Smith, and Vern Bell, this foam treatment provided better coverage against termites than the liquid solution—in a safer and more effective delivery application using a specially designed machine that was especially serviceable in the field. The foam system, eventually embraced by PCOs across the country, penetrates better than liquids and provides "an effective residue on every surface it touches," said Hardy. Even though the system requires more training, expense, and time, Hardy predicted that it would be widely used in order to treat "termites and other pests with less chemicals." He was right.
- Actisol, an ultra-low-dosage piece of pest control commercial service equipment designed to cover a larger area with less chemicals by using air to break the chemicals down into smaller particles. Working with Ted Barrow to develop Actisol, Hardy called it "one of the most broadly used pieces of equipment in the industry."
- The Versa-Tool, a unique treating tip developed with B&G Equipment Company, considered a standard today in termite treatment.
- The Flo-Meter, a device that measures the precise amount of termiticides used on each termite treatment. Orkin was the first company to use this customized device, and developed one that wasn't temperature-sensitive.
- The Perimeter Defense System, an exterior pest control application system designed to stop pests outside, before they could get inside the home.
- The Termiticide Injector System, initiated by Hardy in 1992 and rolled out in the mid-1990s. Involving a compact unit to accurately dispense termiticide, the system eliminates a big holding tank on Orkin trucks and ultimately provides Orkin customers with a better job at less cost to the company.

- Borates (the "fourth" barrier against termites, supplementing the company's "Triple Barrier" termite treatment program).
- The use of global positioning satellite equipment in service vehicles to be able to track the vehicle location, speed, and time spent at an account.
- Handheld computers used by termite technicians and commercial pest control technicians to record customer service activity.

A NEW BUSINESS: PLANTSCAPING

In order to capitalize on the company's extensive commercial customer base and to identify a new service business, Gary Rollins initiated a new commercial interior plantscaping business in 1990. Called Orkin Plantscaping, the division designed, installed, maintained, and serviced decorative plants in business settings, ranging from hotels and shopping malls to office buildings and corporate headquarters. Gary put Gordon Crenshaw and Al Hughes in charge of the new venture, and in 1990, Orkin started an aggressive plantscaping business acquisition campaign around the country, buying plant service companies from such known industry names as Veldkamp in Denver, Botany Center in Knoxville, and Plant Lady in Austin. Within four years, Orkin Plantscaping had grown to $18 million in sales and was the second largest in the United States, behind Tropical Plant Rental owned by Rentokil.

To many, plantscaping was a lot like lawn care—just moved inside. But Larry Spruill, who later became vice president of Orkin Plantscaping, would beg to differ. "Lawn care and plantscaping are very different. Lawn care is highly regulated, due to the strict controls you have for using pesticides; however, the services are pretty routine. Plantscaping is more complex. There are about seventy different plants to know—varieties with challenges in design and keeping it looking good. You never have to worry about scale or fungus or mealy bugs or proper lighting in pest control, but you do in plantscaping. Our biggest challenge is keeping that plant alive. You have to have a person who is capable of caring about that plant. We've hired horticulturists, agronomists, and botanists, with a lot of emphasis on technical training."

Orkin Plantscaping became the fourth division in Rollins, Inc., joining Orkin Termite and Pest Control, Orkin Lawn Care, and Rollins Protective Services. In the early 1990s the services provided by these four divisions meant that Rollins was regarded as one of the nation's largest consumer service companies, servicing nearly 1.4 million residential and commercial customers. Revenues for 1990 reached a record $436 million, an increase of $34 million, or 8 percent, compared to an increase of only 6 percent in 1989; revenues increased another 9 percent in 1991. And there were other improvements, too. Customer and employee retention rates were starting to improve, through Orkin's emphasis on better training, compensation, and benefits. A new computer system at Rollins Acceptance Corporation (RAC) took the finance group from the "Middle Ages to the Space Age," according to collection manager Vance Mason, who supervised the switch from a manual accounting system to a computerized database that improved not only collections but also customer services.

PUBLIC RELATIONS AND MARKETING

When Terminix surpassed Orkin as the nation's largest pest control company, the company decided to launch a "preemptive strike and start marketing Orkin as the World's Best Pest Control Company." And when *Forbes* again recognized the company as the "Nation's Number One Service Company" for the fourth year in a row, Gary and Randall launched an internal quality improvement process, referred to throughout Rollins as the company's "Mission of Excellence." Their goals? To achieve complete customer satisfaction and improve operating efficiency, while building a more professional workforce. "Together," Gary said, "we are making quality the way we do business at Rollins."

And the Rollins executives were adamant about another aspect of Orkin: the company should not be perceived as a threat to the environment. "We've been environmentalists since 1901," Gary often said, and 1990 was the year to emphasize this important message to the public. During the year, the company provided free termite protection to many state and national historical landmarks. Orkin funded an Insect Zoo Interactive Computer (IZIC) at the Smithsonian Institution's rotunda, a display that provided millions of visitors with information about the insect world. This move would begin an association with the National Museum of Natural History that would grow dramatically over the years. The company's annual report stated boldly that "Orkin continues to take an active position as an environmentally responsible company. Because of our professionally designed equipment, tested and proven treatment methods, industry-leading training and research, Orkin has been a long-standing partner with the environment. All materials we use are registered with the U.S. Environmental Protection Agency (EPA). As an additional step toward being more environmentally conscientious, we recently began using recycled paper in customer sales materials. These actions clearly communicate Orkin's ongoing commitment to the environment and our priority of safety for our customers, employees and the general public."

As the company worked to develop its own environmental voice, Gary Rollins started to sound just a bit like Rollins founder O. Wayne Rollins, comfortable and confident enough to hand out his own business maxims and telling stories that not only entertained but drove home a message:

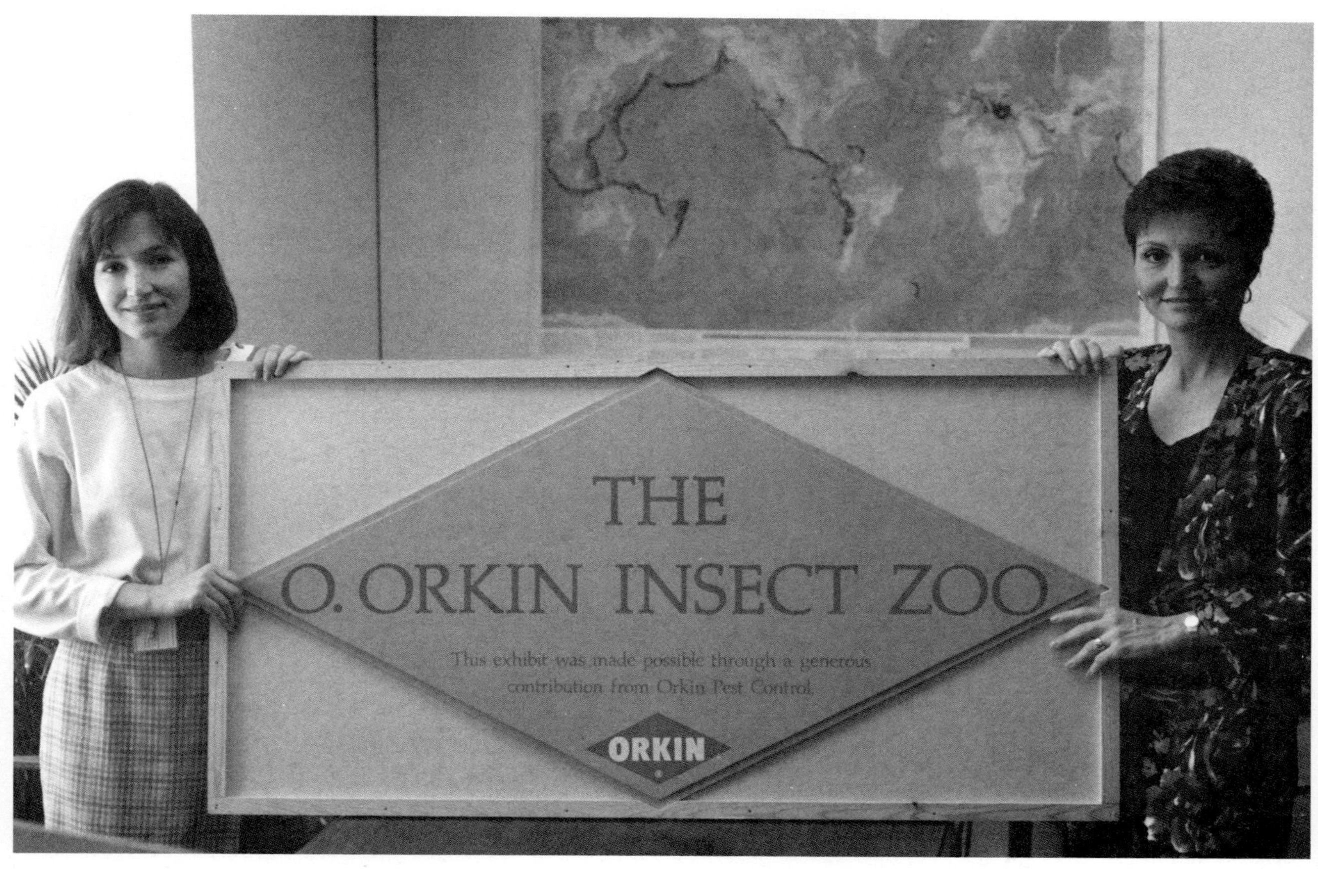

Sally Love, left, developer of the O. Orkin Insect Zoo exhibit at the Smithsonian Institution's National Museum of Natural History in Washington, D.C., and Judy Donner, public relations manager at Rollins, display the temporary sign announcing Orkin's sponsorship of the zoo at its opening in 1993.

Character is the ability to follow through with a good resolution after the mood is gone.

The Number One contributor of our Company's success is the quality of our people.

In a closet in his corporate office on Piedmont Road, Gary began to collect props and Orkin memorabilia that he had used on his annual corporate "Road Shows"—his visits to regional and branch manager meetings held around the country. Wearing his Johnny Carson "Carnac the Great" turban, he predicts the future; his army helmet reminds his troops to "declare war" on customer cancellations; the Orkin White Wash bucket reminds anyone in customer service to "just tell the truth—don't try to cover it up." And in one corner of his office, Gary keeps a three-legged stool, rarely missing an opportunity to explain its significance to his business philosophy. "Each leg represents one facet of our company—our customers, our employees, and our shareholders," said Gary. "You need to give consideration to all three legs equally. If you disadvantage any one of them, the stool will fall. Start with the customer; the employee then benefits, and when they both are served, the shareholders benefit."

The corporate culture of Orkin was now boldly promoted within the organization as three generations of the Rollins family worked to lead the company. Their united message was clear: Work hard. Strive to make Orkin "simply the best, today and tomorrow." Treat your customers and employees the way you want to be treated. And finally, the success of a service industry like Orkin comes down to one thing: people who are dedicated to meeting the needs of the customer.

THE DEATH OF O. WAYNE ROLLINS

As Gary Rollins continued to mentor his own son, he suddenly lost the father who had mentored him. O. Wayne Rollins, the man who taught Gary and Randall Rollins so much about life and everything about business, passed away unexpectedly on October 11, 1991, following a pacemaker implant operation at Emory Hospital. He was seventy-nine years old. By

The O. Orkin Insect Zoo

The tailless whipscorpions, walking sticks, and giant cockroaches hardly make any noise at all. But you can hear the chirp of crickets before you see them, and if you listen carefully you'll hear the low, constant buzz-hum of the honeybees inside the glassed-in hive of their living bee tree. But if it's time for the daily feeding of that scary arthropod known as a tarantula, you can't miss the sounds of children squealing as you approach the O. Orkin Insect Zoo.

Located on the second floor of the Smithsonian Institution's National Museum of Natural History in Washington, D.C., the O. Orkin Insect Zoo is a wonderful maze of insect habitats and interactive learning exhibits that help explain how "over millions of years, insects have managed to flourish everywhere from icy oceans to tropical rain forests, hot deserts to freshwater ponds." The Insect Zoo focuses not only on strange and beautiful insects, but also on the relationships insects have with plants, other animals, and humans.

There's the live bee tree exhibit, where you can watch thousands of busy honeybees in their natural environment, leaving and returning to their hive after foraging on the mall; the fourteen-foot-tall replica of an actual termite mound, where you can crawl in and learn a lot about termites; the "Our House, Their House" exhibit, where visitors can push buttons to light up a part of the house and see what kind of insect is likely to live there (push the flea button and watch the pet dog start to scratch behind his ear!); and when you walk through the tropical rain forest exhibit, you'll start to understand how important this unique ecosystem is to the entire world, and be amazed that it is home to nearly one half of all earth's species of living things.

The Insect Zoo opened in the Smithsonian in 1976 and has remained the only exhibit in the museum to feature live creatures. And when it was renovated and renamed the O. Orkin Insect Zoo in 1993, Orkin became the first corporate sponsor to be associated with the ven-

design and through his life's work, the Georgia farm boy who made business history with his purchase of Orkin left behind a company that could stand completely without him, as strong as the metaphor of Gary's three-legged stool.

"Probably for the last ten years, I had dreaded the thought of my father dying because of the business responsibilities," said Gary, years later, when asked about his father's death. "And when it finally happened, I never thought at all about that, which is a tribute to him in my preparation. I mean, all I could think about was I had lost my father, somebody that no matter what the problem, I could always talk to. I lost my coach and friend. Dad had that saying about, 'Don't worry too much about things because most of the time they don't materialize' or 'Don't worry about everything.' And I thought, 'What irony!' because here was another example of what he said being true. Because when the time finally came, the business concerns didn't worry me at all."

erable Smithsonian Institution, a move that wasn't without some controversy at the time.

By 2002 Orkin had contributed over $4.6 million to support the O. Orkin Insect Zoo and the traveling O. Orkin Insect Safari. The Insect Zoo, the most highly visited exhibit at the Smithsonian, hosts over one million visitors every year. In 2003 Orkin updated the Insect Zoo with new carpeting, restored the insect cases, enhanced video lighting and sound systems, and updated exhibit graphics. The museum is considering moving the Insect Zoo in the future to a larger and more visible space on the first floor in order to better accommodate not only the three hundred live insects who live there but the millions of visitors each year who want to see how these creatures live.

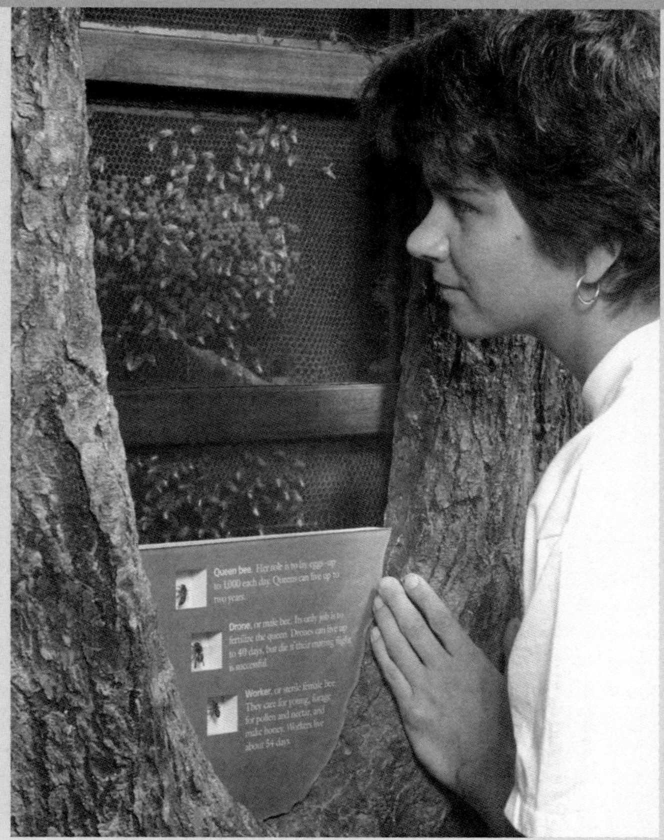

Thanks to Orkin's support and donations over the years, the O. Orkin Insect Zoo has become one of the most visited exhibits at the Smithsonian with more than a million visitors each year.

One of Wayne Rollins's key goals had always been to develop a company that was not dependent on the input of one or two executives. "It's a sign of weakness in a person if the company can't survive without him," he often said. Following his death, his sons were left to test their father's theory, and it held true.

Wayne Rollins: "In my opinion, Otto Orkin was a genius. He didn't have any pattern to follow. He worked hard and built his business by providing excellent service to his customers. Our job was to add our expertise and build upon what he accomplished."

"Following Dad's death, the public companies had to operate," said Randall, who was promoted to succeed his father as chairman of the board of directors and chief executive officer of the company. 'This was the first time we had to prove that we could run them without Dad. And if we didn't know how to do that, we didn't know anything. We had run them a long time. I can't really say that it felt different. We haven't had one crisis or one problem where we've said, 'We wish Dad were here to help us.' We miss him. We've said a thousand times, 'We just wish Dad were here.'"

Gary agreed. "It was a tribute to Dad that there was not any chaos in the organization, there was no panic on Wall Street. People were saddened, but I don't think our stock moved a quarter of a point. Obviously, investors were sorrowful because Dad had died, but people knew that he had two boys who were going to continue doing what they were prepared to do and what they had been taught to do—that although emotionally we had been shattered, there was not going to be a crisis in the company. Our people had been working with Randall and me for many years, and knew their futures were secure."

A few months before he died, O. Wayne Rollins gave an interview to *Rollins Today*, the company magazine that replaced *Orkin Talkin* when Rollins bought Orkin. And in the interview, he reflected both on the company's past and its future. "In my opinion, Otto Orkin was a genius. He didn't have any pattern to follow. He worked hard and built his business by providing excellent service to his customers," said Wayne Rollins. "Our job was to add our expertise and build upon what he accomplished. I consider the past 25 years with Orkin as a real opportunity. Looking forward, we have even further to go in the next 25 years, because I see even greater opportunities if we do our job well."

The opportunities that greeted Orkin in the years immediately following Wayne Rollins's death reflect a company constantly moving forward.

As a service company, there was almost no end to the possibilities. In 1992 Orkin added an agribusiness program to tackle pest control in agriculture, particularly the fly problem that plagued dairy livestock. It also created an Orkin Maid division to bring housekeeping services to existing customers.

Plantscaping expanded to nine major markets in sixteen states, and won the industry's prestigious Grand Award for Christmas Design at the GTE's Telephone Operations Division World Headquarters in Dallas, Texas. The company's income continued to increase as Orkin expanded pest control services in both commercial and residential markets, operating in forty-eight states, Canada, and Mexico. A "Zero Pest" guarantee was offered by Orkin to some upscale commercial accounts, and a PFG (pest-free guarantee) operation was created exclusively to service the entire Winn-Dixie food store chain. The Orkin "Robot" Exterminator advertisements continued to generate a significant increase in telephone leads for the company, and Orkin's marketing executives plotted to have the Exterminator sell Orkin's exclusive termite foam services. The company's aggressive public relations campaign resulted in Orkin becoming the first corporate sponsor at the Smithsonian. By offering Total Quality Management (TQM) training, company officials continued to emphasize job satisfaction and improve its employee retention. *Forbes* magazine responded to Rollins's efforts by listing it the Nation's Number One Service Company for the sixth consecutive year in 1992, and again in 1993 for the seventh consecutive year.

But as O. Wayne Rollins used to say, it's always important to "look behind good news." Beneath the surface of these prestigious accolades and accomplishments, Orkin management was wrestling with some serious issues, issues that would dominate the company until the new millennium—namely, termites, customer retention, termites, employee retention, termites, the changing face of the Orkin customer, termites, commercial versus residential services, termites, and how to expand and keep growing.

THE TERMITE REVOLUTION

No one could ignore the termite issue. Glen Rollins would ultimately call it the biggest challenge Orkin had ever faced. By the mid-1990s, the state of the post-chlordane termite world was clear: the replacement chemicals that had been heralded by the EPA didn't work nearly as well as chlordane; the new chemicals didn't even work as well as the manufacturers initially *stated* they were going to work. Termites were returning with a vengeance and Orkin, which at one point led the industry with its "lifetime guarantee" for its termite offering, was confronted with hundreds of millions of dollars in repair costs due to termite damage. More and more customers were calling Orkin to do repeat termite treatments and make good on Orkin's retreatment and repair guarantees. As a result, Orkin came to realize how effective chlordane had been and how marginal the new termiticides were. One magazine called it the "make or break" time for Orkin—which wasn't news to the Rollins team.

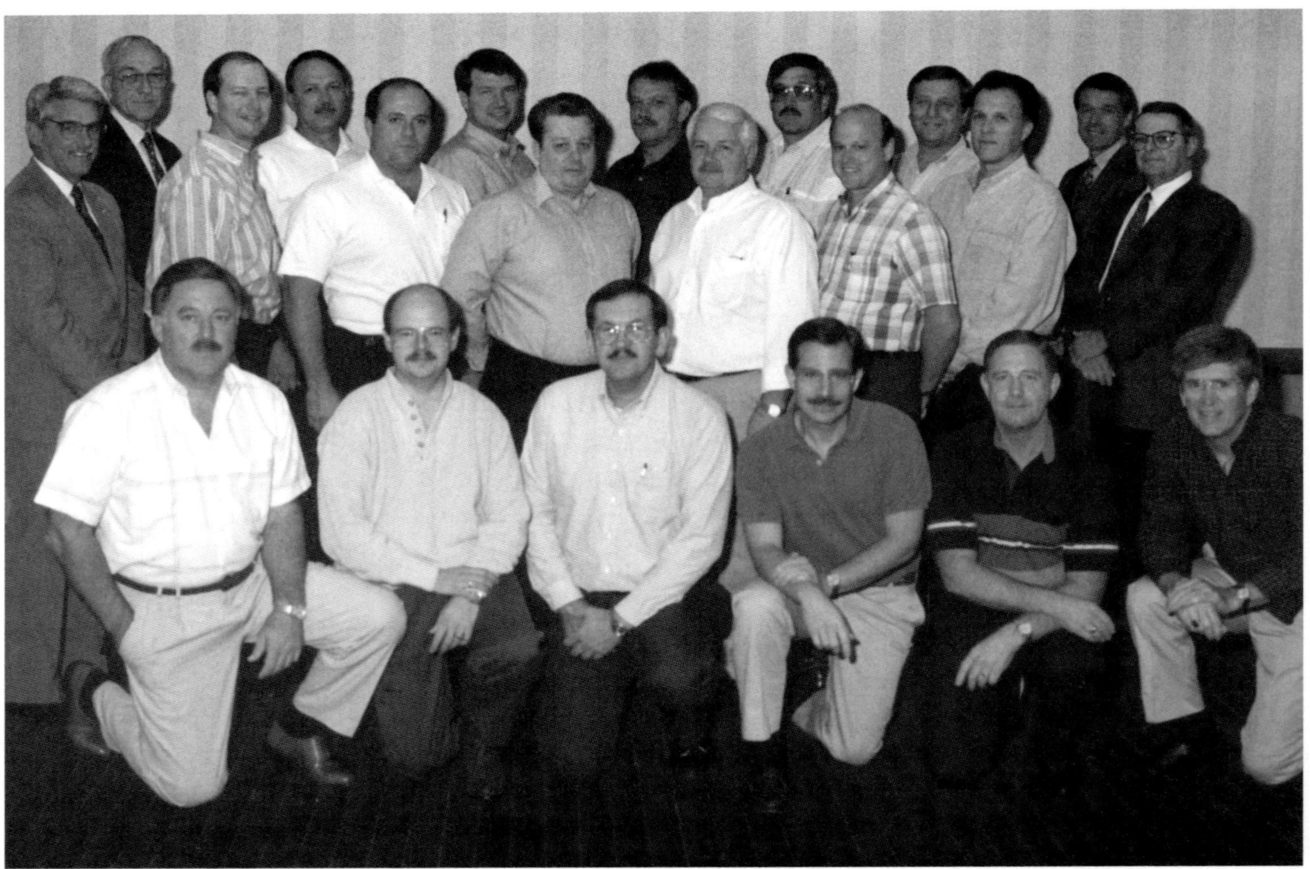

These 1993 graduates were one of many groups that completed Orkin's Quality Training Program. Left to right, front row: Russ Hartman, Tom Gradel, Jay Copen, Larry Miles, Orell Weeks, and Oz Moore (training consultant); second row: Steve Drennan, Ron Kimbell, Larry Gard, Elmer Garee, Ray Underwood, Bill Hackett, T. C. Del Guanto, and John Wilson; third row: Vince Stevens, Mike Connell, Earl Karas, Jay Bordes, Bill Hatfield, John Long, and Clyde Cobb.

"We had to take tremendous steps, and we made conscious decisions to give extra treatments and promptly pay for repairs," recalled Glen Rollins, who was Eastern North Carolina regional manager at the time. "The short-term cost was painful, but it was the right thing to do. We proactively treated thousands of customers with new products that weren't even available when they originally bought their treatment. Again, it was the right thing to do for our customers and for our company."

As Orkin worked to reengineer its termite program, Gary Rollins once referred to it as the "Termite Revolution." First, he said, "There were no more new lifetime guarantees. We offered three-, five-, or seven-year guarantees because that's how long the new termiticides were effective, and developed very extensive treating qualifications and specifications. We advised customers about conducive conditions. If you had a leaky gutter causing excessive water, for instance, we would advise you that the condition made termite control impossible and you were called upon to fix the problem or your termite coverage would be subject to cancellation. This was a real departure from the past. Second, we got very specific on how we wanted termite treatments to be rendered. Potential high-risk jobs were rejected. We created a quality assurance team that traveled across the country checking our termite treatments. We temporarily closed some branches if the work was not being done to meet these standards, and we totally changed what our termite salesmen could sell. Talk about a wet blanket. Our people were used to selling a product that had been relatively easy to sell, and then the very next day it became very challenging to sell. We lost, probably, 80 percent of our termite salesmen in the process."

To provide better termite protection, Orkin developed a treatment approach using borates, precision termiticide application techniques, and wet and dry foam as a termiticide carrier to provide more effective protection. "Whether it was a foam machine, perimeter application, or borates, we had to figure out the best

Once termite control had been relatively easy to sell. Ed Elkins, later president of Orkin, signed this termite service agreement when he was manager of the Knoxville, Tennessee, branch in 1957. With the change in guarantee, the task became more difficult.

ORKIN

Orkin Exterminating Company, Inc.

Renewal: $21.00

Completed:

(A Tennessee Corporation)

BRISTOL CHATTANOOGA CLEVELAND DALTON HARLAN

JOHNSON CITY KINGSPORT KNOXVILLE OAK RIDGE

R 7040

TERMITE CONTROL SERVICE ORDER

Dated at Knoxville, Tenn. (Office) on October 31, (Date) 1957

You are hereby authorized to treat the premises described below for the control of Subterranean Termites, and to make the following necessary repairs to said premises: (If residence property—specify if garage is included)

as per specifications dated October 30, 1957

Owner accepted responsibility of repairing termite damaged hardwood floor.

The cost for this service shall be as follows:

Repairs as above - - - - - - - - - - - - - - $ 38.00

Bonded Termite Treatment - - - - - - - - - - $ 349.00

The total cost of - - - - - - - - - - - - - - - - - - $ 387.00 is due and payable upon completion of work but may be paid as follows:

$96.75 Cash upon completion.

$96.75 Monthly for 3 months as evidenced by a series of ____ monthly notes bearing interest ~~at the rate of 6% per annum.~~

You reserve the right, upon default in any monthly payment to declare the entire unpaid balance instantly due and payable. Upon receipt of full payment as above, you are to deliver the Bonded Termite Control Guaranty to:

Mrs. / Mr. / Miss ____ NAME

Dogwood Ave. (Keith Add) Athens, Tenn.

Street Address City and State

ACCEPTED BY

ORKIN EXTERMINATING COMPANY, INC.

Approved:

By [signature] Manager

By Claude Brant Representative

You are to treat the following premises:

Which is used as a residence

Dogwood Ave. (Keith Add)

Street Address

Athens, Tennessee

City and State

ACCEPTED BY [signature] (Owner—Agent)

This termite control service order shall not be binding upon Orkin Exterminating Company, Inc., until approved by its manager at ____

ORKIN

way to deliver the products and make consumers happy. We resisted blindly jumping on the new termite bait application bandwagon. Orkin did not feel it was totally effective," said Steve Danuser, Orkin's marketing vice president.

It took years for Orkin to turn the corner on its new termite remediation and treatment programs, and the negative impact on employees and costs that the company sustained were substantial. Some high-profile lawsuits were filed against the company by homeowners who sustained termite damage while under contract with Orkin. Orkin settled many cases, and vigorously defended the company in others.

The company's annual report in 1996 reflected the fallout from Orkin's termite revolution. Termite claims, which had been running about $10 million a year, jumped to nearly $20 million. Orkin revenues increased 1 percent to $553.5 million, while operating income and profit margins decreased 49.4 percent and 50 percent, respectively, over the prior year. There was no way to sugarcoat the news, or gloss over the reasons why. "Our financial performance did not meet anticipated results. A decrease in termite sales revenue, escalating insurance costs, and termite claims and retreatment expense negatively impacted operating income."

The same annual report, however, noted that Rollins was committed to "continuing our course of renewal necessary to move our businesses forward through the next decade at a faster and more successful rate." For Orkin this "course of renewal" had already begun and would ultimately include some important new business initiatives in three key areas: keeping customers happy, expanding Orkin's commercial business, and for the first time in Orkin's history, franchising the Orkin brand and systems.

CUSTOMER SERVICE INITIATIVES

If the Rollinses and Otto Orkin have anything in common, it is their insistence that the customer always comes first. They believe that customers are the most important people in every business. That customers are not an interruption to work; they are the sole purpose of it. That customers are the lifeblood of this and every other business, and that without them you would have to close the doors.

To help coordinate their customer service initiatives, the company expanded the Rollins Customer Service Center or RCSC (later named the Rollins Customer Care Center) in 1995.

The service center employees accepted incoming calls generated in part by Orkin's 1-800-800-ORKIN customer awareness campaign, and made quality-control calls to customers. Any complaints and concerns received were electronically forwarded to the service branch for appropriate action. By 1996 Orkin's customer retention rate had reached a modern-day new level, and by 2001 the customer retention rate was better than it had been in twenty-five

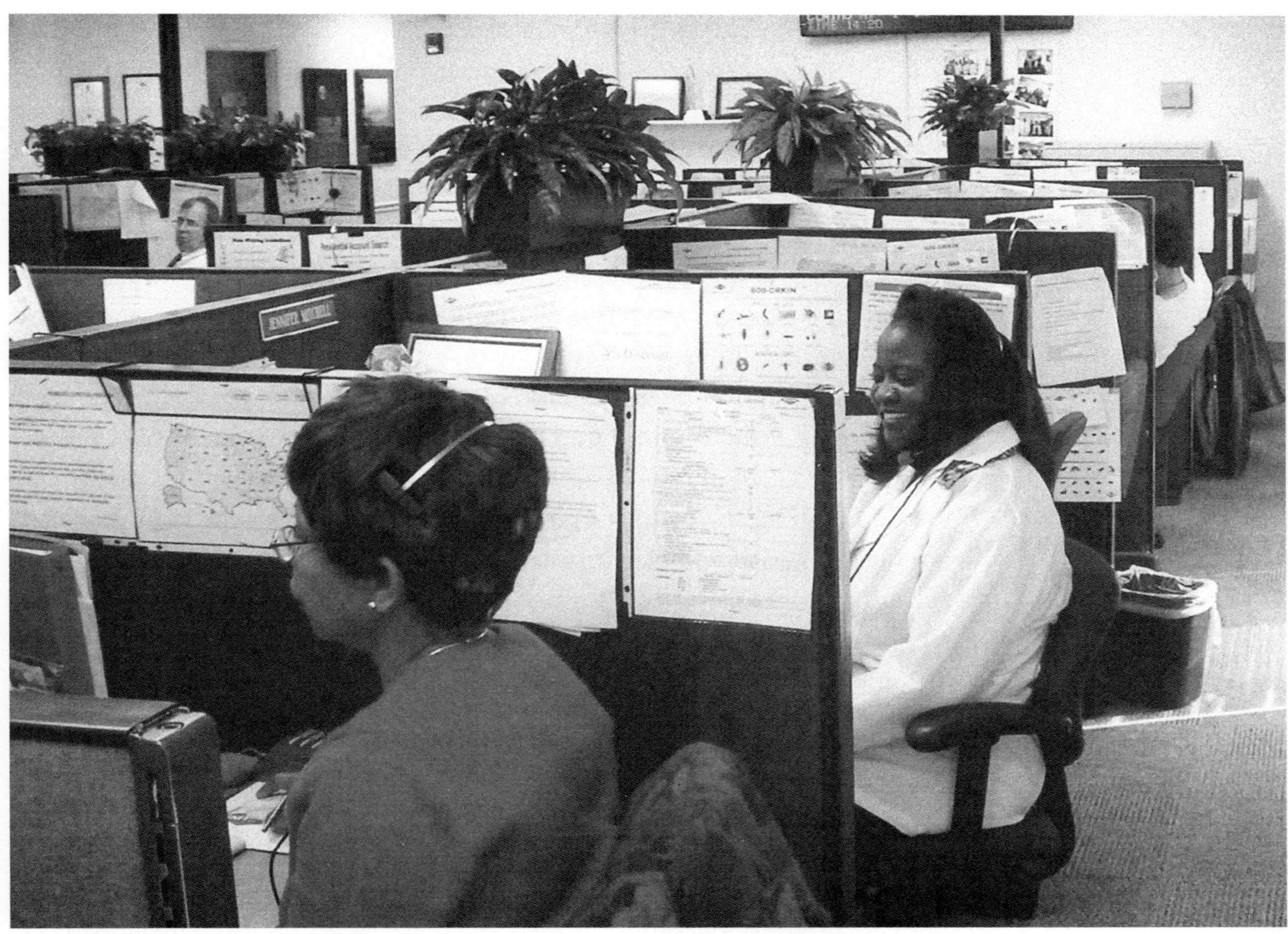

years. Orkin service was further enhanced by periodically calling customers and asking them, "How are we doing?" a step taken to build better customer relationships and to reduce the number of cancellations.

The Rollins Customer Care Center became ISO-certified in 2001, ensuring that its performance is consistent and customer-oriented. Lenna Whyms, left, and Jennifer Mitchell are well trained to assist customers when they call.

The call center reemphasized that Orkin was just as interested in customer service as in sales. According to Vince Stevens, senior vice president, nearly 80 percent of the eight thousand complaints received by the call center in its second year of operation concerned unreturned calls or missed appointments. "We want customers to call us for help, to take their problems up with the organization so they don't cancel." Orkin responded in several ways. It added branch employees where needed to help the servicemen return calls and to keep better track of appointments. And it introduced the 911 Customer Concern Program to make sure each customer phone call is handled by the end of the day. "Just as it would with any of us, unreturned phone calls and missed appointments are guaranteed ways of making customers feel that we don't care about them," said Stevens. "The rewards for this little bit of extra effort are easy to see: more satisfied and loyal customers. We all know that happy customers make for a healthier business."

And there was no denying that the call center also generated important cross-marketing opportunities between the Orkin divisions. For instance, during a call from Orkin about service, a pest control customer might express an interest in termite services. According to Freeman Elliott, who directed the company's cross-marketing program, the ability to solicit customers and share such leads between divisions resulted in over 150,000 leads in one year alone. For instance, in the fall of 1996, the RCSC sold $145,000 in new pest and termite business on a two-month campaign of cold-calling in the Orkin Alabama region. And when the RCSC helped Larry Rufledt, director of operations for the agribusiness program, put together a database of virtually every dairy farmer in the country, over $400,000 in new business was added to the program in a few months in 1996.

In addition, the company had started to recognize a shift in the habits of its consumers, whose busy lifestyles and two-career households made it difficult to schedule home pest control and termite services. As a result, Orkin's service programs underwent some changes. The Orkin Perimeter Defense System (PDS), for instance, provided a continuous barrier of specially formulated materials applied to the exterior of the house to help keep pests out. Orkin could make the application even when the customer wasn't home. Both the company and the customer would benefit, since it was more convenient for the customers as well as for Orkin.

Orkin's new Global Positioning System (GPS) could trace the Orkin service technician's route during the day, which helped the branches document service time, review driving time and speed, and better organize the routes. Inside the homes, the new PestSensor helped monitor insect activity to determine when and where service was needed. And after experimenting with bimonthly service instead of monthly visits, six of Orkin's thirty-five regions began in 1997 to offer every-other-month service, with Orkin adopting this new residential service all over the country by early 2000. "Today's consumer just wants to get it done," said Gary Rollins. "The customer wants you to take care of the bugs, but they don't want to be inconvenienced. Moving to every-other-month service has done everything that we intended for it to do. It has helped improve both technician and customer retention rates, and it has improved the company's profitability."

When asked if Otto Orkin was turning over in his grave, now that his former company had moved away from its trademark monthly service, Gary Rollins laughed. "I think he would be very pleased," he said. "Mr. Orkin's core value was in customer satisfaction. And it just really crushed him to lose a customer. I think that Mr. Orkin was a good enough businessman to understand that if you can do the same job in a different way and the customer likes it better—that's key."

A NEW EMPHASIS ON COMMERCIAL SERVICE

In 1995 Glen Rollins began to concentrate his efforts on learning about the company's commercial pest control services, specifically how to enhance this operation. Though Orkin was the nation's largest commercial pest control provider, growth in commercial accounts had stagnated in recent years. A series of focus groups revealed that the public generally perceived Orkin as a provider of residential pest control and termite services—but not commercial service. This path no doubt seemed contrary to those who remembered the company's early days in pest control for warehouses, food service companies, banks, and hotels. But Clyde Cobb, who remembers when the company "had every commercial account in town," had seen the shift coming.

"From 1966 on, we were on a course of moving away from commercial," said Cobb, who had been with Orkin since 1946 and eventually became vice president of Orkin's Commercial Division. "Television advertising threw so many leads in the offices that we just ran with the leads and didn't try to keep, or go, after the commercial business. It is so easy to pick from the low-hanging fruit. Residential customers were easier to service during the day, not at night like commercial, and it was much easier to sell. Termite business was good and profitable, and the termite and residential pest control leads were coming from the same sources. We just shifted away from the commercial market. However, we were still the largest providers of commercial pest control services in the country, so we had to do something to change those perceptions. What we needed was an advocate for the commercial side."

Glen Rollins became that advocate. After serving as vice president of corporate development, he followed Clyde Cobb and was named vice president of the commercial division and worked in 1996 to accelerate the growth of this division. When Gary Rollins announced in the summer of 1996 that Orkin was going to be "the best pest control provider for commercial customers," Orkin expanded its designated commercial branches to service major commercial markets throughout the country. Orkin started out with ten such commercial branches and, within the next years, grew to over forty.

It was exactly what Cobb had hoped for. "Our commercial branches do a much better job servicing and working as a commercial service team than our residential branches combining commercial and residential work," he said. "That's the reason we need to get as many of our commercial accounts into the hands of commercial technicians and supervisors as possible. We had so many low spots in the country where a residential technician had to service a complicated commercial account. We used to write the book on commercial service, and we just have to put the resources into getting that done as it was before."

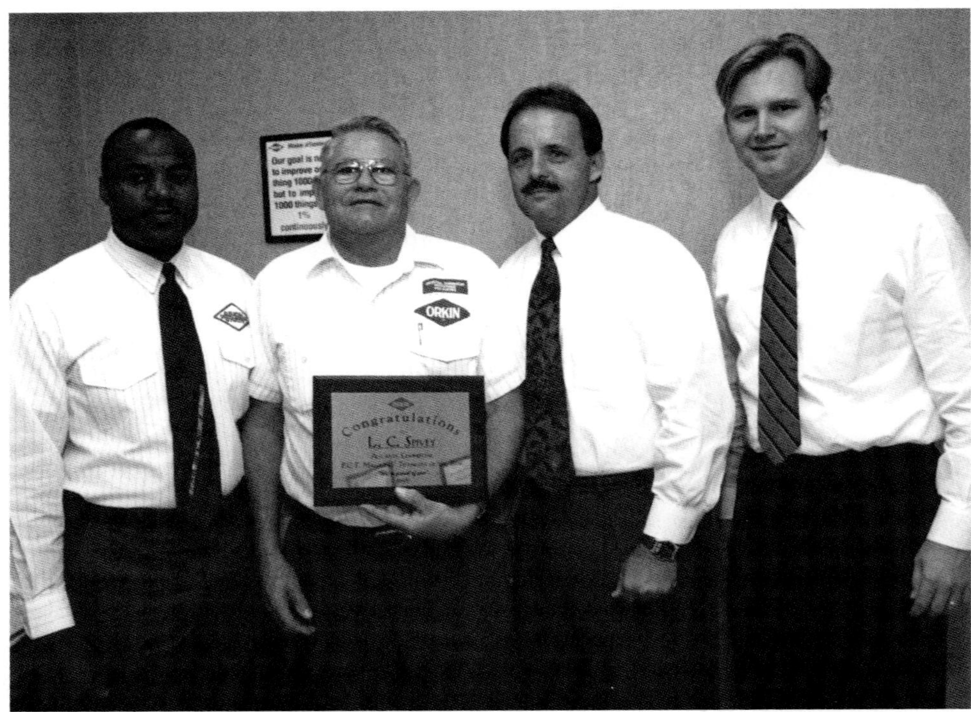

Left to right: Atlanta commercial service manager Willie Banks, commercial technician L. C. Spivey, region manager John Wilson, and division vice president Glen Rollins commemorate L.C.'s winning the national award for PCT Technician of the Year in 1997.

The new commercial division soon anchored an account list that included Kmart Corporation, Delta Air Lines, Taco Bell, Burger King, Tropicana Products, Blockbuster Video, and many others. Orkin's certified commercial technicians were required to take extensive training that included eleven days of classroom work and thirty days of on-the-job training, and to pass the American Institute of Baking and the Purdue University correspondence course. By 1997 Orkin's commercial revenue was growing over 20 percent annually and realizing more than $150 million in business.

And Orkin continued to experiment with some commercial specialties, like Orkin Agribusiness, expanding the Dairy Farm Fly program to many locations in the country and Canada. "I think our success in agribusiness has shown us that there are a lot of good commercial niche markets out there," said Gary Rollins. "We need to provide the resources to reach those markets, while at the same time continuing to serve our residential customers."

Glen Rollins pushed the commercial concept even further two years later when he spearheaded rebranding Orkin Commercial under a new name: *Acurid, a commercial service brought to you by Orkin*. Though the Acurid trademark would later be attached to the company's commercial service training program, the company returned to the name Orkin Commercial Services when research confirmed that the Orkin brand was too powerful to ignore. By 2001 the commercial division provided nearly one-third of Orkin's revenue base, compared with one-fifth in 1991.

THE FRANCHISE PROGRAM

In yet another strategic move to accelerate Orkin's revenue and reach, Orkin announced in 1995 the start of a franchise program that would allow qualified individuals with pest control experience to purchase the rights and systems to provide termite and pest control services under the Orkin name. Almost immediately, veteran Orkin branch manager Don Lackey gave up his position and opened Orkin's first franchise operation with one route and a base of 299 pest control customers in the eastern Atlanta suburb of Conyers, Georgia. During his first year of operation, Lackey predicted revenues of $186,000, but actually realized over $400,000. The association with Orkin was critical. "I like being my own boss and having my own business," Lackey said at the time. "But I don't feel like I'm out here all alone. I still feel like a member of the Orkin family."

Ironically, Otto Orkin and Ted Oser had always insisted that Orkin's reluctance to franchise offered an advantage over the company's competition, which depended heavily on franchise outlets to provide pest control services. But Mark Giglio, Orkin's first director of franchising, said the practice would

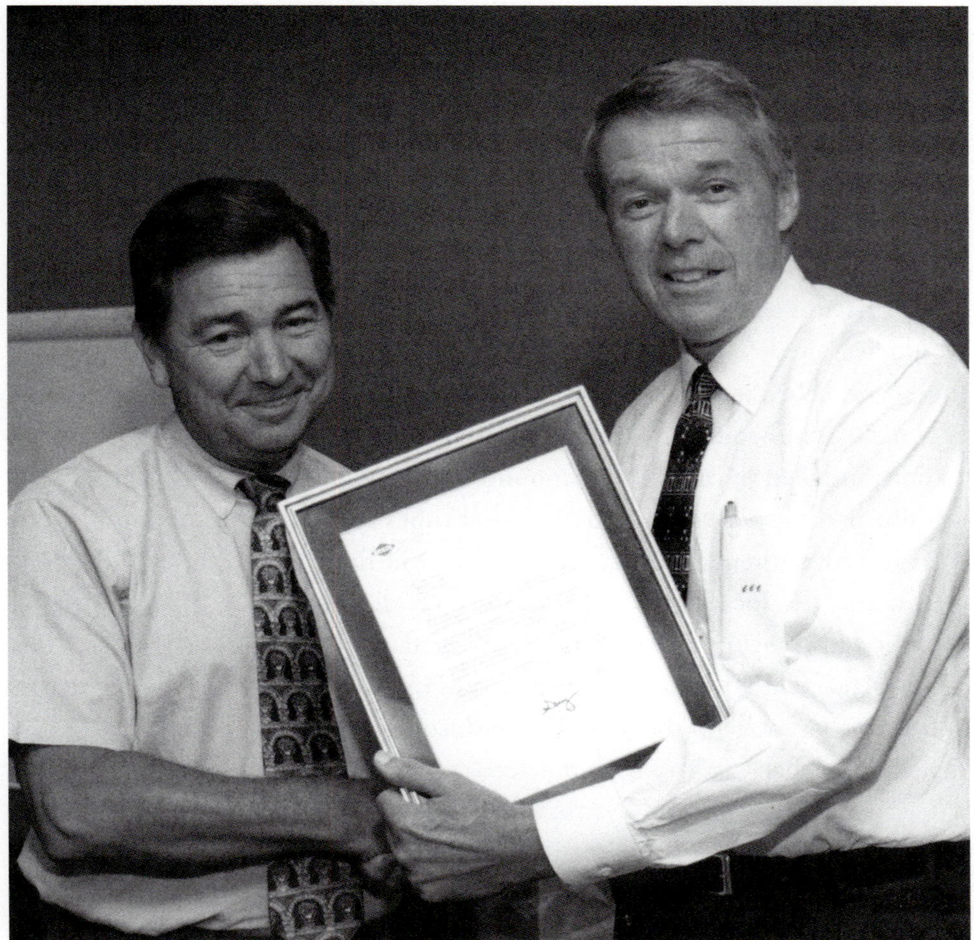

Veteran branch manager Don Lackey, left, became Orkin's first franchisee in 1995. He is shown here with Clyde Cobb, who was vice president of corporate development at the time.

actually help Orkin expand into new markets at a reduced cost—and give Orkin faster exposure in territories that would otherwise take five to ten years to establish. Since the company has a buy-back provision built into the contract, the franchise program also "planted the seeds of future acquisition," said Giglio. From the beginning, Orkin provided each franchise operation an "exit strategy" that would require the franchisees to sell their businesses back to Orkin at Orkin's option once the franchise operations reached certain volume and time milestones. As Orkin reached its hundredth year of business, it began to buy back its initial franchises, an innovative acquisition strategy that would give new meaning to the word "Orkinizing." And interestingly enough, Lackey, who opened the first Orkin franchise operation, was the first to sell his franchise back to Orkin in 2002 for over a million dollars.

TERMITE BAITING

The company had high hopes for termite baiting when it introduced its new OrkinGuard Termite Baiting system in 1996, a system they had been field-testing for over four years. The new termite baiting program was expected to reduce by half the amount of conventional liquid termiticides necessary to safeguard the average home, yet it would add a higher level of protection. Clearly, termite baiting was considered by many in the industry to be the termite control system of the future—the bridge between the "lifetime effectiveness" that earlier termiticides provided and an "environmentally friendly" approach.

Unlike roach or ant baits, which attract the insects to the poison, this program uses specifically designed plastic stations placed in the ground, which contain pieces of specially prepared wood. These monitoring stations have small slits and holes. Technicians place the stations in the ground in termite-conducive areas, for example, near tree stumps, firewood, air-conditioning units, and other areas where wood and moisture combine to attract termites. A two-thousand-square-foot home could have up to twenty baited monitoring stations installed in critical areas around the home. Above-ground bait stations are also used in places where active mud tubes are found on the foundation. This improves the likelihood that termites will find the stations. The technician marks the location of the stations on a diagram of the house to check them for signs of termite visitation or hits. If a monitoring station has a hit, Orkin replaces it with an active baited station. The termites eat the active bait and carry it back to the underground colony. Other termites follow the marked trail back to the bait and feed on it. The bait taken to the colony enters its food supply and eventually disrupts the termites' life cycle. Unlike the rest of the industry, Orkin would sell termite baits only in conjunction with a modified liquid foundation treatment application—a decision that would be applauded by the regulators in five years.

As Orkin rolled out its new bait program, it began to test-market a new animated "Orkin Man" TV commercial to replace the Exterminator robot on television. Studies had shown that when three out of four consumers saw the Orkin Man—still dressed in a crisp white shirt with red epaulets and tan khaki trousers—they immediately thought of pest control. The animated Orkin Man resembled the wildly popular character known as Woody from the popular movie *Toy Story*—only the Orkin Man was extremely buff and remarkably strong, more like Woody's sidekick, Buzz Lightyear. This creative concept was used from 1997 to 2000 in the company's television advertising.

A SINGLE BUSINESS FOCUS

In an effort to strengthen its Orkin brand and return to what Rollins, Inc., called "a single focus," the company decided in 1997 to concentrate its managerial and investment efforts on pest and termite control. Toward that goal, the company sold the Orkin Lawn Care and Plantscaping businesses in July for nearly $37 million, and sold Rollins Protective Services (RPS) in October for over $200 million. "It is fortunate that the timing of these two independent transactions occurred when the Pest Control business requires a substantial amount of attention and investment," both Gary and Randall Rollins reported together in the year's annual report. "Selling these companies will enable our top management to focus their resources on our core business." At the time of the divestitures, Gary noted that Orkin provided 98 percent of the company's profits, and approximately 85 percent of its revenue. To squash rumors that had started to circulate among the company's eight thousand employees, Gary reassured them that these moves were "not an indication of more events to follow. Orkin Exterminating Co., Inc., *is not for sale.* The ability to be singularly purposed in creating the World's Best Pest Control Company will be beneficial to all of our employees, customers and shareholders."

Though publicly his words were optimistic, by mid-1997 Gary was in the throes of grappling with the realities of the pest control industry in general and the termite crisis in particular. To wit: the company's drop in revenue and its waning profit margins, Orkin's difficulties with termite property damage claims, and both customer and employee retention were challenging issues faced by corporate management every day. Financial reports told the story of the company's economic decline: in 1994 Rollins reported the highest earnings per share in the history of the company, at $1.39 per share; just three years later, in 1997, earnings had dramatically skidded to $0.04 per share and for the first time in the company's history, it reported a net operating loss. In an internal memo written in July 1997, Gary Rollins noted that "June was

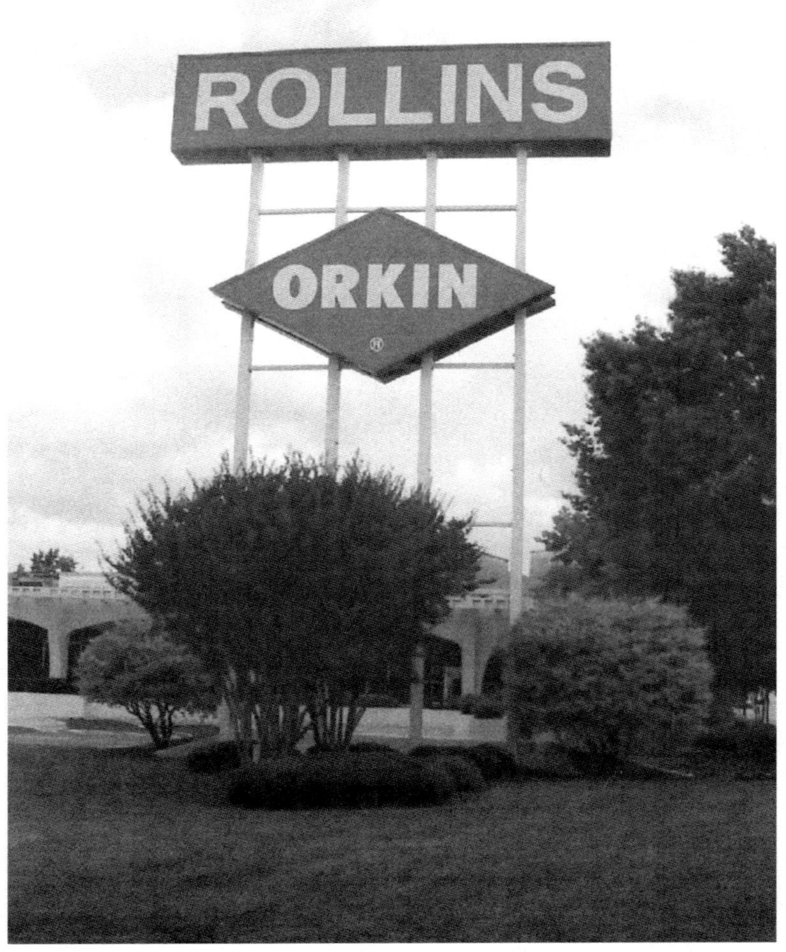

With the sale of Orkin Lawn Care and Plantscaping divisions and Rollins Protective Services in 1997, Rollins focused on the core business operations of Orkin Pest Control.

a disappointing month for all pest control divisions of Rollins. We did not have a division that made its Revenue plan for the month. . . . **Keep in mind: it's always darkest before the dawn.**"

In the face of this business dilemma, the company took a decidedly bold and proactive step in 1997 to take care of its termite customers and, at the same time, to try to protect Orkin shareholders and customers from further expenses related to termite liability. From profits related to the sale of RPS, Rollins established a $117 million termite reserve designed to cover the "anticipated costs of reinspections, repair obligations and associated labor, chemicals and other costs incurred relative to termite work performed prior to December 31, 1997." This Provision for Termite Contracts, reported in the company's 1997 Annual Report, meant that literally thousands of Orkin termite customers would have their properties retreated—and, if necessary, repaired—by Orkin for free. The company hired additional employees and fanned out all over the country to voluntarily retreat homes that Orkin identified as "at risk" for future termite damage in these uncertain post-chlordane years.

When Michael W. Knottek joined the company as senior vice president in June 1997, he was impressed by the fact that the company had created this fund to provide termite insurance for its customers. Granted, the creation of such a fund would enable Orkin over time to keep its termite liability costs down. But what Mike immediately saw in this unusual termite reserve was the company's remarkable commitment to do right by its customers.

"One of the reasons that I came with Rollins was because of this kind of action. It really showed a commitment to the customer," Knottek remembers. "We retreated a huge number of homes before there were any complaints. The company had over $100 million in cash that could have been used for new buildings, extra dividends for shareholders, or bonuses to management. But they said no, we want to take this money and we want to protect our customers. I was stunned at the time by the corporate responsibility that Rollins showed. There are not a whole lot of companies that would do that."

DIVIDE AND CONQUER

It's probably safe to say that not a whole lot of companies would embark on the next step that Gary and Randall had in mind for Orkin. In the summer of 1997, the Rollins brothers initiated a bold, somewhat controversial plan to rejuvenate the company and help Orkin realize again the financial success it had experienced in the past. Effective July 1, 1997, Orkin's residential branch network was expanded from four to six residential divisions. Essentially, it was announced, the company would be split under two leaders: Randall Rollins would be in charge of two of the divisions: Mid-Atlantic and West Central, with David Downing and Robert Stevens as division vice presidents, respectively; Gary Rollins would be in charge of the remaining four residential Orkin divisions, namely Southeast, with Vince Stevens as vice president; Northeast, with Bill Hackett, vice president; Midwest, with Steve Drennan, vice president; and West Coast, with Gary Rowell, vice president.

"To me," said Randall, when asked to describe how he and Gary developed such a strategy, "if you are not doing as well as you should, something's broken. Orkin has been a good company all the time, but what happens with a company and specifically Orkin, we get out of focus and we have to bring it back into focus. Everyone is working hard every day, and they are working on whatever they are working on—but that doesn't mean they are working on the right things in the right way. And I think it's my job to get them into focus."

Years later, Gary would describe this period and his partnership with Randall as the "Divide and Conquer" era at Orkin. Translated? Divide the work and conquer the problems. The premise, Gary and Randall always maintained, was really simple: two heads are better than one. By doubling the top management horsepower, the likelihood of fixing the financial and operating problems quickly would be dramatically improved. In some ways, it was an expanded version of what Randall and Gary did when they went to Memphis with the region managers in 1979, and the various experiments and operational programs that followed in the Decatur branch. Without having to test every new procedure throughout the company, results could be realized more quickly.

What's more, this new initiative would provide opportunities to address some home office weaknesses while identifying new business procedures and approaches. Said Gary: "There was no time for egos or pontificating. The company had a crisis, and it was time to act." Randall agreed: "Gary and I had always worked well together. There was no reason to think that this would be any different."

The Divide and Conquer experiment had one goal: get the company back on track, and restore it to profitable and efficient levels. As they had done in the past, Gary relied on Randall's efforts to effect change and to explore new ideas and methods; he respected Randall's opinion that if you are a good manager, you can run any kind of business. In turn, Randall trusted Gary's judgment as to what ultimately would and would not work in the bug business.

But to many outsiders, and to many of the rank and file within the company, it was the ultimate sibling competition—six Orkin residential divisions allocated to two brothers, both working to improve revenue and increase profits, streamline procedures, and provide better customer service. The sense of competition increased when Randall, in an effort to invigorate the company with new ideas and techniques, hired several top management executives from service industries outside of Orkin. The long-term Orkin insiders on Gary's team occasionally bristled because so many new managers came from the linen service industry.

Mike Knottek on the Divide and Conquer strategy: "It was a laboratory for change. . . . It allowed each group to undertake its own initiatives to improve profitability. It allowed for twice as much experimentation and progress."

"It was a laboratory for change," said Knottek, one of the "Linen People" hired by Randall just as the company reorganization was initiated. "Orkin was clearly on the skids, for all of the reasons we've listed: the chlordane change, the increase in termite claims brought about by this and the guarantees, Orkin's insistence on retreating threatened homes. Orkin was proactive. But that was one of the main reasons for the decline in profitability. It was looking bad for the company. When Gary and Randall said, 'Let's split the company,' it allowed each group to undertake its own initiatives to improve profitability. It allowed for twice as much experimentation and progress."

Robert T. Stevens was hired by Randall in 1997 to run one of his two divisions. One of the first things he noted about Randall was his "sincere and deep concern as to the direction that the company was taking. Randall is a very, very tough businessman, and he has high expectations, and he expects his people to have those high expectations also. I believe that he felt like he owed it to the shareholders, the employees of the company, the customers, and to his family to do what he and Gary believed would be necessary to put the company back on what was the right path."

The path taken by the brothers, however, wasn't necessarily embraced by the company ranks, Stevens readily admits. "The Orkin people did feel that they were in competition with us," he said. "I think it was more that they felt threatened, and it had to be a traumatic time for some. I'm sure they had to look on it as, 'Why are those guys being brought into this company at the same level I've worked twenty-five years to get to?'"

Clarence E. "Butch" Thress Jr., now regional manager for Tennessee who worked for Orkin as a branch manager during the Divide and Conquer years, felt immediately like he "had a target on my back" when his region was taken over by Randall. "No one doubted Randall's sincerity, but his mere presence in the field was a shock," said Thress. "As far as the field people were concerned, Gary was our boss. Randall was never visible. He was The Man, and you just never saw the CEO of the company. But one of the most positive things I got out of this was getting to know Randall Rollins. We all knew and respected Gary, and during this period of time, we got to know Randall and it was just an honor to work for him, too."

In April 1998, Harry J. Cynkus, a former colleague of both Knottek and Downing, was hired to be the new chief financial officer for Rollins. The "division years," he later recalled, were all about "restoring profitability to the company. The business model was broken. The company had for a number of years been very successful. It may have become complacent—it's hard to say. But the termite business and their guarantee program almost put Orkin out of business. For many years, the claims ran about $6 million a year. And then, at one point, we were paying out $40 million a year to retreat and repair homes and settle the claims. I joined the company saying, 'Here's a challenge.'

"But there was a misperception of what Gary and Randall were doing when they divided the company," Cynkus continued. "Gary and Randall never felt that they were competing. By running two divisions, Randall had

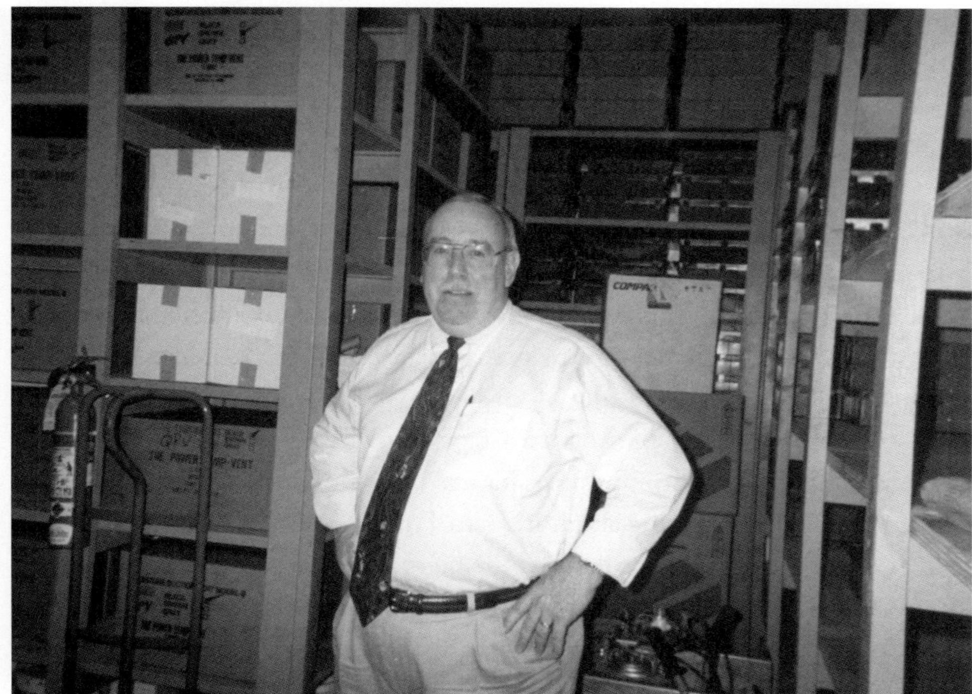

Clarence E. "Butch" Thress, region manager for Tennessee, was surprised when Randall took over two divisions of Orkin, because he had not been very "visible" in the field before.

the chance to say, 'I want to try something different and break some paradigms. Let's experiment. If some things work, we can use them; if others don't, you can say, 'I told you so.' Gary and Randall knew what they were doing. They were finding the best things for the business, and then they would put it back together. They didn't see the strife, but people misperceived it. There was even a posting on the Internet that Gary and Randall has been spotted in the parking lot, duking it out!"

During the Divide and Conquer era, Gary Rollins asked longtime Orkin employee Steven Drennan, who joined Orkin in 1970 as a pest control technician and was now vice president of the Midwest Division, to take over the Southeast Division in January 2000. Drennan recalls that at the time, the "company just absolutely had to get a stranglehold on the termite issues. A new person coming in will see a whole new area of concern that maybe you may have failed to see. Randall allowed us to attack a number of issues using different methods. He brought in a lot of outside people. And yes, I have to agree. It was 'divide and conquer.' Everyone can have their own opinion as to why things were done when they were done, but certainly seeing what's been accomplished through the changes can help everyone see that the concept was a good one."

To Gary, fixing Orkin was "personal, professional, and financial. I guess as a major shareholder and stakeholder in the business, we kind of 'bleed' Orkin red. The consequences of the termite issues were substantial, and at the same time, we had other issues to address—the company had to address Y2K in anticipation of the year 2000 and its impact on computer systems, employee and customer retention were ongoing challenges, every-other-month service was getting close to being launched. There were a number of priorities. We just said, 'Gee. It's going to take both of us working together to get this thing fixed.'"

The new Orkin divisions had the full support of the board of directors. Director Henry Tippie, a former Rollins, Inc., executive and chairman of the board and chief executive officer of Tippie Services, Inc., noted that the Divide and Conquer years really showcased and capitalized on the very different but very complementary business styles of two extremely astute businessmen. There's Randall Rollins—brilliant when it comes to probing and discovering the details, obsessed with facts and known to ask a lot of questions, never without a little piece of paper. "If something comes up that is of interest, he will make a note about it," said Tippie. And there's Gary Rollins—brilliant when it comes to looking at the big picture, able to see the the broad scope of business and the domino effect business decisions have on subsequent steps, someone who connects easily to employees. "He thinks things out carefully," said Tippie, "and he knows the business."

"It was a good move, to split it up a bit," said Tippie. "That way, you get the benefit of two approaches in half the time. It worked. Each quarter showed progress."

James B. Williams, a board member since 1978 and former chairman of the board of SunTrust Banks, Inc., remembers that the company wasn't in a crisis. "We saw the numbers," he said. "They were never in trouble. Other companies would have seen the numbers, which were starting to deteriorate, and would have said it's a business cycle and played right through it. But Randall and Gary don't let things alone. They knew that this company could make more money than it had been making. It was like, 'We need to do better.' And they solved it. The difference here is that they didn't hire outside consultants—they solved it themselves. Randall and Gary got in there and rolled up their sleeves, and their sleeves were already pretty much rolled up. They just added another layer."

James B. Williams: "Other companies would have seen the numbers, which were starting to deteriorate, and would have said it's a business cycle . . . . But Randall and Gary don't let things alone."

And how was the Divide and Conquer strategy presented to the board? "Gary wanted it, and Randall wanted it," said Williams. "That wasn't awkward. They always presented it as 'We did this, we built a team.' It was not an 'I did it' kind of proposition." Presenting a united front to the board of directors was one thing; maintaining that sense of camaraderie throughout the company was altogether different. Each team had its marching orders and was challenged to achieve certain objectives. Occasionally, said Knottek, the process "developed into a 'we' and 'they' within the company. Within the individual groups, it was fine. But at times, there were hard feelings that developed between the two groups. As an example, they didn't necessarily follow the same procedures or the same training schedules. And when they interacted, there was naturally some jealousy, some contempt and hard feelings, a sense of competition. All of those emotions were there at one time or another. Clearly both sides were driven to do better, and to upstage each other. And you lost certain synergies when it wasn't one company; however, the end result was worth the sacrifice."

Randall Rollins was genuinely surprised at the level of animosity and competition the division created. "I didn't think about that happening," he said. "But that was just naive on my part. I felt like everyone would buy in, but change is threatening to people, so they dug their heels in a little bit. But that's natural. I don't think there's anything unusual about that."

Gary Rollins readily admits that one of the greatest challenges of the Divide and Conquer years was "for me to keep the people out of the rumor and gossip business, to understand that this decision was not based on some ulterior motive on my part or Randall's part, or that it was based on a lack of confidence in my abilities or a slap in the face to the more senior Orkin people. The people who really knew us said immediately, 'Hey, get off of that. You're not going to split them up.' Randall and I have never been competitive. We've always been close. I was still doing some of my annual company-wide Road Shows and talking to branch managers, on both sides, Randall's as well as mine. But the questions always came up with both sides. And I explained that we have an ox in the ditch, and we need to get it out. Clearly, the need is there, and I had asked for his help. But as soon as the ox is out of the ditch, I reassured them that Randall had no designs on staying involved with Orkin to the present extent."

The Divide and Conquer years, which stretched from July 1997 to June 2001, resulted in some critical and business-saving initiatives within Orkin.

Said Randall: "We've just been fortunate. Dad and Gary and I got along great, and after Dad passed away, Gary and I continued to get along great. And you know, three people can just decide things better than one, and two people can make better decisions than one. We've kind of carried that tradition and way of operating along. It was always intended that the divisions would eventually go back into the same operation. The separate operation of the two divisions gave us the opportunity to look at some different business models and try some different programs, and some programs that are now being used company-wide have come out of that. I want to make it very clear that they weren't just *my* ideas—but ideas from Gary and Gary's team, from the Orkin folks and the people who came in from other areas. All those people contributed greatly."

When the two companies went back together, Ray T. Smiley, Kentucky Region manager, remembers that "there was as much fear when we were ready to merge back as there was when we separated. Herman Borel, the new division vice president of the area where I worked, made that transition very, very easy. Certainly Gary Rollins wanted to make sure that everyone understood that it was the same company, and we were all going to be doing the best things that we had learned through the separation."

And though the separation did not last very long in retrospect, it resulted in some, well, surprising emotions and lasting friendships. After the reorganization was announced, Thress remembers watching David Downing say good-bye. There was hardly a dry eye in the room. "At the very first, I didn't have very good feelings about these Linen Guys. But I'll tell you what, I was emotionally affected by watching David. He had found out that us Orkin guys were pretty good guys. He was a little choked up. He was going to miss us. That sent a message to me that we had become coworkers, and that we were all headed in the same direction." The Divide and Conquer years, which stretched from July 1997 to June 2001, resulted in some critical and business-saving initiatives within Orkin. Though each brother is loathe to take individual credit, their joint accomplishments were nonetheless highlighted by some very distinct achievements driven by each brother's unique business passions: Gary, it turned out, excelled at creating innovative service initiatives and turning them into new company-wide policies that brought about improved profits and customer retention; Randall, on the other hand, focused much of his energy (and, at one point, his own financial resources) on improving the company's training programs, resulting in a new training center that led to improved employee retention.

In many ways, the operational split of Orkin for those four years—with all of its inherent or perceived competition, its accomplishments, and its failures—deserves its own Harvard Business School case study, as unique in many respects as the purchase of Orkin by Rollins some forty years ago. Imagine: one company run as two companies by two different people, competing to see who can come out ahead in specific areas and then putting it back together. And while people continue to differ on the strategy of the experiment's execution, no one doubts the achievements these years produced. Consider the introduction of the following policies and programs:

- Every-other-month pest control service, which would become the company's primary residential pest control service offering, positively impacting productivity, pay, and customer retention.
- GPS, the Global Positioning System for service trucks and cars, which resulted in significant improvement in accident rates and employee accountability; and TruckStops, the computerized routing and scheduling program. Combined, these two technologies were designed to improve the timeliness of customer service while improving technician efficiency and reducing fleet operating costs.
- A computer software program for a handheld device developed and tested for commercial pest control and termite technicians.
- A new Termite Quality Assurance program, which initiated compliance audits in residential branches company-wide under the new Termite National Quality Control Department. Called "QAs" in the field, the new Termite Quality Assurance program required field inspectors, as well as branch and region management staffs, to make monthly inspections to ensure that customers receive the treatments and service specified in their contracts. "It just forced people to do a better job," said David Downing, Randall's assistant during and after the Divide and Conquer years. Said Butch Thress: "That business could not be charged as new business until the QAs were completed."

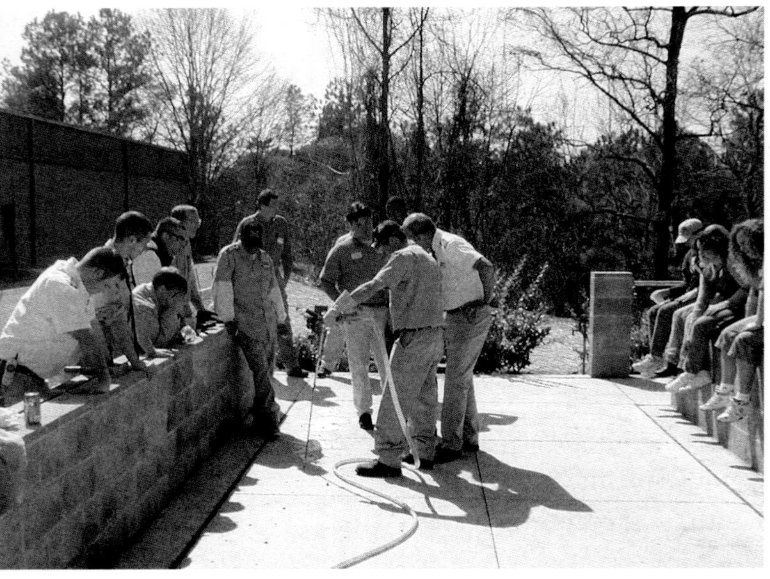

- Termite service guarantees changed from lifetime to three-, five-, and seven-year term agreements. An actuary was engaged to compile termite damage claims statistics by the year of initial treatment.
- Changes in compensation bonus programs and benefit plans were made to better reward and motivate employees.
- Centralized administrative offices and service centers as a new form of field organization.

Orkin trainees and visiting University of Florida students look on as training specialist Doug Lambright discusses drilling techniques.

The Training Center

Since the post–World War II days of Herman L. Fellton, Orkin has placed a premium on training and professional expertise. Hired as the company's first technical director in 1946, Fellton began a series of training courses for branch managers and supervisors, and developed the company's first printed instructions for handling and administering chemicals in all locations.

Those early days of training, however, no doubt consisted of lectures, printed materials, chalkboards, and eventually watching filmstrips in front of a Dukane projector. But over the years, Orkin developed a series of professional training materials and began to work with leading universities and organizations to deliver pest management techniques and training on new service techniques, the latest technological advancements, and equipment. As the company approached its first century of service, it enjoyed technical and training relationships with such leading universities as the University of Florida, Virginia Polytechnic Institute, the University of Georgia, Purdue University, and California Polytechnic Institute. Orkin's most recent educational partnership was formed through its association with Texas A&M University, which developed an advanced university-certified termite training correspondence program exclusively for Orkin.

And in the summer of 2000, Orkin officially opened the new Orkin Training Center, a remarkable facility just outside Atlanta that quite literally brings the problems and pests of the pest control industry right inside, all for the purpose of training.

A tour of the new facility speaks volumes. The large classrooms are often packed with Orkin Men and Women learning the entomology ropes from Training Center manager and entomologist Ron Harrison. Ron's refrigerator is always packed with the necessary show-and-tell items as he explains the biology and habits of pests, and how to recognize evidence of infestation without seeing bugs. Additional training personnel provide lectures on Integrated Pest Management; how to crawl under a building or a house for a termite inspection; and how to manage that unique aspect of being an Orkin Man that training specialist Doug Lambright calls "the secret of the confessional: you can't share what you've seen."

- The new Atlanta Orkin Training Center and new and improved technical training materials. The new training center not only has a full-sized house, but also other structures where technicians can see the connection between pests and home construction and where they can simulate pest treatments under the supervision of qualified instructors.
- Improved university alliances and training materials provided by leading research institutions and universities such as Texas A&M University, one of the nation's leading termite control schools.
- Improved customer service and employee retention rates (the results of better training and pay).
- The addition of new executives and managers who brought experience and perspectives from other service industries; when the Divide and Conquer experiment was over, most moved into important positions within either Orkin or Rollins.

After completing course work in the training facility classrooms, participants head outside to the modern, one-story brick house with a two-column front portico and a one-car garage, complete with furniture and linens, dishes and food in the pantry, and attractive landscaping. But this house is actually a home laboratory designed to provide hands-on training for Orkin Men. Throughout the home, wall sections and floors containing plexiglass panels expose pipes, floorboards, beams, wires, and any number of unseen areas where pests traditionally live. The kitchen pantry is stocked with food that reveals the presence of pests, like the saw-tooth grain beetle in a container of rice or a packet of grits that shows rodent damage. The plexiglass panel on the wall between the bathroom and bedroom allows trainees to see how normally unseen plumbing moisture can draw pests inside. The doggie bed next to the fireplace serves as a reminder to check for fleas, and even the basement windows are designed to show different types of soil that may be adjacent to the foundation walls. From this unique vantage point, Orkin students can easily see how termiticides penetrate clay and sand soils differently.

And there's more. Not far from the Orkin training house is a concrete slab where students practice drilling for application of termiticides. An outdoor pavilion exhibits several different types of home construction foundations and structures—including bricks, concrete blocks, and wood—and the various concrete slabs and crawlspaces technicians may encounter. Future plans for the Training Center include the construction of a fifteen-thousand-square-foot addition that will be used for commercial service and sales training. Craig Goodwin, director of training, is quick to point out, "This new facility will have a restaurant kitchen, a hospital room, a motel room, a supermarket layout, and a warehouse space so our trainees can get hands-on experience."

Every year thousands of Orkin technicians and managers travel to Atlanta to take part in the varied programs offered by the Training Center. "Our business is constantly changing," Ron Harrison notes. "We will have to develop training on new techniques and new tools when they come along, but the one constant is that we are in a people business—people delivering a service. So the teaching of people skills will always be needed."

- An array of new sales and services programs that benefited not only the Orkin customer but also the Orkin financial bottom line. The new bait and directed-liquid termite treatment became the company's newest defense against termites; the combined treatment offered immediate relief from termite infestation that bait-only services often lacked, while the termite bait and monitoring stations provided ongoing protection.
- Improved financial and operational reporting (the result of the Y2K computer and financial system conversion).
- Improved national customer service center (RCCC).
- The development and introduction of FOCUS, Orkin's new branch and home office computer system, a $28 million investment in the company's future.

The list could go on. Granted, none of these results were achieved overnight. And while the 1999 Annual Report hinted that the "strategic initiatives launched in 1997 and 1998 have begun generating results," Randall and Gary's message in the 2000 Annual Report didn't mince words:

> Since 1997, Rollins, Inc. has taken steps to focus attention on its core business, Orkin Exterminating Company, divesting businesses less central to our new direction, launching new sales and service programs and taking other initiatives designed to promote pest control growth while making our operations more efficient. We are pleased that our efforts are paying off, as evidenced in part by our improved market share and financial results. The Company continues to concentrate on enhancing stockholder value by building recurring revenue, with emphasis on Orkin's commercial pest control business and containment of termite claims costs. . . . Fiscal Year 2000 was an excellent year in many respects. Among the highlights were: Revenues grew by 10.7%, the highest annual growth since 1993; Net Income improved 33.6% over prior year; Basic and Diluted Earnings Per Share increased by $0.08 or 33.3% over 1999.

Gary was quick to point out that "we are not back to where we were in the mid-90s, but we will be. Because through this initiative, so many things that were negative drivers began to change. It was obvious to everyone that we had this thing on an upward trajectory, and we could see these key indicators confirming that things were on the mend, that we had positive momentum."

And Stevens would argue that while not every improvement can be credited to the Divide and Conquer strategy, "I believe that if we had continued to lose money after 1997, then everyone would have blamed it on that." Did one side win at the other's expense? No, he said emphatically. "I felt like the company won." Has he ever heard of another company trying such a strategy? No, he said equally emphatically. "And I'm not sure I'd want to go through it again."

When Downing revisits the years of the experiment, he argues that it would be shortsighted for anyone to say, "I wish we hadn't done it." "The best interests of the company were at heart. And you could see the wisdom of the decision in the results of the total company."

Scenes from the Orkin Training Center, Spring 2002

If Herman L. Fellton, Orkin's first training specialist, had walked into the Orkin Training Center on a spring day in 2002, here are just a few of the activities he would have witnessed:

- Training specialist Doug Lambright outside on the ground, working with a group of students to collect and identify various ants and insects from the landscaped areas and adjacent woods. Lambright urges branch managers and branch service managers to communicate with the Training Center staff about their training needs, which can vary widely. For instance, the Southeast and Midwest divisions have different climates and different pest problems. "Although our general training must be standardized to a degree, we have been creating specialty schools in a region or in a branch when a particular problem exists in that location," said Doug. "For example, we have developed special classes on fire ants, on carpenter ants, and on drywood termites."
- Training Center manager and entomologist Ron Harrison inside the first floor of the red brick professional classroom building, pulling out bugs and rodents to prepare for a lecture in pest identification and control for the Commercial Service School, a class designed for new technicians assigned to a route with at least 40 percent commercial customers.
- Lisa Metcalf from the Orkin training department, coaching the participants of Orkin's Management Development School on the ins and outs of communication, hiring, legal and financial issues, and management skills. Today's exercise is to make a paper airplane, and see whose team can make it fly the longest distance in the Training Center parking lot.
- Carol Molnar from the home office's Corporate Communications staff, snapping photos of a group of state regulatory officials touring Orkin's state-of-the-art training facility in order to see why it's being touted as among the best in the industry.

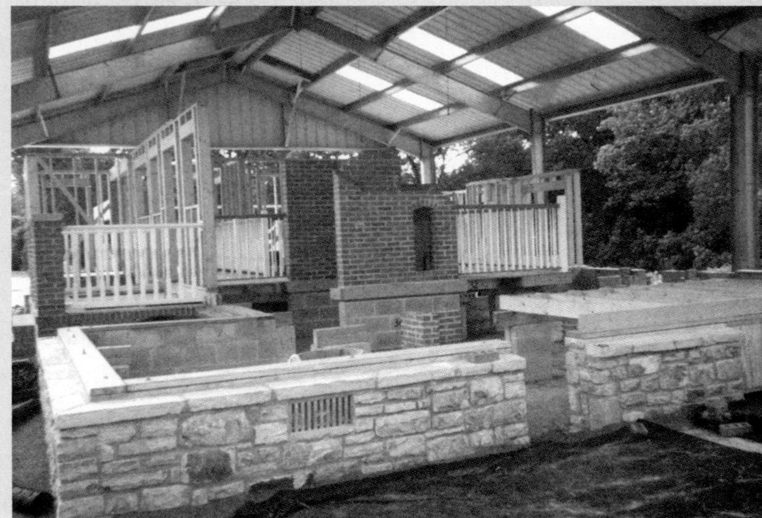

Orkin's Training Center has a specially built area to demonstrate various construction types. Trainees can see where insects are able to enter structures and what has to be done to exclude them.

Downing chuckled. "At the beginning, Randall used a cartoon to get his message across. It was a bathtub, with a trickle of water going in that said 'revenue' or 'sales.' And then there were three holes, with water pouring out that represented lost business and cancellations, termite damage claims, and employee turnover—just gaping holes. And you could just see people's eyes light up when Randall said, 'It's bigger than you realized. The money is pouring out of the tub faster than you realized. Fellas, if we don't change, we are going to be in serious trouble.'"

The Divide and Conquer era ended quietly in 2001, when the six divisions (now joined by a separate commercial division) came together under Glen Rollins, who was named Orkin executive vice president. "He was the common denominator, and it was a nice way to put Orkin back together under a third person," said Gary.

The company divisions came back together in 2001 under the leadership of Glen Rollins with a reshuffled top management team he calls "the best . . . we can remember in the company."

Glen was clearly delighted that the company was back as one. He was never a fan of a long-term Divide and Conquer strategy, for one simple reason: "It's very hard to turn around a company, and it's especially hard to turn around a service company," he said. "A service company is all about people and morale, and morale affects the level of service. Even though my father and uncle got along very well, the competition between the divisions got blown out of proportion. Candidly, a number of people tried to manipulate that situation. It was harmful at times."

But Glen admits that the experiment that began in 1997 allowed the company to identify problems and move forward, to reshuffle the management team in order to get "the best top management team we can remember in the company. The process caused a lot of innovations and changes—some that didn't work, but plenty that did. It takes a lot of energy to focus on businesses or new processes that may or may not add value to the company, and we were able to do that and move on with the best," said Glen.

When the divisions rejoined, Glen emphasized that there would be no immediate, major changes for the Mid-Atlantic and West Central divisions, though some changes were inevitable. "We are focused on reaching our employee retention, customer retention, profit, and growth goals," said Glen. "Clearly, our operating diversity is a strength."

WHAT'S OLD IS NEW AGAIN

In many ways, the events of 1997 created an Orkin pest control company in which what was old gradually became new again during the next several years.

With no plantscaping and lawn care or maid services to concentrate on, top management returned with renewed commitment to focus on the company's core business—pest and termite control services, training programs for its sales staff and its service people, sales and marketing programs, and improving customer service. When the company decided to replace the flash of the highly successful Orkin Exterminator robot, it brought back a new and improved animated Orkin Man, but one that was reminiscent of many uniformed, professional Orkin Men from the past. In an effort to provide better customer service, Orkin once again expanded its commercial division and later began to establish separate termite control branches, which Gary Rollins admitted "reminds me of the way we did business when I came to Atlanta thirty-five years ago." And with growth strategies that made possible Orkin's claim that it operated from "coast to coast," Orkin began to expand again by making three important pest control company acquisitions. The first two were PRISM (the number-three U.S. commercial pest control company) and PCO Services (the leading pest control provider in Canada, with 35 percent of that country's market share), both subsidiaries of S. C. Johnson Professional Services. The third acquisition was REDD, a leading pest control company in Mississippi and in the southeastern United States.

There were a few new twists, however, to the return to the past. According to Glen Rollins, Orkin was no longer interested in buying small companies and totally revamping them or "Orkinizing" them to duplicate Orkin's style. Rather, acquisitions now represented an opportunity for Orkin to adopt the "specialties and strengths of the companies we've purchased." The PCO purchase in the fall of 1999, for example, caused Orkin to "become more proactive with our commercial customers by utilizing our service technicians to increase our commercial sales." When Orkin later purchased R&S Exterminators in California, it was privy to this company's strategies for dealing with the California termite market; it adopted them—without changing them to fit previous Orkin molds. The company had learned that its former competitors had good ideas and programs as well. When it came to PRISM and PCO Services, Orkin benefited from these companies' connections to retail and commercial markets. "It was really a matter of combining the strengths of Orkin and S. C. Johnson and creating a win-win situation for both companies," said Harry J. Cynkus.

TELESELLING

One more modern twist on a familiar theme involved changing how Orkin sold its services. Since the days when Otto Orkin sold rat poison door-to-door, Orkin salesmen had been coached on the importance of meeting face-to-face with each client in order to carefully explain the Orkin service and what the customer could expect. But as Orkin approached its one hundredth birthday, Orkin executives realized that the pest control customers no longer wanted or needed this particular Orkin method of personal on-site presentation. Why? Gary Rollins explained.

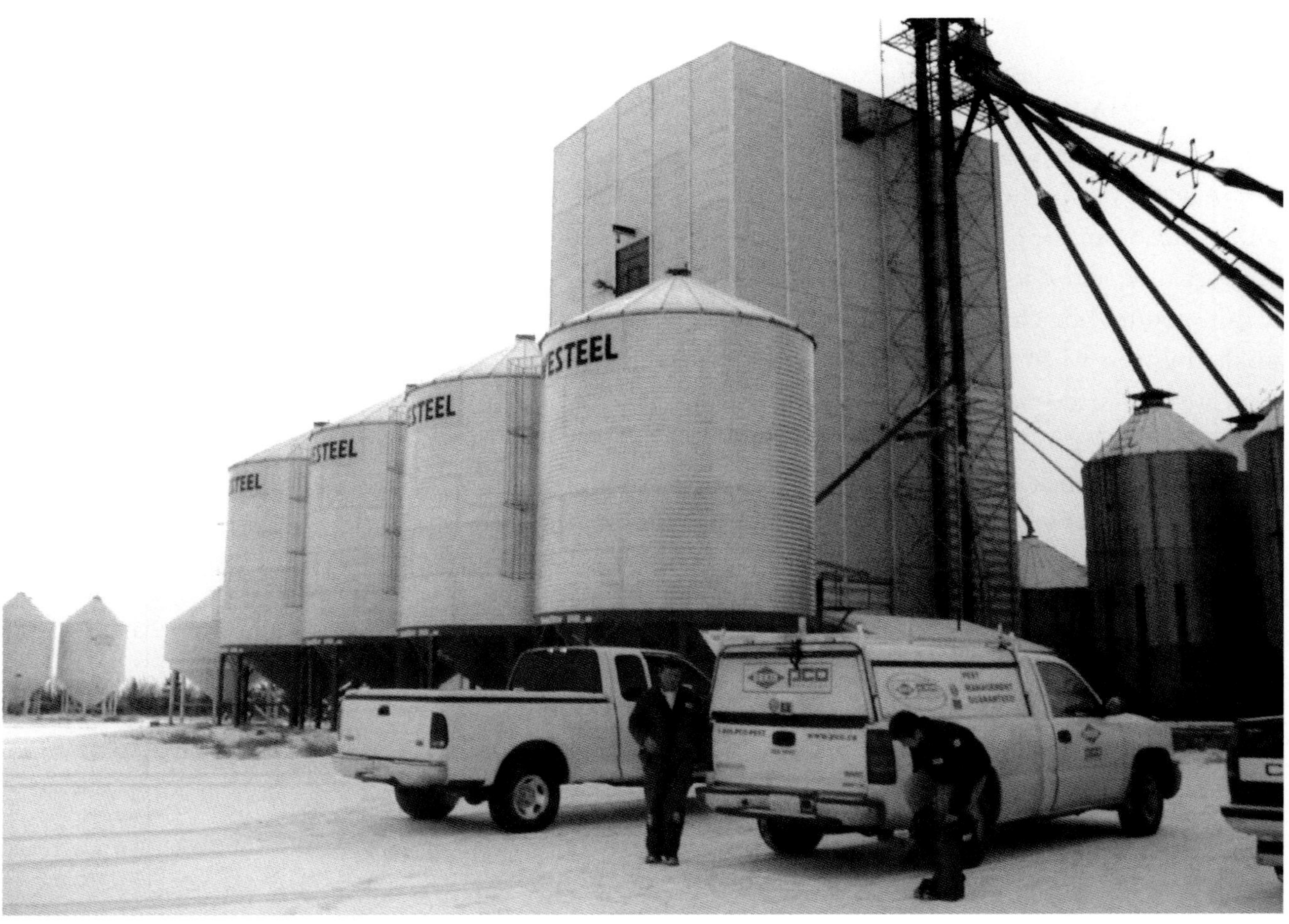

The purchase of PCO in the fall of 1999 caused Orkin to become more proactive with large commercial customers.

"There was a time when you called Orkin for pest control services, we would want to send someone out to your house, to look under the kitchen sink, go into the basement and other areas, and then sit down with you and make a full presentation," he said. "Our position was, 'We need to distinguish ourselves . . . the guy in the uniform, the professional appearance, the inspector, and the point of sales material. But the change taking place with the consumer was to an attitude of, 'My time is valuable. Just tell me what I need and how much it is going to cost.' Today's consumer just wants to get it done. So we started selling over the telephone. Our costs went down, and our closure went up."

Following the trends noted during Orkin's phone sales initiative in five states in the late 1990s, the company gradually replaced 1,600 pest control outside salespeople with 380 customer service representatives. Many of the displaced employees moved into other positions in termite sales or commercial sales, and the transition was successful and financially beneficial for the company. Research confirmed that people didn't have time to sit down and have an appointment; through their telephone inquiry, they basically wanted to know, "How much will it cost to kill my ants, and how will you do it?" As it turned out, Orkin could give them an explanation and answer over the telephone *and* close the sale.

The realization also helped expand the Rollins Customer Care Center (RCCC, formerly the Rollins Customer Service Center), which today handles incoming calls from Orkin's customers in the United States and Canada as well as prospect calls from Orkin's 1-800-800-ORKIN phone number that appears on the company's television advertising.

Along with Orkin's dedicated commercial pest control branches, the RCCC earned the prestigious ISO 9002 certification, an internationally recognized quality standard that validates the quality process for companies throughout the world. Orkin may be unique in having the only customer service center with this distinction in the United States.

SURVIVING AND THRIVING

As Orkin approached its hundredth year of service in 2000, the company made advertising news and continued a tradition of cutting-edge promotional techniques when it featured a new television commercial—one that quickly became one of the most talked-about commercials in the advertising industry. The television commercial appears at first to be a fabric softener advertisement . . . until a cockroach suddenly appears and darts across the television screen. The ingenious "Fake Out" campaign was so real that many people thought the cockroach was real; one woman called Orkin to say she had bashed in her television set with her motorcycle helmet because she was so disgusted by the sight of the cockroach as it scurried across the screen. Orkin added a feature to the company's Web site called "Orkin Got Me" to help capitalize on the advertisement's frenzy and to have customers log on and tell how they got fooled.

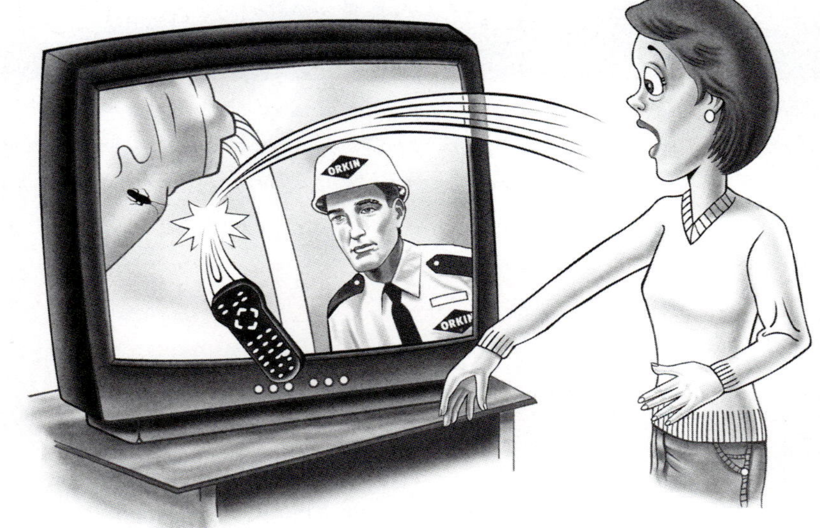

The "Fake Out" commercial, in which a roach appeared to be crawling on the screen of the viewer's television set, received a huge amount of media coverage.

To celebrate its one hundredth birthday in 2001–2002, Orkin literally took to the road. Once again joining forces with the Smithsonian, Orkin created a traveling insect exhibition called the Smithsonian O. Orkin Insect Safari that visited schools and communities throughout the United States. Fun, innovative, and packed with entertaining information about the world of insects, the traveling safari reminded many of Otto Orkin's Bug Bazaar, the interactive open house he coordinated to celebrate the company's move to new headquarters in 1952.

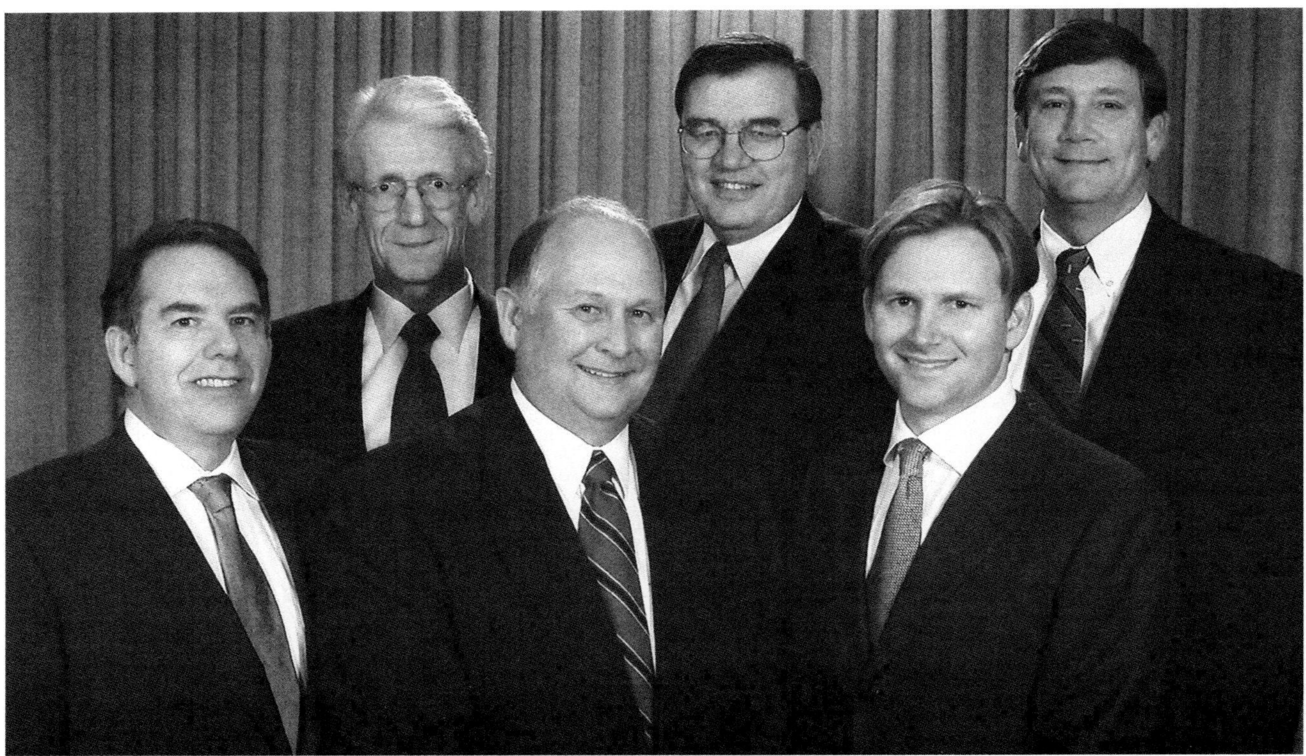

The Rollins, Inc., Executive Steering Committee pictured on the pages of the 2002 Rollins Annual Report has something to smile about: the company had recovered from the problems caused by termite guarantees and was once more doing well. Left to right, top row: Mike W. Knottek, William E. Newton, and L. Thomas Porter; bottom row: Harry J. Cynkus, Gary W. Rollins, and Glen W. Rollins.

Advertising through the Ages: *The 1990s*

In 1990 Orkin introduced a new Orkin Man in the form of a futuristic, robotlike Exterminator. The message was clear: "The idea is to position Orkin as the ultimate high-tech exterminator," marketing manager David Murphy said at the time. "We're the professionals." Though the new campaign appeared to be a takeoff on Arnold Schwarzenegger's successful *Terminator* movie, the new Orkin image was based on Orkin's technical superiority, not the popularity of the movie images. The Exterminator could eliminate any pest problem.

Indeed, the Orkin Man Exterminator's futuristic image communicated the message that Orkin is the best, most innovative, and technologically advanced company in the industry. The 1990 campaign was so successful that it was carried over for several years, and Orkin updated the commercials periodically to feature such unique bug-busting devices as the Flo-Meter and OrkinFoam.

And in 1994, a new twist was added to the Exterminator. The Orkin Man became the Orkin Lady. An article in the *Wall Street Journal* suggested, "She gives a whole new meaning to the phrase, 'If looks could kill.' In the ad, after a pest-killing spree, the lady exterminator sheds her shiny body armor and flashes an alluring smile. 'One call destroys them all,' goes the voice-over." The female Orkin Exterminator was a nod

And during Orkin's centennial anniversary, the company had reached some impressive milestones, serving approximately 1.6 million residential and commercial customers, through four hundred locations and seventy-five hundred employees.

In 2001 Gary W. Rollins, fifty-six, was named to the additional post of chief executive officer of Rollins, succeeding R. Randall Rollins, who would continue as chairman of the board of Rollins, Inc. Glen W. Rollins was named Rollins executive vice president, responsible for managing Orkin's field operation through the company's divisional vice presidents representing the Northern, Southeast, West Coast, Midwest, West Central, Mid-Atlantic, and Commercial divisions.

But the "icing on the cake," perhaps, was the company's latest financial figures. In 2001 Orkin reported that its net income had increased 77 percent over the year before, with a net income of $16.9 million on revenues of $652.3 million; the company's profit margin improved 76 percent. "Our sales and service programs have enabled us to increase customer retention, as well as make our operations more efficient," management reported. "This was evidenced by the improvement in financial results in a slowing economy. The Company will continue to focus on enhancing stockholder value by building recurring revenue and controlling expenses, with special emphasis on expanding Orkin's commercial pest control business."

to Orkin's growing female customer base, and the fact that over 10 percent of Orkin's employees who make house calls are female.

The female Exterminator never really caught on, but the Exterminator campaign proved to be one of the company's most successful lead-generating campaigns ever. It played until the end of the 1990s, when it was replaced by something totally different. The "Fake Out" campaign in 2000 created the illusion that cockroaches were running across the viewer's personal television screen. Orkin enjoyed a barrage of media attention with this campaign.

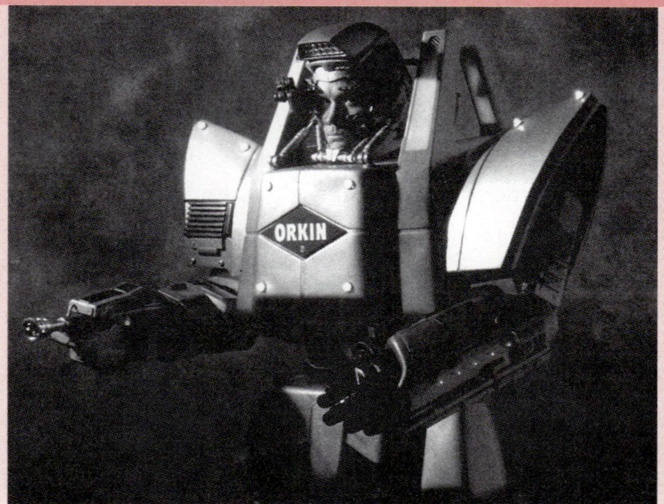

The Orkin Exterminator was a very successful advertising icon for many years.

When more than two hundred of Orkin's top performers and their guests gathered in Lake Tahoe, California, for the 29th Annual President's Club festivities in September 2002, the group did more than tour Squaw Valley, or go horseback riding, or take a trip back in time to the hit TV show *Bonanza* set by visiting the legendary Ponderosa Ranch. Together, Gary Rollins and Glen Rollins discussed the value of customer retention with their outstanding employees, and the numbers were impressive.

Gary Rollins spoke first. "I want to show you the tremendous progress we've made since 1999—two and one half years ago. If you went back to Orkin's 2000 strategic plan, as well as our 2001 and 2002 plans, you would see a pretty simple but challenging list of strategic objectives: First, to improve employee retention. Next, improve customer retention and satisfaction; then revenue generation, and finally, improving our profitability. Let's see how we've done on the first objective. For the past thirty months, we've had a 22 percent improvement in employee retention. . . . We had a 20 percent annualized improvement in our pest control customer retention, and we improved our termite customer retention 12 percent.

Up Close and Personal with the O. Orkin Insect Safari

How often do you get to literally walk through a hornworm caterpillar and enter a fifty-three-foot tractor trailer with a giant grasshopper sitting on top? If the Smithsonian O. Orkin Insect Safari rolled into your town, the experience was not one to miss.

To celebrate its one hundredth anniversary in 2001–2002, Orkin launched the Insect Safari, a one-of-a-kind traveling insect exhibit that moved from Atlanta to El Paso to Seattle to Washington, D.C., to Toronto, Canada in order to educate hundreds of thousands of visitors on the important roles that insects play in our environment.

Inside the giant ocean-blue rig, four very creative learning areas emphasized life from an insect's perspective and covered everything from insect body parts to the role of dung beetles in the environment. Through cartoons, videos, interactive displays, and visual tools designed just for kids, visitors moved through the exhibit and answered these important questions: How do insects thrive and survive? What role do insects play in the environment? Where do insects live? And how do arthropods live with human beings?

For two years the O. Orkin Insect Safari was staffed with a group of safari-clad tour guides who called themselves the "oldest second graders in the world." Nick Canzano served as tour coordinator for two years, traveling with the giant rig to over a hundred schools and cities, parking on the mall in front of the Smithsonian's O. Orkin Insect Zoo and even stopping by when the prestigious Orkin President's Club met in 2001 in Montreal. It made its last tour around the country in 2002.

Combined, the O. Orkin Insect Safari and the O. Orkin Insect Zoo served to remind the public that Orkin is "dedicated to educating Americans about insects and the vital role they play in our environment," said Gary Rollins. "The Smithsonian O. Orkin Insect Safari expanded the message advanced by Washington, D.C.'s

Our pest control revenue is up over 5 percent; termite control revenue is up almost 4 percent, so our total revenue is up approximately 5 percent. Although we were not as successful here as we wanted, we should be proud that we have increased our revenue when many companies have had no growth during this same period. To put things in perspective, our revenue target for this current year is $660 million. That represents a tremendous number of mouse, ant, roach, and termite services."

When it was Glen's turn to speak, his projections created an equally detailed picture of customer retention and why it is so important. "We aim to retain residential customers an average of four years or longer, business customers eight years or longer, and termite customers ten years or longer," he said. "This means canceling fewer than 2 percent of our homeowner customers each month and fewer than 1 percent of our business or termite customers each month. . . . We must continually look for ways to help customers make Orkin a part of their lives year after year. Whether they are homeowners or businesses, old or young, with or without children, working or retired in the city or in the country, we want to make it easy for Orkin to be a part of their lives."

permanent O. Orkin Insect Zoo, enabling our education messages to reach Americans one city at a time."

Over the years, Orkin's role as educator has grown significantly—ranging from impromptu school visits by Orkin Men to an official Orkin Speaker's Bureau that helps promote environmentally sound pest control as a benefit, and not a threat, to society. The insect road show, which cost nearly $2 million a year to operate, was a popular and successful addition to the company's educational initiatives—and one that was highly respected by its peers. In 2002, Martha C. Craft, Orkin's director of public relations and corporate communications, accepted the prestigious Silver Anvil, the public relations industry's equivalent of the Oscar, on behalf of the Insect Safari.

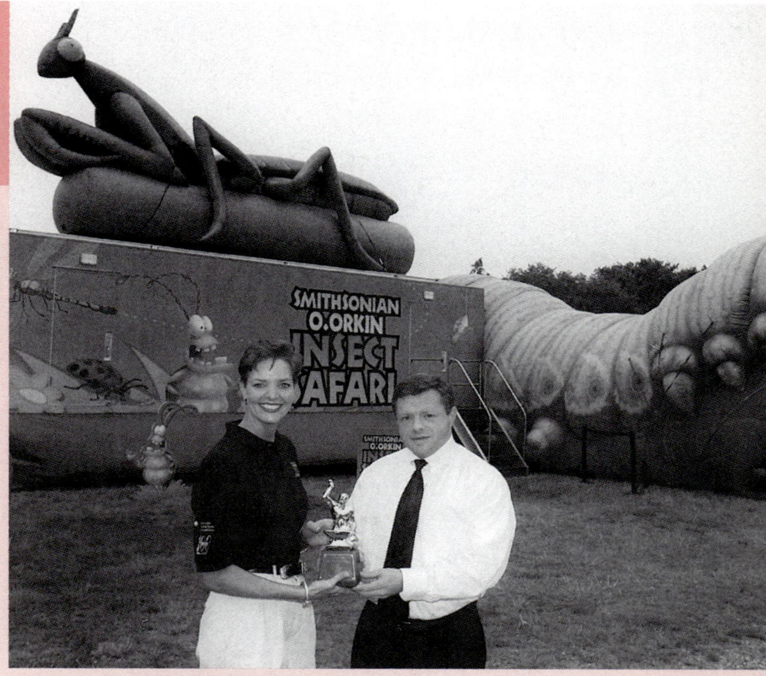

Public relations director Martha Craft and Charles Katzenmeyer, associate director of development and public affairs for the Smithsonian, in front of the Smithsonian O. Orkin Insect Safari exhibit with the Silver Anvil Award Orkin won for the program.

"I think Orkin's support of the O. Orkin Insect Zoo and the O. Orkin Insect Safari has been important, both within the company and the community," said Glen Rollins. "It has been a source of pride. It was groundbreaking for both of us. The aesthetic quality of both exhibits, as well as Orkin's association with the name 'Smithsonian,' has been unequaled from a visibility and credibility standpoint."

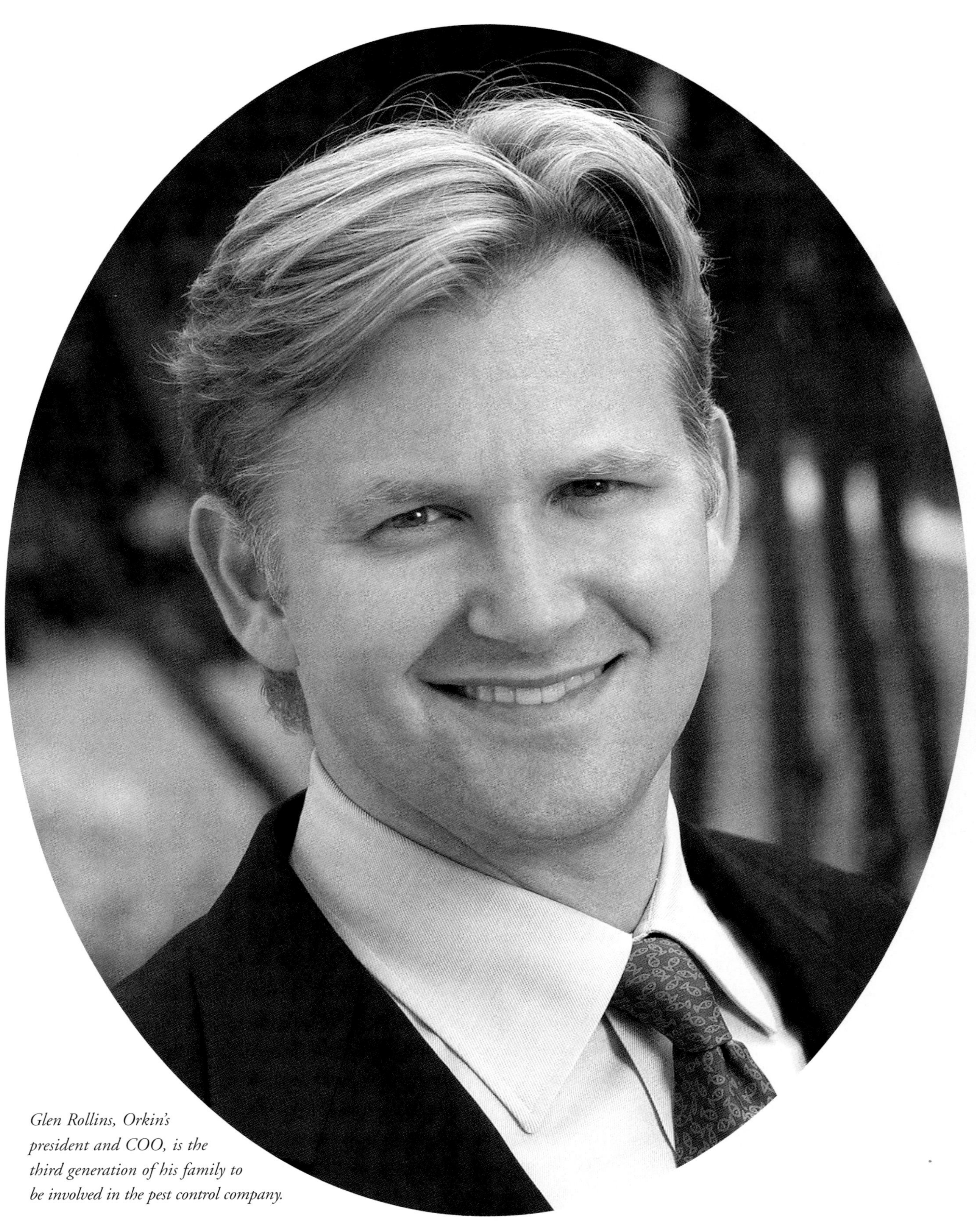

Glen Rollins, Orkin's president and COO, is the third generation of his family to be involved in the pest control company.

Chapter 7

The Future

Every morning in Africa, a gazelle wakes up. It knows it must run faster than the fastest lion or it will be killed. Every morning a lion wakes up. It knows it must outrun the slowest gazelle or it will starve to death. Lesson: Whether you are a lion or a gazelle, when the sun comes up, you'd better be running.

—Quoted by Glen Rollins
President's Club, Lake Tahoe, 2002

When Glen Rollins thinks about the future of Orkin, this energetic young executive barely recognizes the company that began over a hundred years ago. In fact, Glen, who represents the third generation of his family to be involved in the pest control company, readily admits that the Orkin he envisions taking into the next century is far different from the company that Rollins purchased nearly forty years ago.

"When Rollins purchased Orkin back in 1964, Orkin was not just the leader in the industry: *no other pest control company even approached our size or our power in the market,*" Glen noted in a spring 2003 column in *Rollins Today.* "Our resources, compared to those of other pest control companies, were staggering. In essence, we had no serious competition. And, over the almost 40 years since then, we have not only retained our market share, but improved it."

However, in the meantime, the market has matured. Other PCOs have also distinguished themselves from the hundreds of small companies that make up the industry. Orkin is no longer alone in the lead with a multitude of lesser rivals running behind them. They are shoulder-to-shoulder with their competitors in a race for the market's pest control dollars.

Which is why the story of the gazelle and the lion that Glen first shared with the President's Club in Lake Tahoe in 2002 so appropriately describes Orkin's current competitive environment.

"We dare not stop to rest," Glen cautioned. "We dare not stumble and fall. Survival depends on keeping running—no matter how successful we appear to be."

If there's any theme to mark the beginning of the second century of Orkin—and if there's any answer to the question of what's in store for Orkin's future—it lies in the cautionary tale favored by O. Wayne Rollins's grandson: keep running.

As the Rollins family leads the company into the future and continues its steady recovery from the financial doldrums of the mid-1990s, there are plenty of signs that Orkin is doing just that. From a reorganization of the home office to constantly striving to improve customer retention, services, and coworker productivity, the Orkin leadership appears committed to following Glen Rollins's insistence that they not rest. Even the beloved Orkin Man is being reevaluated, with a corporate goal to make the industry icon more reflective of the company's core values. And this push for constant review and improvement continues even though significant achievements were realized in 2002. At the end of the fiscal year, Orkin revenues were 13.9 percent higher than the end of the 1990s; coworker retention had improved by 17.6 percent, pest control customer retention was up 13 percent; and termite technician productivity had increased by 72.2 percent with an average pay raise of 39.5 percent.

Glen Rollins: "We dare not stop to rest. We dare not stumble and fall. Survival depends on keeping running—no matter how successful we appear to be."

"We can't relax and slacken our pace just because we had a good year," cautioned Glen, echoing, perhaps, O. Wayne Rollins's adage to "always look behind good news." "On the contrary, we must let our momentum lengthen our stride, and build on our success."

MOMENTUM ON EVERY FRONT

Orkin's second century of operation began on a firm footing. After a reorganization reduced a number of positions, the Orkin home office is now both leaner and better positioned to address the future. And along the way, FOCUS, the company's primary computer system and a somewhat painful reminder of corporate stumbles in the late 90s, finally came into, well, focus.

In June 2002 L. Thomas Porter joined the company, the most recent hire in a long list of chief information officers who would wrestle with the challenges associated with FOCUS, the company's highly touted proprietary branch computer system. This system was designed to replace OSCAR, the company's computer system that went into operation in 1993. Initially FOCUS was scheduled to be introduced company-wide in 2001, but there was just one small problem, according to assistant vice president Cindy Bordes. FOCUS was a disaster. Or as Porter diplomatically put it, "They flipped the switch, and it didn't work as advertised."

Designed to consolidate customer information in branches throughout the country—and provide organization processes for managers—FOCUS was supposed to do everything that the slow, labor-intensive, and difficult-to-change OSCAR couldn't do—namely, track sales, billing, receivables, customer service, technician productivity, and many other elements of the business, with the ultimate goal being increased sales and reduced costs. It was touted as being far more sophisticated and advanced than OSCAR, with a myriad of applications designed to enhance Orkin's services. But when the conversion from OSCAR to FOCUS began in selected branches in 2000, there were so many problems with the new system that the company's Technology Support Center (TSC) was inundated with calls and complaints; more than half of the eight thousand calls each month to the TSC Help Desk involved FOCUS problems. In an attempt to get a grip on the issues and handle the calls, the TSC established a "branch mentoring" program to help implement FOCUS during the five rollout/conversion months in 2001. The mentoring branches tried to answer business-related questions and how-to questions and cover issues related to procedure or policy; the TSC Help Desk tried to focus on hardware or software issues that were more technical in nature. But as the four FOCUS software releases took place (1.18, 1.19, 1.20, and 1.21), the problems were clear to everyone. If something could go wrong with FOCUS, it did, Bordes said.

After FOCUS was deployed, everyone eventually realized that it was an unfinished project. One by one, the problems experienced within the system would have tremendous operational impact in various modules—for deposits, service postings, acknowledging revenue, customer accounts, billing, routing, scheduling. The branches couldn't process their work. And so the screaming started, and Orkin stopped converting new branches in May 2001.

Millions of dollars were spent trying to fix the problems. Finally, to begin to resolve the issues, Gary and Randall developed a FOCUS Advisory Council and hired a company called Solution Resources, Inc., not only to help them fix FOCUS but to reorganize the company's Information Technology Department. These independent consultants enabled Orkin to take a step back from the FOCUS problems and come up with a method to identify and fix the problems, and to begin to add system enhancements.

When FOCUS was introduced—and later, when the company dared once more to deploy FOCUS through additional branches in December 2001—people were so frightened of the application's penchant for losing information that they continued to maintain manual records. But today, the true operational benefits of FOCUS are obvious. For the first time in sixteen years, the company's technology resources are exceeding the business requirements of the branch and region managers, division vice presidents, and the home office. New releases are now standard every ninety days that are primarily new process enhancements. One such enhancement, the credit card payment program, as an example, has improved customer retention and added millions of dollars to the cash flow. At the same time, FOCUS is becoming more of a customer relationship management application, providing the ability to better track customers while enabling Orkin to better respond to their needs.

The company's goal is to continue to make information technology (IT) more closely aligned with the nature of the work at Orkin, and to focus on process efficiency. The time line between getting a new customer and that customer's first payment for service, for example, consists of a myriad of steps that can be analyzed by IT in conjunction with the business in order to eliminate inefficiencies and make the customer happier. Other technology goals

Rollins Today

When O. Wayne Rollins introduced a new company magazine called *Rollins Today* in 1966, the bimonthly black-and-white publication immediately lived up to its mission to "increase the general understanding of our Company, our people, our services, products and policies."

Through stories and photographs, this well-crafted magazine presented important company news about such diverse topics as new insecticide techniques, health-care benefits, and quarterly earnings. And it also included the genre of stories that might best be described as "water cooler" features—those tidbits of information first heard through conversation with fellow employees.

Like the story of Art Kilponen, an auditor in Orkin's Waukegan, Illinois, branch who became known as "The Friendly Stranger" for waving to drivers as he walked to work each day in the 1960s and 1970s. Or the story of pest control technician Kerry Cox and what happened when he stopped at a customer's home in the fall of 1980. According to a feature in *Rollins Today*, "An Orkin customer had more than a pest control treatment to be thankful for after Kerry Cox, pest control technician in Orkin's Somerset, Kentucky, branch, stopped at her home. On his arrival, Kerry found the sliding glass door open and entered to begin servicing the house. He soon discovered the customer lying unconscious on the floor. When he was able to rouse her, the customer asked him to make her a cup of tea with plenty of sugar in it. Kerry did so and then helped her to a couch. He stayed with her until a daughter-in-law arrived. On being asked to make the cup of tea, Kerry realized what had happened to the customer. Like his own father-in-law, she was a diabetic and had passed out due to a lack of sugar." Kerry's quick action no doubt helped avert a tragedy.[2]

Over time, the company magazine became a quarterly publication, acquired color, and picked up many awards—including a 2001 and 2002 APEX Award for Publication Excellence. It still includes many familiar original features—"Milestones" for employee service anniversaries, "In Brief" messages about employee accomplishments—but it also tackles in-depth stories on Formosan termites, the impact of the events of September 11 on the company, and the ISO certification of all dedicated commercial branches.

for the company include implementing and integrating internal applications to improve management reporting and business methods, and to help process operational data as soon as possible—ideally linking the information from the customer call center to the branches to the home office. For the customer, the future no doubt includes online or Web-based billing and payment, service scheduling and reporting, plus the ability for the customer to request service, and handheld computer applications.

When a final division reorganization in December 2002 officially closed the books on the Divide and Conquer years, financial and retention figures pointed out just how successful the experiment turned out to be. In 2002 annual revenues totaled $666.425 million, with a net income of $27 million and earnings per share of $0.90. By April 2003 the stock price was within thirty-five cents of hitting an all-time high. Rollins stock was recommended by analysts as a "Buy" again.[3]

Under editor Carol Molnar, the magazine is carefully put together to reflect what Molnar compares "to the role of the chorus in a Greek drama."

"The chorus helps the audience focus on what's important so they can follow the twists and turns of the plot and understand the playwright's message," said Carol. "Even more important, the chorus represents the collective values of the community, so the audience has a baseline against which to judge the actions on the stage."

With each issue of *Rollins Today*, Carol tries to create a Rollins/Orkin in miniature for the people who work for the company. Not only does she try to present articles that focus on trends or programs that are important to the company, but she also attempts to include stories that reflect the values of the company and the desirable characteristics of coworkers.

She thinks that the magazine's "Superstars" column, which consists of letters from customers praising employees and their professionalism, is one of the most important features in the magazine. The column "means people who matter—our customers—are judging our performance and finding us successful. And the actions and characteristics that customers praise are the same ones we want to encourage in other employees."

Though many corporate communications experts don't approve of the use of service anniversaries in company publications, Carol adamantly does. "I think a list of people, some of them with thirty-five or forty years of service to the company, says something about the kind of company we are—a company that cares, a good place to work. That's something for all of us to think about."

Carol also insists that human-interest stories go into every *Rollins Today*. Why? "The magazine is sent to the homes of employees, people on leaves of absence, and retirees. We hope that the families of those people read the magazine, too." She argued. "Now the wife or husband of an employee may not be interested in a new treatment protocol we are using, but they very well may be interested in a child of another employee whose mother made him an Orkin uniform for his Halloween costume. We hope it makes the reader feel part of the Orkin/Rollins family."

2. For more stories of Orkin Men's heroism, turn to Appendix C.
3. For a five-year financial summary of Rollins, Inc. (2000–2004), turn to Appendix B.

And the many field improvements—such as a new-generation GPS tracking system that allows 24/7 monitoring and reporting of vehicle speed, location, and seatbelt usage (which helped reduce accidents and identify employees with poor driving practices)—actually helped the company in its ongoing effort to improve employee retention. As committed as Orkin is to using state-of-the-art pest and termite control techniques and materials, the organization now appears equally if not more committed to improving and maintaining an excellent workforce. Henry F. Anthony, who was hired in 2002 to head up the company's Human Resources Department, made employee retention a major goal for the new Human Resources Service Center (HRSC). The HRSC provides a convenient, one-call-and-you're-done approach to helping employees get answers about such issues as their benefits and payroll. Anthony and his Human Resources staff will track important employee statistics that include not only turnover, cost-per-hire, and retention, but employee complaints and the time it takes to resolve those complaints, improving employee benefits and salaries. And there's a proactive program called the Rollins Business Abuse Program, which allows employees to confidentially report directly into a Business Abuse hotline any indications of unacceptable business practices.

"Corporate governance" and "ethics" are not just words at Orkin.

For this company, "corporate governance" and "ethics" are not just words. Orkin/Rollins reinforces this message in all forms of communication, and even includes the message on employee pay stubs. "This is your company. If you see anything inappropriate, we want you to feel comfortable calling us, without fear of retribution." Behind the corporate governance program is a systematic investigation of employee complaints, and resolutions that are fair.

Is attaining a 75 percent employee retention rate realistic? Glen Rollins argues that it is. During an interview in his office, where framed prints of insects hang on the walls, the young executive's self-confidence and business skills are readily apparent. As he recalls past business debates and discussions he has enjoyed with his grandfather, father, and uncle, it's clear that Glen's interests in the pest control business transcend the nuance of day-to-day operations or the latest entomology discovery. Rather, bugs and termites are his medium for testing various business paradigms and indulging what he readily calls a "hobby that's become a passion. Business is something that I love, and pest control is a great business." And while Glen has a global vision of what he and Orkin are trying to accomplish, he has the Rollins gift for describing what that is in very simple terms.

"The number-one factor we need to pay attention to is to be able to attract and keep the best people," said Glen, who now prefers to call employees "coworkers" to reflect his emphasis on how valuable they are to the success of

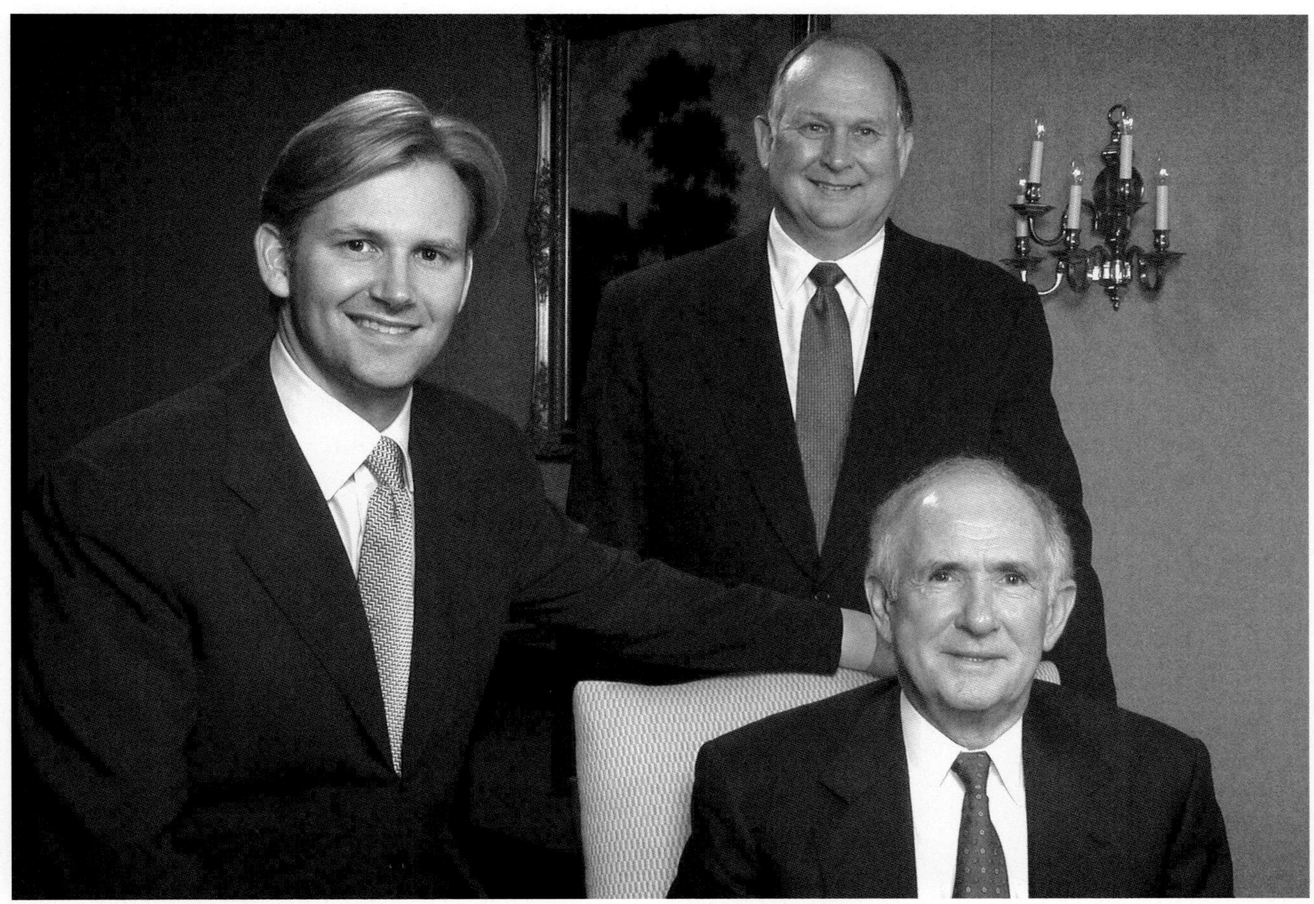

Left to right, Glen Rollins, Gary Rollins, and Randall Rollins on July 30, 2002, a few months before management of all the Orkin divisions was passed from Gary and Randall to Glen—a new generation.

the company. "I try to be very attuned to that. Turnover has gone down double digits for seven years in a row—it obviously used to be astronomical—but it needs to improve more. But getting great people is really what it's all about. We have to put courteous experts on business doorsteps and on homeowners' doorsteps. When the customer is confident and pleased, then business is good."

Everyone agrees that reaching 75 percent employee retention is a realistic goal only as long as the caliber and stability of Orkin management remains intact. The corporate culture of Orkin now includes an emphasis on finding and keeping the right kinds of people in key positions such as region managers and branch managers, a corporate philosophy that Orkin executives believe will lead directly to improved employee retention, which drives customer retention. This goal is very much a part of the culture of the company. From home office to regional meetings to branch managers, there is a real effort to reinforce the culture and to give it more value.[4]

4. For the stories of a few of the many Orkin Men who invested many years of their lives in the company, turn to Appendix C.

One of the key factors in employee retention is exceptional training, a long-standing corporate tradition that was reemphasized during the Divide and Conquer years when Randall made training and the new training facility one of his main objectives. Those efforts quickly earned national recognition. In 2003 and 2004, Orkin University was selected by *Training* magazine as one of the Top 100 training programs in the country. Orkin was also tapped as one of only six companies chosen for an "Editor's Choice" distinction, based on criteria such as training practices, evaluation methods, and outstanding training initiatives. The Rollins/Orkin Training program, with its twenty-seven performance improvement specialists, operates under the acronym SERVE (speed, execution, ROI, versatility, and excellence) to support employee development. And by the end of the 2003, Orkin had received yet another prestigious training award when it earned the 2003 BEST Award from the American Society of Training and Development. The first-place ASTD BEST Award, which Orkin shared with Delta Air Lines, recognizes

Advertising through the Ages:
One Hundred Years and Counting

Orkin's hundred-year-plus history of self-promotion and innovative advertising has resulted in an astonishing statistic: according to recent marketing research, nearly 70 percent of consumers recognize the Orkin brand name. And as American icons go, the Orkin Diamond and the Orkin Man rank as high as Ford, Oscar Mayer, and Motorola when it comes to brand recognition.

As the Orkin Man campaign heads solidly into the twenty-first century, the Orkin Man is back—but with a difference. In 2003's "Local Expert" campaign, the Orkin Man is technologically savvy and the consummate, caring professional, but he's somewhat kinder and gentler. Kevin J. Smith, the company's vice president of sales and marketing in 2004, is using part of his department's \$29.9 million budget (nearly \$13.3 million of which is devoted to television and radio advertising) to perform a minor—not extreme—makeover on the Orkin Man. "We think that what we really want to do is develop his brand personality," said Smith. The Orkin Man "is knowledgeable, dedicated, determined to solve your problems. He will be approachable. You will be comfortable talking to him, having him come into your home. In his uniform, he is all about being someone you can trust to solve your problem. Television advertising sets an expectation for the consumer. 'This is what you should get, this is what you should see when the Orkin Man comes.'"

Today, the advertising challenges are obviously more complex than they used to be. "The media market is so fragmented, one of our challenges is how do we identify and reach our market?" said Smith. "And the second challenge is to try to determine what message will compete in the marketplace and get the customer to choose Orkin."

But after more than a hundred years of branding and promotion, the company's advertising goal is nearly identical to the goal Otto Orkin envisioned when he handed out customers' letters. Said Smith: "We absolutely want them to call Orkin."

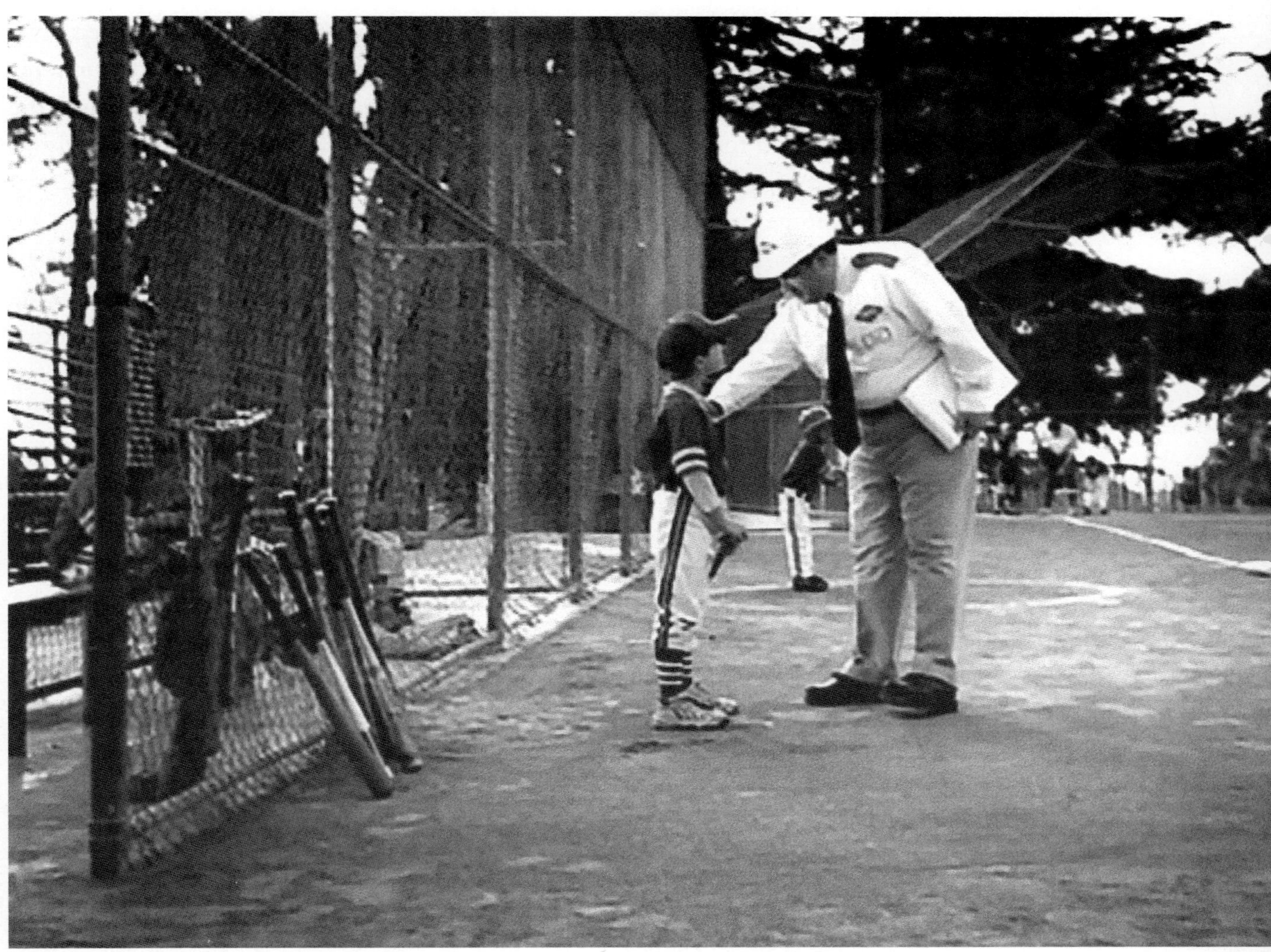

The new Orkin Man—the kinder, gentler Ned—is the ultimate expert . . . and approachable.

organizations that demonstrate success as a result of excellence in training and human capital development.

The scrutiny that Orkin gives its employee training programs did not bypass one very important corporate representative—the Orkin Man. In 2003 this celebrated industry icon went back to the drawing board, so to speak, when Orkin hired Kevin Smith to be the company's new vice president of sales and marketing.

Smith recognized that the Orkin Man is an amazing advertising icon—the face of the brand to millions of consumers, able to deliver the brand promise to the consumer. But as someone new to the company, Smith was struck by one facet of the Orkin Man campaign: Every time he saw the Orkin Man, he felt a little different. Was he a robot or a cartoon character? A man or a machine? Warm and fuzzy, or technologically advanced and cold? For such an important icon, Smith felt that it was critical for the consumer to have a better concept of exactly *who* the Orkin Man is. "When *I* think of the Orkin

Man, I think of him as the ultimate expert who is only there to keep your home bug-free," said Smith. "But the key question for us is what do *you* want him to be? We want to build the image of the Orkin Man around the demands of the consumer, to see if we can excel even more in the pest control market." To make him relevant for the next generation, the Orkin Man may need some tweaking.

Toward that goal, Orkin's marketing department recently conducted some extensive market research based on two questions: Why do people select a professional pest control company? And why do they select Orkin? Along the way, they discovered five distinct customer segments: the *National Branders*, pest control customers who believe that a national brand will do a better job than anyone else; the *Safety First* consumers, those concerned primarily with the safety of their environment, families, and pets but who recognize that pest control must be factored in; the *Relationship Seekers,* customers who select a pest control service based entirely on whether or not they are responsive, flexible, courteous; the *Bug—EEEK!* customers, who can't stand the sight of bugs and want the first person they call to get rid of them; and last, the *Service Demanders,* those customers who would really rather do it themselves, but they haven't been successful and they want to solve the problem.

How does the company plan to position the Orkin Man in order to meet the needs of all five consumer categories? By developing his brand personality. According to Smith, the Orkin Man is knowledgeable and dedicated to solving your problems, but also approachable—someone you can feel comfortable asking questions.

Which means no more robots. The Marketing and Sales Department has softened the Orkin Man a bit by de-emphasizing technology, striving to be consistent, enhancing the strong image and personality of the well-known Orkin icon in the new "Local Expert" television commercials. After all, the Orkin brand has had a wonderful association with the customer for over a hundred years, and Orkin doesn't want that to change.

THE FUTURE: PEST CONTROL AND ORKIN

As the Orkin Man begins his second-century makeover, the pest control industry is not immune to world headlines, those that tell the stories of Iraq military action, the decline in investor confidence, corporate accounting scandals, and an economy struggling to recover from high unemployment and low interest rates.

But Gary Rollins has a saying: "Rats and roaches don't read the *Wall Street Journal*. Fear of insects is the third greatest fear of mankind." Which means that no matter what the economic indicators, Orkin realizes that customers are going to need pest and termite control in their homes and businesses. And it's Orkin's job to provide these services for them.

And if bugs and mice and roaches could read national headlines, that wouldn't necessarily be a problem for the pest control industry. First, there's the renewed emphasis on rodents and insects and their connection to serious disease, as witnessed by the West Nile Virus and the SARS outbreak in the spring of 2003. Even the Orkin Web site announced the link when it went online with this "Health Spotlight" story: "Recent reports indicate a possible link between Severe Acute Respiratory Syndrome (SARS) and cockroaches. While there have been no confirmed reports that cockroaches spread SARS, researchers are continuing to investigate how the disease is spread." Another press release in the spring of 2003 noted that cockroaches are linked to "50 known pathogens in pneumonia, food poisoning, salmonella and typhoid." By the end of the year, a household pest once thought to be eradicated was back in the news—the blood-sucking bedbug, reported in thirty-five states. A survey by Orkin found that reports of bedbug infestations had increased 300 percent between 2000 and 2001; 70 percent between 2001 and 2002; and

The Longest Customer

James M. Coker has been an Orkin customer for over fifty-three years. According to Orkin's records, that makes him the longest-running, continuous Orkin customer in the history of the company. His rural home on Peeks Pike, just outside Charleston, South Carolina, has been protected against termites ever since it was built in 1950. And Coker still has the Orkin bond to prove it.

In 1950, according to Coker, Orkin treated the ground the house was built on and then treated the small, two-story house in order to protect it from termites. Decades later, when termites and termite damage showed up around the front door jamb, Orkin honored its original lifetime guarantee and repaired every bit of the termite damage, which had extended into the second-floor joists. "They came back," Coker said of Orkin. "It's just a sheet of paper, but it guarantees lifetime service."

Over the years, Coker has had many Orkin termite technicians come into his home. He readily admits that he liked the services provided by some Orkin Men better than others. But he stayed with the company for one simple reason: "Orkin had a good reputation," said this retired mechanic. "Orkin still has a good reputation. With the choice of companies that's around here, I'd still take Orkin."

Two years ago, Coker, a widower, moved from his home on Peeks Pike into the home of his new second wife in Goose Creek, South Carolina. He left his original Orkin-protected home to his two daughters ("I hope they keep up the termite treatment") and continued his Orkin service at his new address. So far, the Orkin Man only comes to treat for termites, but Coker is considering some pest control services, too. "Oh, yeah," he said. "If you live in Charleston, you've got roaches."

70 percent from 2002 to 2003, according to Frank Meek, national pest control technical director for Orkin.

Second, there are changes afoot in pest control management, reflecting everything from pesticide-resistant insects to growing demands from consumers for better health protection. Scattered reports from Orkin's branch offices throughout the United States have noted that German cockroaches are no longer "taking the bait"—which means that in some markets they are becoming resistant to standard bait treatments. As pest control operators and researchers study the issue and decide not only why it's happening but also what to do about it, other termiticide and rodenticide issues are sure to come up. When it comes to termites, the use of a new category of nonrepellent liquid termiticides to either supplement or replace baits is suddenly a burning topic in the pest control industry (Orkin already uses a combination termite treatment that includes liquids and baits), despite the industry and the consumers' affinity for termite bait in the very recent past. And the future of termite baits as a sole solution becomes even more clouded as the EPA begins its re-registration process.

Randall Rollins: "We basically ask two questions. Is it good for the customer? Is it good for the employees and the company? You have to have both."

Apparently, this possible change of heart also applies to rodenticide. Paul Hardy, now Orkin's technical director for termites, has noted that consumers who call the company's "Ask Orkin" help line have more questions about rodenticides and safety than any other issue. "If they are concerned about rodenticides," said Hardy, "it's an important consumer issue."

For the Rollins and Orkin team, the changing trends in the pest control business—from liquids to baits, from residential to commercial—do not distract from their basic business goals and commitments, the very business principles that allowed them to create the world's best pest control company. "I believe the best thing for us to do is to run our business, run it with integrity, go out there and see those customers and sell them our services," said Randall Rollins, chairman of the board of Rollins, Inc. "We basically ask two questions. Is it good for the customer? Is it good for the employees and the company? You have to have both—or you don't do it. It's not a complicated thing, really. It's the way we've always done it. And it should work for another one hundred years."

For Glen Rollins, the past, the present, and the future of Orkin are always intertwined. As much as he wants to move the company forward and "keep running" to outdistance the competition, Glen does not want Orkin and its executives to misinterpret those business moments when sales are down or profits don't meet expectations. Why? Because Glen is constantly reminded of his grandfather's wisdom and his remarkable business skills, and his ability to learn from adversity.

This was obvious at an executive meeting of division vice presidents during the spring of 2003. During a very challenging economic period, first-quarter results had just been announced, which showed that Orkin's first-quarter revenue had increased 1.2 percent to $155.1 million for the period ended March 31, 2003, compared to $153.3 million for the prior-year quarter; and net income had increased 47.2 percent to $7.3 million, compared to $4.9 million for the same period in 2002; and coworker

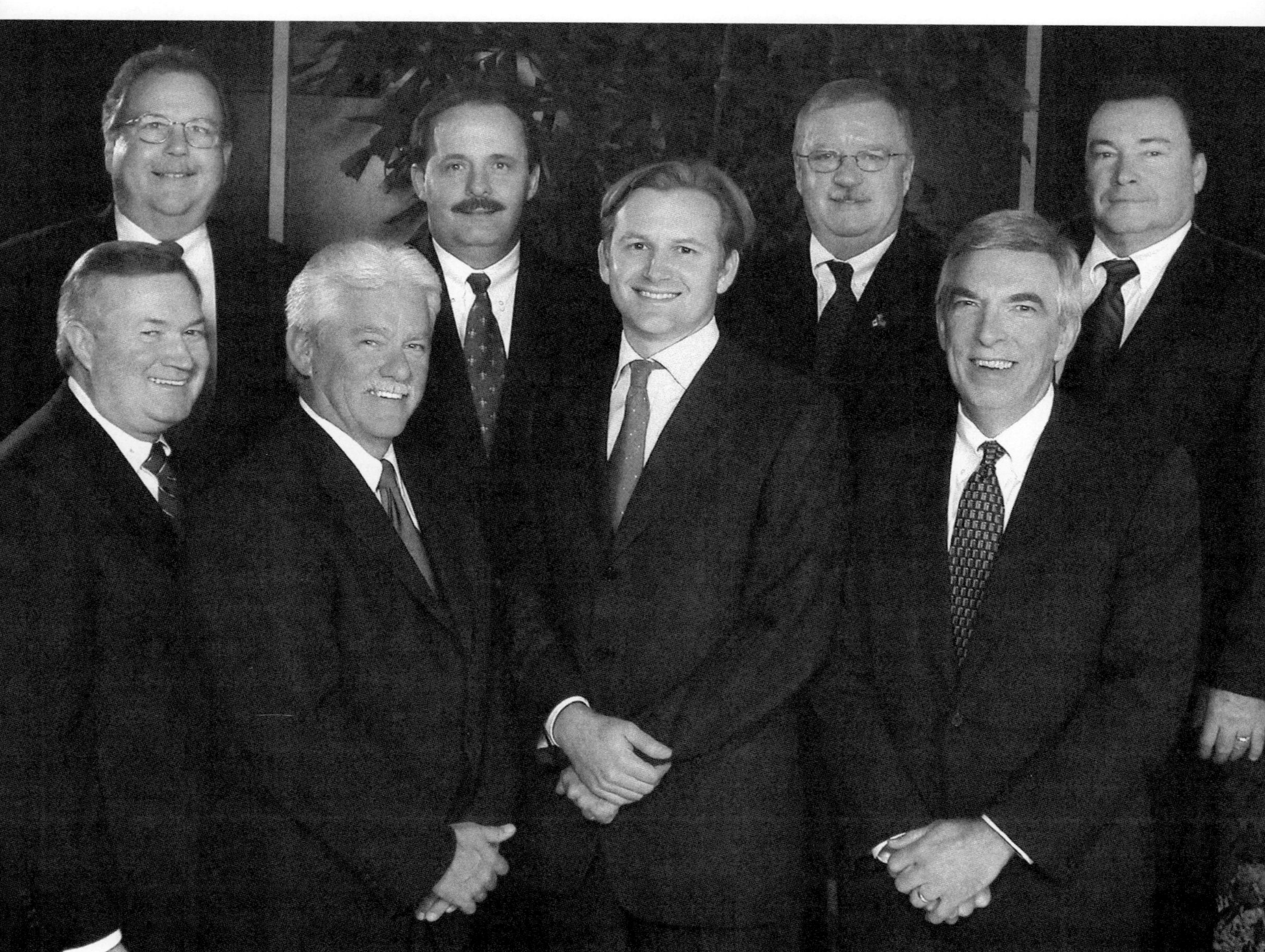

As the company entered its second century, experienced division vice presidents under the leadership of executive vice president Glen Rollins made sure Orkin was on the right pathway to growth. Left to right, top row: Gary Rowell, John Wilson, Gary Muldoon, and Herman Borel; bottom row: Robert Stevens, Steve Drennan, Glen Rollins, and Harry Sargent.

turnover had been reduced by double digits once more, down another 20 percent from the year before. Everyone from Gary and Randall to Glen and outside financial analysts emphasized that improvements in productivity, and customer and employee retention were responsible for the company's strong financial performance.

But as he stood before the division vice presidents, Glen had to temper the good news with the not so good. Though nearly every business indicator was basically solid and improved, one was off: sales were down.

And although he quickly moved to put the news into perspective, the fact remained: "Our culture is changing," said Glen. "We used to focus on sales and not on long relationships. Life was different. Today, our emphasis is really very much on having long relationships with coworkers and customers. As we've laid out this strategy and reinforced it every chance we've got, it has improved our profitability and customer service. And yet, our sales are down."

And in a very simple spin of both thoughts and words, Glen delivered the message he wanted everyone to hear. "We are off to a slow sales start," he repeated. "And I'd like to change that. The only reason we haven't added as many customers as we want to is because we didn't ask enough people to be customers. That's an irrefutable law: if you ask more, some will say yes and become your customers. If you didn't add as many customers in April, it's because we didn't ask enough people to enjoy the benefits of Orkin's services."

A few days later, Glen was asked about his comments, to explain why he presented the disappointing sales issues in such a manner. He didn't hesitate. "I know that we have built—and I hope that we continue to build—a company that can swim well in any current, that can swim a bit harder when the current is coming against us. And I drew inspiration for that from my grandfather. A lot of the great things he did, and the things that he learned, were lessons learned from adversity, from when times were tough. I really believe that this is a great time for us to be a greater company, to meet the challenges of our future knowing that we have the skills to learn how to be a better company, even if things do go wrong.

"Because adversity is a great teacher. And Orkin," Glen Rollins said, "is a great company."

The pest control industry would seem to agree that Orkin and its leaders are exceptional. When the National Pest Management Association (NPMA) gathered for its national convention in Dallas in October 2003, Gary Rollins had no idea that members of his extended family were secretly waiting in the wings to congratulate him. Why? To the thunderous applause of a standing ovation, Gary W. Rollins received the Pinnacle Award, the association's most prestigious distinction, honoring Gary's lifetime of dedication and commitment to the pest management industry. The award "is symbolic of the pinnacle of success in the pest management industry," said Donnie Blake, NPMA president. "Throughout his career, Gary Rollins has demonstrated his support for the entire pest management industry. Without that support, our industry would not be what it is today."

Glen Rollins: "We used to focus on sales and not on long relationships. . . . Today, our emphasis is . . . on having long relationships with coworkers and customers."

Gary was beaming, completely surprised by the award and the family members who joined him on stage—Glen and his wife Danielle, Gary's daughters Nancy and Ellen, and his wife, Ruthie. "I am honored to receive this award," he said. "As one of the nation's oldest and largest pest control companies, Orkin prides itself on our mission of excellence, and leadership within the industry. The NPMA's Pinnacle Award is another powerful endorsement to the strides that Orkin has made over the past 102 years."

Gary wasn't the only Orkin employee singled out for special honors during the year. In 2003 Glen Rollins and Frank Meek, one of Orkin's technical directors, were named two of *Pest Control Technology* magazine's "40 Under 40." Orkin was one of only two companies with more than one representative to receive this special award for leaders under the age of forty. The award also reflected Glen's growing expertise and leadership in the pest control industry and his role as a founding member of the Board of Directors of the Professional Pest Management Alliance, an arm of the National Pest Management Association established in 1997 to increase awareness among consumers of the value of professional pest management services.

By the end of 2003, both Glen and Gary Rollins were more than pleased with the efforts of the entire Orkin team. The company's renewed focus on long-term customer and employee relationships resulted in a steady increase in pest control customer retention rates, climbing from 65 percent in 2002 to nearly 72 percent in 2003. With a nod to greater efficiency, a smaller and better workforce, and improved employee leadership, Glen reported that coworker turnover continued to drop dramatically, down from nearly 58 percent in 2000 to just under 37 percent in 2003. Though Glen admitted that the "tail of termite liability is fairly long," he cautiously noted that the number of claims and customer retreatments had steadily dropped since 2000, a "trend that helps explain why I'm excited about our future. We have been paying more money to get these things behind us, but if the number of redos and claims are going down, eventually these dollars are going down. I hate to tempt fate, but I think 2003 is the high-water mark."

With improved revenue and earnings for Orkin in 2003, Glen predicted even better results for the coming year. "I think in 2004 and beyond, our revenue will begin to grow quickly."

At its annual January meeting, when the issue of succession was on everyone's mind, the Orkin board of directors threw its support and vote of approval behind Glen W. Rollins and named him the new president and COO of Orkin. He replaced his father, Gary Rollins, who was named chairman of the board for Orkin and continues as president and CEO of Rollins, Inc. The father was thrilled for the son. "He had a passion for the business from the very beginning," said Gary, reminded that Glen began his career with Orkin in 1979 when he was fourteen, working during that first summer as a termite technician and eventually joining the company full-time in 1990. "He loved the business and people loved him. I would get letters from customers, telling me what a great experience they had with Glen. But my thinking all along was that he needed to build a record. I wanted other people to think that he deserved it—to the extent that people would say, 'This guy has paid the price. He has been an influence on the direction of the company, an advocate for the customers and an advocate for the employees. I did not want a situation where a large group of people would say, 'Well, he's the boss's son—go figure.' Glen has done a wonderful job of establishing himself not only at Orkin but in the industry as well."

The company's corporate culture of hard work, integrity, and dedicated employees who put the needs of customers first has sustained Orkin throughout its history.

But what appears to make Glen Rollins a remarkably natural choice to be the new Orkin president lies in something that goes beyond his last name or his burgeoning industry expertise. For Glen, becoming president of Orkin was never about family duty or responsibility. It was *his* choice, a career path. "I was allowed to choose," he said.

Somewhere along the way—in Virginia in 1994 to be exact—Glen actually made the decision to enjoy this career path, no matter what his last name might be and regardless of the fact that the Rollins family is the majority shareholder in the parent company. "I had a time in my career when I felt like I was scrutinized. I tried to be Mr. Everything—the first one at the office, the last one to leave, the one who never made a mistake," Glen recalled a few days after being named the new Orkin president. "I was so scrutinized, and everyone was so curious about me, I concluded that I am not going to carry the burden of trying to be perfect. Much to my amazement and relief, my performance probably improved. It was a great weight off—to just be myself."

The story of Orkin, Glen Rollins believes, "is a fabulous story"—but not because of its colorful past or Otto Orkin or O. Wayne Rollins's role in orchestrating the first leveraged buyout in American business history.

"I'm not inclined to focus so much on the past," said Glen. "I think it's a fabulous story that we had a company that had a lot of trouble, and because of the ethics and determination of my father and my uncle, we, in the grand scheme of things, rebuilt this company in an effective and successful way. I think it has been exciting. But more importantly, we have such an exciting future. And because of that, Orkin is poised for success in another century."

THE WINNING TRADITION

After more than a hundred years in business, the company known to almost everyone as simply "Orkin" officially changed its name from Orkin Exterminating Company, Inc., to Orkin Inc. in June 2003. And when it passed this important milestone, it joined a select group of American businesses that have managed to operate successfully for over a century—a category that includes such American business titans as Coca-Cola, Harley Davidson, and Ford Motor Company. The fact that this hundred-year-old-plus public company is still primarily family-owned and operated gives it further entry into a select group. According to Loyola University's Family Business Center in Chicago, only a handful of the 18 million family businesses in America ever make it to the hundred-year milestone.

The company's corporate culture of hard work, integrity, and dedicated employees who put the needs of customers first has sustained Orkin throughout its history—and particularly since it was purchased by the Rollins family in 1964. And these pervasive corporate values were never more evident than on a particularly muggy day when all of the Rollins and Orkin employees in the Metro Atlanta area and beyond were invited to Zoo Atlanta to attend Orkin's Hundredth Anniversary Celebration on October 6, 2002. The entire zoo was open without charge to employees all day long, with special attention given to the formal dedication of the new Orkin Children's Zoo, funded by the Gary W. and Ruth M. Rollins Foundation. The first phase of the children's zoo had just been completed—including a building to house the zoo's golden lion tamarin primates and two-toed sloth, nestled close to the set of three "Camp Discovery" canvas cabins designed to give young zoo patrons an overnight educational experience, sleeping among animals from around the world.

The overcast, slightly muggy day bothered no one, and the zoo was soon filled with hundreds of Orkin employees wearing special anniversary T-shirts and "Orkin 100 Years of Service" badges, along with an occasional "Orkin" and "Acurid" baseball cap. There, near the black and white ruffled lemurs, was Cindy Pitts, an Orkin telecommunications financial analyst for two and a half years, enjoying the zoo with her two sons. Janet Childs, a twenty-two-year veteran, who works in administration for Orkin's law department, watched the early-morning cleanup crew work around the tamarins in the Children's Zoo. John Wilson, vice president of the Northern Division and an Orkin employee for six years, his children Sydney and Jay, and his wife, Alison, roamed around the petting zoo, which would soon be scheduled for Phase 2 of the Children's Zoo renovation. Kathy Gray, a Rollins employee for twenty-four years and currently executive assistant to Gary Rollins, had made her way over to the giant pandas, where she was joined by Marie Waters, another long-term Rollins employee with twenty-nine years with the company. Ellen Kinnon, who's been with RAC for twenty-three years, was on her way to see Yang Yang and Lun Lun, the pandas, followed closely by Pam Barker, an RCCC field support officer with the company for five years, and Lynetta Graves, also with RCCC for four years, and their families. Gary and Ruthie Rollins had arrived with various grandchildren in tow, and Glen Rollins and his wife, Danielle, holding their third child—a new infant son—would soon join them.

Gary Rollins: "It makes me very proud that Orkin is the kind of company where we haven't just survived—we have thrived."

Around noon, the Orkin families made their way to the big white tent known as the Ford Pavilion, just down the hill from the giant pandas, for a barbecue lunch and awards ceremony. Against a backdrop of tables with red and white tablecloths and white chairs, Mike Knottek, Rollins senior vice president, welcomed everyone to a "100th Anniversary Celebration that is truly a remarkable accomplishment, achieved by very few companies in today's environment." When it was time to introduce Gary Rollins to the crowd, Mike said simply, "This is a man who needs no introduction. He has thirty-five years of service to Orkin, a long-term employee who started out as an Orkin Man, and that makes a difference. Mr. Gary Rollins."

As the company president began talking to the Orkin employees about the zoo and Orkin's sponsorship of the new Children's Zoo, it seemed so clear that Gary had avoided what he once referred to as the "burnout. Your people will have heard all your stories, all your jokes, and all your management lessons. You can run a few good years, and if you don't keep yourself up and your people up, you find yourself winding down." For this crowd and this presentation, there was no hint that Gary Rollins was winding down. Even with his designated successor seated at the same table, Gary appeared to relish the day, working through his prepared comments with the ease of a good speaker in front of a welcoming and admiring audience.

"This is an accomplishment that few companies achieve, and it's a tribute to the people who work for Orkin," said Gary Rollins of the company's one hundredth anniversary. "It makes me very proud that Orkin is the kind of company where we haven't just survived—we have thrived."

He then recognized six employees who together had accumulated 252 years of service to Orkin, each accounting for more than 40 years with the company in an employee retention record few could match: J. D. Burger, 49 years of service, ranging from bookkeeping to heading up Dettelbach; Paul Hardy, 41 years of service, the technology and termite specialist who once said he "took a job with Orkin until I could find something better, and I'm still looking"; Carolyn Harrison, 41 years with Orkin, who started out processing

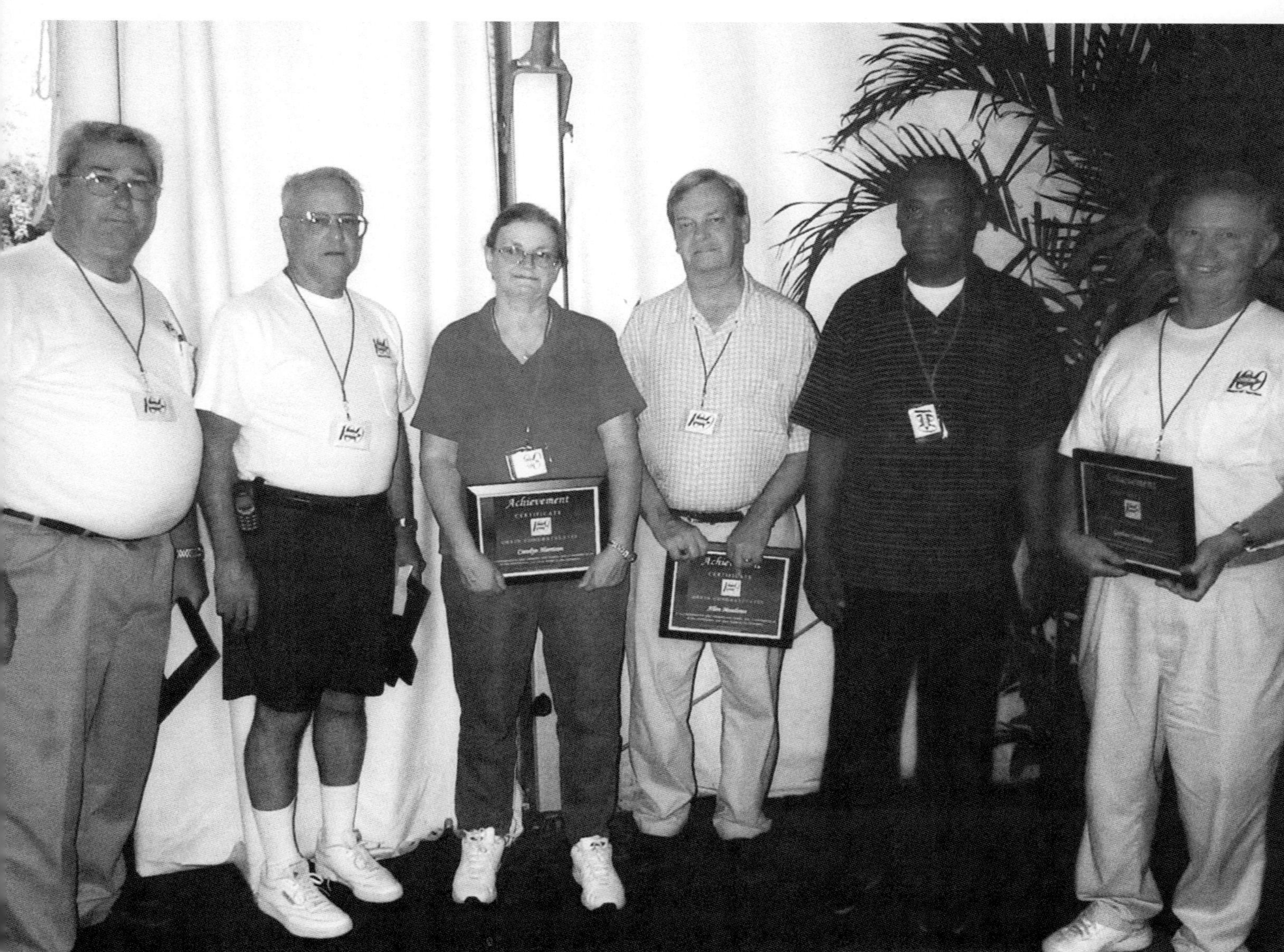

At the Orkin Centennial Celebration held at Zoo Atlanta on October 5, 2002, employees with the most years of service were honored. Left to right: Paul Hardy (41 years), J. D. Burger (49 years), Carolyn Harrison (41 years), Allen Meadows (41 years), Glenn Martin (42 years), and Gordon Crenshaw (39 years).

the Orkin guarantees and checks; Allen Meadows, hired by J. D. Burger 41 years before to work in the original payroll department; Glenn Martin, 42 years with the company mail room and delivery crew, who became a star player in the Rollins Bowling League; and Gordon Crenshaw, described by Gary as someone who "has worked in every division of Rollins for the past 39 years and 5 months."

As the six individuals made their way to the podium and received their forty-year recognition awards, Gary shook their hands and posed for pictures, just as he has done with countless Orkin employees for over three decades and previous presidents have done for over a hundred years. Today, the only pest worth worrying about seemed to be the occasional yellow jacket flying around under the pavilion's tent. Gary Harris, an Orkin termite inspector from the Gainesville branch, wasn't even thinking about swarm season as he sat with his wife and twin daughters, enjoying his barbecue platter and sweet iced tea. For Doug Lambright and Ron Harrison, it was good to see everyone away from the new Orkin Training Center, where they both teach entomology and pest control techniques to the Orkin servicemen. Glen Rollins seemed to be keeping a low profile, greeting coworkers and enjoying the day with his family.

Paul Hardy on his more than forty years of service at Orkin: "I took a job with Orkin until I could find something better, and I'm still looking."

Indeed, it just wasn't the kind of day to talk about succession planning, growth, and revenue projections. The zoo seemed a safe haven from the world of pest control concerns, call centers, commercial branches, core services, borates, foam, customer retention, stock prices, and the company's constant concern with how to better follow up on customer leads. As Gary Rollins frequently reminded the staff, "Orkin has reigned for a century as the leader in the pest control industry—twenty-six years longer than our largest competitor. Congratulations to each of you, and happy birthday, Orkin! We look forward to the next hundred years."

For now, it was enough just to enjoy the cookies and the face-painting activities, and then walk back to the Orkin Children's Zoo for another look at the golden lion tamarins, which weren't too far from the carousel. There, the various members of the Rollins family gathered to ride around and around on the carousel horses, while some chose to sit with Gary Rollins on a nearby bench and watch. The sun came out, and so did the bugs. It was a wonderful Orkin day.

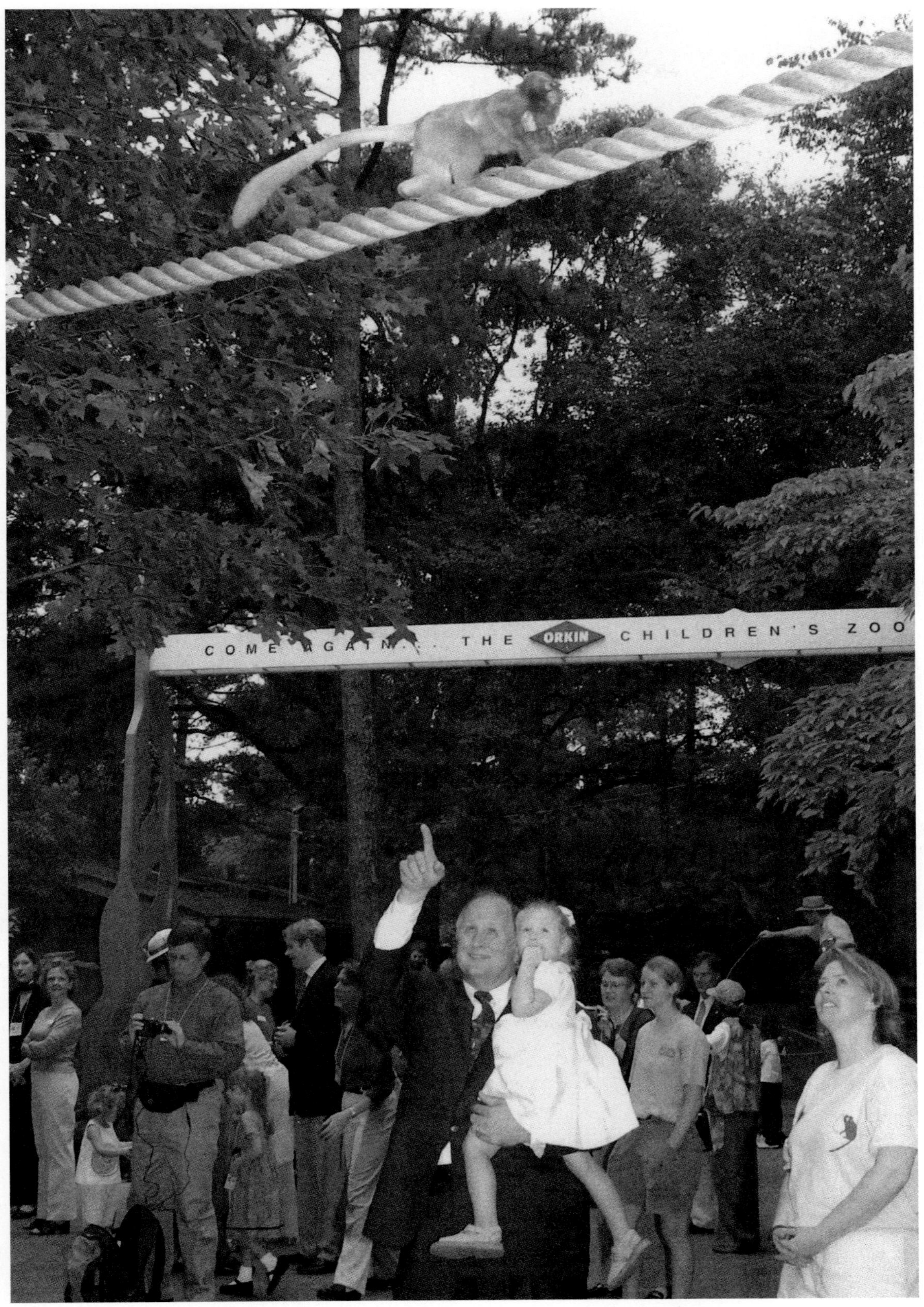

Gary Rollins and granddaughter Carlyle spot a golden lion tamarin at the Orkin Children's Zoo opening September 19, 2002.

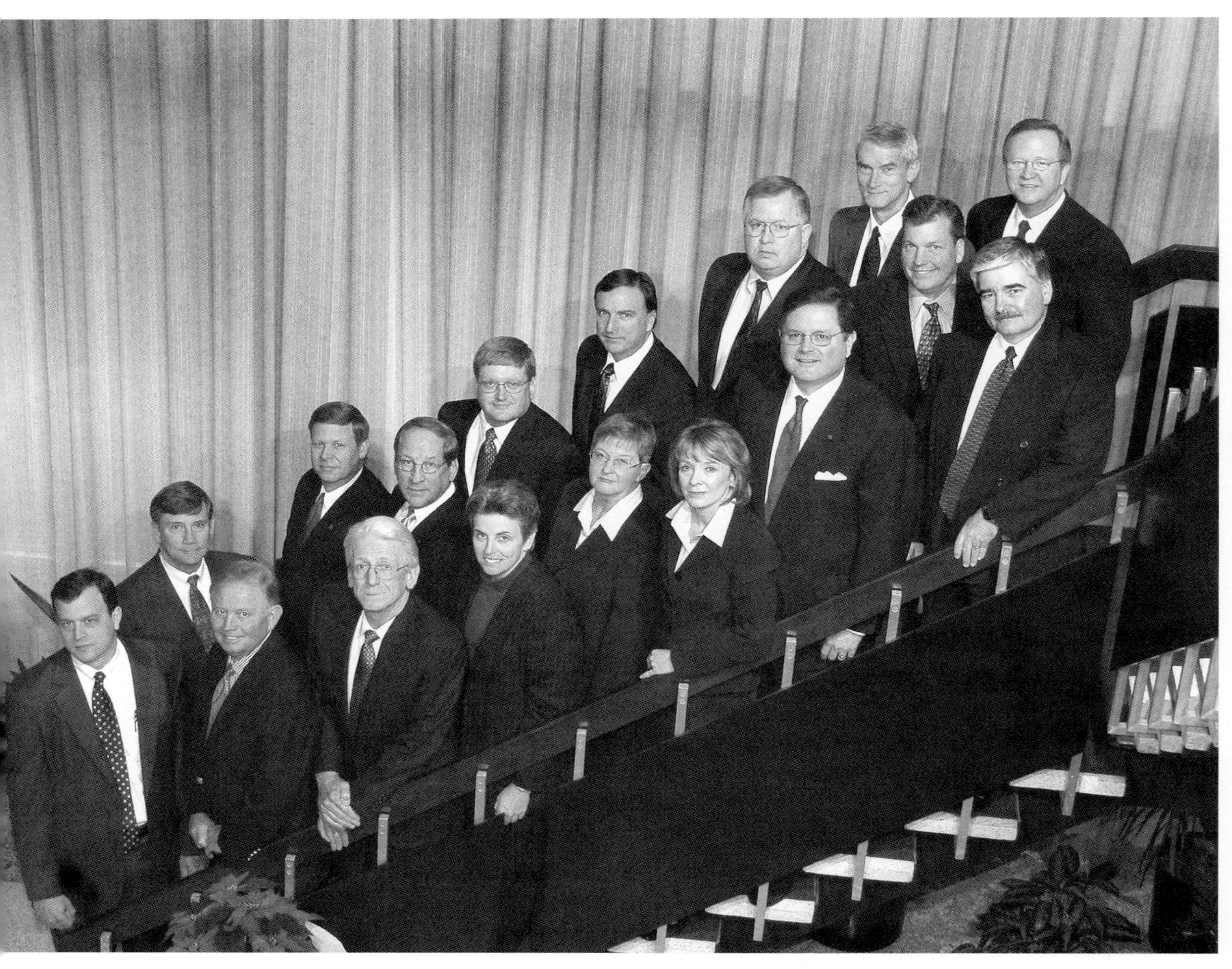

Home office vice presidents at Rollins at the end of 2004. Left to right, first row: Gordon Crenshaw, vice president, special projects; Mike Knottek, senior vice president, corporate administration; Carran Schneider, vice president, financial services; Vye Ladd, assistant vice president, human resources; Kathleen Mayton, vice president, law; Henry Anthony, vice president, human resources; and Jack Mackenzie, vice president, RCCC. Middle row: Nelson Jackson, vice president, internal audit; Tom Diederich, vice president, government relations and environmental stewardship; Kevin Smith, vice president, sales and marketing; and David Lamb, vice president, training. Back row: Tom Porter, chief information officer and vice president, ITC; Chris Gorecki, vice president, termite quality assurance and claims; Alan Ariel, assistant vice president, ITC networks; Tom Luczynski, vice president, RSI, technical services, and real estate; Ben Carroll, assistant vice president, ITC operations; and Fred Emry, vice president, ITC applications and development. Not present for the photograph were Bill Newton, vice president, Orkin operations support; Harry Cynkus, chief financial officer; Mike Sullivan, vice president, finance; Cindy Bordes, assistant vice president, field administrative support; Karen Dunn, assistant vice president, credit and collections; and Pope Nash, assistant vice president, tax.

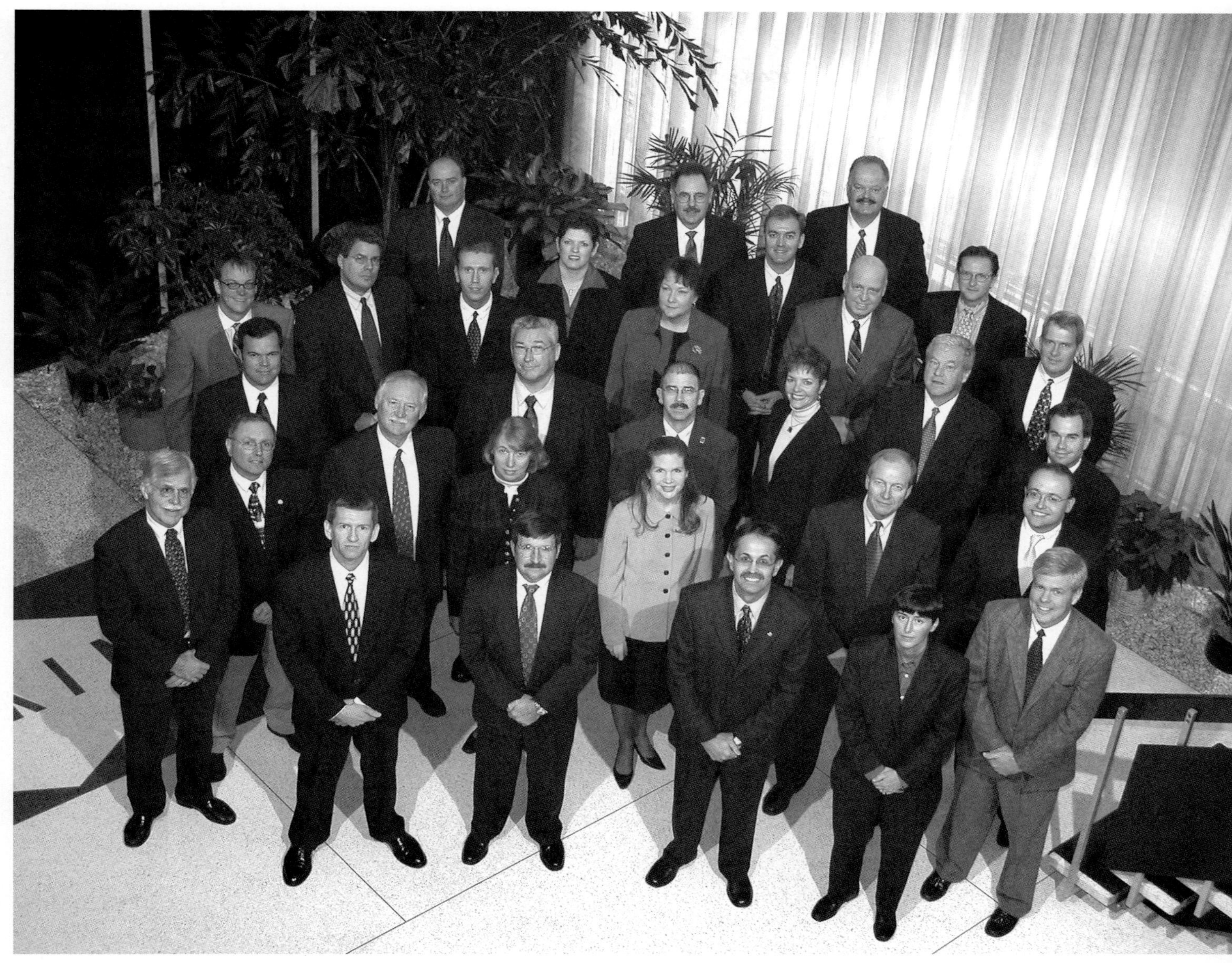

Directors/controllers at Rollins at the end of 2004. Left to right, front row: James Greutert, division controller; Peter Jepson, director of strategy and innovation; Barry Noll, assistant corporate controller; Ramiro Banderas, director of media services; Melody Davis, director of instructional design; and Mike Gibney, director of claims. Second row: Paul Bello, RSI technical director; Dan Steedly, director of termite claims; Evelyn Morris, assistant director of real estate services; Marylynn Parker, director of compensation; Ron Kimbell, director of corporate services; and Kim Gilbert, director of ITC networks. Third row: Jeff Seibert, director of ITC project management; Paul Hardy, technical director; Frank Meek, technical director; Martha Craft, director of public relations and corporate communications; Ron Buchanan, director of real estate; and Stacy Wiggins, division controller. Fourth row: James Ward, director of internal audit; Ken Nagy, director of finance and administration; Dan Buzzard, corporate controller; Pat Crowe, director of systems; Bob Hines, director of corporate development; and Pat Murray, division controller. Back row: James Lossick, director of ITC applications/integration and architecture; Pam Foulis, director of ITC system development; Craig Goodwin, director of training; Mark Wyan, division controller; Charles Bowen, director of fleet services; and Brian Greene, director of planning and analysis. Absent for the photograph were Amy Manno, director of benefits; Bill Anderson Jr., director of RAC administration; Debbie Roberts, director of payroll; Fran Griggs, director of accounts payable; JoAnne Thomas, assistant director of benefits; Marcia Christman, director of employee services; Mark Stevens, director of business development; Roxanne White, director of Orkin human resources; Stan Thompson, director of ITC branch services; and Stefanie Smith, director of marketing.

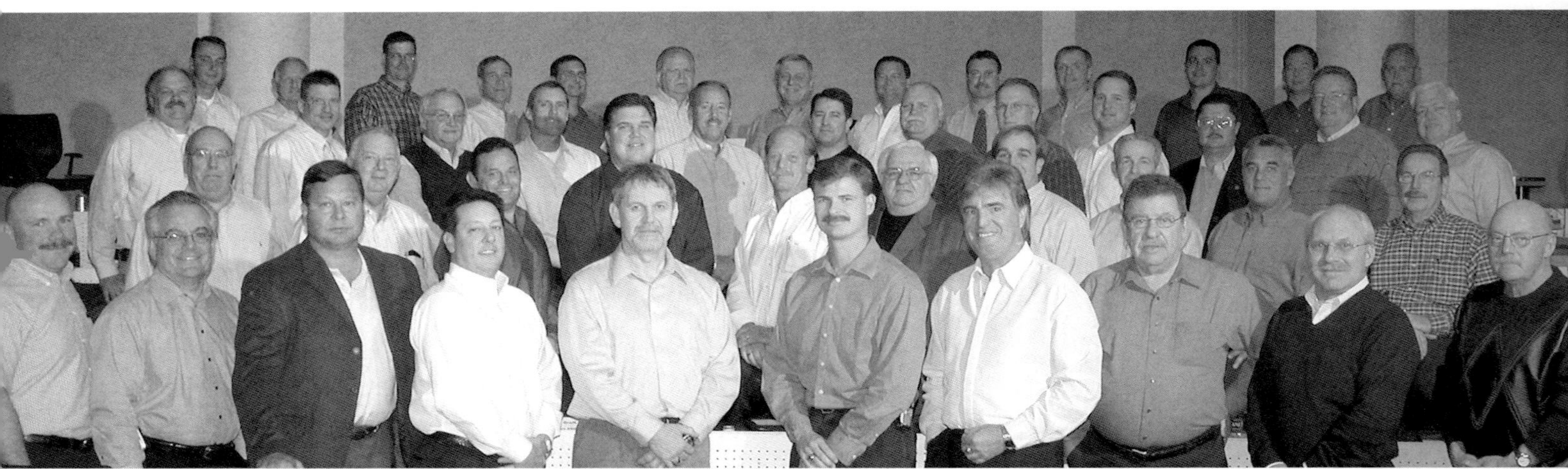

Region managers at annual meeting January 2005, left to right, front row: Mark Male, Pacific Termite; Tom Pedersen, New York, Northern New Jersey; Bill Sadler, Southern Commercial; Jeff Zeigler, Indiana/Ohio; Norm Doiron, Canada Atlantic/Quebec; Dave Bridge, Virginia; Steve Vaughn, North Florida (assistant region manager); Joe Emanueli, Philadelphia/Southern New Jersey; Mark Mumm, Wisconsin; Ernie Meadows, Iowa; second row: Butch Thress, Tennessee; Ted Whittaker, North Carolina; Jose Rodriguez, South Florida; Stephen Vey, Northern Commercial; Bruce Steinke, Michigan; Marv Leavitt, Northwest; Steve Leavitt; Southern California; Steve Breitweiser, Southwest; Gene Iarocci, Louisiana; Norman Cowger, South Central; third row: Kim Boltz, Maryland/Virginia; Gary Dady, Illinois (assistant region manager); Ray Smiley, Kentucky; Kevin Sullivan, Florida/Atlanta; Lee O. Savage, South Florida (assistant region manager); Freeman Elliott, Northern Commercial; Charles Self, Kentucky (assistant region manager); Tiziano Del Guanto, Delaware; Terry Groft, Delaware (assistant region manager); Mike Turki, Georgia; Chris Mally, Central Commercial; Michael Smith, Northern California; fourth row: Bill Minahan, New England (assistant region manager); Bill Melville, Canada Prairie; Jay Keating, North Florida; Darrel LaVigne, New England; Glen Genther, Michigan (assistant region manager); Ray Glover, South Texas; John Long, Oklahoma; John White, North Texas; Craig Tweedale, Wisconsin (assistant region manager); James Earl Thomas, Alabama; Darren Dougherty, Central Commercial (assistant region manager); Craig Stephens, South Carolina; John Laughner, Maryland.

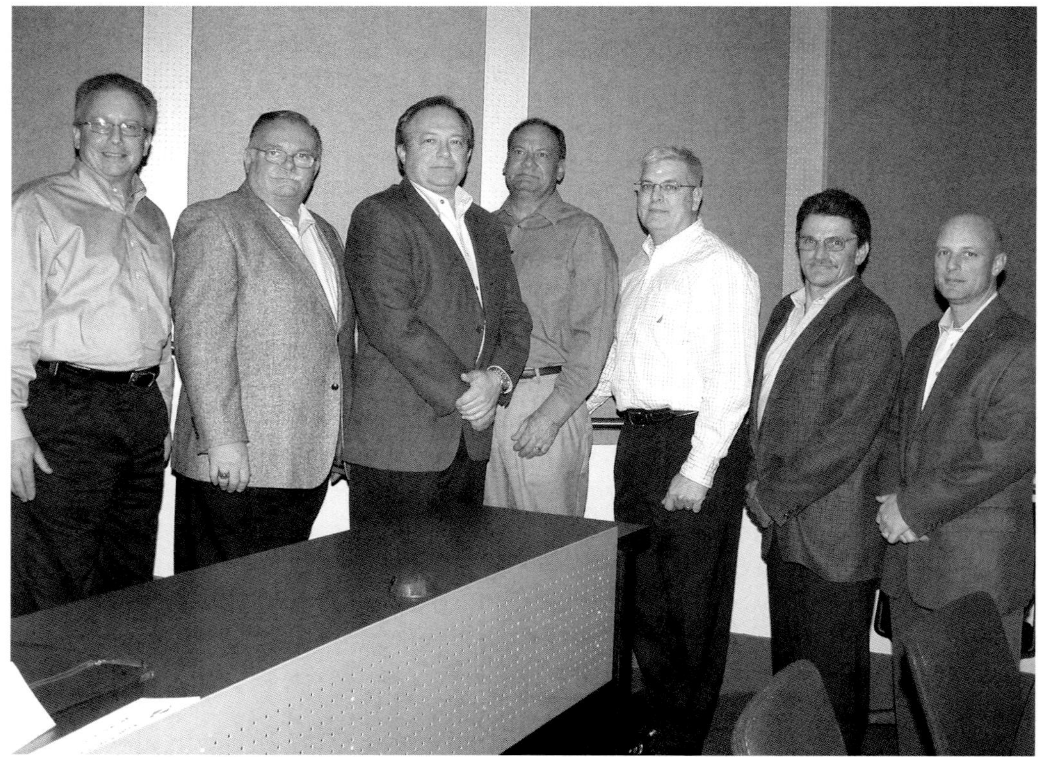

Assistant division vice presidents at Region Managers Meeting in January 2005, left to right: Gary Strumlauf, Atlantic; Ken Keup, Midwest; Paul Youngpeter, Southeast; Randy Baumgartner, South Central; Bill Sullivan, Western; Tom Heard, Pacific; Ken Stieren, Commercial.

Appendix A: Origin of Pest Control

Oh, rats!

Ever since people have had homes, rats have invaded them. Rats have been around since the Stone Age, apparently pestering Paleolithic humans and threatening their survival and their meager food supplies. Archaeologists have found the remains of rats and other pests in cave dwellings. Combs designed to remove lice have been dated to 10,000 B.C., and the Egyptians carved locusts feasting on leaves in their bas-relief friezes about 2400 B.C. The Bible is filled with stories of plagues and famines, which were no doubt due in part to insects and rodents.

It took thousands of years for man to fully understand the role that insects and rodents played in transmitting plagues and disease. But it appears that they always had a clue. Hebrew laws, such as those stated in Leviticus and Deuteronomy, forbade people to eat, or even touch, certain animals, including rats, insects, and crawling things. The Mosaic Code required cleanliness, and noted that any animal sacrificed for eating should be "without blemish," thus preventing illnesses caused by diseased animals. Ancient writings from the Chinese, Hebrew, Arabic, and Byzantine cultures associated rats with the spread of plague. For instance, an ulcer found on the mummy of the Egyptian pharaoh Ramses V, about 1000 B.C., may have been caused by fleas from infected rats. In China, rats and health risks were clearly reflected in the household caution to throw away any rice if rats happened to run over the family rice baskets.

The Egyptians, however, had a true love-hate relationship with rodents, particularly rats. Historians have noted that in Egypt the rat symbolized utter destruction, but it also stood for wise judgment because it "always chooses the best bread." The Egyptians drew the line, however, when rats attacked their grain warehouses along the Nile, and they introduced the cat to control the problem. When cats died, these highly regarded animals were embalmed and buried with great ceremony; a few embalmed rats were even buried with them, a tasty treat in the afterworld. In 150 B.C. the cat was imported from Egypt to Rome and became an important element in controlling that city's rodent problem, too.

It's important to understand that plagues and famines were often viewed as miraculous interventions from God or as punishment for transgressions. For these reasons, the earliest attempts at pest control were considered the domain of diviners, priests, and witch doctors who used various kinds of magic in their efforts to prevent sickness, restore health, and destroy the pests. And in their work, they were the first to turn to poisons for pest control.

The logic couldn't have been more practical: if certain plants, minerals, and elements such as sulphur made people sick, why couldn't their toxic properties be harnessed to kill pests?

And so pest control by poisons began. The Egyptians, Greeks, and perhaps other civilizations nearly four thousand years ago practiced "fumigation by burning sulphur." Homer referred to a "disinfectant sulphur . . . to make a fire so that I can fumigate the house." Hippocrates, the leader of modern medicine, regarded sulphur fumigation as an antidote against plagues. First-century Romans treated animal wool with sulphur to guard against pests, and used sulphur in street fires that were lit in public places affected by diseases.

The toxic effects of various plants and berries have also long been noted. The oldest rodenticide called red squill, an ancient rat poison known to rat killers since at least 1500 B.C., comes from a flowering plant (*Urginea* or *Scilla maritima*) native to countries that border the Mediterranean. Another plant once employed inadvertently against rats was rue, a strong-scented plant used in the Middle Ages. Rats hated rue, which people used to hang in their windows to protect their houses against the plague. Although rats were not suspected to be carriers of the Black Death until as late as

Appendix A: Continued

1894, this practice probably helped keep rats, and the disease, at bay.

Arsenic, the original poison of choice by young Otto Orkin in his fight against farm rats, is one of the oldest poisons known to man. This brittle white powder is deadly and has been used since the Middle Ages. Phosphorus, another poison used by Orkin, wasn't discovered until 1669, and it's not known when it was first used to control pests. However, a formula for poison that included phosphorus was authorized by the Prussian government and dated April 27, 1843:

Phosphorus	8 parts
Warm water	180 parts
Mix in a mortar and add:	
Rye meal	180 parts
When cold, add:	
Butter or lard	180 parts
Sugar	125 parts
Mix the whole thoroughly together.	

Prior to 1860 there were only occasional references made in scientific literature about the use of chemicals for insect control in the United States. For instance, in 1850 two important natural insecticides were introduced: rotenone from the roots of the derris plant and pyrethrum from the flower heads of a species of chrysanthemum. In 1867 a copper arsenite was introduced as the insecticide Paris Green—the very same poison used some forty years later on the Orkin farm. The first U.S. patent for phosphorus paste was issued in 1878, claiming to be a useful improvement in vermin-destroying compounds. The original formula consisted of boiling syrup, adding flour for the proper consistency, and then adding the required amount of phosphorus. Otto Orkin used this deadly, gritty substance, mixed with arsenic, in his sandwich rat bait to kill the rats in the family's attic.

Appendix B: Five-Year Financial Summary, 2000-2004

Rollins, Inc. and Subsidiaries

Earnings per share and dividends per share for 2004, 2003, 2002, 2001, and 2000 have been restated for the three-for-two stock split effective March 10, 2005, for all shares held on February 10, 2005.

(in thousands except per share data)	2004	2003	2002	2001	2000
OPERATIONS SUMMARY					
Revenues	$750,884	$677,013	$665,425	$649,925	$646,878
Net Income	$52,055	$35,761	$27,110	$16,942	$9,550
Earnings Per Share–Basic Net Income	$0.76	0.53	0.40	0.25	0.14
Earnings Per Share–Diluted Net Income	0.74	0.51	0.40	0.25	0.14
Dividends Per Share	0.16	0.13	0.09	0.09	0.09
FINANCIAL POSITION					
Total Assets	$418,780	$349,904	$318,338	$296,559	$298,819
Noncurrent Capital Lease Obligations	0	0	0	0	256
Long-Term Debt	1,700	1,734	2,913	4,895	4,656
Stockholders' Equity	167,549	138,774	90,690	85,498	78,599
Shares Outstanding at Year-End	69,060	69,356	67,198	67,657	67,581

Appendix C: The Orkin Man in a Starring Role—Hero

The Orkin Man is universally recognized as someone who can protect homes and property from all kinds of pests and termites, providing home and business owners with the state-of-the-art service and peace of mind. According to a 1990 list of customer service tips, the Orkin Man should be respectful, interested, courteous, understanding, informative, and responsible.

The list didn't mention, however, that the Orkin Man is also often a hero.

As constant as the red epaulets on the uniform, Orkin-Man-as-Hero stories have been a part of the company landscape as long as anyone can remember. From lifting cars out of ditches to fixing flat tires to true life-saving efforts, the Orkin Man just seems to have a knack for being in the right place at the right time.

- **Meridian, Mississippi:** Orkin Men Ray Lott and Hubert Harris happen upon a woman whose car is stuck in a muddy ditch. Ray—6 foot 6 and 287 pounds—lifts the rear of the car right out of the mud and sets it free.
- **Homestead, Florida:** Orkin Man José Montes is on a routine service call when he hears a scream from the area of a nearby swimming pool. He rushes outside, leaps over a fence and helps pull a child from the water, then performs CPR on the child, who is not breathing. Thanks to José, the child survives.
- **Decatur, Georgia:** Orkin Man Lamar Perkins discovers that an elderly resident is very ill when he arrives at her home for a routine service call. He helps her to her bed, puts the telephone beside her, and helps her call both her doctor and her children. "Because of this nice young man, my mother was taken care of," wrote her daughter, Mrs. C. R. Elliott.
- **Pompano Beach, Florida:** Orkin Man William (Bud) Hoffmann discovers a horrific sight during a routine home visit—a small child, bound and gagged and lying on the floor of a dark closet because, his parents said, "he was being punished." After intense soul-searching, Hoffman contacts the proper authorities; child-neglect charges are brought against one parent, and the child is placed in foster care. After extended therapy and treatment, the parents and child are reunited.
- **Valdosta, Georgia:** "My husband and I had a flat tire on I-75 near Valdosta. We were handicapped in that my husband had just left a Ft. Lauderdale hospital following abdominal surgery and I had a broken wrist in a splint.... After an hour in the 94-degree temperature, my husband was on the verge of collapse, so I persuaded him to let me try to stop someone for help. I had about decided that was a lost cause when this BEAUTIFUL ORKIN MAN stopped." The Orkin Man was service representative Raymond Futch.
- **McLean, Virginia:** Orkin Man Roger Smith hears his customer yell "Fire" and rushes up from the basement to find a kitchen stove filled with flames and the oven on fire from a burning roast. Smith first grabs a box of baking soda, throws it on the flames to put out the fire in the oven bottom, then carries the roast to the sink and douses it with water. "I fully believe that he saved the house from going up in flames," wrote Mrs. Grace McLean Moses.
- **Winston-Salem, North Carolina:** Standing in the basement of a home he has serviced for eight years, Orkin Man Kenneth Floyd looks up to find a poisonous copperhead snake. He safely captures it and gets it out of the house, once again making the basement safe for two little boys, ages two and six, who play there. "It certainly is gratifying to know that our home is protected by a company with men of Mr. Floyd's stature," wrote the homeowner and father, J. R. Baker of Goff, North Carolina.
- **Washington, D.C.:** Orkin pest control service representative James Letcher was an Orkin Man Hero—twice. He rescued a woman from a fire that was burning on the second floor of a house on his service

route, called the fire department, and returned to save the family dog! And on another occasion when he found a stolen wallet filled with important papers and photographs, he returned it to its proper owner in Florida.

- **Annandale, Virginia:** Orkin Man Ron Rush barely had time to think during his service run to a day care center, when he saw a little four-year-old girl dangling from the rafters of a built-in playhouse; her head had lodged on the beams when a stool had overturned and her feet didn't touch the floor. Ron could see that she was strangling—her faced had turned purple and she wasn't breathing. Ron immediately got her down and began CPR, which he continued until the rescue squad arrived. The little girl recovered completely, thanks to this Orkin Man.
- **Columbia, South Carolina:** Termite service technician Tom Anderson saved a customer's life when he found a gas leak under her home and told her to call the gas company—which described the leak as a "one-in-a-million accident with a regulator" that would have blown up the house.
- **Jackson, Mississippi:** Orkin Men are even heroes at Orkin. Acting service manager Paul Sumrall and his wife saved the branch office, files, and equipment when they risked their lives during a flood to enter the Orkin building, turn off the electricity, and secure important documents. For three hours, they moved equipment and even Orkin vehicles to higher ground. The next morning, the water in the office was up to three feet. "Catastrophic loss of records, vehicles, and equipment was avoided due to the loyalty and unselfish attitude of Paul Sumrall," his manager said.
- **Bristol, Tennessee:** Though they briefly considered turning around, Orkin Men Ron Shoenholz and Irwin Wyatt continued through six inches of snow to make their last sales call of the day on a narrow country road. When they got to the door, a little girl answered and pointed to a sofa where a woman lay face down, an empty pill bottle by her side. The Orkin Men managed to get the woman up and help her regain consciousness, and stayed with her until the emergency rescue unit arrived. Her family credited both men with saving her life.
- **Tyler, Texas:** The *Marshall News Messenger* called Orkin Man Benton Ratcliff a hero when he saved a two-year-old from drowning. "The people in Marshall don't even want to deal with any other Orkin man but Benton," said his branch manager Bob Preast. "He knows everybody, he's good at his job, and because of that he's been on the route for a long time," twenty-two years.
- **Decatur, Georgia:** Orkin Man Horace Clarington was on his service route when he noticed a lawnmower running in a yard and a man stretched out behind it. "All I knew was to stop the truck and get out and help," he said. The man was unconscious. Horace immediately started CPR and saved the man's life.
- **St. Louis, Missouri:** Orkin Man Mike Wilhelm had just pulled into the gas station lot to turn around when an explosion shattered the glass in his truck and Mike watched in amazement as the service station collapsed, trapping an employee. Reacting quickly, Mike jumped from his truck and began lifting roof rafters to free the man, just before flames engulfed the entire area. Police said that the man would have died in the flames if Mike had not been so quick to act.
- **Hudson, Florida:** Jack Archambo, then a sales inspector for Orkin, was working to secure a service contract with the Links of Bernadette when a member stumbled against a window and cut her arm badly. Jack immediately placed a tourniquet above the gaping wound and worked to control the bleeding, which prevented the woman from going into shock and kept her stable until the emergency

Appendix C: Continued

medics arrived. "We just wanted you to know what an outstanding employee you have and how pleased we were that he was at our clubhouse when this near tragedy occurred," wrote manager Frank Wilmath. "Needless to say, he got our contract!"

- **Near Charleston, West Virginia:** Two carloads of Orkin termite inspectors were headed home through a real snowstorm when they came upon a horrible accident between a car and a pickup truck. Orkin Man Dave Jacobs of the Braddock Hills branch rushed to help a young Marine in the car who was badly injured, while Clark Loffredo of the Pittsburgh branch assisted the driver of the truck and flagged down a motorist to help call for police and firemen. Orkin Men John Schacter, Bob Weiderstein, Bill Siegel, and Arron Trapuzzano helped direct traffic and did whatever they could to help make the injured drivers comfortable.
- **Orlando, Florida:** Orkin Man Marshall McCallum quickly realized that an accident between a car and truck was horrible: the driver of the car and one of her sons was killed, but Marshall was able to pull a little girl out of the car. For thirty minutes, Marshall performed CPR to keep the little girl alive until the paramedics arrived. His heroic efforts saved her life.
- **Worthington, Ohio:** Orkin termite inspector Joe Temesvary just had a feeling that something wasn't right. The person who answered the phone during Joe's routine call to schedule an appointment didn't say anything, but Joe detected something odd, a "funny noise, sort of like heavy breathing, but odd sounding." He called the police and asked them to check out the customer's residence, and they found a man who was almost choking to death. Paramedics performed an emergency tracheotomy on the man as they rushed him to the hospital. Authorities credited Joe's quick action with saving the man's life.
- **Marietta, Georgia:** All in a day's work? Orkin Man Norman Reid was servicing a customer's home when the harried mother inadvertently locked her baby son in the car with the engine running. In a rush to get to work, the woman had also forgotten to secure her baby in the car seat; he promptly climbed out and fell backwards, trapping his leg in the seat and his head between the door and car floor, crying hysterically. Norman stayed calm and called 911. Then he worked to get into the car by prying open the rear window and finally unlocking the door. "I'm thankful to Norman who acted above and beyond the call of duty to rescue my son," wrote the mother. "He is truly an asset to Orkin and the community."
- **East Los Angeles:** Orkin Man Ed Mullaney wasn't thinking about himself when he helped a police officer apprehend a violent hit-and-run suspect and in the process helped save the officer's life.
- **Marion, Illinois:** Orkin Man Keith Pritchett was a hero in the eyes of two customers for actions that Pritchett would never describe as heroic: he merely brought them food. "We never had much money," the customers wrote, "and Keith was our salvation on more than one occasion. He made trips on his own time to bring us fish and game for meals, which we wouldn't have had if not for Keith. But he never made us feel like a charity case. He always had 'too much' and wanted to 'share' with us. If you didn't know, Keith is an employee you can be proud of."
- **Dayton, Ohio:** Orkin Man Jeff Copeland was traveling on a rural road during sub-zero temperatures when he spotted a car on the side of the road with two elderly women inside. They had a flat tire. Jeff changed the tire and, noting the poor condition of the spare, suggested that the women stop and have it replaced as soon as possible. "Words cannot adequately express our appreciation to Jeff for coming to our aid on such a cold day," the ladies wrote.
- **Charlottesville, Virginia:** Orkin Man Brian Lading was a most unassuming hero to a pest control customer. Instructed by her doctor to walk daily, Brian

realized that the woman wasn't walking because she had fallen twice and was afraid to walk alone. Brian called several volunteer associations to find a walking partner for her. "I am touched by Brian's thoughtfulness," she wrote. "Other people heard me say I wanted someone to walk with, but he helped me find a solution to my problem. All businesses try to build goodwill, and employees like Brian certainly help Orkin's image."

- **Riverside, California:** Orkin Man Rhon Walker foiled a holdup at a Long John Silver's restaurant by alerting the staff that two suspicious-looking men were lurking outside, and then called police. The employees knew not to open the door until help arrived, even when the robbers started banging on the drive-through window. "All ended well, thanks to the wisdom, alertness, and concern for our safety by Rhon Walker."
- **Anderson, South Carolina:** Orkin Man Jeffrey Bearden knew that his customer was home—he had just spoken with her on the telephone—but no one was answering the door. He looked in and could see that someone had apparently fallen in the hallway. Bearden went to house after house in the neighborhood until he found someone who could call a family member and an ambulance. And then he waited outside the house to make sure his customer was going to be fine. Bearden checked in the next day, too.
- **Brooklyn, New York:** Orkin Man Patrick Dicicco stopped his truck when he noticed the frantic woman trying to flag someone down on the side of the road: She had just run her car off the road and hit a tree, and she couldn't open the back door to reach her three-year-old daughter. Patrick broke the window and pulled the child to safety just before the car was consumed by flames. Patrick refused to accept any reward, saying simply that he had to rush to his next appointment.
- **Brewer, Maine:** Orkin Man Ryan Simpson slammed on his brakes when he saw the AT&T truck flipped onto its side, flames flicking from under the metal body. He grabbed the fire extinguisher in his truck, scaled the guardrail, and helped the driver out of the truck as he worked to put out the fire. "On behalf of AT&T, please accept my most sincere thanks for the heroic efforts of Ryan Simpson. Most people would have passed by, but he risked his own safety to help a stranger in need."

Orkin has the world's best people! There are numerous heroes among us, and these are just a few who had an opportunity to show it.

Appendix D: Real-Life Orkin Men

Take a ride with any Orkin Man in the twenty-first century and you're in the company of two distinct individuals—a seasoned professional who knows every detail of Orkin's modern pesticide application systems and someone who's not above changing a lightbulb or putting out the trash for someone who needs a helping hand.

Symbolically, the Orkin Man has always stood for the consummate professional with the heart of gold. And over the years, these real Orkin Men have done their part to live up to the Orkin Man myth. Just listen to their stories:

* * * *

"I don't think I've ever been bored in my entire working career," said Paul Hardy, who started working for Orkin as a termite technician in 1961 and still worked for the company forty-three years later. "Some people go to work for a company and work real hard for the first year and learn everything, and then repeat it thirty-nine more times. Or you can have the opportunity to learn something new every year. I choose the second option. If you are doing today what you were doing yesterday, you are actually backing up. We are in a changing world, and you should not get up in the morning with the intent to do what you did yesterday."

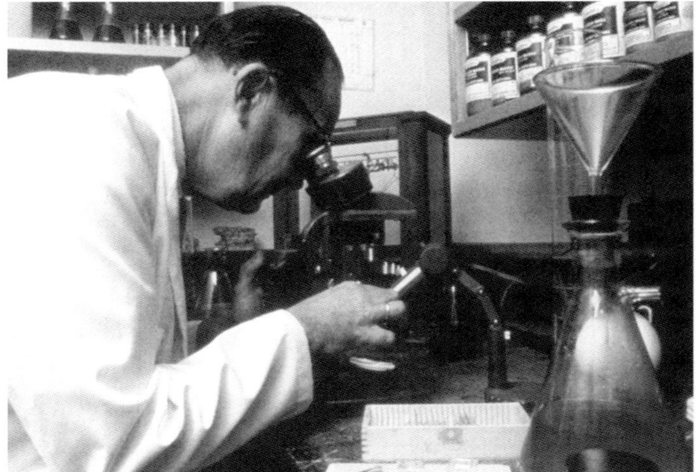

C. W. Marshall, the longtime technical director in Orkin's National Service Department, was nicknamed "Doc" because he could diagnose problems like a physician and always seemed to find the right answers.

In 1995 Hardy was named one of the top ten pest control industry leaders by *Pest Control Technology*; in 2001, *PCT* named him Professional of the Year, citing his pioneering work for Orkin in application techniques, equipment development, and termiticide and pesticide treatment systems.

"I do the things I do because they're the right thing to do," said Hardy, who always credited Orkin Man Sam Walkup with being his original teacher and mentor. "My first responsibility is to the field. I spend most of my time answering customers' questions, writing service alerts, and interacting with technicians. I've crawled many a house and tented many a structure. If I ever lose the understanding of the field, that's the time to get out of the business."

Orkin does not seek patents on most of its equipment developments. "I brought that up once, and the response was, 'We're not in the equipment business; we're in the service business.' We have not taken advantage of the equipment we have helped develop, but we use it for the benefit of the industry. We believe that anything you do that helps the industry actually helps you. The more we can do to develop our competition, the better we are. I can't think of any direct instance where helping the competitor has hurt Orkin. And I can give you a whole host of times where helping the competitor benefited Orkin."

* * * *

C. W. Marshall was nicknamed "Doc" because he could diagnose problems like a physician and always seemed to find the right answers. As a longtime technical director in Orkin's National Service Department, Doc Marshall had a special fondness for rats and was considered one of the best rat control experts in the country. "I especially enjoy difficult rat jobs," he once said. "They're the toughest of all." The largest job he recalled was for a feed mill in Missouri. Using a fast-killing agent, Doc Marshall said that they eliminated almost three thousand rats in two days. Killing rats, he admitted, was no easy task, a theory once shared by company founder Otto Orkin. "You see, rats are smart—some people believe they can even think. All I know is that you have to use your brain to fool them. So I've always found it challenging to discover the baits and traps to use. And I've yet to be defeated."

* * * *

Vince Stevens started with Orkin in 1962 and was thirty-two years old when he was assigned to be the branch manager of Richmond, Virginia. "I had ten employees who had been with Orkin longer than I had been living," he remembers. "Richmond is where Mr. Otto Orkin started selling his services in the commercial business area, and a lot of these employees had worked right with Otto Orkin. They were true, true Orkin People. There was Dorsey Hall, he was the termite service manager. James Wesley Hall was a salesman in my branch. Floyd Hall was a route technician, and they had another Hall in Norfolk, Virginia. They were like a little Orkin family of their own, and sometimes it was spooky. But they were the most enjoyable people to work with."

Stevens stayed with Orkin for thirty-eight years, retiring in June 2001. He is amazed at how the industry has changed. "It became a science," he said. "When I was servicing as a route technician, I mixed chemicals myself. It was nothing to mix three or four chemicals together, knowing that if one ounce would kill them, two will kill them deader. And that all changed during my time. Everything had to be very specific. And that's so much better."

Stevens's funniest story involves his days as an Orkin Man in Swansea, South Carolina, when he went to service a home and found a pig under the kitchen sink. "I went to move back a curtain from underneath the kitchen sink, and a pig ran out! The customer had a pig in the house! It scared the fool out of me! But I did say, 'Excuse me,' to the pig, and kept on servicing the home."

* * * *

Vice president of franchising and acquisitions Gordon Crenshaw started as a pest control technician for Orkin in Memphis, Tennessee, in 1963, shortly after graduating from the University of Tennessee. Over the next forty years, Gordon would work in almost every level of the company, but some of his favorite stories come from his days as an Orkin Man from 1963 to 1977. "In 1963, in Memphis, Tennessee, I was Elvis Presley's Orkin Man. He had just bought Graceland, and we were out there about a week doing termite treatment on those buildings. One day, I saw Elvis sitting there, and I asked him, 'You want me to show you how your rival, Jerry Lee Lewis, does it?' My brothers always said I played like Jerry Lee Lewis, so I showed him a couple of piano licks, just a certain way to do the bass. After that, every time I saw him, he would say, 'Come in here a minute. I want you to show me something.' I was twenty-three years old. And I still have a matchbook, with a gold 'E.P.' on it.

"There were thirteen branches in the Tennessee District divided up into East, Middle, and West Tennessee. Lamar Culbreth was my branch manager. They came out with the Skil Hammer, a drill used for termite work that Paul Hardy called the 'man killer' because it was so hard to use. I remember taking that hammer under a church and got it all hooked up and told everyone to stand back and let me show them how to drill a hole! The drill bit hit a piece of steel and whipped me around—like to half beat me to death! After that, I was ready to quit, except for what Mr. Culbreth said: 'I didn't think you could make it, college boy!' I had to prove I could."

Crenshaw was in Nashville in 1971. He remembers, "Orkin had been working with Micro-Gen to come up with a machine that treated large spaces in commercial accounts with the least amount of chemical. We came out with a new machine that broke down the chemical into such fine particles it was like smoke. It would go behind cracks and flush the roaches out. It was particularly good in restaurants. I remember we were trying to get the Shoney's account, and they wouldn't even talk to us. I called the head guy and had him meet me at his best Shoney's, early in the morning.

Appendix D: Continued

"I want to show you this new equipment." He agreed, and we met at his very best restaurant at 2 A.M., and he brought his engineer and I brought my sales manager, Jim Purdue. After we got the customers out, we went in the kitchen and we cranked up this Micro-Gen machine and it started this smoke, back in the corners. In a few minutes, roaches were coming out, and in fifteen minutes that kitchen was absolutely crawling with roaches. I just amazed him. Five minutes later, a rat about half as long as my leg jumped out and ran across the kitchen. He said he had seen enough. "Be in my office at ten o'clock tomorrow morning." So we signed Shoney's—about 110 stores. I think that was one of the first national accounts we sold. We were rolling."

* * * *

Steven Drennan, who worked for the company for more than thirty years, joined Orkin in 1970 as a pest control technician, just after he returned from military duty in Vietnam. "I drove past the Orkin office and noticed a lot of cars, and figured that might be a good place to work. I didn't have any idea what Orkin was. I had been raised on a farm and knew about rats, but I was surprised to find that people were actually killing insects and rats for a living. When I started, I worked on the route about four and a half weeks, and decided it was easier to sell pest control that it was to service, so I started selling pest control as I was doing the route. The one thing I realized very quickly was that if you could talk earnestly about a product and had the facts to back up what you said, it's not a big deal to sell. Orkin had everything in black and white; there was no mystique about what we did. You had bugs and rats, and we got rid of them.

"I believe that if you provide the service you say you're going to do, you don't have to worry about your sales. In smaller towns, word of mouth got around and if you didn't do what you said you would, everybody knew about it. If you mess up one account, you may not get the rest of the relatives and neighbors.

"Even though we emphasize sales, we are a service company first. The challenge is to be the best service company in the world. You learn in the service business that you have to be the one who changes—you are not going to change the customer. You have to adapt to what they want, how they want it, how you deal with them, talk or listen to them. That is the challenge. And from a corporate philosophy, the customer is always right."

* * * *

Clyde Cobb came to work for Orkin in 1966 as one of the company's first manager trainees. In four and a half years, he was named a district manager, claiming at the time that he had climbed up the management ladder faster than anyone in the history of the company. "We were the only company advertising on TV in 1966. The advertising was changing from the comedy cartoon type to more professional, such as a consultant talking about sanitation and how dirty roaches were. There were celebrities in our advertisements, like Miss America, Bess Myerson. We were the innovator in advertising, and it wasn't long before our competitors were copying our advertising, point-of-sale material, everything.

"We didn't have staff positions. It was all line management. We made one report on Friday—the Old B & A (Business and Addressograph) Report. It was the only report I ever did for my first ten years with the company. I would hear from Taft Pierce, then operations vice president when I was hired, on the phone about once or twice a month. My job was hiring, working in the field, doing work myself. Everything was sales driven—like the King Bee contest. Claims were not too much of a problem then, but I remember the first lawsuit we had in our district, in Xenia, Ohio. It was a termite lawsuit. They wanted seven thousand dollars to settle at the court house steps. When I called Taft, he hollered, "Seven thousand dollars!! Are you crazy? You'll have to call Earl Geiger." He had the same reaction, but we settled it for seven thousand dollars. A couple of years later, the worst tornado came through Xenia and blew the house down."

* * * *

Fresh out of high school in 1956, Lowell Buckingham was hired by Orkin to work in Miami at a branch run by Bernard Kolkana. "They were looking for someone to check in route technicians ahead of the supervisor. I was to go over the route sheets, and if a technician didn't get all of his stops, I was to send him back to complete his route. The technicians were much older than I was, a kid right out of high school, and they would sometimes give me a hard time. I was tempted to leave, but then Taft Pierce came at the end of 1956. He was very positive and made you want to continue working and doing your best for the company. The Miami territory covered a big area, including a sub-office in Key West. The office was in an old filling station–garage on the Causeway at Thirteenth Street. The front door was right on the street, so when it rained, cars splashed water through the door into the office. And the wet floor would conduct electrical charges from anything that was plugged in. We typed the B&As on old manual typewriters, but we did have electric ten-key adding machines, which caused the electrical charges when it stormed."

* * * *

In 1962 J. D. Burger hired a Georgia State accounting graduate named Allen Meadows to work in the company's payroll department. He worked for Orkin for forty-two years. "I was in payroll for six to nine months, then Joe Cantrell hired me for the accounting department," Meadows remembered. "My first job was to conduct an inventory on the company vehicles. Everything was manual, so it was a long, drawn-out process. I finally narrowed it down to two or three vehicles, one of which belonged to the old North Georgia area. We identified it as a pickup truck assigned to a man who used to chauffeur Mr. Otto Orkin, Frank Cofer. Neither Cofer nor Mr. Orkin admitted they knew anything about the truck, but finally, it was identified as a truck Mr. Orkin had sold for two hundred dollars to a young, aspiring entrepreneur. Mr. Orkin said it was his truck and he could sell it if he wanted to. Billy Orkin took the money from his pocket to take the vehicle off the books. Then, I understand, the amount was deducted from Mr. Orkin's paycheck.

"Every Monday morning, Mr. Orkin would come by Joe Cantrell's desk and ask how much money we had in the bank. Joe would pull out his P&L (profit and loss report) and Mr. Orkin would say, 'No, I don't want to know about that paper. I want to know how much money we have in the bank.' He didn't care what the details on the P&L were, just what the collections were in the bank.

"All accounting was done manually or put on IBM punch cards and sent to an outside source until the Rollinses bought Orkin. The main thing I remember was Rollins's willingness to provide what we needed to improve the manual posting system. The company was growing at geometric proportions, and the old system just couldn't keep up. The Rollinses saw that the company needed a more sophisticated accounting system. The Rollinses took what Orkin was and turned it into a very smooth-running corporate entity."

* * * *

After four years in the service, John Wilson tried several different jobs and ended up being a sales-service representative with Orkin as of January 1960. "I loved working for Orkin from the beginning," said Wilson, who would one day become vice president of the Southeast Division. "My first training was working with a serviceman for a few days then I started selling. I thought our material was pretty good back then. We had the little 'Who's Who in

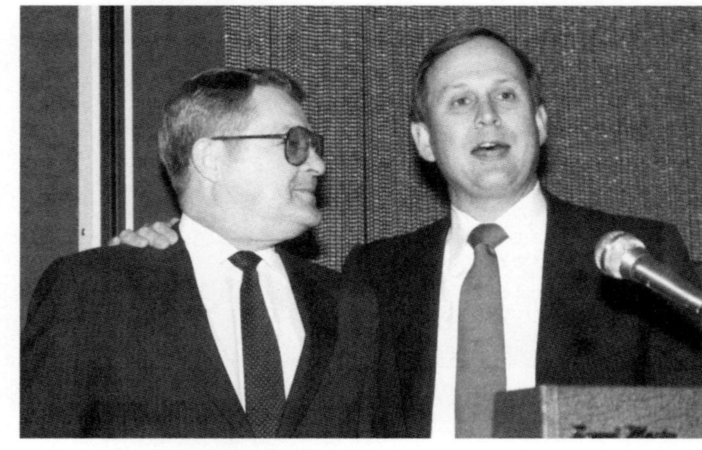

John Wilson, left, Orkin Southeast Region vice president, and Gary Rollins, Rollins, Inc., president, at a 1985 district managers' meeting.

Appendix D: Continued

Pests,' which I thought was excellent. We didn't have the proposals like today. We made up our own termite proposals. We used to get our own staff together. We had sheets you put together and more emphasis was placed on the graph—you sold a lot from the graph itself. If you found an article in the paper—i.e., mouse had chewed electrical cable—you cut that out and put that in your 'evidence book.' But the best marketing we ever had was Otto the Orkin Man. That went over well.

"Lamar Culbreth, then Memphis manager, was a master at motivation and working people, and I worked under him as a salesman in the branch. And when he was made district manager in Tennessee, I became his sales manager from November 1963 to November 1965. The branch-level accountability from salespeople was considerable. We were in the office about 7:30 in the morning and started the sales meeting by 8 A.M., and by 9 A.M. we would be out of the office. We called the office several times a day for messages and leads. Every morning, the manager would meet with each one about the previous day's activities. Lamar had us prelist our prospects. We knocked on doors in the area where we were treating, but it may not have been called cloverleafing. A tremendous amount of our business came from referrals—satisfied customers who refer our service. Referrals were where we got our greatest growth. In rural areas, the word-of-mouth is the biggest difference.

"But I believe it's the administrative portions of the business that make our people successful, such as having their route productive, knowing how to set up a day. I try to teach the branch manager the basics. The good manager is there to meet the pest control technicians as they come in the door, to see what kind of day they had yesterday, to see what kind of attitude they have about today. Are they prepared to be successful? Do they have a good day planned? So many managers don't realize how important attitude is with their productivity.

"I didn't have a lot of education," Wilson said. "I just outworked everyone I was ever around. And the only advice I ever had for anyone is to work hard, be honest, and do your job well. Then you'll be all right."

* * * *

Robert Edward Lee, Gary Rollins once said, owned Louisiana. Or at the very least, this longtime Orkin pest

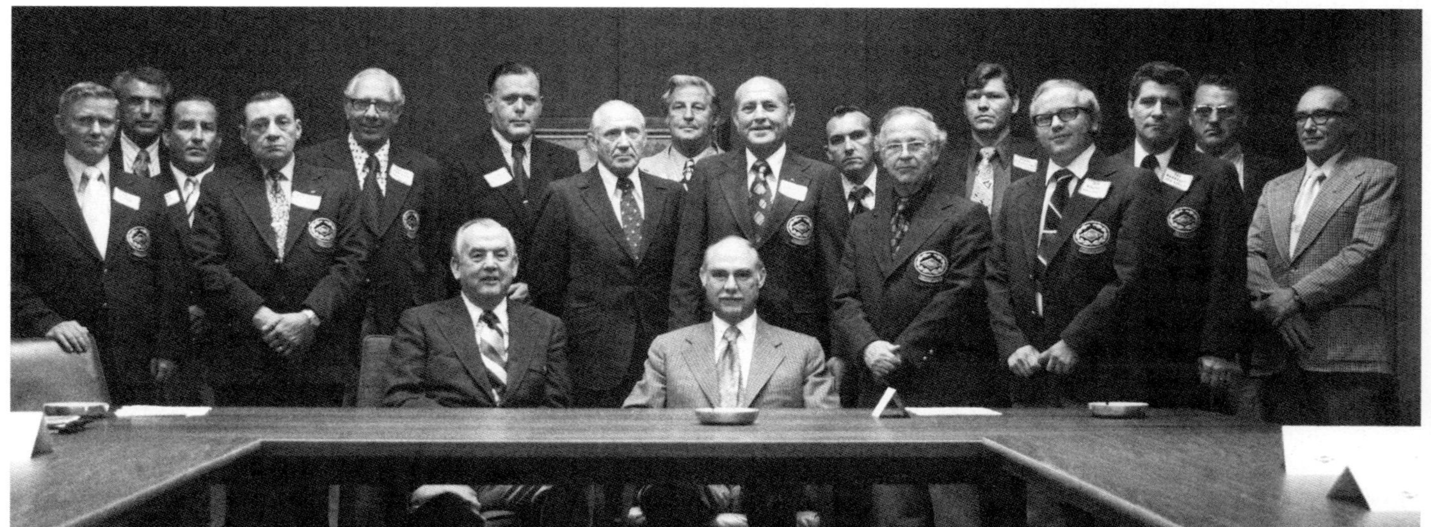

Some charter members of the President's Club, composed of the leading Orkin sales representatives for fiscal 1973, are shown with corporate and division executives. Standing, left to right: Ed Dutton, Bob Rominger, Frank Sodupe, Herman Runtenelli, George Davidson, Jack Hoey, Bernie Kolkana, C. C. White, Gerald Ellerbee, Paul McBrayer, Harold Yaffe, Buddy Strickland, Roy Bulley, Pat Barberot, Bill Bishop, and Ed Elkins. Seated are chairman and president O. Wayne Rollins and executive vice president Earl F. Geiger. Robert E. Lee was not present for the photograph.

control salesperson owned Houma, Louisiana, where he started as an Orkin Man in 1955 and counted generations of the same families as his customers. He was one of the charter members of Orkin's President's Club, developed in 1972 to honor top salesmen. "I just liked the business, and they treated me like a king," Lee said in an interview in late 2003. "I feel like the Orkin family is part of my family. I started out as a pest control operator, and that was for Otto Orkin himself. He was just a fine, fine fella. Then the Rollins family bought it in 1964, and Mr. O. Wayne Rollins had a lot of guts, excuse the language. He put the company on the stock market. All of the Rollins people have very positive attitudes. They do not accept 'No.' I picked that up from them, and went on from there.

"I worked out a system of deciding where to go and which people to see, and it was very successful. I would get referrals from the people where I would go, and use them. They brought me to Atlanta one time, around 1971, and they questioned me on how I was so successful. I said, 'First of all, you have to know where you're going to go before you can expect to do any work. There has to be a system to your day. One day, I got the phone book, got some referrals, and from that day on, I planned out my day.'"

Lee claimed that he was the first Orkin employee to ever sell over two hundred thousand dollars worth of business in one year. "Mr. O. Wayne Rollins himself said to me, 'Is it possible to sell two hundred thousand dollars a year?' At the time, it took one hundred thousand dollars to be in the President's Club, but I knew that Mr. Rollins didn't take no for an answer. And I made it!"

His secret as a salesman? "Just being me. Just being completely honest. Always be 100 percent honest. Never make a problem that's not a problem. You know, I've even offered to tell all of my customers, 'If you want to try to treat your property yourself, here's all the details.' I drew up a finished graph of the house, showing everything in detail. Some would take me up on it, and I didn't consider it a big deal because I would sell another contract down the street."

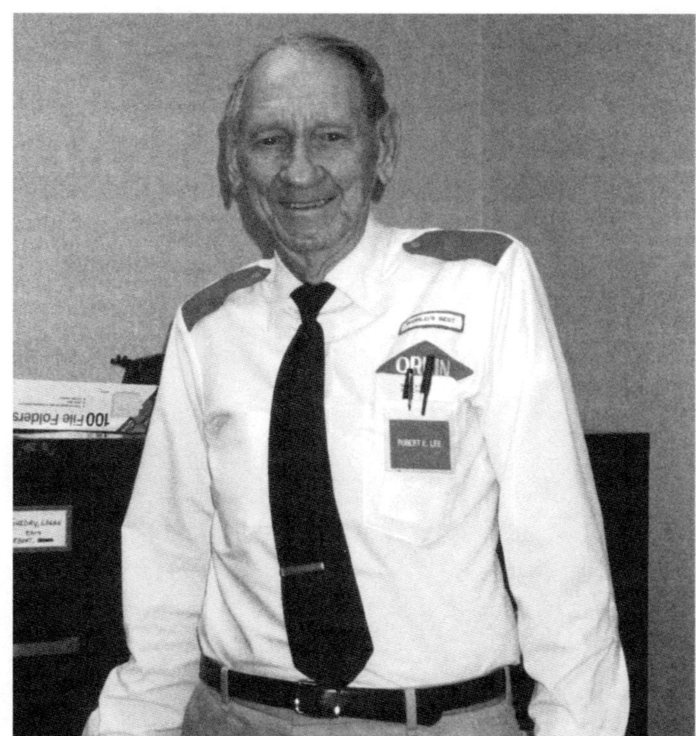

Robert E. Lee spent more than forty-seven years at the Houma, Louisiana, Orkin branch and attended President's Club for each of his last thirty years there.

Lee retired on January 1, 1987, just a few years ahead of the retirement of two other long-term Orkin employees in the Houma branch: Lloyd Robichaux, a termite technician for forty-three years; and Gert Byrd, an office manager who was a thirty-eight-year employee. But Lee continued to work as an Orkin Man for several more years on a part-time basis and attended every President's Club as an honorary member until 2002. After bouts with heart disease and cancer, he still went to work in an Orkin office file room, a few days a week. "But I liked sales the best. I was my own boss. I made a good living, oh yes, indeed, I made a good living. I never even talked about being a branch manager, and I never was. I believe that they threatened one time that they were going to let me go if I didn't take a branch manager's job, and I said, 'Well, then I guess I'll have to be an exterminator elsewhere.' And that was the end of that!"

One of the most treasured, devoted, and successful Orkin Men in the company's history, Robert Edward Lee passed away on April 10, 2004.

INDEX

Numbers in *italics* indicate photographs.

S

T